MEDICAL IMAGING

Dedication
For those who have loved or inspired us.

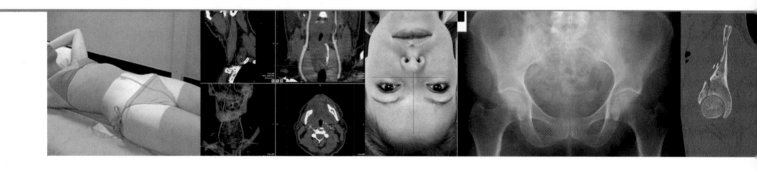

For Churchill Livingstone

Commissioning Editor: Sarena Wolfaard/Dinah Thom

Project Development Editor: Dinah Thom

Project Manager: Joannah Duncan

Designer: Judith Wright

Illustration Manager: Bruce Hogarth

Illustrations: Graeme Chambers

MEDICAL IMAGING

Techniques, Reflection & Evaluation

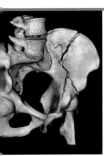

Edited by

Elizabeth Carver BSc(Hons) DCR FAETC

Undergraduate Course Director, School of Radiography,
University of Wales, Bangor, Wales, UK

Barry Carver PgDipCT PGCE DCR(R)

Director of Postgraduate Studies, School of Radiography,
University of Wales, Bangor, Wales, UK

FOREWORD BY

Patrick Brennan PhD DCR HDCR CTC

Senior Lecturer and Director of Research, School of Diagnostic Imaging,
University College Dublin, Dublin, Ireland

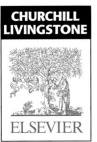

CHURCHILL
LIVINGSTONE

ELSEVIER

Edinburgh   London   New York   Oxford   Philadelphia   St Louis   Sydney   Toronto   2006

CHURCHILL
LIVINGSTONE
ELSEVIER

First published 2006

ISBN 0 443 06212 9

British Library Cataloguing in Publication Data
A catalogue record for this book is available from the British Library

Library of Congress Cataloging in Publication Data
A catalog record for this book is available from the Library of Congress

Notice

Knowledge and best practice in this field are constantly changing. As new research and experience broaden our knowledge, changes in practice, treatment and drug therapy may become necessary or appropriate. Readers are advised to check the most current information provided (i) on procedures featured or (ii) by the manufacturer of each product to be administered, to verify the recommended dose or formula, the method and duration of administration, and contraindications. It is the responsibility of the practitioner, relying on their own experience and knowledge of the patient, to make diagnoses, to determine dosages and the best treatment for each individual patient, and to take all appropriate safety precautions. To the fullest extent of the law, neither the publisher nor the editors and contributors assume any liability for any injury and/or damage.

The Publisher

Working together to grow
libraries in developing countries

www.elsevier.com | www.bookaid.org | www.sabre.org

ELSEVIER   BOOK AID International   Sabre Foundation

ELSEVIER   your source for books, journals and multimedia in the health sciences

www.elsevierhealth.com

The publisher's policy is to use **paper manufactured from sustainable forests**

Printed in China

CONTENTS

CONTRIBUTORS

Julie Burnage DCR DMU CertMamm FETCI&II
*Director, Ultrasound Now Ltd, St Asaph, Denbighshire,
Wales, UK*

Philip Cosson BSc(Hons) PGCE PGC DCR(R)
*Senior Lecturer in Radiography, School of Health and
Social Care, University of Teesside, Middlesbrough,
Cleveland, UK*

Mark Cowling BSc MBBS MRCP FRCR
*Senior Lecturer in Radiology, University Hospital of
North Staffordshire, North Staffordshire NHS Trust,
Stoke-on-Trent, UK*

Susan Cutler MSc BSc PGCE HDCR
*Senior Lecturer in Medical Imaging, School of Health
and Social Care, University of Teesside, Middlesbrough,
Cleveland, UK*

Patricia Fowler MMEd BSc(Hons) DCRR CertCI
*Senior Lecturer, Faculty of Health and Social Care,
London South Bank University, London, UK*

David Wyn Jones MSc DCR(R) DRI
*Superintendent Radiographer, Wrexham Maelor Hospital,
Wrexham, North Wales, UK*

Andrew Layt DCR(R)
*Superintendent Radiographer, Neuroradiology,
King's College Hospital, London, UK*

Margot McBride PhD MSc DCR
*Enterprise Fellow, Royal Society of Edinburgh,
George Street, Edinburgh, UK*

Jonathan McConnell MSc PgCert(image interpretation) CertRes
BSc DCR(R)
*Head of Medical Imaging, Faculty of Health and Applied
Science, Christchurch Polytechnic Institute of Technology,
Christchurch, New Zealand*

Julian MacDonald PhD MSc BSc
*Medical Physicist, North Wales Medical Physics Service,
Wales, UK*

Susan Penelope Nash BA(Hons) MA PGCE HDCR
*Head of School of Radiography, University of Wales,
Bangor, Wales, UK*

Tim Palarm MSc DCR(R) SRR ILIM
*Ultrasound Sales Specialist, Toshiba Medical Systems,
Crawley, Sussex. Formerly Senior Lecturer in Diagnostic
Imaging and Programme leader MSc in Medical
Ultrasound, University of the West of England, Bristol, UK*

Rita Philips MSc DMU DCR FAETC
*Senior Lecturer (Programme Leader), Medical Ultrasound,
Faculty of Health and Social Care, University of the West
of England, Bristol, UK*

Amanda J. Royle BSc(Hons) DCR(R) CTCert
*Director, Compass Medical Ltd, Westbury, Shrewsbury,
Shropshire, UK*

Joanne Rudd MSc (GI Reporting) BSc(Hons)
*Lead Radiographer Practitioner in GI Imaging,
Radiology Department, West Suffolk Hospitals NHS Trust,
Bury St Edmunds, UK*

Michael Scriven HDCR(R) DMS(OU) PgC MedicalUltrasound
*Superintendent Paediatric Radiographer, Department of
Paediatric Radiology, Southampton General Hospital,
Southampton, UK*

Mike Stocksley MSc CertEd MDCR DMU
*Senior Lecturer (Programme Leader) Clinical Ultrasound,
Department of Allied Health Professions, Faculty of
Health and Social Care, London South Bank University,
London, UK*

John Talbot MSc
Senior Lecturer, Anglia Ruskin University, Cambridge, UK

Catherine A. Williams BSc(Hons) CertEd DCR(T) FAETC
*Lecturer, School of Radiography, University of Wales,
Bangor, Wales, UK*

Linda Williams HDCR IHSM(Cert) LHE(Cert)
*Lead Tutor for Clinical Education, School of Radiography,
University of Wales, Bangor, Wales, UK*

Darren Wood DCR(R)
*Senior Radiographer, Department of Medical Imaging,
Leighton Hospital, Crewe, Cheshire, UK*

FOREWORD

Health service provision, particularly departments of diagnostic imaging, are undergoing unprecedented change. Equipment and procedures are developing rapidly and this, along with national initiatives on clinical excellence, international radiation legislation and greater patient awareness, means that radiographers must not only be aware of the best methods of imaging, but must regularly reflect on their practice to ensure that the best possible service is offered to individuals requiring radiological examinations. This book provides for these requirements.

In the current context of radiographers taking more responsibility for their role, the book should serve as a catalyst for optimum practice. Often radiographers have relied on well-established procedures to examine patients, based on texts published many years ago. However, with the advent of more powerful X-ray tubes, newer methods of imaging and alternative methods of image acquisition, this acceptance of traditional practice will become increasingly displaced. Practitioners must question the way they do things and this book, with contributions from the radiographic, medical and industrial communities, provokes such questions in an effective way.

The approach taken by the authors is unique. In the chapters provided, there are reviews of techniques for an array of investigations encountered in radiographic practice. These reviews, however, are cleverly combined with well-referenced discussion of issues that will affect how radiographers deal with patients and are likely to impact on image quality. Even consideration of relatively unknown agents such as the impact of evolutionary change on patient length is evident, and the impact of such factors on positioning the patient is fully explored. Some of the intriguing topics raised should inspire imaging undergraduates and postgraduates in their search for research topics to complete their degree.

In the wake of European and national radiation legislation, it is encouraging to see that justification for individual examinations is well emphasised. Using research findings and the latest professional guidelines, clear indications for specific procedures are shown and reference to methods of optimising specific procedures is included. A clear description of what is expected in an image for specific examination and conditions is shown and supported by relevant images, and causal agents for less than optimal images are presented. The information is comprehensive so that commonly encountered examinations are included along with the most recent developments in interventional radiology.

The authors have been comprehensive, thorough and innovative. This well-presented book should be adopted by schools of diagnostic imaging in Europe and elsewhere and be a constant companion to the reflective radiographic practitioner.

2006
Patrick Brennan

PREFACE

The role of practitioners in medical imaging has been developing for many years and professional practice now requires an evidence-based approach to this practice. In a rapidly expanding field this can seem overwhelming, especially for the undergraduate or newly qualified radiographer. No one can hope to reach advanced or consultant status as a diagnostic imaging professional without a reflective attitude.

Before even considering these requirements, professionals in medical imaging are required to acquire and implement skills that provide a safe, caring and efficient diagnostic service. Basically, we cannot expect professionals to be reflective if they do not first have access to information regarding the core requirements of medical imaging techniques. They have to know what their choices are before making their final choice on appropriate clinical practice, whilst considering the challenges that present themselves in a variety of guises: patient condition, the clinical question, image quality, dose from ionising radiation and related legislation, contraindications related to use of pharmaceuticals, contraindications related to the imaging modality in question and imaging principles. This list names but a few of the most relevant considerations, yet the concept of the reflective approach becomes even more complex when we realise that each one affects others in this important list and often we must consider a trade-off of one important consideration against another.

In order to cultivate this evidence-based approach we can no longer apply our skills without questioning the suitability of the techniques we employ. Most educators in medical imaging attempt to promote the reflective, evidence-based approach to all aspects of diagnostic imaging but it is often difficult for undergraduates, and even graduates, to continue this approach, especially during independent clinical practice or study.

Having considered these points it became clear to us that we needed to produce a resource which addressed these issues by providing information on a core of knowledge, sensibly presented and related to medical imaging techniques, whilst promoting the reflective approach. The result is this text, a project which has brought together contributions from radiographers, radiography lecturers,

radiologists and other experts from the commercial sector of medical imaging, all selected for their clinical and academic expertise.

The first section of the book provides the basic information that is required to understand and initiate diagnostic imaging techniques, including implications for image quality and radiation dose related to exposure factors and image recording systems. Information is not merely descriptive; at times the authors consider and discuss published sources and relate this information to the concepts they present.

The next section has familiar aspects in that it offers descriptions of radiographic positioning and provides images of suggested patient positions and resulting radiographs, which also bear anatomical labelling. A step-by-step approach is used, making the requirements of each position easier to follow. Often a radiographer or student will only need to check a centring point or angle of central ray rather than read the whole position descriptor, and for this reason these sections are clearly identified under separate headings after the position descriptor. Often there are several methods described for one position requirement. These chapters are supplemented by a range of approaches:

- There is discussion, or even questioning, regarding suitability of projections or methods related to patient condition, practicality of the position used, radiation dose and imaging principles. References are used, either as a basis for reflection or to present an argument. At times questions are raised to promote further reflection by the reader.
- Tips for improved practical implementation are provided where relevant.
- Full image quality criteria for all radiographic projections are provided.
- Advice on causes and correction of common errors is given.

As an additional note, it should be mentioned that 'general radiography' is often considered as a non-specialist area, yet it relies so heavily on high level skills such as an understanding of human anatomy and related surface markings, an intuitive approach to communication which ensures patient concordance and compliance, and an understanding of the use of ionising radiation and its impact on image quality and human tissue. The editors acknowledge that general radiography still provides the higher proportion of a medical imaging service and stress that medical imaging professionals must not exclude general radiography as a specialist area in itself. By emphasising the reflective aspects of this section we hope to highlight this most clearly.

Moving on to other sections in the text, other non-contrast radiographic imaging is also covered in sections on mammography, accident and emergency, and paediatric imaging. A descriptive and reflective approach continues in these sections, which are again supported by references.

In the contrast examinations chapters, the descriptive and reflective philosophy continues. Improved imaging via complementary imaging methods posed a problem regarding what to include in this section; many angiographic examinations have been replaced by other methods such as computed tomography (CT) and magnetic resonance imaging (MRI) contrast studies and this is considered alongside descriptions of techniques used.

The final section on comparative imaging considers the basic principles and clinical applications associated with these techniques, also with some reflective content and considerations for future developments, thus complementing the other sections of the text to provide an all round medical imaging approach. Every attempt has been made to ensure that the information provided in this section is as up to date as is possible in the rapidly developing areas it covers, but the authors acknowledge that even the time in production between manuscript submission and publication may see developments beyond those described.

It would have been unrealistic to hope to provide a text which was all things to everyone, and for this reason the editors would urge that further reading is undertaken via up-to-date specialist texts or journal articles relating to physics, radiation science, imaging recording, CT, MRI, radionuclide imaging (RNI), ultrasound, accident and emergency, paediatrics, interventional radiology, gastrointestinal and genitourinary investigations, mammography and health psychology. However, we believe that this text will provide a good basis for a core of knowledge, leading to safe and holistic practice that is based on evaluation and reflection.

We conclude by mentioning that production of this text would not have been possible without a large number of people and institutions. The authors feature as key to its success and their names will obviously be associated with their chapters but others have helped with this project in various ways: provision of images or permissions to reproduce images from other authors' work, use of equipment in hospitals, modelling, providing advice or undertaking administrative tasks. A separate list of those we wish to acknowledge is given after this preface.

Stoke on Trent 2006   *Elizabeth M. Carver*
                                              Barry Carver

ACKNOWLEDGEMENTS

The editors and authors wish to acknowledge the following for their help or inspiration:

Bill Bailey, Neil Barker, Pam Black, Ken and Alma Carver, Mary Casey, Margaret Cliffe, Jacqui Coals, Sheila Copeland, John Copeland, Timothy Cox, Neil Deasy, Joanne Fairhurst, GSDS Ltd, C Chris Hale, Mark Hitchman, Mark Holmshaw, Hospital for Neurology and Neurosurgery, London, Lynn Gilman, Peter Groome, Leighton Hospital, Crewe, Julie Mead, Penny Nash, Neuroradiology Department, King's College Hospital NHS Trust, Carl Pavey, Oncology Systems Ltd, Gillian Phillips, Graham Plant, Jack Reese (Tomotherapy Inc), Meryl Rogers, Anne Scard-Jones, Claire Shackleston, Andrew Shaughnessy, Sandra Skeoch, Christine Smith, Neil Staff, Graeme Stow, Mike Tatlow, Alice Turner, Alexandra Unett, University Hospital of North Staffordshire, University of Wales, Bangor, School of Radiography, Ysbyty Maelor, Wrexham, students of the BSc(Hons) Diagnostic Radiography and Imaging course at the University of Wales, Bangor, students of the BSc(Hons) Diagnostic Radiography and the BSc(Hons) Physiotherapy courses at St Martins College, Carlisle.

For reproduction of images:

Phillip Ballinger and Eugene Frank, Stephen Eustace, Christine Gunn, Professor P Lauterbur, Linda Lee, Michelle McNicholas, Stephanie Ryan, Verdi Stickland, Robin Wilson, Andrew Evans, Professor Sir Peter Mansfield, Eric Whaites, Philips Medical Systems, Toshiba Medical Systems, Xograph Medical Systems.

The editors wish to offer special thanks to Alexandra Unett for her patience and commitment during modelling sessions.

ABBREVIATIONS

^{57}Co	Cobalt 57
^{18}F-FDG	Fluorine 18 – fluorodeoxyglucose
^{131}I	Iodine 131
^{99}Tc^m NaTcO$_4^-$	Sodium pertechnetate
^{99}Tc^m	Technetium-99m
2D	two-dimensional
3D	three-dimensional
4D	four-dimensional
A&E	accident and emergency
AC	abdominal circumference
ACR	American College of Radiology
ADC	analogue to digital conversion
AEC	automatic exposure chamber
AED	automatic exposure device
AFM	after fatty meal
ALARA	as low as reasonably achievable
ALARP	as low as reasonably practical
AO	anterior oblique
AP	anteroposterior
ARAS	atheromatous renal artery stenosis
ARSAC	Administration of Radioactive Substances Advisory Committee
ASIS	anterior superior iliac spine
ATLS	advanced trauma and life support
AVM	arteriovenous malformation
Ba FT	Barium follow through
BIR	British Institute of Radiology
BPD	bi-parietal diameter
BPH	benign prostatic hyperplasia/hypertrophy
BPP	biophysical profile
Bq	Becquerel
CAD	computer aided detection
CBD	common bile duct
CC	craniocaudal
CDH	congenital dislocation of the hip
CEMRA	contrast-enhanced MRA
CFA	common femoral artery
CPR	cardiopulmonary resuscitation
CPC	plexus cysts
CR	computed radiography
CRL	crown rump length
CRT	cathode ray tube

CSE	conventional spin echo
CT	computed tomography
CT	cardiothoracic
CTA	computed tomography angiography
CTDI	computed tomography dose index
CTLM	computed tomography laser mammography
CTPA	computed tomography pulmonary angiography
CVA	cerebral vascular accident
CVC	central venous catheter
CVP	central venous pressure
CVS	chorionic villus sampling
CZT	cadmium zinc telluride
D	density
D&C	dilatation and curettage
DAP	dose area product
DAS	data acquisition system
DCIS	ductal carcinoma in situ
DDF	direct digital fluoroscopy
DDH	developmental dysplasia of the hip
DDR	direct digital radiography
DGH	district general hospital
DLP	dose length product
DNA	deoxyribonucleic acid
DOBI	dynamic optical breast imaging
DP	dorsipalmar or dorsiplantar
DPO	dorsipalmar oblique or dorsiplantar oblique
DPT	dental panoramic tomography
DQE	detective quantum efficiency
DR	digital radiography
DRL	diagnositc reference level
DSA	digital subtraction angiography
DTPA	diethylenetriamine penta-acetic acid
DVT	deep vein thrombosis
DW	diffusion weighted
EAM	external auditory meatus
EBCT	electron beam computed tomography
ECG	electrocardiogram
EDD	estimated date of delivery
EDE	effective dose equivalent

EFOV	extended field of view
EOP	external occipital protuberance
EPI	echo-planar imaging
ERCP	endoscopic retrograde cholangiopancreatography
ESD	entrance surface dose or entrance skin dose
EUS	endoscopic ultrasound
EUS-FNA	endoscopic ultrasound – fine needle aspiration
ESWL	extracorporeal shockwave lithotripsy
FAST	focused abdominal sonography for trauma
FB	foreign bodies
FDG	fluorodeoxyglucose
FET	field effect transistor
FFD	focus film distance
FISH	fluorescence in situ hybridisation
FL	femur length
fMRI	functional MRI
FNA	fine needle aspiration
FNAC	fine needle aspiration cytology
FNST	fetal non-stress test
FO	frontooccipital
FOOSH	fall onto out-stretched hand
FOV	field of view
FSE	fast spin echo
FWHM	full width half maximum
GCS	Glasgow coma scale
GI	gastrointestinal
GIT	gastrointestinal tract
GOJ	gastrooesophageal junction
GOR	gastrooesophageal reflux
GSV	gestational sac volumes
HC	head circumference
hCG	human chorionic gonadotrophin
HDP	hydroxymethylene diphosphonate
HIDA	hepatobiliary iminodiacetic acid
HIV	human immunodeficiency virus
HLA	horizontal long axis
HOCM	high osmolar contrast media
HRCT	high resolution CT
HRT	hormone replacement therapy
HSG	Hysterosalpingography
HU	Hounsfield unit
HyCoSy	hysterosalpingo contrast sonography
IAM	internal auditory meatus
IARC	International Agency for Research on Cancer
ICH	intracranial haemorrhage
IOFB	intraocular foreign body
IV	intravenous

IVC	intravenous cholangiogram
IVC	inferior vena cava
IVF	in vitro fertilisation
IVU	intravenous urogram or urography
KeV	kilo electron volt
KUB	kidneys, ureters and bladder
kVp	kilovoltage peak
LAO	left anterior oblique
LBD	light beam diaphragm
LCD	liquid crystal display
LCR	low contrast resolution
LOCM	low osmolar contrast media
LNT	linear no threshold
LPO	left posterior oblique
lppm	line pairs per millimetre
LSJ	lumbosacral junction
LSO	lutetium oxyorthosilicate
MAA	macro-aggregated albumin
mAs	milliampere seconds
MCU	micturating cystourethrography
MDP	methylene diphosphonate
MI	mechanical index
MIP	maximum intensity projection
MIRD	medical internal radiation dose
MLO	mediolateral oblique
MRA	magnetic resonance angiography
MRCP	magnetic resonance cholangiopancreatogram
MR	magnetic resonance
MRI	magnetic resonance imaging
MRM	magnetic resonance mammography
MSD	mean sac diameter
MSP	median sagittal plane
MSS	maternal serum screening
mSv	milliSievert
mT	milliTesla
MUGA	multiple gated cardiac acquisition
NAI	non-accidental injury
NCEPOD	National Confidential Enquiry into Perioperative Deaths
NHSBSP	National Health Service Breast Screening Programme
NICE	National Institute for Clinical Excellence
NM	nuclear medicine
NMR	nuclear magnetic resonance
NMV	net magnetic vector
NOF	neck of femur
NRPB	National Radiological Protection Board
NST	non-stress test
NT	nuchal translucency
OF	occipitofrontal
OFD	object film distance

OGD	oesophagogastric duodenoscopy	SC	sternoclavicular
OI	osteogenesis imperfecta	SFA	superficial femoral artery
OM	occipitomental	SFDM	small field digital mammography
OMBL	orbitomeatal baseline	SID	source image distance
OPG	orthopantomography	SI	sacroiliac
OPT	orthopantomography	SIJ	sacroiliac joint
PA	posteroanterior	SMV	submentovertical
PACS	picture, archiving and communication systems	SNR	signal-to-noise ratio
		SOL	space occupying lesion
PCA	phase contrast angiography	SPET	single photon emission tomography
PCNL	percutaneous nephrolithotomy	SPECT	single photon emission computed tomography
PD	proton density		
PE	pulmonary embolism	SPR	scan projection radiograph
PET	positron emission tomography	STIR	short tau inversion recovery
PID	pelvic inflammatory disease	SUFE	slipped upper femoral epiphysis
PGMI	perfect, good, moderate, inadequate (system)	SVC	superior vena cava
		SXR	skull X-ray
PMT	photomultiplier tube	T	Tesla
ppm	parts per million	TAS	transabdominal scan
PSA	prostate specific antigen	TE	time to echo
PSIS	posterior superior iliac spine	TFT	thin film transistor
PSL	photostimulable luminescence	TI	thermal index
PSP	photostimulable phosphor	TIA	transient ischaemic attack
PTC	percutaneous transhepatic cholangiography	TLD	thermo-luminescent dosimetry
		TMJ	temporomandibular joint
PW	perfusion weighted	TOF	time-of-flight (angiography)
QDE	quantum detection efficency	TPN	total parenteral nutrition
RA	rheumatoid arthritis	TR	time to repetition
RCR	Royal College of Radiologists	TS	transabdominal scan
RF	radiofrequency	TVS	transvaginal scan
RNI	radionuclide imaging	UAE	uterine artery embolisation
RAO	right anterior oblique	US	ultrasound
RPD	renal pelvic dilatation	UTI	urinary tract infection
RPO	right posterior oblique	VDU	visual display unit
RSD	reflex sympathetic dystrophy	VLA	vertical long axis
SA	short axis	VENC	velocity encoding
SAH	subarachnoid haemorrhage	V/Q	ventilation/perfusion lung scan
SBE	small bowel enema	w/v	weight to volume

IMAGING PRINCIPLES

FILM/SCREEN IMAGING

Susan Penelope Nash

INTRODUCTION

This chapter is not intended to be a comprehensive account of screen and film technology as there are many excellent resources available for students in this field. However, students cannot be expected to evaluate new digital technologies without an understanding of the contribution of film/screen technology to medical imaging during the last century, so with this in mind, a summary of the history and main developments follows for background information.

IMAGING PLATES

The first medical radiographic image receptors were silver halide coated glass plates, which were placed in light-tight envelopes or cassettes. Junior staff often had the task of waxing the edges of the plates to prevent the emulsion from slipping off![1]

Although the value of photographic film was recognised, it was used sparingly prior to the 1920s. Once in regular use, however, the X-ray film soon proved its worth. It was quickly recognised that, unlike the early glass plates, a film could be coated on both sides. This had obvious advantages – particularly when used with intensifying screens. Since only about 1–2% of incident radiation was absorbed by the X-ray film alone, it was soon apparent that this wastefulness could be reduced by utilising light rather than X-rays to create the latent image on the film.[2]

INTENSIFYING SCREENS AND FILM EMULSION TECHNOLOGY

The introduction of fluorescent intensifying screens proved to be a significant development, enabling more of the incident X-rays to be absorbed by the phosphor material and emitted as light. In addition, the use of two intensifying screens meant that double emulsion films could be used – instantly doubling the light absorption. However, the increase in density and contrast was partially counterbalanced by a decrease in resolution, and an increase in quantum noise in faster film/screen combinations. As always in radiography, there is a choice to be made when balancing image quality and patient dose.

During the remainder of the 20th century, screen and film technology continued to develop. Intensifying screens became more efficient when 'rare earth' phosphors were introduced in the 1970s, while the familiar globular silver halide crystals in the film emulsion were superseded by the 'tabular' variety.

The introduction of asymmetric film screen combinations with anti-crossover features provided greater visualisation with reduced image blur. In recent years, there have been further developments in emulsion technology, but the undoubted success of the new digital technologies has mounted a serious challenge to traditional practices. Nonetheless, cassettes, films and screens still have an important role in medical imaging – at least in the short term.

THE X-RAY CASSETTE

The cassette is essentially a light-tight, protective container for the film and intensifying screens. It is also designed to maintain a uniform contact between the film and screens. A foam pressure pad behind the back screen helps to ensure this.

Various cassette materials such as aluminium and plastic laminate have been used in the past. However, the ideal low attenuation material for the cassette front is carbon fibre, since it represents a considerable reduction in patient dose. It is lightweight, durable and relatively comfortable for the patient, but rather more expensive than other materials. The cassette back is lined with lead foil to reduce scattered radiation. A sliding aperture and lead blocker is incorporated into the design for use with patient identification systems.

Whilst the film/screen cassette is still relatively commonplace, older cassette types are less familiar sights in a modern imaging department. These include the multisection cassette, the formatter cassette and the photofluorographic cassette.[3]

RADIOGRAPHIC FILM

Film technology depends upon certain materials undergoing changes when subjected to electromagnetic radiation such as visible light or X-rays. The main light-sensitive materials used are the halogens, e.g. bromine, iodine or chlorine. In radiographic film these are combined with silver to form, e.g. silver bromide or silver idobromide.

■ Film manufacture

The manufacturing process is extremely stringent as there must be no variation between batches of film. Solutions of silver nitrate ($AgNO_3$) and potassium bromide (KBr) are added to liquid gelatine. Potassium nitrate, which is soluble, is washed away in the process.[4]

There are usually four stages in the preparation of the emulsion layer. It is during the latter stages that the characteristics of the film are determined. For example, the speed and contrast of the film depend upon the size of the silver halide grains. A high contrast, narrow latitude film has a narrow range of grain sizes, while relatively large grains will produce a film of greater speed. In the final stage, various additives are introduced such as sensitisers, colour sensitisers, hardener, plasticisers, fungicide, anti-static agent, wetting agent and antifoggant.[3]

Impurities such as sulphur are deliberately added during the process in order to create imperfections in the crystal lattice. These imperfections create areas known as electron traps or sensitivity centres. These centres, coupled with excess bromine added to the mix create the conditions necessary for the formation of the latent image.

■ Film construction

In order that it can be used as a photographic material, the silver halide needs to be prepared in a form that can be coated on to a support or base (Fig. 1.1).

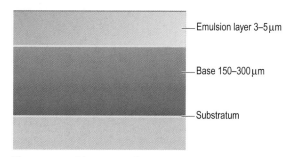

Figure 1.1 Diagrammatic representation of film structure, not to scale

Emulsion layer 3–5 μm

Base 150–300 μm

Substratum

Base

The material for the base is usually polyester. It has all the necessary characteristics required as it is:

- strong but flexible
- dimensionally stable
- non-flammable
- unaffected by processing chemicals and high temperatures
- impermeable to water
- uniform in colour tone and thickness.

Photographic emulsion

The silver halide crystals have to be suspended in a suitable binder to form a photographic emulsion. Gelatine has the properties required to act as a binding agent and suspension medium. It allows the silver halide crystals to grow. Gelatine is transparent and can exist as either a liquid or a solid; therefore it allows the crystals to be suspended evenly within the emulsion. It does not react chemically with the silver, but it allows the processing chemicals to penetrate the emulsion.

The emulsion layer is coated on to one or both sides of the base. A thin adhesive layer (substratum) binds the emulsion layer easily to the base. A supercoat or protective layer of clear gelatine protects the emulsion during processing and handling.[3,4]

■ Effect of exposure on silver halides

Silver halide crystals or grains may consist of a variety of shapes, although modern grains are likely to be tabular in X-ray applications. Tabular grains are flat and provide a greater surface area available for latent image formation.

The latent image

The latent image is the hidden image that is created as a result of an interaction between X-ray or light photons and the silver bromide crystals. There are two theories of latent image formation – the Gurney-Mott and the Mitchell theories. The theories are the subject of some debate but the Gurney-Mott theory seems to be preferred in radiographic imaging.[5]

The silver and bromine atoms are fixed in the crystal lattice in ion form: positive silver ions and negative bromine ions. In simple terms the interactions between X-rays or light photons and bromine ions cause electrons to be released. These electrons migrate to the electron traps. The interstitial silver ions are attracted to the electrons in the electron traps (or sensitivity centres), and they combine to form silver atoms.

As the process is repeated, other silver ions are attracted to the sensitivity centre and more silver atoms are created. The latent image centre is not visible – even microscopically; it is the developer which renders the image visible by acting as a chemical reducing agent and transforming the silver atoms into visible metallic silver.[5]

Types of film

Duplitised or double emulsion film is the standard film used for general applications. The vast majority of these films are used with two intensifying screens. The exceptions are the intraoral dental film, which is a direct exposure film, and the radiation monitoring film which is coated with two different emulsions and is used with various filters.

Single emulsion film is used in mammography where high resolution is the primary requirement. Laser imaging and duplication film are also coated with a single emulsion. Less frequently one may see subtraction film and 100 mm photofluorographic single emulsion film.

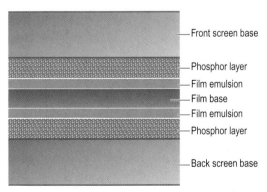

Figure 1.2 Cross-section of a duplitised film/screen combination

Labels (top to bottom): Front screen base; Phosphor layer; Film emulsion; Film base; Film emulsion; Phosphor layer; Back screen base

INTENSIFYING SCREENS

In many ways, the intensifying screen represents the most important component of the film/screen/cassette combination. Although X-rays do interact with the film emul-

sion, they only contribute approximately 1–3% to the latent image in a typical screen/film combination. On the other hand, about 30% of the incident X-rays interact with the screen.[4] Even though a considerable amount of the incident energy is lost, the process is much more efficient if intensifying screens are used. This results in a considerable dose reduction for the patient.

Screen construction

Base
The base or support consists of cardboard, plastic or polyester. It is usually up to 1 mm thick. Obviously the base must be robust and moisture resistant.

Substratum
The substratum layer is a bonding layer between the base and the phosphor layer. This may be reflective, absorptive or transparent. A reflective layer will reflect light back towards the film for maximum effect in faster film/screen combinations. Titanium dioxide is often the material used. The increase in speed, however, is achieved at the expense of increased image blur or unsharpness.[4]

Alternatively an absorptive layer contains a dye that will absorb light and therefore may be used in high resolution screens. More commonly there may be a coloured pigment or carbon granules within the phosphor layer which serve the same purpose. Greater resolution is achieved at the expense of some loss in speed.[3,5]

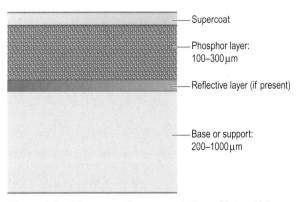

Figure 1.3 Diagrammatic representation of intensifying screen structure, not to scale

Labels (top to bottom): Supercoat; Phosphor layer: 100–300 μm; Reflective layer (if present); Base or support: 200–1000 μm

Phosphor layer
The phosphor layer contains fluorescent crystals which emit light when bombarded by X-ray photons. The crystals are held in a clear binder such as polyurethane. This material protects the phosphor material from moisture. This is important since many phosphor materials are hygroscopic.

LUMINESCENCE

A luminescent material emits light as a result of external stimulation. The process is similar to the emission of characteristic radiation, but involving outer-shell electrons. There are many different types of luminescence but in radiography only three are of relevance: fluorescence, phosphorescence and thermo-luminescence. Thermo-luminescent materials emit light when stimulated by heat. This process is used in thermo-luminescent dosimeters (TLDs).

■ Fluorescence

This occurs almost instantaneously and the emission of light ceases within 10^{-8} seconds.

Within the phosphor material there are three energy levels known as the conduction band, the forbidden band and the valence band. Incident X-ray photon energy is absorbed within the phosphor material by the photo-electric effect or Compton scattering. In the process, high energy secondary electrons are emitted. These collide with other electrons knocking them from the valence band to the conduction band. Electrons already in the electron traps and electrons in the conduction band can fall into the holes created in the valence band, emitting light as they lose energy.[5]

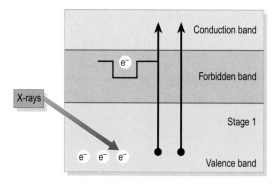

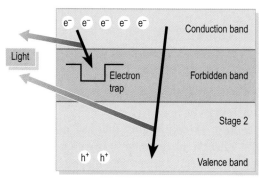

Figure 1.4 Fluorescence. Stage 1: X-rays remove electrons from the valence band. Stage 2: the electrons drop into the electron traps, or directly into the conduction band, emitting light energy as they do so

■ Phosphorescence

If the phosphor continues to emit light after irradiation has ceased, then the process is called phosphorescence. This is called afterglow or image lag and is not desirable in an intensifying screen for obvious reasons. Afterglow, however may occasionally be observed in older image intensifiers.

Types of phosphor

Until the 1970s the most popular phosphor was calcium tungstate ($CaWO_4$). It was known as the universal phosphor and emitted ultraviolet light. Other phosphors included barium strontium sulphate and barium lead sulphate. Then rare earth phosphors were developed such as gadolinium oxysulphide and lanthanum oxybromide. Small quantities of activators such as terbium are added during manufacture. The combination of phosphor and activator determines the colour and intensity of light emitted. These phosphors combined with activators had distinct advantages over $CaWO_4$ – in particular higher quantum detection efficiency and improved conversion efficiency.

Quantum detection efficiency (QDE or absorption efficiency)

Rare earth phosphors are kVp dependent to a certain extent, but if used within recommended limits, the QDE of rare earth phosphors is superior. The QDE is proportional to the atomic number of the rare earth phosphors. Consequently these phosphors are usually more efficient at absorbing X-ray quanta – particularly between the K-shell absorption edge for rare earth elements and tungsten (Fig. 1.5).

The energy range extends from approximately 30 keV to 70 keV. For example, Gd_2O_2S:Tb has an absorption efficiency of 51% at 60 keV compared with $CaWO_4$ at 13%. However, at 80 keV there is very little difference at 27% and 28% respectively. Energy levels above or below

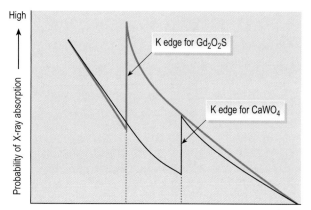

Figure 1.5 X-ray absorption spectra for calcium tungstate and gadolinium

this range will result in decreased QDE in rare earth phosphors.[3,4]

Conversion efficiency

The rare earth phosphors have an even greater advantage when X-ray photons are converted to light. Approximately 15–20% of X-ray photons are converted to light compared with 3–5% for $CaWO_4$.[3]

SPECTRAL SENSITIVITY AND SPECTRAL EMISSION

Films are sensitive to all wavelengths of light but during the manufacturing process certain types of X-ray film are designed to be particularly sensitive to certain wavelengths of light. Radiographic films are either monochromatic (blue/violet sensitive), orthochromatic (green sensitive), or panchromatic (red or infrared sensitive).

It is essential to match the spectral sensitivity of the film to the spectral emission of the intensifying screens. Calcium tungstate is known as a broad band emitter as it emits a continuous spectrum with a peak emission of approximately 440 nanometres (nm). Many rare earth phosphors emit narrow bands of wavelengths with peak emission of approximately 550 nm in the green area of the spectrum (Fig. 1.6).

Spectral mismatching will occur if, for example, a green-emitting screen is used with a blue sensitive film. The peak emission in the green region of the spectrum will be undetected by the film and this will result in a considerable reduction in speed.[4]

▇ Factors affecting screen performance

Crossover

The crossover effect can be detrimental to image quality due to the increased image blur caused by light crossing

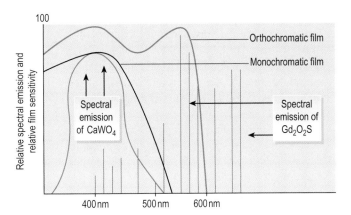

Figure 1.6   Relative spectral emission and spectral sensitivity

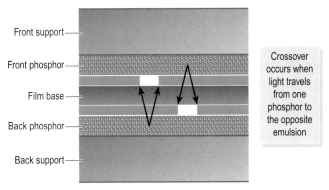

Figure 1.7   Crossover

from one screen as far as the opposite emulsion layer. The increased distance involved results in greater divergence of light and reduced sharpness (Fig. 1.7).

Other factors

Speed will be increased if the following factors apply:

- larger phosphor crystal size and greater coating weight
- use of a reflective layer
- greater QDE
- greater conversion efficiency
- no anti-crossover layer.

The above factors will, however reduce the sharpness of the image. Conversely, reducing the phosphor crystal size and coating weight, and adding carbon granules or a dye to the phosphor layer, will reduce speed and increase sharpness.

COMPARISON OF FILM/SCREEN SYSTEMS

It is useful to be able to easily compare different systems in terms of speed, contrast and latitude. Manufacturers attach a number to their products in the same way as photographic films are identified. Par-speed $CaWO_4$ screens are assigned a value of 100. High resolution screens are usually between 50 and 100, while others range from 200 to 1200.

The speed of a film/screen system is inversely proportional to the exposure required to produce a given density. Therefore a 200 speed system will require half the mAs of a 100 speed system to produce the same density on the film (all other factors being constant)

Image quality deteriorates with very fast systems because quantum noise becomes unacceptable.

Purchasers of film/screen combinations do not make their choice on speed alone however. Film contrast and latitude also need to be considered carefully before a system is selected for general or specialist use. In addition, processing requirements must not be forgotten.

Asymmetric screen/film systems

A dual receptor system uses asymmetric screens and dual emulsion films. The back screen contains a thicker phosphor compared with the front screen. The film has a high contrast emulsion on the front surface and a wide latitude emulsion on the back surface, and the film base is coated with an anti-crossover layer. This essentially means that two different images are superimposed (Fig. 1.8).[2]

The result is that the final image has enhanced visualisation of the posterior mediastinum of the chest for example, without losing detail of the lung fields. Asymmetric systems are not universally used, but are valuable in chest and paediatric imaging in particular. Research suggests that greater visualisation of anatomical structures is possible although there do not seem to be particular advantages in identifying chest pathology.[6]

LATEST DEVELOPMENTS

Manufacturers have been continuing to refine their products, particularly in relation to emulsion technology. For example, Kodak have produced the X-SIGHT system which uses smaller phosphor particles to reduce image noise while maintaining speed.[7] In addition zero crossover asymmetric screens reduce light scatter. The latest development, however, is 'visually adaptive contrast', which provides additional contrast in areas of increased optical density. This contrast is achieved with the use of different emulsion layers. At the same time it is claimed that film latitude is not reduced.[7]

The Kodak Min-R EV mammography screen-film system uses similar 'contrast-enhancing emulsion grains' and also maintains contrast in high density areas. Again, improved phosphor structure emits more light than earlier intensifying screens.[8]

THE FUTURE

In Western Europe and North America, in particular, the advance of digital imaging technologies would appear to be irresistible, and although screen/film technology still appears to offer some advantages in mammography,[9] in other areas computed radiography (CR) has gained a strong foothold, while digital flat panel systems are gaining ground. In the UK, for example, this is driven by the nationally funded programme for the installation of Picture Archiving and Communication Systems (PACS) in the National Health Service.

Although the spatial resolution of CR systems is generally lower than film/screen – typically 3–7 lp/mm compared to

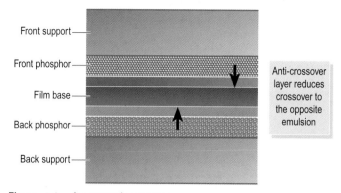

Figure 1.8 Asymmetric systems

Front support
Front phosphor
Film base
Back phosphor
Back support

Anti-crossover layer reduces crossover to the opposite emulsion

7–10 lp/mm, the potential savings in dose more than compensate for this.[10,11] Therefore, in the long term it is difficult to see how an analogue film screen system can survive in the face of such rapid technological advance.

In the final analysis, film/screen technology is still the gold standard against which all other technologies must measure themselves. Digital installation is not cheap and in the developing countries such investment is certainly not feasible at present. Therefore it is probably safe to say that films and screens will not be consigned to history just yet.

References

1. Thomas A, et al. The invisible light: 100 years of medical radiology. Oxford: Blackwell Science; 1995.
2. Pizzutiello R, Cullinan J. Introduction to medical radiographic imaging. New York: Eastman Kodak; 1993.
3. Ball J, Price T. Chesney's radiographic imaging. 6th edn. Oxford: Blackwell Science; 1995.
4. Bushong S. Radiologic science for technologists. 7th edn. St Louis: Mosby; 2001.
5. Gunn C. Radiographic imaging: a practical approach. 4th edn. Edinburgh: Churchill Livingstone; 2002.
6. Greaney T, Masterson J. Comparison of an asymmetric screen-film combination with a conventional screen-film combination for chest radiography in 51 patients. British Journal of Radiology 1997; 70:929–932.
7. Eastman Kodak Co. Kodak X-SIGHT imaging system. 2002. Online. Available: www.kodak.com/go/health
8. Eastman Kodak Co. Kodak MIN-R EV screen-film system. 2003. Online. Available: www.kodak.com/go/mammo
9. Skaane P, et al. Population based mammography screening: comparison of screen-film and full-field digital mammography with soft copy reading. Radiology 2003; 229(3):877–884.
10. Khalifa K, Brindhaban A. Comparison between conventional radiography and digital radiography for various kVp and mAs settings using a pelvic phantom. Radiography 2004; 10(2):119–125.
11. Lau S-L, et al. Reject analysis: a comparison of conventional film-screen radiography and computed radiography with PACS. Radiography 2004; 10(3):183–187.

CHAPTER 2

DIGITAL IMAGING

Philip Cosson

INTRODUCTION

Film/screen systems are predictable as physical and chemical principles govern the exposure response of these systems. Digital systems, as a consequence of the technologies involved, do not have simple exposure response relationships. It is not easy to transfer the old 'rules of thumb' to the new systems, causing difficulty in the use of these technologies within the radiography department.

There are two main types of system available currently, which can be considered as computed radiography (CR) and digital radiography (DR).

IMAGE STORAGE

Digital images can be stored as graphic files in a number of formats. Radiographs are generally stored as bitmap graphics and common formats are 'bmp' and 'jpeg'. Bitmapped graphics are stored as a series of numbers, rather than being described in terms of formulae as used in vector graphics (e.g. 'gif' files). Bitmaps are usually larger than vector graphics because areas of empty space must be recorded as well. Uncompressed they are the exact same size no matter what the image content.

A bitmap can be visualised by considering a chessboard pattern, each square ('pixel': picture element) is allocated a colour (in a bitmap this will be a numerical value to represent each shade) which best represents the contents of that square. The quality of the image produced will depend on the size of the 'chessboard', the number of squares (matrix), and the colours available (in radiography this will be shades of grey).

Changing the size of the image ('chessboard') will change the outer dimensions of the picture, but not add any detail to it, just make each square bigger. When the squares are big and noticeable the image is said to be 'pixelated' (Fig. 2.1).

Increasing the number of pixels (squares on the chessboard) causes each to be smaller and therefore less noticeable. The Nyquist theory suggests that the smallest detail visible in any bitmap is twice the size of a pixel. This limit is referred to as the extended Kell factor.[1]

A smaller pixel size also makes the selection of the allocated 'colour' easier as each pixel is representing a smaller area of the image. As there can only be one colour covering each pixel, the closest match to the average colour in that area of the image must be used. The smaller the area of the image and the more extensive the available colour selection (greyscale), the easier the choice and the more accurate the copy (stored image) (Fig. 2.2).

A standard chessboard has 8 rows and 8 columns of squares that form an 8×8 matrix, or array. The total number of pixels is 64. Each pixel is 50 mm square[2] and is adjacent to its neighbour, therefore a pixel pitch of 50 mm. A computer represents the colour of a pixel by storing a number, called the pixel value. In computing, numbers are stored in binary form, i.e. a series of 0s and 1s. Each numerical value is termed a bit; the number of values the computer can use for each pixel (i.e. number of bits) is called the bit depth. For example if 6 bits were used, then binary values from 000000 to 111111 (0 to 63) would be available, that is 64 grey shades (pixel values). Computers generally group bits into units of 8 (8 bits = 1 byte), hence images are generally stored as 8, 16, 24, or 32 bit files.

There are three ways to generate a radiological bit-map:

- Computed tomography (CT), positron emission tomography (PET) and magnetic resonance imaging (MRI): the pixel values are found using a mathematical compu-

Figure 2.1
Standard
chessboard: 8 × 8
matrix

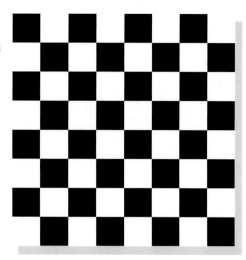

Figure 2.2
32 × 32 matrix

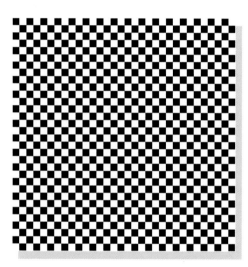

- detector (changing the CR plate size, or choosing DDR)
- zoom or electrostatic focus of an image intensifier
- FOV variable in CT and MRI.

RESOLUTION

Matrix size is very important to resolution. Up to a point, the more squares on the matrix, the better the image will look and the more the image can be modified. Of course, each additional square takes additional computer memory, but an unlimited amount of memory would not remove all limits to size of matrix. The Royal College of Radiologists (RCR) do not quote a limit for 'large matrix' images in their guidance on teleradiology. They state that any system must be able to resolve 2.5 lppm.[3] Applying a Kell factor of 0.5, this would require a matrix size of 1760 × 2140 for a 35 × 43 cm chest radiograph, but only 1000 × 1255 for an 18 × 24 wrist radiograph: however, would a 2000 – 2510 matrix wrist radiograph be any better quality?

In PSP CR, the thickness of the phosphor layer is also a limit to resolution, as is the size of the laser that reads them. In most DR the size of the electronics required to amplify and transmit the signal from each pixel is finite and no pixel can be any smaller than this size. With either technology, to some extent, the display technology limits the usefulness of very high definition images as radiographers and radiologists cannot work with small, zoomed, areas of a large image.

By far the biggest problem with minimising pixel size, however, is reduced signal strength, and hence problems with signal to noise ratio. As resolution is affected by noise as well as pixel size, increasing the matrix size often does not improve resolution, without an increase in signal strength, i.e. an increase in the number of photons, and consequently radiation dose.

COMPUTED RADIOGRAPHY

PSP technology underpins CR. First introduced in 1983,[4] it is now the dominant method of acquiring digital radiographs. Analogous to the rare earth phosphor screen technology of 1970-1990, CR uses new alkaline-earth halides and alkaline halides as PSPs to record a latent image of any irradiated structure. These include salts of barium (Ba), strontium (Sr), caesium (Cs) and rubidium (Rb) combined with halides such as chlorine (Cl), bromine (Br), iodine (I) and fluorine (F). These are then 'doped' with an activator, usually europium (Eu), but cerium (Ce), thallium (Tl), indium (In), lead (Pb) and samarium (Sm) are also used.

tation called Fourier back projection; the matrix is fixed (128, 256, 512, 1024). A variable called 'field of view' (FOV) determines how much of the scan area is used in the calculations and therefore displayed in the bitmap.
- Analogue to digital conversion (ADC): the pixel values are found by scanning across a detector. The matrix size is fixed in the factory by the engineers who design the scan system, not the detector. Image intensifier fluoroscopy, ultrasound (with computation for radial scanning), photostimulable phosphor (PSP) CR, transmission radiographic film scanners.
- Direct digital radiography/fluoroscopy/scintillation detector (direct digital radiography (DDR)/direct digital fluoroscopy (DDF)/gamma camera): the pixel values are directly detected within a fixed matrix, and are hardwired by the manufacturer of the detector.

Although there are fixed matrix sizes (as mentioned above), radiographers can alter the matrix size relative to the patient by altering the:

One of the design considerations when selecting a PSP is the colour of the laser light the PSP is most stimulated by. Some lasers are cheaper, smaller, more powerful and easier to use in a scanning system. For example BaFBr:Eu is stimulated best by yellow/orange light (590 nm). It would be beneficial to shift the stimulation spectra more towards red or near infrared since very powerful (>20 mW) and small red (670 nm) lasers (GaAlAs) are available and well-suited for reading out imaging plates. Fuji launched new imaging plates with the incorporation of iodine to allow these new lasers to be used. Konica recently launched a BaFI:Eu imaging plate that also provided a higher attenuation coefficient.[5]

■ The structure of an imaging plate

The PSP layer is coated onto a substrate and covered with a protective layer. A powder phosphor consists of crystals evenly distributed in a binder. The technology is very similar to intensifying screen construction with the possibility for the inclusion of pigments in the binder and anti-halo layers to reduce the effect of noise due to scattered light. This layer is generally thicker than intensifying screens of the same 'speed class'. The thickness of the PSP layer and the flatness of the surface are factors associated with noise noticed as mottle.[5] (Fig. 2.3)

■ 'Flying spot' imaging plate reader

Ionizing radiation penetrating an object will excite electrons in many substances, and does so in an image plate. An unusual mechanism of photostimulable luminescence (PSL) is that the irradiation also creates storage centres in the halide crystal structure that the ionised electrons can get trapped in. These storage centres are termed 'colour centres' and in German they are known as 'Farbzentren' hence they have become known as F-centres. A typical BaFBr:Eu imaging plate will form approx 400 F-centres for every one photon of X-radiation absorbed in the normal diagnostic range. Absorption depends on photon energy and phosphor thickness, but is approximately 50% for this plate.

The process of PSL in a plate as above has been described as:[6]

1. One X-ray photon absorbed
2. Formation of 400 F-centres
3. Laser stimulation produces light photons in 30%
4. 50% emerge at the photomultiplier side of the phosphor
5. 30% of these are collected by optical fibres and guided to the photomultiplier
6. 25% of photons received are recorded by the photomultiplier.

Between stages 2 and 3, the trapped electrons have more potential energy. This is the state of an irradiated imaging plate prior to being read; if the plate was left in this state, over time, the electrons would receive energy by random events such as background radiation, and the number trapped would gradually drop. At 1 hour only 76% would be trapped; consequently it is important to read the plate within 5 minutes.[7]

The speed of movement is critical to the plate read time. In a busy department the radiographer would like the plate as quickly as possible to engender speedy workflow. CR typically reads at approx 3 line pairs per millimetre. This is not the limit of the technology, but there is some trade off between resolution and plate read time. The reason only 30% of the trapped electrons are liberated is in part due to the speed and power of the laser and the thickness of the phosphor. The faster the flying spot moves, the less time it can stay over a particular area of the phosphor, the less stimulation can occur at the deeper levels of the phosphor, and the less signal is collected. Those that do get stimulated recombine and luminesce in all directions.

In stages 4, 5 and 6, those light photons that are travelling in the direction of the light guide can be collected and a quarter of these are recorded by the photomultiplier that converts the luminescence into a weak electrical signal.

A new technique is to use a transparent base with the phosphor coated onto it. This then allows optical collection of photostimulated light from both sides of the plate simultaneously. This can increase the number of light photons collected.

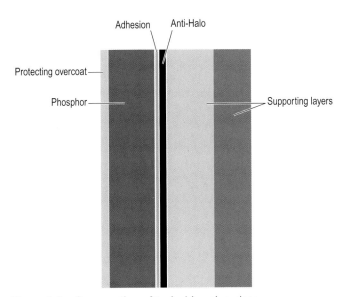

Figure 2.3   Cross-section of typical imaging plate

Once the plate has been through this process, the remaining 70% of trapped electrons must be liberated prior to the imaging plates reuse.

Up to this point, there is nothing computed or digital about this process. It is fundamentally analogue, where the electrical signal can take any value. The process termed 'ADC' must now take place to allow the latent image to be captured and represented by the computer.

Analogue to digital conversion: the 'flying spot' approach

The analogue signal in this case is a weak variable electrical signal from a photomultiplier tube or similar device. The conversion of this signal into a bitmap requires quantitisation and sampling of the signal. Quantitisation can simply be understood as the choice of palette (greyscale), and deciding the pixel value according to the signal strength. Sampling is about deciding the matrix size. This is a choice of the number of lines that the imaging plate will be scanned, and the corresponding number of pixels sampled along each line, to ensure the pixels are square. The size of the laser spot, the power of the laser beam and the plate read time are all critical to this choice.

To scan the picture, we would systematically move from top left across, then 'fly back' to the next row and scan again across. This produces a fast scan direction across the imaging plate and a slow scan direction down the imaging plate. These scan directions are important and radiographers should have an understanding of them in relation to the use of the cassette in practice.

We have therefore converted our analogue signal to a digital array that can be displayed as a bitmap. One can see that the choice of matrix size is dependant on the mechanical scanning process, as each scan line is represented by one line of data. Therefore, the closer the scan lines, the smaller the laser beam and the narrower the scan line width, the larger the possible matrix size and the more pixels possible.

The future for CR

The next generation of image plate readers may feature a line scanner (as opposed to the 'flying spot' approach) to increase dwell time without delaying the plate read time. Together with the use of high-powered lasers, this will increase the percentage of deep F-centres stimulated.[8] This linear scanner can be miniaturised to fit inside a radiographic table or wall stand. The imaging plate will no longer have to be flexible to be handled by the reader, and needle crystal CsBr:Eu phosphors could be used in commercial systems for the first time.

A needle phosphor leads to better image quality than a powder for two reasons. The needles act as light guides, thereby strongly reducing light spread in the phosphor layer. In addition, no binder is present in a needle screen, which implies a higher phosphor packing density, higher X-ray photon absorption, and therefore greater signal-to-noise ratio.

FULL FIELD DIGITAL RADIOGRAPHY

For a direct digital detector, as the name implies, the image is captured directly to a bitmap instantly within the detector itself. There is no latent image to decay, nor any mechanical moving parts. Limitations on the size of the bitmap do exist however. There are also at least two different technologies worth describing in detail here and these are amorphous silicon full field (CsI:Tl phosphor with a-Si/TFT array) and amorphous selenium full field.

Amorphous silicon full field (CsI:Tl phosphor with a-Si/TFT array)

This system uses a phosphor, much as CR does. The CsI:Tl needle phosphor converts X-ray photons to visible light in the green spectrum. This gives it its other name: indirect DR.

An ultra thin (2 μm) film of amorphous silicon, sensitive to this light, is attached to the thicker CsI:Tl phosphor. Commonly, phosphor thicknesses of up to 1000 μm are used, with 500 μm being common. The silicon is laid out in a fixed matrix of pixels - each pixel is a photodiode 'sensor' which acts as a receiver for electrons and records a separate signal. The thin film transistor (TFT) or field effect transistor (FET) behaves as a pixel switch to access the associated photo-diode.

When a TFT is conductive, the corresponding photo-diode can be charged. The TFT is then turned off prior to exposure. Light photons create electron-hole pairs in the photo-diode causing it to partially discharge. The TFT is then turned back on and the photo-diode is recharged. The amount of charge required is measured by the readout electronics and converted to a digital value (binary number) by the analogue to digital converter attached to each column. It is transmitted to memory and recorded at the required bit depth (usually 14). The advantages to this system are the high sensitivity of CsI:Tl needle phosphor to X-rays and the relatively stable properties of amorphous silicon. These systems have the highest detective quantum efficiency (DQE) of all digital systems. CsI:Tl is also used in fluoroscopy systems, as it has a fast decay time, allowing for updated images at 30 plus frames per second without noticeable lag.

Arrays have been made with pixel sizes from 100 µm to 400 µm.[9] The standard pixel design has a ratio of sensor to TFT known as the 'fill factor'. This approaches 50% at 100 µm, making this a practical limit, e.g. in mammography applications. A new full fill factor design is required for these applications.

Amorphous Selenium Full Field

Selenium is a photoconductor, most sensitive to energies in the lower X-ray range. It is therefore able to directly convert X-ray photons to signal without a phosphor stage. The a-Se is laid onto a predetermined matrix of TFTs, one for each pixel and each pixel area records its signal on a capacitor. The pixel size is not determined by fill factor, as the a-Se layer is continuous. Normally pixel pitch is 140 µm, but 70–85 µm pixels can be used for mammography.

The advantage to this system is the lack of any light scattering in a phosphor layer. This system has a very high modulation transfer function (approx 80% at 2.5 lp/mm). The a-Se layer can be thick without the risk of increased noise, however, the thicker the layer the larger the voltage required across it to capture the electrons. A practical limit would be 1000 µm as this would require 10 000 volts. For lower photon energies, i.e. mammography, 200 µm thick detectors achieve 100% absorption with less than 5000 volts. However, the requirement for a high voltage system makes the detector relatively complex and bulky (Fig. 2.4).

Digital image display

Having captured a radiographic image, some form of display is required. It can be argued that in the future this may become an unnecessary step due to the development of computer aided detection (CAD). This technology allows 'rules' written in software to be applied to the numerical data held in the image file. On comparing pixels with others and 'normals' in a database, abnormalities may be detected by the computer. Bitmap location, pixel value and other variables can predict, with varying accuracy, the presence of disease.

CAD is already used in some centres to second and third read mammograms. However, currently the 'gold standard' in image interpretation is the human reader of the displayed image. The fidelity of the display is as important as the quality of the image capture technology. It should always be remembered that the reader is human and the characteristics of the display should be designed for the human visual system, both physical and psychological.

The first characteristic of the visual system is that its performance is affected by the environment and changes over time: ambient lighting, fatigue and distraction are important factors. It is a mistake to specify a display technology without considering the whole reading environment. For example, the distance the eye is from the image will affect the resolution perceived. The angle at which the image is viewed can change the perception of patterns, and the background noise and heat of computer cooling fans can increase fatigue and distraction. There are two types of display technology currently used: cathode ray tubes and liquid crystal display (LCD) panels.

Cathode ray tube (CRT)

CRTs have been the dominant display technology, but are fast being challenged by active matrix LCD panels. The diagnostic CRT is a monochrome monitor, i.e. it only displays shades of grey. It has a high luminance of 700+ cdcm^{-2} but this still does not approach that of a light box. It requires a special video card to drive the monotone output instead of the standard RGB output of a computer video card.

Disadvantages of CRTs are that they are large, heavy, have a high power (and hence heat) output, and a high quality assurance (QA) burden because luminance varies and deteriorates over time. There have also been fears regarding radiation output from workstations, although for a typical CRT there is no penetration of the glass screen front.

The use of a CRT reverses the process of ADC in order to create an analogue signal from the digital data held in the computer; this extra step may produce signal distortion.

LCD panels

An active matrix LCD panel utilises similar technology to a DR detector, a thin film semiconductor covers the surface with a pre-defined bitmap of pixels etched into it; these displays have a set maximum resolution. They are inherently digital devices and therefore require no normal

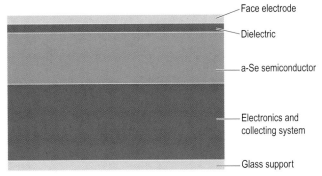

Figure 2.4   Structure of a typical amorphous selenium detector

Face electrode

Dielectric

a-Se semiconductor

Electronics and collecting system

Glass support

video card, but a simpler digital 'CDI' card. There is now no loss in signal. This technology does not require the size and space of a CRT.

Although luminance is variable, the backlight can be changed and restored to original values very simply. Many systems have auto-calibration to account for this variability second by second. These systems are much simpler to site several together to view many images at once.

Disadvantages of LCD panels are:

- Fixed resolution: zooming, etc requires resampling, which can cause aliasing artefacts
- Angle of view can be limited or only single axis
- Initial cost is greater than for CRT.

DIGITAL IMAGE MANIPULATION

Perhaps the greatest advantage of digital imaging is the ability to duplicate, store, search and manipulate the acquired data.

In acquisition and display, the emphasis is on fidelity. Recording the radiographic contrast emerging from the patient as faithfully as possible is paramount, which means displaying the pixel values and locations accurately and consistently. The number one benefit of all digital projection radiography systems is the ability to deal with changing radiographic exposure parameters, even incorrect ones! In this case we want to change the data coming in before displaying it because the pixel values are either too high (overexposed) or too low (underexposed). The computer achieves this adjustment by adding or subtracting an array from the stored bitmap before display.

This is a simplified example to show the benefit of changing the data in a controlled way. The initial data acquired is stored in a file called the RAW Data. Any manipulation should be on a copy of this data, leaving the original intact. In some systems, after manipulation, only the new data is sent across the network to be viewed and stored; this can be with a reduced palette (14 becomes 12 bit). Although this might be seen as a disadvantage, it does emphasise the radiographer's role in QA informed by clinical indications. Poor decisions at the QA station can cause loss of diagnostic information.

Digital image processing

Different manufacturers have different names for certain processes; they may carry out tasks in a different order and some have patented processes that are unavailable for scrutiny. This situation is a major cause for confusion in digital projection radiography at present, but there are several basic principles which should allow understanding of these disparate systems; these are:

- Histogram analysis
- Exposure control
- The characteristic curve and inherent response of the CR and DR systems
- Digital system response and LUT
- Multi-frequency processing.

Histogram analysis

Typically, one imagines a digital image as data that is displayed in a matrix that locates each pixel value in an X and Y location, but data does not have to be ordered in that fashion, it is just numbers. Another way to order data might be in size order. Consider an aerial view of a crowd at the Glastonbury festival; we can allocate each individual on the image a number representing their shoe size. We can then draw a graph of this data, but in size order rather than based on location (Fig. 2.5).

This representation of the data is called a histogram. Some educated guesses may be made using this data representation. For example, Glastonbury is an adult only festival and the mean shoe size of the female UK population is 7. From this it may be inferred from the graphical data that this is a mainly adult female population, as the mean of the histogram is 7. This highlights the problem with histogram analysis. As with all assumptions, there is a risk that it is incorrect.

In DR, the first process that occurs is a histogram analysis. Various assumptions are made about how the radiographer exposed the PSP. Each manufacturer has a method of analysing the histogram assuming various ways in which radiographers are likely to use the system, but this can be fooled by unusual exposure situations, e.g. using a large detector for a small object, failing to collimate, exposing several areas on one detector (splitting the field), gross over- or underexposure, and posi-

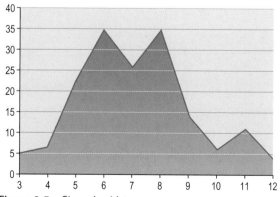

Figure 2.5 Shoe size histogram

tioning the area of interest on an outer edge of a detector (because some systems use a combination of area and histogram analysis).

Manufacturers' software is becoming more and more sophisticated; some systems take note of the identity given to the image prior to histogram analysis, i.e. chest X-ray or hand. Errors are becoming fewer but this is still a major cause of confusion for radiographers when using CR and DR applications. Radiographers frequently have to 'recollimate' or 'reoutput' the image to provide guidance to the system on which area of the exposed plate to base the histogram on. When an apparent error has occurred this should be the first step to rectify it.

Exposure control

In digital systems a figure for exposure control must be indicated somewhere in the system. Much has been made of the potential for over- and underexposure due to digital systems. Several systems aim for a value of 2.0 (antilog 2.0 is 100, i.e. 100% of the expected value). Radiographers who get a value of 2.3 seem within limits, but the antilog of 2.3 is 200%, i.e. double the expected value and this is a considerable overexposure.

With such a system, a recent audit of pelvic examinations showed that 28% of images accepted had exposure levels of 2.6–2.8 possibly indicating endemic 400–600% overexposures.[10] Having said that the exposure index or sensitivity is vital, but it may also be misleading.

The value is unpredictable depending on collimation, positioning, time taken to develop image and background scatter present before exposure. Lehning et al,[11] showed a variation of up to a factor of 2 in sensitivity index values for the same exposure depending on conditions prior to and after exposure and prior to reading of the plate.

The characteristic curve and inherent response of the CR and DR systems

Radiographers should be familiar with the HD exposure response curve. Each film/screen system has a characteristic curve, this representation of exposure response is seldom used by engineers or physicists, as any exposure response is energy dependant and this is not represented on the graph. It is therefore difficult to find an exposure response graph in the literature for CR and DR systems. Most systems are said to have linear exposure response.

In some ways, the inherent response of the digital detector is not as relevant as with a film/screen system, but radiographers are used to the appearance of an image using a detector that has a typical HD 'S shaped' response curve. This type of response to radiation differs from a linear response in its poorer sensitivity to low energy radiation. Scattered radiation and extra focal radiation are both likely to be low energy and therefore are more likely to be detected by any CR/DR system. It is vital that all collimated areas are screened with lead and that CR plates are erased daily and used in strict rotation.

Digital system response and LUT

In the case of over- or underexposure of the imaging plate, the pixel value histogram will be shifted along the exposure axis. With a conventional film screen system, the HD curve is fixed, and the optical density histogram will therefore be severely affected. With the digital system, another HD curve can be created with the aim of matching the pixel value histogram with the desired optical density histogram.

Modern systems can alter the response depending on the area of the image, enabling an effect similar to dual windowing in CT. This is useful to visualise C7 through the shoulders on a large patient, or view the lungs through the heart.

Multi-frequency processing

Many systems now aim to reduce the complex content of the digital image into its constituent parts. Areas of mottle and noise are all very high frequency. Areas of clinically important detail, e.g. bony trabeculae, are said to be medium frequency harmonics. Areas of subtle shading over the whole image are said to be low frequency harmonics.

The low frequency elements of the image can be digitally suppressed, as they are generally not felt to be helpful in image interpretation. This leads to an image with special properties that enhance fine details. Edge enhancement can be achieved through transforming the acquired data by applying a mathematical function to accentuate the difference between adjacent pixel values where one exists currently. This has the visual effect of enhancing any boundaries. These are high frequency structures: statistical variation, such as noise, is also high frequency so becomes much more apparent. The most unsatisfying digital images visually are those with low exposure and high edge enhancement. However, this is what is preferred in situations such as central venous pressure (CVP) line, long-line or chest drain location; hence this is another important consideration for the radiographer who must match appropriate manipulation to the clinical indication for the examination.

QUALITY ASSURANCE (QA)

Windowing, orientation, shuttering, manual collimation and annotating are the functions performed by radiographers at the 'QA station'. A well set up system run by well trained, meticulous radiography staff does not require much technical image manipulation. The time spent at the QA station should really be about positional adequacy which is the largest reason for re-takes, and first line image interpretation. Nevertheless QA features do exist and can be used to correct earlier errors or overcome particularly challenging exposure circumstances that have confused the ordinary histogram analysis.

Orientation

Orientation is applicable to all systems, but particularly to CR or portable DR. Needless to say, changing orientation is very dangerous on an image without a correct anatomical marker irradiated on it. CR cassettes have a right and a wrong orientation. These rules need to be posted clearly. Situations such as axial projections and tangential projections must be considered. In some cases the orientation feature can be an aid to image interpretation, but should be set back to the standard setting prior to sending the image to archive or print.

Shuttering

Shuttering is time consuming and should never be an excuse for poor collimation. Automatic shuttering to the edge of the collimation is beneficial for readers, to eliminate ambient light around the image. Collimation edges are a fundamental record of the radiographer's compliance with IR(ME)R and should be indicated on the image.

Manual collimation

Distinct from shuttering, manual collimation is often required when several collimated areas are on the same receptor (CR) or where there is a large amount of scatter/extra focal radiation due to histogram analysis failure. In certain cases a radiographer unaware of this feature will be presented with an image that appears completely undiagnostic. This is often due to the absence of lead between two areas of exposure on a CR plate. The system may see the 'image' produced by extra focal radiation as the true image, with the real exposed areas as primary beam. The result could end up being repeated if manual collimation is not used.

Annotation

Question: where do you put a red dot when you have no film? Answer: it depends! Annotation on a digital screen is more distracting than stickers, simply because stickers do not transmit light, but white text is a source of glare.

It is still important to document time and position, but irradiating markers are still preferable to annotation applied after the event. In a court of law an image is no longer a diagnostic tool, it is a piece of evidence. Different standards of veracity are required. In many cases an image with annotation applied will not stand up as opposed to one with irradiated markers.

CHANGING RADIOGRAPHIC TECHNIQUE: 'THE REAL QUALITY ASSURANCE'

There seem to be two schools of thought: those that have adopted CR into their departments without much thought about changing their techniques: and those who have instigated major changes in their technique on the basis of trying to get CR to work properly, or to improve radiation dose to their patients. It seems quite early to find any evidence that would support large scale changes in radiographic technique but a few pointers that seem to make some sense follow.

Exposure orientation and annotation

It is very important to use orientation correctly, especially when splitting a film as you cannot cut films in two or turn monitors upside down! The same rigour is required regarding irradiated annotations (but the use of lead markers between grids and CR cassettes can cause grid artefacts).

Exposure factor selection

CR systems and DDR systems are not inherently dose reducing except for the reduction in re-takes.[10]

In low tube voltage examinations, it has been shown that CR (with a fixed pixel size of 200 μm), and a-Selenium compare well with 200 class film screen systems when exposed with equal mAs.[12] DDR amorphous silicon systems using CSI:Tl phosphors have been shown to have higher DQE than film/screen, BaF(X) PSP, and a-Selenium systems. The thickness of these phosphors may allow lower than 400 class system exposure.[13] For all these systems, reducing exposure further will increase the appearance of noise and reduce image quality.

Some CR manufacturers offer specialist thin layer 'extremity' PSPs, and others reduce the pixel size of smaller imaging plates to 100 μm. These have been shown to definitely require a minimum dose equivalent to a speed class of 200.[14] The adoption of CR for extremity radiography therefore can be a complex decision. The choice open to departments is to continue to use the mAs values associated with previous 'extremity' optimized film/screen systems, or to reduce the mAs values to levels broadly similar to 400 class 'regular' film/screen values. Although it would appear logical to harmonise exposure with a particular 'exposure index' value, it would be advantageous to maintain higher extremity exposures when using smaller PSPs to maintain adequate signal to noise ratio.

Automatic exposure chamber (AEC)/device

The calibration of any automatic exposure chamber device fitted to a table or vertical Bucky is very important; it is often omitted. A recent survey of 150 AEC chambers throughout the UK found wide variations in mAs (a factor of five) and optical density.[15] The implementation of CR with uncalibrated AEC chambers can cause serious problems of overexposure or poor image quality. Due to the marked energy dependence differences between ionisation chambers and PSP plates, the use of exposure index is not an optimum method of calibrating these devices.[16]

kVp

Selection of kilovoltages has been debated by several authorities. Theoretically, any difference in the energy absorption spectra of CR and DDR detectors compared with film/screen systems could result in a different optimum kVp.

Data from Hubbell and Seltzer[17] and Nakano et al[5] for BaF(X) based CR PSPs and A-Si/CsI:Tl indirect digital systems, suggests broadly similar responses to that of film/screen. a-Selenium detectors, however, are highly kVp dependent and should always be used in the lower kVp range (<80 kVp). The ability to use signal processing techniques to amplify contrast can compensate for the reduced subject contrast available with high kVp techniques. This has led some authors to suggest increasing kVp to reduce patient dose. A thorough study of contrast detail detectability over the 60–120 kVp range concluded that BaF(X) based CR PSPs performed slightly better than 400 class film/screen systems in demonstrating low contrast detectability, but only when receiving a 200 class exposure level. This study concluded that patient dose savings could be made, but only through use of increased tube filtration.[18]

Source image distance (SID)

Thicker detectors have a severe image quality penalty associated with off axis radiation at the extremities of the detector. Hajdok and Cunningham[19] measured reductions of 70% in DQE 13 cm from the central ray in mammography. These angles are most acute at lower SIDs and larger detector sizes. With 500 μm thick detectors, a longer SID may be appropriate.

Extra focal radiation

Not to be confused with scatter, there is also a requirement to reduce extra focal radiation reaching the receptor *and* preferably the patient. Simple use of lead rubber sheeting alongside the area that is collimated can help and sometimes use of tube head collimators commonly referred to as 'cones' can help as well. Failure to control this will cause histogram analysis errors.

Scatter control

CR and Digital Direct Radiography seem to demand higher standards in scatter control. This includes use of collimation and reducing the collimated area to reduce the volume of tissue irradiated, therefore controlling scatter produced. Field and Blower[10] reported the use of lead rubber to block back scatter behind a CR cassette as beneficial.

Selection of grids or air gaps

Grid selection is complicated by the potential for aliasing artefact patterns with bitmap graphics and scanning systems that operate line by line. New detectors and display sizes may alter the choice of grids and the type of grid, but grids cannot be eliminated from practice. Radiographers must continue to make choices about grid use based on patient size and anatomical area, not modality. It is never going to be appropriate to radiograph a hand with a grid even if the DR system has one built in.

Conversely it is currently not acceptable to use a detector alone when examining L5/S1 in a large adult. Several studies have suggested that grids can be eliminated in certain situations, e.g. skull radiography, but use is more preferable than not in most cases, particularly with the larger patient. The use of air gaps for scatter reduction, with a consequent low patient ED is documented for chest radiography.[20] Some researchers have advocated the use of thin copper or aluminium sheets with uniform attenuation. As the distribution of scattered photons is predominantly at lower energies, this technique will remove scatter preferentially without the difficulties of using a grid.

There are currently efforts underway to analyse the image data to pinpoint 'scatter' and remove it in software. The use of double sided PSP plates and even two plates in a single cassette allows for 'energy subtraction' imaging.

This technique would also greatly assist in identifying scatter and eliminating it.

■ Techniques to avoid grid artefacts

- *Grid resolution.* Select a grid that has a resolution that is not similar to the spacing of the CR scan lines, the size of the phosphor crystals or the size of laser spot. Current wisdom is to use a grid of high line rate (7–9 lpmm^{-1}/ 180–210 lpi^{-1}) and low ratio (4:1 or 6:1) at the correct focal distance, or long focal distance if it is parallel.[21]

- *Orientation of grid to laser scan lines.* In CR, grid orientation should be perpendicular to the fast scanning direction of the laser; it is important to mark these line orientations on stationary grids, and fast scan direction on CR plates.

- *Grids in trolley trauma and bedside radiography.* This is not strictly a 'digital problem', but the use of high line rate grids causes it. The use of high line rate grids in these cases requires extreme care with centring and grid angulation. The lowest ratio possible is required (4:1) and long SIDs. Even the use of radiographic markers between the cassette and the grid has been reported to cause artefact.

- *Resampling artefacts.* Sometimes grids are blamed for aliasing artefacts, which are not grid caused. When an image is moved from one bitmap size to another, the data has to be resampled. This commonly occurs when images are viewed on monitors with different native resolutions, e.g. the QA workstation and the diagnostic workstation. This can introduce aliasing artefacts. This, and variation in luminance, make it possible for a digital image to look poor on one monitor and good on another.

References

1. Benson K, Fink D. HDTV: advanced television for the 1990s. New York: McGraw-Hill; 1991.
2. Federation Internationale des Echecs Chessboard standard size. http://www.fide.com/official/handbook.asp?level=C02
3. Jarvis D (ed.) Clinical radiology and electronic records. London: Royal College of Radiologists; 2002.
4. Sonoda M, et al. Computed radiography utilizing scanning laser stimulated luminescence. Radiology 1983; 148:833–838.
5. Nakano Y, et al. Improved computed radiography image quality from a BaFl:Eu photostimulable phosphor plate. Medical Physics 2002; 29(4).
6. Leblans P, et al. A new needle-crystalline computed radiography detector. Journal of Digital Imaging 2000; 13(20)(suppl 1):117–120.
7. Mackenzie A. Effect of latent image decay on image quality in computed radiography. Proceedings of UK Radiological Congress. BIR: London; 2004:21.
8. Schaetzing R, et al. New high speed scanning technique for computed radiography. Proceedings of SPIE 2002; 4682:511–520.
9. Weisfield R. Amorphous silicon TFT X-ray image sensors. IEDM Technical Digest International 1998; 21–24.
10. Field S, Blower C. Moving to CR – impact on radiography practice. Proceedings of UK Radiological Congress. BIR: London, 2004:41.
11. Lehning L, et al. Exposure indicators in digital radiography: What is their relation to exposure? Proceedings of the European Congress of Radiology 2002; C-0746.
12. Zähringer M, et al. Detection of porcine bone lesions and fissures. American Journal of Roentgenology 2001; 177:1397–1403.
13. Borasi G, et al. On site evaluation of three flat panel detectors for digital radiography. Medical Physics 2003; 30(7):1719–1731.
14. Peer R, et al. Storage phosphor radiography of wrist fractures: a subjective comparison of image quality at varying exposure levels. European Radiology 2002; 12(6):1354–1359.
15. Ward M, et al. Assessment of automatic exposure control (AEC) systems. Proceedings of UK Radiological Congress. BIR: London, 2004:26.
16. Athanasiou C, Mackenzie A. Methodologies for automatic exposure control calibration of computed radiography systems. Proceedings of UK Radiological Congress. BIR. London, 2004:25.
17. Hubbell J, Seltzer S. Tables of X-ray mass attenuation coefficients and mass energy-absorption coefficients (version 1.4), 2004. Online. Available: http://physics.nist.gov/ xaamdi [6 Feb 2005]. National Institute of Standards and Technology, Gaithersburg, MD.
18. Lu Z, et al. Comparison of computed radiography and film/screen combination using a contrast detail phantom. Journal of Applied Clinical Medical Physics 2003; 4(1):91–98.
19. Hajdok G, Cunningham I. Penalty on the detective quantum efficiency from off-axis incident x-rays. Physics of Medical Imaging, Proceedings of SPIE. 2004; 5368:109–118.
20. Bernhardt TM, et al. Digital selenium radiography: anti-scatter grid for chest radiography in a clinical study. British Journal of Radiology 2000; 73(873):963–968.
21. MXE. Anti-scatter CR grid. Medical X-Ray Enterprises Inc, 2003. Online. Available: http://www.mxe.com/XRayGrids/ cr.asp [accessed 1 Jan 2004].

CHAPTER 3

EXPOSURE FACTORS, MANIPULATION AND DOSE

Barry Carver

IMAGE QUALITY

For accurate diagnosis we require high quality radiographic reproduction of the patient area being examined. What is a high quality image? Many factors need to be included in the assessment of an image to determine its quality; patient positioning and compliance will affect the resultant image, as will the image receptor and exposure used.

Density and contrast are the photographic properties that affect the resultant image quality, commonly combined (inaccurately) by students to form 'exposure'. Whilst density and contrast are inextricably linked they can be differentiated on the image and the effects of each manipulated to optimise image quality. Unsharpness includes many aspects of image geometry which also contribute to the quality of the result. Taken together these three factors may provide a means by which a radiographic image can be evaluated for 'technical quality'; other contributing factors, such as acceptability of positioning, will be discussed in the relevant chapters for each body part/technique.

DENSITY

Density may also be referred to as optical density, or radiographic density. Density in radiography is a measurable quantity, in its simplest sense it is the degree of 'blackening' seen on the image. When thought of in this way density is easy to evaluate and correct: is the film too dark (decrease exposure) or too light (increase exposure).

The density perceived on an image will vary from black to almost clear; the degree to which the film may appear clear is governed by the amount of base fog present. Base fog is the combined density of the film base plus the density of the unexposed film emulsion. Base fog varies with the age of the film, storage (but storage fog, due to exposure to safelight, should nowadays be negligible due to the prevalence of daylight processing), and film speed (generally faster film will exhibit higher base fog levels than a slower film). Unexplained variation in base fog may indicate problems with the development cycle of processing.

In the case of a radiographic film the density we can measure is the transmitted density (D), this is defined as the base 10 logarithm of the ratio of the light incident upon the film (I_o) to the light transmitted through the film (I_t):

$$D = \frac{I_o}{I_t}$$

The use of a logarithmic measure is appropriate as the response of the eye to visual stimulation is itself logarithmic.[1,2]

In order to be useful, the range of densities demonstrated on the image needs to be within the range for visual perception and differentiation, usually considered to be approximately the range D = 0.25 → 2.50.[3] Whilst a density of >2.5 may not be immediately differentiated by eye, densities of up to 4 may be recorded on film.[4] In effect, too much information has been recorded; it is sometimes but not always possible to use and view this information by use of increased illumination ('bright light') or photographic reduction. In the case of digital imaging, the 'dark' image can be manipulated to produce an acceptable image; this is one of the perceived strengths of digital imaging techniques which can lead to a reduction in population dose due to eliminating the need to repeat 'overexposed' images.

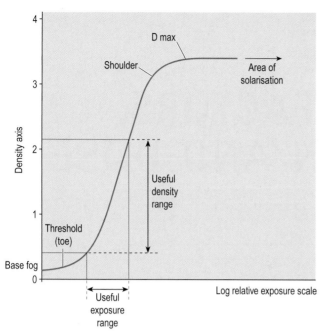

Figure 3.1 Characteristic curve

The radiographic image which is 'too light' is, however, more problematic as it does not contain enough inherent information; manipulation of the image is unhelpful.

This leads to the advice 'if in doubt use the exposure that will produce a darker image'.[3] Whilst this is potentially good advice, care needs to be taken as clearly the greater exposure will result not only in a darker image but also more dose to the patient. The temptation, especially when using digital techniques is to overexpose, as the safety net of image manipulation will prevent the necessity of a repeat examination, however this practice leads to each individual exposure being higher than is necessary for the individual patient. Clearly this is a temptation to be avoided and professional standards in application of the 'as low as reasonably achievable' (ALARA) principle need to be maintained: give the right exposure for the individual patient, but if in doubt apply the principle above.

Variation of applied mAs is often given as the controlling factor for density,[5] although the effect of variation of kVp on intensity, and therefore density, must also be considered. However in general it is considered better to use a fixed kVp for each examination, using variation of mAs to control required changes in density.[6]

CONTRAST

Image contrast is a combination of subject contrast which is the contrast produced due to the anatomical area under examination; the receptor (radiographic) contrast which is

the contrast produced as a result of the image receptor being employed; and may be influenced by subjective contrast which is the effect on contrast perception due to the observer or observing conditions.

The image itself is produced by means of differences in the attenuation of the X-ray beam within the patient. The differences thus produced in the transmitted beam are due to anatomical variations within the patient part under examination, in turn producing visible differences in density and contrast in the resultant image.

The contrast formed on the image in this way is termed 'subject contrast', due to the inherent 'contrast' which is the result of varying tissue types and densities of the body part under examination. Subject contrast can be influenced and manipulated by use of positive and negative contrast media, and application of varying kVp techniques as described below.

Contrast can be shown to be inversely proportional to the applied kVp, hence in general at lower kVp values greater subject contrast is obtained. This is because, in the diagnostic range, the main interaction processes responsible for attenuation are photoelectric absorption and Compton scatter. Photoelectric absorption for a given beam energy is proportional to the cube of the atomic number and directly proportional to the density of the structure imaged, hence using the exposure ranges where photoelectric absorption is the dominant process (lower kVp) will maximise subject contrast.

There is again a dose trade-off, as use of low kVp may increase skin dose. Indeed, current guidelines for paediatric radiography recommend use of 55–60 kVp, even for extremity work,[7] however the increase in kVp will reduce subject contrast and hence image definition.[8] Commonly forgotten in departments who have adapted this technique for adult use, is the requirement for additional copper filtration to optimise the useful spectrum.

kVp is the exposure factor by which contrast can be manipulated. If an image has adequate density but lacks contrast then kVp should be reduced, however as kVp reduction will also reduce the number of photons reaching the image receptor, and hence density, an appropriate increase in mAs is required to maintain the final image density.

For intrinsically high contrast examinations such as the chest, the use of high kVp enables better visualisation of lung structures despite reduction in overall image contrast. This is because at low energies the high subject contrast of the thorax together with high radiographic contrast produced makes the overall image contrast such that all structures cannot be demonstrated within the useful density range.

High contrast can be referred to as 'short scale',[5] i.e. fewer shades of grey are represented within the image;

consequently fewer are available to represent the structures to be demonstrated. Use of a high kVp (120+)[9] reduces the radiographic contrast but enables all structures to be visualised within the useful density range. Low contrast produces a 'long scale' image,[5] with more shades of grey available for image depiction; the result is a 'flatter' image but with greater detail particularly of lung parenchyma.

The 'flat' or grey appearance of such images does not suit all subjective tastes, and as such the technique is not universally accepted, however this subjectivity is difficult to reconcile with accepted best practice, both in terms of image quality and dosimetry. Film readers need to educate themselves to accept these changes and embrace best practice.[7]

Subject contrast will be affected both by pathological processes, which may change the appearance from the expected 'norm', and the effects of scatter which are discussed below.

Subjectivity in image viewing, as mentioned above, can be an important factor when considering image contrast, and 'subjective contrast' requires some consideration.

Not to be confused with subject contrast as described above, subjective contrast is due to the observer rather than inherent in the image,[10] but nonetheless is important to consider. The observer needs to be considered: eye strain and fatigue can have an effect on perception; several short viewing (or reporting) sessions are preferable to a single extended session; aids to visual acuity should be utilised as required (e.g. spectacles should be worn if they are needed!).

Viewing conditions need to be optimal. A dim viewing box in high ambient lighting, or holding a radiograph up to a window, are not ideal viewing conditions, and will not enable accurate appreciation of either the radiographic density or contrast demonstrated on the image. Viewing boxes should be matched for brightness and colour of illumination, checked on a regular basis, and used in appropriate conditions, i.e. in low ambient lighting.[11]

Radiographic contrast can be defined as the difference in density values between two defined areas on an image. As density is measurable using a densitometer, it is possible to produce a measure of radiographic contrast.

When using film, the manufacturer controls the inherent film contrast by altering the range of silver halide grain sizes and types used to produce the film emulsion, and similarly the type of intensifying screen used.

The radiographer will select the most appropriate film-screen combination for each examination from those available. Most departments will use only one film type with a choice of two or perhaps three intensifying screens.

The use of one intensifying screen or another will not appreciably affect the contrast produced. The screen speed will determine patient dose and have an effect on image sharpness, but the effect on contrast is minimal. Some authors state there is no effect,[3,12] others that there is a linear relationship between screen speed and contrast.[13,14] Experimentally it has been shown that whilst there is some effect, it is neither linear, nor perceptible to the human eye and can therefore be ignored.

For skeletal radiography where we are examining areas with a relatively high subject contrast, a fairly low contrast film can be used to demonstrate the majority of structures within the useful density range. This selection will also provide a reasonably wide exposure latitude, which can lead to fewer repeats due to exposure errors.

However, it should be carefully noted that if a repeat is required and a wide latitude film is being used, small increments of changes in exposure factors are to be avoided. This is because small incremental changes (the 1 or 2 kVp change by the supervisor which so infuriates students, and is anyway useless) have no effect on the resultant image. A wide latitude means that within that range of exposures a similar resultant image is produced. For example, if film is considered too dark and a repeat is required then consideration should be given to halving the mAs to produce a more reasonable density.[3] Similarly changes in kVp should be of the order of 15%.[5] If only a small change is required the question must be asked – should the film be repeated at all?

As already stated, the amount of scatter reaching the image receptor will also affect image contrast. An increase in scatter reduces radiographic contrast by contributing a general increase in the overall image density, without any positive contribution to image definition.

Unfortunately, all examinations in the diagnostic range result in the production of scattered radiation, some of which inevitably reaches the image receptor. Consideration needs to be given to the most effective means by which scatter can be prevented from reaching the receptor in all circumstances.

Limiting scatter production can only be effectively achieved by use of appropriate collimation; minimising the irradiated volume minimises the scatter produced. Maximum use of appropriate collimation should be applied to *all* projections undertaken as there are also clear dose implications.

Given that some scatter will be produced, shielding the unused part of the image receptor by the use of lead rubber should be routine practice. This is particularly true when using film as the unexposed area is rendered more sensitive when irradiated by scatter, further degrading the image when scatter from a second view is incident, which will then have a more severe effect on the final image.

For larger body parts where higher beam energies are utilised, hence more forward scatter is produced which is more likely to reach the film, consideration should be given to the use of a grid. Placed between the patient and image receptor, the grid will absorb scatter, but also to a degree primary radiation, leading to a requirement to increase exposure factors, and consequently patient dose.

Careful thought needs to be given as to whether utilisation of a grid is required to produce the image quality required, for example when undertaking fluoroscopy, use of a grid should not be automatic.[15]

UNSHARPNESS

Having the 'correct' density and contrast on the resultant image is important, but if the image produced is unsharp then detail is lost and the diagnostic quality of the image reduced.

Such unsharpness may be due to several causes, which include system geometry (penumbra, photographic) and lack of patient cooperation due to voluntary or involuntary movement.

As the anode target produces a finite effective focal spot size rather than the ideal point source, there is inevitably some penumbral effect produced as shown in Figure 3.2.

The penumbra causes geometric unsharpness within the resultant image. There are three ways in which this effect can be reduced:

- Select the smallest useful focal spot size, which will minimise the size of the penumbra. Choice is limited in practice by tube loading considerations, but in general, the smallest focal spot that enables the choice of the required exposure without compromise to tube life, should be selected.
- Minimise object to film distance; as seen in Figure 3.2 increasing object to film distance increases the size and therefore the effect of the penumbra.
- If a broad focal spot is required and a large object film distance cannot be avoided, e.g. when imaging a thick body part, consideration may be given to increasing focal film distance. Again this will lessen the penumbral effect due to the increase in focus object distance.

Unsharpness due to penumbral effects (geometric unsharpness) can be expressed as:

$$\text{Geometric unsharpness} = \frac{\text{OFD} \times \text{FocalSpotSize}}{\text{FOD}}$$

Photographic unsharpness is inherent to the receptor system resolution; it depends on the size of the detector

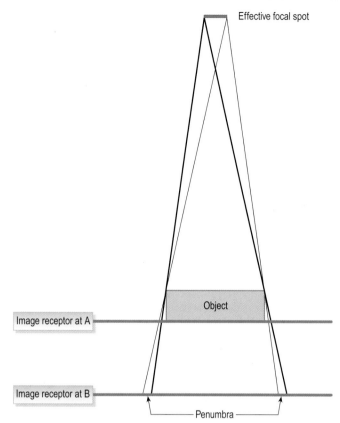

Figure 3.2 Penumbral effect: as OFD is increased the size of the penumbra produced can be seen to increase

and detection technique. For a film screen system this will depend on the size of the light emitting crystals in the intensifying screen and their distance from the film. Large crystals produce an image made up of large 'blocks' of information, and smaller crystals use smaller 'blocks' to build the image which therefore appears sharper due to its superior resolution.

As the distance between the crystals and the film increases, the light emitted will diverge causing a loss of resolution in the same way as described for the penumbral effect. Therefore the requirement is for thin screens in good contact with the film.

Fine grain screens with smaller crystals produce a sharper image but once again with a cost in terms of dose to the patient, so for most imaging, a system with sufficient resolution produced with a reasonable dose is chosen.

Movement produces a blurred, unsharp image, hence steps should be taken to minimise patient movement. The risk of voluntary movement should be minimised by adequate explanation of the procedure, rehearsal of manoeuvres such as breath hold, and appropriate use of aids to immobilisation, such as radiolucent pads. The effect of involuntary movement should be minimised where appropriate by selection of the shortest available exposure time.

Density, contrast and unsharpness are distinct elements which should in all cases be individually assessed and manipulated in order to produce images of optimal quality.

DOSIMETRY

A full discussion on dosimetry is beyond the scope of this text. There are many resources, particularly for students, that discuss the issues of dose measurement and radiation protection.[1,2,3,4,6,9] The commonest measures used are effective dose equivalent (EDE quoted in milliSievert), entrance surface dose (ESD quoted in milliGray), and dose area product (DAP quoted in milliGray).

Optimisation of patient dose is a requirement of both European directive,[16,17] and UK law[18] each requiring doses to be kept 'as low as reasonably practicable'. IR(ME)R requires the setting of diagnostic reference levels; readings from DAP meters are often used to provide information for establishment of DRLs. ESD and EDE can also be used but require calculation from exposure factors or measurement with dose meters.

The current system for radiation protection uses the linear no threshold model (LNT) for assessment of the risk from medical exposures. This assumes a linear relationship between the exposure received and the risk of cancer induction. At high exposure levels (>200 mSv) there is evidence from epidemiological studies to show that this is the case, however below this threshold there is little hard evidence. Current legislation, based on LNT, is a 'safe' approach assuming harmful effects from low doses in order to provide maximum protection to the public.[19]

It has been argued that individual molecular lesions may[20,21] or may not[22] induce cancer. There is a rising tide of opinion in favour of radiation hormesis; the argument being that there may in fact be beneficial effects associated with low doses. Our bodies have very efficient repair mechanisms which cope with the ever present effects of background radiation, as well as the more significant effects of deoxyribonucleic acid (DNA) damage from biological sources. Feinendegen argues that the stimulation of these processes at low doses may in fact be beneficial.[23]

Deterministic effects encountered in radiotherapy, are also found in diagnostic imaging, e.g. erythema has been observed,[24] and lens opacities may be induced in children from doses as little as 0.1 Gy[25] (a CT head scan can be 0.03 to 0.06 Gy in paediatric patients).[26] Consequently these effects must also be taken into account when considering protection policy.

This is an extremely complex argument which is likely to continue for some time. Until proven otherwise application of the LNT model as required by current legislation would seem to be a sensible approach. Research should continue – with an open mind: as Arthur Conan Doyle pointed out 'premature assumption results in a tendency to interpret data to agree with the assumption'.[22] An appropriate quotation for application by all researchers at whatever level.

References

1. Farr R, Allisy-Roberts P. Physics for medical imaging. London: Saunders; 1997.
2. Graham D, Cloke P. Principles of radiological physics. 4th edn. Edinburgh: Elsevier; 2003.
3. Carlton R, Adler A. Principles of radiographic imaging. 2nd edn. New York: Delmar; 1996.
4. Bushong S. Radiologic science for technologists. 7th edn. St Louis: Mosby; 2001.
5. Bontrager K, Lampignano J. Textbook of radiographic positioning and related anatomy. 6th edn. St Louis: Mosby; 2005.
6. Dowd S, Tilson E. Practical radiation protection and applied radiobiology. 2nd edn. Philadelphia: Saunders; 1999.
7. Cook JV, et al. Guidelines on best practice in the X-ray imaging of children. Bristol: Ian Allan Printing; 1998.
8. Pizzutiello R, Cullinan J. Introduction to medical radiographic imaging. Eastman Kodak; 1993.
9. European Guidelines on Quality Criteria for Diagnostic Radiographic Images, Rep. EUR 16260, 1996, Office for Official Publications of the European Communities, L-2985 Luxembourg.
10. Whitley AS, et al. Positioning in radiography. 12th edn. London: Hodder Arnold; 2005.
11. McCarthy E, Brennan P. Viewing conditions for diagnostic images in three major Dublin hospitals: a comparison with WHO and CEC recommendations. British Journal of Radiology 2003; 76:94–97.
12. Wallace J. Radiographic exposure: principles and practice. Philadelphia: FA Davis Company; 1995.
13. DeVos S. Basic principles of radiographic exposure. Philadelphia: Lea and Febiger; 1990.
14. Fodor J, Malott J. The art and science of medical radiography. 6th edn. St Louis: The Catholic Health Association of the US; 1987.
15. Lloyd P, et al. The secondary radiation grid; its effect on fluoroscopic dose-area product during barium enema examinations. British Journal of Radiology 1998; 71:303–306.
16. European Union. Council directive 97/43 Euratom on health protection of individuals against the dangers of ionising radiation in relation to medical exposure. Official Journal of the European Communities 40; 1997.
17. European Commission Directorate-General for the Environment 2000. Referral guidelines for imaging. Radiation protection 118.
18. The Ionising Radiation (Medical Exposure) Regulations. Statutory Instruments 2000, no. 1059. London: HMSO; 2000.

19. Martin C. UKRC 2004 debate: the LNT model provides the best approach for practical implementation of radiation protection. British Journal of Radiology 2005; 78:14–16.

20. Chadwick K, Leenhouts H. UKRC 2004 debate: radiation risk is linear with dose at low doses. British Journal of Radiology 2005; 78:8–10.

21. Anoopkumar-Dukie S, et al. Further evidence for biological effects resulting from ionising radiation doses in the diagnostic X-ray range. British Journal of Radiology 2005; 78:335–337.

22. Cameron J. UKRC 2004 debate: moderate dose rate ionising radiation increases longevity. British Journal of Radiology 2005; 78:11–13.

23. Feinendegen L. UKRC 2004 debate: evidence for beneficial low level radiation effects and radiation hormesis. British Journal of Radiology 2005; 78:3–7.

24. Mooney R, et al. Absorbed dose and deterministic effects to patients from interventional neuroradiology. British Journal of Radiology 2000; 73:745–751.

25. Wilde G, Sjöstrand J. A clinical study of radiation cataract formation in adult life following gamma irradiation of the lens in early childhood. British Journal of Opthalmology 1997; 81:261–266.

26. Shrimpton PC, et al. Doses from computed tomography (CT) examinations in the UK – 2003 review. NRPB W67.

SECTION 2

SKELETAL RADIOGRAPHY

INTRODUCTION TO SECTIONS 2 AND 3: SKELETAL, CHEST AND ABDOMINAL RADIOGRAPHY

Elizabeth Carver

To avoid repetition within the text, some safety and technical issues can be addressed by the use of initial statements regarding patient preparation, selection and use of image recording media, dose reduction methods, image identification and anatomical markers. Coverage of this information is found in this section:

PATIENT PREPARATION

For all examinations, patient preparation includes:

- employing appropriate and effective communication methods which will ensure patient compliance or cooperation
- removal of items of clothing or artefacts overlying the relevant examination area; in cases of severe trauma it may not be advisable or even possible to remove some items
- accurate identification check
- assessing justification for request
- assessment of possibility of pregnancy for examinations where this is required.[1]

IMAGE RECORDING (CASSETTES AND DIGITAL PLATES)

With the current situation of image recording, where there is a combination of computed radiography (CR), digital radiography (DR) and film/screen systems in use, it has been difficult to select a method of description that accurately embraces the use of all of these methods. Since CR uses cassette sizes that are similar to conventional film/screen systems, there should be little or no confusion, however some notable differences regarding DR exist. It has therefore been decided that the term 'image receptor' will be used as an umbrella term. This is intended to include any of the recording systems which may be used by the radiographer; when necessary, the term 'cassette' will be used as clarification, since some projections may not be possible with less versatile DR systems. Cassette size is referred to, usually at the start of the positioning description, for those who do use cassettes. It should also be noted that use of lead rubber for masking is not advisable for CR and DR systems, although some of the positioning images do demonstrate this on a film/screen cassette.

At the time of writing, there has been development of DR plate sizes, which improves the flexibility and range of uses for these digital plates. Initially plate sizes were limited and there was also limited or no availability of plates which were remote from the table assembly. This reduced the range of examinations and projections for which DR could be utilised. DR plates are now available in:

- large (43^2) sizes for use in the table and erect tray (with or without scatter reduction device)
- 43^2 for use remote from the table unit; e.g. is useful for erect anteroposterior (AP) chest radiography; these are now available for connection to mobile radiography units

- smaller size (around 24 ×30 cm) for more versatile positioning for extremities
- Dental sizes for dedicated dental systems.

(See Figs 4.1–4.4 for examples of digital plates.)

DR plates do not require the centre of the body part to be placed coincident with the middle, unlike cassette radiography. For this reason, the positioning descriptors provided in this text assume that the radiographer will always ensure that the centre of the body part lies at the middle of the cassette, or within an unexposed section if the cassette is used for more than one projection. At times it will be necessary to centre the body part to the middle of the DR plate, e.g. when that body part is large (as in chest or abdomen radiography) and this will be advised in descriptors for some sections, in order to ensure the whole of the body part is included in the image.

When the technique descriptor refers to placing a cassette in a bucky, at the start of the description, it should be assumed that digital plates will be used in conjunction with an anti-scatter device, which can be deselected if not required.

FILM/SCREEN COMBINATIONS

For cassette examinations of the upper and lower extremities (areas that require high definition screens and are defined as the following: thumb, fingers, hand, elbow, toes, foot and ankle), film/screen combinations that provide definition high enough to demonstrate fine trabecular patterns should be selected. These are most often referred to as 'high definition' film/screen combinations, although they are often, colloquially, called 'extremity cassettes' or 'detail cassettes' by many. Film/screens of this type are essentially of a slower speed than standard systems used for examination of other body areas; their use requires

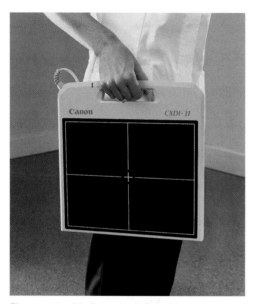

Figure 4.1   Medium sized digital image receptor. Reproduced with permission from Xograph Imaging Systems

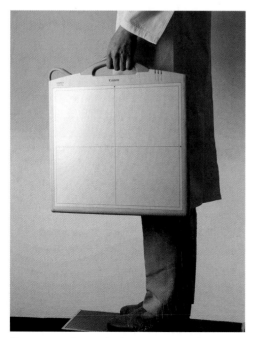

Figure 4.2   Large size image receptor. Reproduced with permission from Xograph Imaging Systems

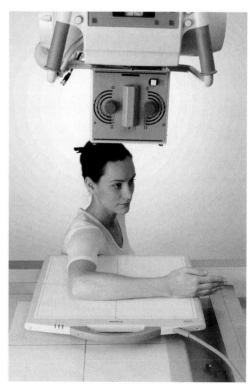

Figure 4.3   Extremity radiography. Reproduced with permission from Xograph Imaging Systems

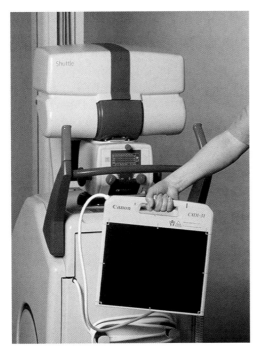

Figure 4.4 Mobile direct digital equipment. Reproduced with permission from Xograph Imaging Systems

selection of exposure factors (namely mAs) higher than those that would be selected for examination of the same area using standard screens. However, these should not be confused with specialist screens which provide very fine detail such as that required for intraocular foreign body (IOFB) demonstration.

For all other examinations, film/screen speeds used are usually known as 'standard', 'medium' or even 'fast' and these are selected for all other body areas.

SPLITTING THE CASSETTE FOR MULTIPROJECTIONAL USE

Splitting the cassette is suggested most frequently in the descriptions of projections for the extremities of the upper and lower limb. When it is recommended that a cassette is used for more than one projection, lead rubber should be used to mask off the sections which are not utilised during a particular exposure. Although it is not advisable to split DR or CR image receptors with lead rubber in this way, splitting CR cassettes is not actually necessary, as two images can be displayed on a single hard copy without both images having to be actually exposed onto the original cassette. Similarly, DR image receptors do not need to be split for multiprojectional use.

Returning to the matter of splitting conventional cassettes, despite claims that modern collimators are accurate enough

to negate the use of lead rubber in this way, it must be remembered that an already exposed section of film will have increased sensitivity to radiation and the light emitted by intensifying screens. This can potentially lead to fogging of these areas during subsequent exposures made on the same cassette and film.

ANATOMICAL MARKERS

It is assumed that anatomical markers will *always* be placed within the field of primary beam, clear of the essential area of interest. Therefore instruction for this will not be included for every description of projections. Unless otherwise specified, it will be assumed that AP markers will be applied. Use of posteroanterior (PA) markers will be referred to but the authors do acknowledge that some imaging departments do not use PA markers. Anatomical markers do not always appear in positioning images as often they are too small to reproduce on a small photograph.

It will also be assumed that the radiographer will always check accuracy of anatomical markers on resulting images; therefore the image quality criteria will not refer specifically to this requirement.

IMAGE IDENTIFICATION

Correct identification on the image will be assumed to be an area that the radiographer need not be reminded to assess during image quality assessment. This, therefore, is not included in the image evaluation lists in the text.

DOSE REDUCTION METHODS

This refers to physical mechanisms for protection during the examination, rather than precautions such as avoidance of unnecessary irradiation of patient, fetus or personnel. Use of lead rubber will be specifically referred to in projection descriptors. Collimation is also commented upon, to:

- ensure the required area of interest is definitely included on the image
- limit the radiation field to the area of interest as a dose limitation method
- reduce scatter in order to maintain image quality and reduce radiation dose.

The philosophy of the authors is that application of lead rubber, wherever and whenever possible, must be a consideration for every patient and projection. Observations have shown that it is tempting to omit the use of lead rubber for extremity examinations that are low-dose and well-collimated. However, since the only safe dose is *no* dose, the authors will *always* recommend use of lead rubber for protection. Consistent and habitual use of lead rubber, for every examination, will ensure that the radiographer never forgets to use it. Lead rubber protection will not always appear in positioning images as, at times, its application may mask demonstration of the body position.

Other recommendations for dose reduction are listed as follows:

- The patient's head should be turned away from the primary beam and examination area during exposure, if possible in the position described, in order to minimise radiation dose to the radiosensitive lenses of the eyes and thyroid.
- Legs are never placed under the table, to clear the femora and gonads from the primary beam, edge of collimation and scattered radiation.
- Lead rubber can be used under the cassette, during examinations of the limbs, to absorb a significant proportion of primary beam and thus reduce the amount of scatter.

SPECIFIC NOTES FOR SECTION 2: SKELETAL RADIOGRAPHY

Radiographic examination of the human skeleton may identify a range of pathologies or appearances that identify traumatically induced changes. Many of the conditions identified in this section are found generally throughout the skeleton or its articulations and, for this reason, are listed before all sections describing skeletal examination techniques. Information related to specific areas of the skeleton will be included at the beginning of the appropriate section, or related to individual projections if more appropriate. Not all conditions listed are necessarily justification for plain radiographic examination, nor is plain radiography necessarily the initial imaging method of choice for each condition. The pathologies given here are by no means exhaustive but comprise those conditions most commonly encountered.

COMMONLY ENCOUNTERED PATHOLOGIES THAT AFFECT THE SKELETON AND ITS ARTICULATIONS

Acromegaly

Overproduction of growth hormone due to a pituitary gland tumour may result in increase in the size of the skeleton, even after full normal adult growth has been completed. The soft tissue of the heel outline shows an enlarged fat pad, whilst there is apparent increase in joint spaces, increase in vertebral height, possible pituitary fossa enlargement and early arthritis.[2] It is very likely that cassettes used for patients affected by acromegaly will need to be of greater dimensions than those suggested within this text. Modern diagnostic methods have resulted in earlier detection of pituitary tumours, thus reducing the number of people suffering from increased growth.

Ankylosing spondylitis

Most notably referred to as 'bamboo spine' in its advanced stages; inflammation of the fibroosseous junctions leads to calcification of fibrous tissue. Eventually, vertebral bodies appear fused, with dense calcification which is wider than the bodies themselves. This gives the ridged appearance of the vertebral column, which is likened to a bamboo stick.

Bone age

Although not technically seen as skeletal pathology, epiphyseal appearance and fusions will determine bone age.[3] This type of assessment is requested when a child's physical development or size does not fall within the range considered to be within normal limits. Amongst areas included in bone age surveys are hand and wrist, knee, elbow and iliac crests. Bones selected for the bone age survey vary according to the chronological age of the child.

Chondrosarcoma

This aggressive lesion is the third most common primary bone tumour and arises from cartilaginous tissue. There may be a soft tissue mass at the site, usually with cortical destruction. Slow growing lesions will show cortical thickening.[2]

Enchondroma

Enchondroma consists of hyaline cartilage found as an island in bone. A noticeable lesion, with some sclerosis and containing small calcifications, may be accompanied by pathological fracture. There may be some soft tissue outline changes, especially if accompanied by a visible mass. Often the lesion is asymptomatic and findings may thus be incidental.

Gout

Crystals of monosodium urate monohydrate are deposited in synovial fluid, which results in inflammation and erosion of cartilage and articular surfaces of bone. Radiologically there are likely to be narrowed joint spaces, soft tissue outline indicative of swelling around the joint and small, localised erosions over the bone surface.

Metastases

Metastases are malignant secondary tumours, which spread to bone from primary malignancy. They affect other tissue types in addition to the skeleton. Appearances in the skeleton: lesions appear as lytic, in some cases sclerotic (metastatic deposits from carcinoma breast and prostate); pathological fractures may be present.

Myeloma

This is a neoplastic condition arising from bone marrow. Lesions show as low density lytic areas; they may appear as multiple lesions seen as clusters, which have a scalloped edge appearance.

Osteoarthritis

This wear-and-tear disease displays: narrowed joint spaces which may show as asymmetry in weight-bearing joints; osteophytes; sclerosis and erosions. Bone density is likely to be preserved unless the patient is generally osteoporotic.[2,3,4]

Osteochondritis

Osteochodritis is a condition affecting primary and secondary centres of ossification, leading to avascular necrosis of a portion of bone due to a cut in the blood supply. In children this is idiopathic; in adults it can be due to trauma or inflammation.[4,5] Appearances vary according to locality of disease; these include loose bodies apparent in joints, sclerosis of epiphyses, collapse of affected bone and soft tissue swelling.

Osteomalacia

This is low bone mineralisation causing low bone density, which may or may not be apparent radiologically. Vertebral bodies may collapse, causing a kyphosis seen on lateral spine radiographs. Small linear radiolucencies (Looser's zones) may appear and can develop into fractures that follow the same linear direction.

Osteomyelitis

Osteomyelits is inflammation of the bone and bone marrow following soft tissue infection or, occasionally, injury. It most commonly affects children. In the acute stage, radiological signs are not likely to appear for up to 10 days but, when present, will likely show as metaphyseal bone destruction and periosteal reaction. Radionuclide imaging is effective in early detection of the condition. More long-standing osteomyelitis can be very aggressive, leading to changes in the periosteum and even deformity of the bone.

Osteoporosis

Osteoporosis is bone demineralisation which mainly affects elderly females, however some elderly males may also suffer from this condition. Diagnostic route does not use plain radiography as first choice, since a significant percentage of demineralisation (approximately 30%) must occur before loss of bone density is shown on plain X-ray. Early diagnosis is made by osteoporosis screening methods. In addition to loss of bone density, plain images may reveal noticeable loss of cortical width and wedge appearance of vertebral bodies. Patients with known osteoporosis will require a reduction of exposure factors for skeletal radiography.

Osteosarcoma

Osteosarcoma is an aggressively malignant tumour which most often affects the young patient. Soft tissue swelling is often seen on plain radiography of the area.

Paget's disease

Increased bone density, which is a result of this disease, is often referred to as having a 'cotton wool' appearance. The inexperienced can confuse the signs with the moth-eaten appearance of metastatic deposits in bone but the mottled appearance of both can be distinguished thus: metastases erode (reducing density of areas of bone by comparison to normal bone) whilst Paget's disease has areas of increased density when compared to normal bone.

Perthes

This condition is categorised as an avascular necrosis at the head of femur. It affects children. Radiologically there will be increased joint space at the hip, changes in the convexity of the femoral head which appears flattened, sclerotic appearance of the femoral epiphysis and areas of low density over the metaphysis.

Rheumatoid arthritis (RA)

This is a condition of unknown origin, which may affect any of the synovial joints, most commonly in the hands and wrist. RA results in synovial inflammation, joint articular destruction and deformity. Radiologically significant appearances include: soft tissue outline which indicates swelling at joints, osteoporosis, narrowing of joint spaces, joint deformity, subluxation and marginal erosions.[4,5,6]

Trauma

Most positive diagnoses involve fractures or dislocations, which are categorised as follows:

Avulsion fractures

These fractures occur as a result of hyperflexion, hyperextension or unnaturally forced lateral movement of a joint; they are often seen in examinations of the fingers and thumb.

Comminuted fracture
The fracture site consists of several fragments.

Compound fracture
The fracture site is accompanied by an open wound onto the surface of the body part affected by the fracture.

Complicated fracture
Complication arises due to the involvement of the fracture with important functional sites of the body, usually a joint, vascular supply/drainage or nerves.

Dislocation
Articulating surfaces of bones are no longer normally aligned and within the normal joint capsule, showing disruption of the normal radiographic appearance of the joint. This appearance varies according to joint type. Dislocation may occur at the site of any joint. Most commonly affected are the shoulder, hip and elbow. Incomplete dislocation is known as subluxation.

Depressed fracture
The fracture is caused by impact or forced pressure onto the vault of the skull. The fragments are forced to lie under the normal position of the dome of the vault (calvarium). Fragments may overlap and appear as hyperdense at sites of overlap. There may be a stellate appearance of fracture lines radiating from a central point.[7]

Displaced fracture
In this fracture, fragments are separated, usually in more than one direction.

Epiphyseal injuries
Fracture and/or separation of the epiphysis can occur, with varying severity which ranges from the most simple (Salter Harris class I), involving fracture along the epiphyseal line to Salter Harris V where the epiphysis is crushed.[8]

Salter Harris Type I	The fracture line passes along the epiphyseal line, or physis. If there is no displacement of the epiphysis, effusion may be the only indication.
Salter Harris Type II	The fracture line runs along the physis and then obliquely, taking a triangular fragment of metaphysis (this is the most common Salter Harris classification injury found).
Salter Harris Type III	The epiphysis is split in a vertical direction with a fragment displaced along the epiphyseal line.
Salter Harris Type IV	The fracture extends through the metaphysis, the epiphyseal line and through the epiphysis.
Salter Harris Type V	This is compression or crush of the epiphyseal plate, which may not be noticed radiologically. Axial load injury typically causes this type of fracture. It is rare in occurrence and causes interruption or cessation of normal growth at the site. It is often undetected and only investigated after growth disturbance becomes apparent. Prognosis is poor.

Types VI - IX are extremely rare and include injuries to the periosteum which affect membranous growth, and injury to perichondral structures and injuries which may affect endochondral ossification.

Greenstick fracture
Greenstick fractures are almost exclusively found in the long bones of children and are frequently seen in the radius and ulna. This type of fracture does not completely traverse across the bone, which may appear bent rather than broken. A buckled appearance may be seen instead of an incomplete fracture; this is known as a torus fracture. A torus fracture is most commonly found near the metaphysis of the bone; the most commonly affected bone is the radius.

Hairline fracture
This is a fine fracture which has no displacement or separation of the fragments.

Simple fracture
A simple fracture is a fracture of the bone, usually into two fragments, with no involvement of other structures and no displacement.

Spiral fracture
This is a fracture which travels along a bone shaft in a spiral direction. The fracture may be seen apparently travelling obliquely on each individual radiographic projection, rather than obviously demonstrated as a spiral.

Torus fracture
See 'greenstick fracture' above.

References
1. The Ionising Radiation (Medical Exposure) Regulations 2000. London: HMSO
2. Burnett S, et al. A-Z of orthopaedic radiology. London: Saunders; 2000.
3. Ryan S, McNicholas M. Anatomy of diagnostic imaging. London: WB Saunders; 1994.
4. Helms CA. Fundamentals of skeletal radiology. Philadelphia: WB Saunders; 1995.

5. Burgener F, Kormano M. Bone and joint disorders. New York: Thième; 1997.

6. Manaster BJ. Handbook of skeletal radiology. 2nd edn. St Louis: Mosby; 1997.

7. Heller M, Fink A (eds). Radiology of trauma. Berlin: Springer; 2000.

8. Scally P. Medical imaging. Oxford: Oxford University Press; 1999.

FINGERS, HAND AND WRIST

Elizabeth Carver

Descriptions of projections of the upper limb refer to aspects of the arm in relation to the human body in the anatomical position (i.e. with arms abducted and palms facing anteriorly). This means that the aspect of the limb which would normally be orientated outwards (laterally) in this position will be referred to as the lateral aspect, even when the hand is in pronation. The aspect of the arm which is normally nearest the trunk in the anatomical position (medial aspect) will always be referred to as the medial aspect, even for projections with the hand in pronation.

THUMB

A common fracture affecting the thumb is the *Bennett's fracture*, an oblique fracture at the base of the first metacarpal effecting dislocation of the 1st carpometacarpal joint. The mechanism of injury is usually due to forced abduction.

Anteroposterior (AP) thumb

Traditionally the AP thumb projection has been described with the patient seated,[1] however these positions create difficulties when trying to clear the hypothenar eminence from the field. Method 1 described in this text uses a position considered to be significantly more comfortable and achievable than other methods. The idea was originally researched with the patient in an erect position[2] with the later suggestion that radiation protection and immobilisation might be more effective if the patient is supine.[3]

It is clear that the patient's thyroid and lenses of eyes are close to the primary beam and edge of collimation in method 1; if the head is turned away efficiently, the cassette is placed as far away as possible from the trunk, and lead rubber is used effectively, risks can be minimised.

If a cassette is used for examinations of the thumb, two projections can be undertaken on an 18 × 24 cm cassette divided transversely into two sections by the use of lead rubber.

Positioning
Method 1: Patient supine (Fig. 5.1A,B)
- The patient is supine with the affected arm flexed at the elbow and the dorsum of the hand in contact with the table-top. Lead rubber is applied to the trunk
- The fingers are extended and separated from the thumb
- The anterior aspect of the thumb is placed in contact with the image receptor and adjusted until the long axis of the thumb is parallel to it; the hypothenar eminence is cleared from the thumb and thenar eminence
- Since the dorsum of the hand is not in contact with the image receptor, a radiolucent pad is used under the dorsum to aid immobilisation
- The head is turned away from the primary beam

Method 2: Patient seated alongside table (Fig. 5.2)
- The patient is seated with the affected side next to the table; lead rubber is applied to the waist
- The affected hand is externally rotated and the thumb cleared from the fingers
- The anterior aspect of the thumb is placed in contact with the image receptor; it may be necessary for the patient to lean towards the table in order to facilitate this
- A radiolucent pad is used under the dorsum of the hand to aid immobilisation
- Care must be taken to clear the hypothenar eminence from the 1st metacarpal
- The head is turned away from the primary beam

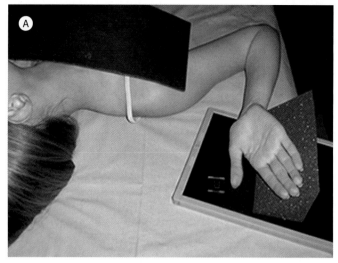

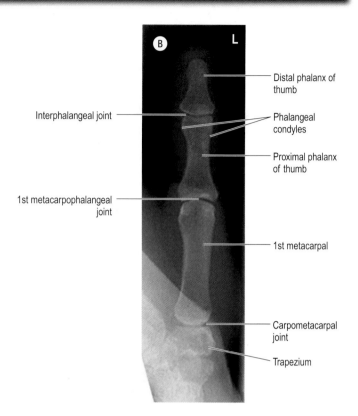

Figure 5.1   AP thumb with patient **(A)** supine; **(B)** AP thumb

Distal phalanx of thumb

Interphalangeal joint

Phalangeal condyles

Proximal phalanx of thumb

1st metacarpophalangeal joint

1st metacarpal

Carpometacarpal joint

Trapezium

Method 3: Patient seated with back to table (Fig. 5.3)
- The patient is seated with their back to the table, with a lead rubber apron fastened behind the waist
- The affected arm is abducted posteriorly and medially rotated
- The anterior aspect of the thumb is placed in contact with the image receptor; the hypothenar eminence is cleared from the thumb and thenar eminence
- A radiolucent pad is used under the dorsum of the hand to aid immobilisation
- Care must be taken to clear the hypothenar eminence from the 1st metacarpal

For patients who are unable to achieve any of these positions, the posteroanterior (PA) projection should be used. Principles of radiographic imaging indicate that there will be some magnification of the thumb with this projection, thus increasing unsharpness. However, an increase in the focus film distance (FFD) will compensate for and reduce the effects of this. An increase in mAs will be necessary in order to account for reduction in radiographic density due to the inverse square law. However, this is likely to be minimal and the balance of benefit versus risk should be considered.

Popular opinion would suggest that creation of an air gap between the thumb and film also requires an increase in mAs, in order to effect further film blackening as compen-

sation for the reduction in scatter. For denser body areas requiring higher exposure factors than the thumb, this would be a relevant consideration. However, since this projection is performed with the selection of a relatively low kVp, the dominant interaction process is one of absorption rather than production of scatter. Thus this negates the requirement for an increase in mAs (see Section 1, Ch. 3). Possible other disadvantages of using the PA projection are possibility of poor maintenance of position and immobilisation; use of immobilisation aids therefore becomes of paramount importance.

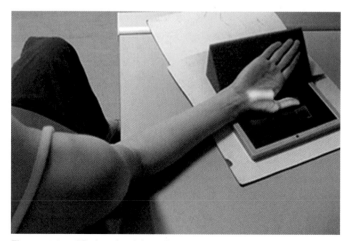

Figure 5.2   AP thumb with patient seated next to the table

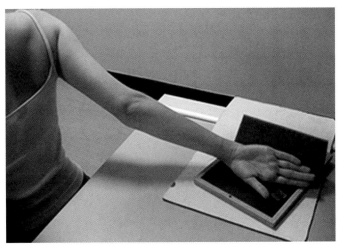

Figure 5.3   AP thumb with patient's back to the table

PA thumb (Fig. 5.4)

Positioning

- The patient is seated with the affected side next to the table; lead rubber is applied to the waist
- From a dorsipalmar (DP) position, the hand is externally rotated through 90° and the lateral border of the wrist placed in contact with the table
- The fingers are extended and superimposed vertically; the thumb is extended and cleared away from the fingers
- If a cassette used, the 1st metacarpophalangeal joint lies over the middle of the available space
- The long axis of the thumb is supported in a horizontal position by a radiolucent pad
- The thumb and thenar eminence are cleared from the hypothenar eminence and palm of the hand

Beam direction and FFD (all AP methods and PA method)

Vertical, at 90° to the cassette
100 cm FFD

Centring point

Over the 1st metacarpophalangeal joint

Collimation

All phalanges, 1st metacarpal, trapezium, soft tissue outlines including that of the thenar eminence

Criteria for assessing image quality (all AP methods and PA method)

- All phalanges, 1st metacarpal, trapezium and soft tissue outline are demonstrated and clear of the hypothenar eminence

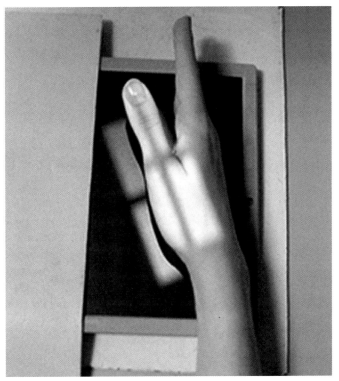

Figure 5.4   PA thumb. The immobilisation pad is removed to show position more clearly.

- Clear interphalangeal and metacarpophalangeal joint spaces; symmetry of the phalangeal condyles
- Sharp image demonstrating soft tissue margins of the thumb and thenar eminence, bony cortex and trabeculae; adequate penetration of thenar eminence to demonstrate 1st metacarpal and trapezium

Common errors	Possible reasons
Interphalangeal joint space not clearly demonstrated	Long axis of thumb may not be parallel to image receptor
Asymmetry of phalangeal condyles	Transverse axis of thumb may not be parallel to image receptor
AP Methods 1–3 Shadow of hypothenar eminence superimposed over 1st metacarpal and trapezium	Inadequate rotation of hand; rotate hand further to clear
PA Shadow of thenar and hypothenar eminence superimposed over 1st metacarpal and trapezium	Thumb may be positioned too close to the rest of hand; clear thumb and 1st metacarpal from hand and fingers

■ Lateral thumb (Fig. 5.5A,B)

Positioning

- The patient is seated with the affected side next to the table; lead rubber is applied to the waist
- In the DP position, the thumb is cleared from the fingers and the hand is medially rotated until the thumb lies lateral with its phalangeal condyles superimposed. The long axis of the thumb is parallel to the image receptor
- Since the medial aspect of the hand will be raised to achieve the correct position, a radiolucent pad is used under the palmar aspect of the hand to aid immobilisation
- An alternative method for immobilisation is to flex the fingers into the palm of the hand, whilst maintaining separation of the thumb, and use the fist to support the dorsum in the required position

Beam direction and FFD

Vertical, at 90° to the image receptor
100 cm FFD

Centring point

Over the 1st metacarpophalangeal joint

Collimation

All phalanges, the 1st metacarpal, trapezium, soft tissue outlines including that of the thenar eminence

Criteria for assessing image quality

- All phalanges, 1st metacarpal, trapezium and soft tissue outline are demonstrated
- The thumb, 1st metacarpal and trapezium are cleared from the fingers and hand
- Superimposition of phalangeal condyles to clear interphalangeal and metacarpophalangeal joint spaces
- Sharp image demonstrating the soft tissue margins of the thumb and thenar eminence, bony cortex and trabeculae. The thenar eminence should be penetrated to adequately demonstrate 1st metacarpal and trapezium

Common error	Possible reason
Poor joint space visualisation and non-superimposition of phalangeal condyles	Hand has not been rotated adequately; medial or external rotation of the hand will facilitate superimposition of phalangeal condyles

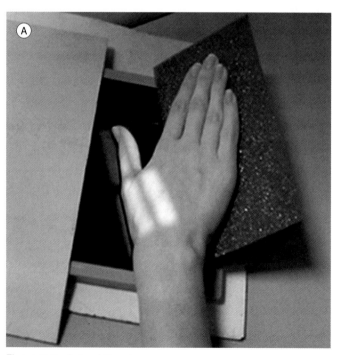

Figure 5.5   Lateral thumb

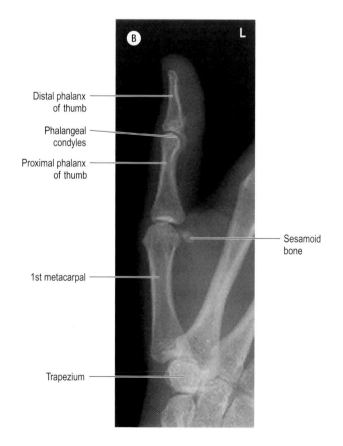

Distal phalanx of thumb

Phalangeal condyles

Proximal phalanx of thumb

Sesamoid bone

1st metacarpal

Trapezium

FINGERS

The most frequent reason for imaging of the fingers is to demonstrate the results of trauma to the area. Avulsion fractures, such as those accompanying *mallet finger*, are often seen, as are dislocations and foreign bodies.

Opinions on centring points and area for inclusion in the primary beam vary for finger examinations. The radiographer has a medicolegal responsibility to ensure that the correct digit has been examined and that there is evidence to support this.

One way to ensure this is to include the adjacent finger or border of the hand in the field of collimation; comparison of size of other fingers will ensure correct identification of the finger. Unfortunately this does involve irradiation of areas not required for examination and could theoretically be deemed to be in contravention of IR(ME)R 2000.[4]

Centring points also vary, according to the area of interest required to be included in the field of radiation (see variation in descriptive section).

If a cassette is used for finger examinations, two projections can be undertaken on an 18 × 24 cm cassette divided longitudinally into two sections by the use of lead rubber.

DP fingers (Fig. 5.6A,B)

Positioning
- The patient is seated with the affected side adjacent to the table; lead rubber is applied to the waist
- The affected hand is pronated and the finger under examination is placed with (a) the proximal interphalangeal joint or (b) the metacarpophalangeal joint centralised in the middle of the cassette, if used. The fingers are extended to facilitate visualisation of interphalangeal joint spaces, and slightly separated

Beam direction and FFD
Vertical, at 90° to the image receptor
100 cm FFD

Centring point
Method (a): over the proximal interphalangeal joint *or*
Method (b): metacarpophalangeal joint

Collimation
Centring method (a): All phalanges of the finger under examination; the metacarpophalangeal joint; adjacent finger/s to facilitate correct finger identification
Centring method (b): As above but to include associated metacarpal

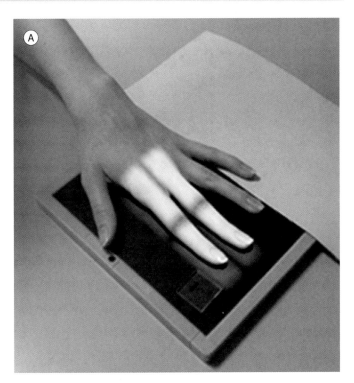

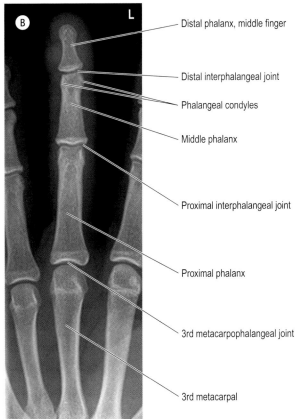

Distal phalanx, middle finger

Distal interphalangeal joint

Phalangeal condyles

Middle phalanx

Proximal interphalangeal joint

Proximal phalanx

3rd metacarpophalangeal joint

3rd metacarpal

Figure 5.6 (A) DP finger; (B) DP middle finger

Criteria for assessing image quality
- *Centring method (a):* All phalanges and the metacarpophalangeal joint are demonstrated

- *Centring method (b):* All phalanges, the metacarpophalangeal joint and the metacarpal are demonstrated
- Adjacent finger/s and soft tissue outline of the affected and adjacent fingers are demonstrated
- Symmetry of the phalangeal condyles
- The interphalangeal and metacarpophalangeal joint spaces are clearly visible and open
- Sharp image demonstrating the soft tissue margins of the finger, bony cortex and trabeculae

Common error	Possible reason
Interphalangeal joint spaces not clearly demonstrated	Fingers may be flexed; extend to clear

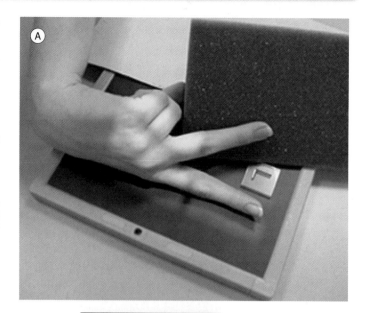

Lateral fingers

Lateral projections of some fingers can prove difficult to achieve and maintain, especially when attempting to separate and immobilise middle, ring and little fingers. The injured or arthritic patient may be even less cooperative. Small wedge-shaped radiolucent pads may be used to separate fingers for radiographic examination.

Positioning

1. Index (1st) finger (Fig. 5.7A,B)
- From the DP position the hand is internally rotated through 90° and the 3rd and 4th fingers flexed and held in position by the thumb
- The index finger is extended and positioned with its lateral aspect in contact with the image receptor
- The long axis of the index finger is parallel to the long axis of the image receptor and separated from the palmar flexed middle finger with a radiolucent pad

2. Middle finger (Fig. 5.8)
- From the DP position, the hand is internally rotated 90° and positioned as for the lateral index finger projection
- The middle finger is extended and aligned with the long axis of the image receptor, and separated from the index finger with a radiolucent pad
- The middle finger is supported in a horizontal position by a radiolucent pad

3. Ring and little finger: method 1 (Fig. 5.9)
- From the DP position the hand is externally rotated through 90°
- The index and middle fingers are flexed and held by the thumb; the little finger remains extended as does the ring finger

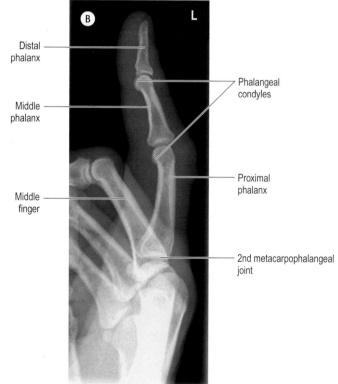

Figure 5.7 Lateral index finger

- The medial aspect of the 5th metacarpal is in contact with the image receptor
- The finger under examination is aligned with its long axis parallel to the long axis of the image receptor
- The ring finger is slightly dorsiflexed to clear it from the little finger
- If under examination, the ring finger is supported in a horizontal position; in any event it is separated from the little finger by a radiolucent pad

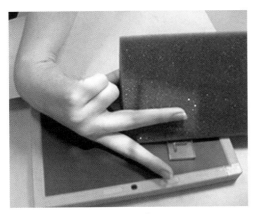

Figure 5.8 Lateral middle finger

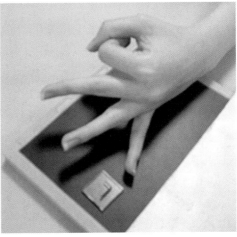

Figure 5.10 Ring and little finger – method 2

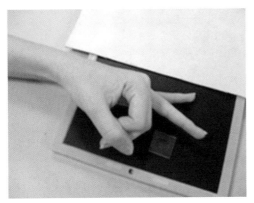

Figure 5.9 Ring and little finger – method 1

4. Ring and little finger: method 2 (Fig. 5.10)
- From the DP position the hand is externally rotated through 90°
- The index finger is flexed and held by the thumb, the remaining fingers are slightly dorsiflexed and fanned out, whilst remaining with their long axes horizontal
- The finger under examination is aligned with its long axis parallel to the long axis of the cassette, if used
- If under examination, the ring finger is supported in a horizontal position; in any event it is separated from the other fingers by radiolucent pads

For all the fingers and positions

Beam direction and FFD
Vertical, at 90° to the image receptor
100 cm FFD

Centring point
(a) Over the proximal interphalangeal joint of the finger under examination *or*
(b) metacarpophalangeal joint of the finger under examination

Collimation
Centring method (a): All phalanges, soft tissue outlines and the metacarpophalangeal joint. Evidence of the adjacent finger for confirmation of identification of the finger under examination
Centring method (b): All phalanges, soft tissue outlines and the associated metacarpal. Evidence of the adjacent finger for confirmation of identification of the finger under examination

Criteria for assessing image quality
- *Centring method (a):* All phalanges and the metacarpophalangeal joint are demonstrated, with the outline of adjacent finger/s
- *Centring method (b):* All phalanges, the metacarpophalangeal joint and the metacarpal are demonstrated with the outline of adjacent finger/s
- Clear interphalangeal and metacarpophalangeal joints are demonstrated, with phalangeal condyles superimposed
- Sharp image demonstrating the soft tissue margins of the finger, bony cortex and trabeculae of phalanges under examination

Common error	Possible reason
Poor joint space demonstration with non-superimposition of phalangeal condyles	Long axis of finger may not lie parallel to image receptor; reposition and support more effectively *or* angle beam to coincide with angle of interphalangeal joints if patient cannot comply

HAND

The Boxer's fracture (or *punch fracture*) is frequently seen on imaging requests from the A&E department. Mechanism of injury is that of impact on a clenched fist, hence the name of this fracture, which usually occurs in the 5th metacarpal. Usually there is anterior displacement of the distal bony fragment, particularly if the fracture occurs through the neck of the metacarpal (which is most common). Less commonly, the 4th metacarpal can be affected.

■ DP hand (Fig. 5.11A,B)

If a cassette is used, two hand projections can usually be undertaken on a 24 × 30 cm cassette divided transversely

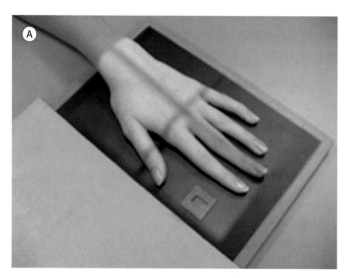

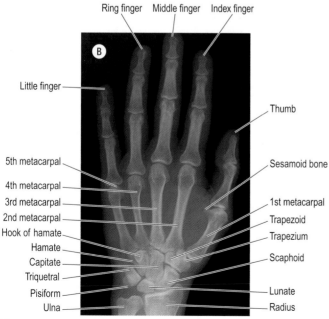

Figure 5.11   DP hand

into two sections by the use of lead rubber. A commonly encountered error is to mask off a distal phalanx with the patient's identification area. To avoid this, always orientate the cassette with its identification area next to the wrist.

Positioning
- The patient is seated with the affected side next to the table; lead rubber is applied to the waist
- The hand is pronated and its palmar aspect placed in contact with the image receptor
- The fingers and thumb are extended and slightly separated

Beam direction and FFD
Vertical, at 90° to the image receptor
100 cm FFD

Centring point
Over the head of the 3rd metacarpal

Collimation
All phalanges, soft tissue outline of the hand, wrist joint

Criteria for assessing image quality
- All phalanges, the wrist joint and the soft tissue outline of the hand are demonstrated
- The fingers are separated, and the interphalangeal and metacarpophalangeal joints are clear
- Symmetrical appearance of the heads of metacarpals 2 to 4
- Obliquity of thumb and the heads of metacarpals 1 and 5
- Sharp image demonstrating the soft tissue margins of the hand, bony cortex and trabeculae. Adequate penetration to demonstrate the hook of hamate whilst showing distal phalanges

Common errors	Possible reasons
Superimposition of soft tissue outlines of fingers	Fingers are not separated adequately
Poor demonstration of joint spaces	Fingers may not be extended; extend fingers *or* examine with hand in supination to utilise obliquity of rays around centre of beam, to 'open out' joints

In this position it is to be noted that the 5th metacarpal and little finger are externally rotated into an oblique appearance. The concept of reducing this obliquity and the impact of this on the image has been discussed in the past,[5] yet it does not appear that there has been a widespread adoption of the measures suggested. Could this be that reporting radiographers and radiologists find that the projections of the 5th metacarpal provided by the DP and DPO positions are at sufficiently different angles? Or, is familiarity with these more usual appearances enough to inspire confidence in outlining a report?

Dorsipalmar oblique (DPO) hand (Fig. 5.12A,B)

Positioning

- The patient is seated with the affected side next to the table; lead rubber is applied to the waist

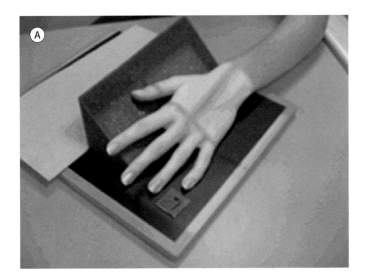

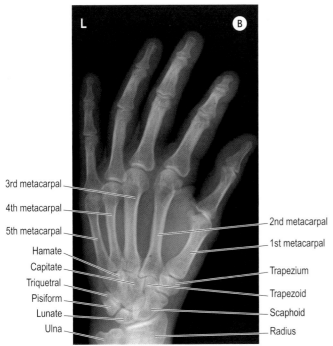

Figure 5.12   DP oblique hand

- From the DP position the hand is externally rotated through 45°; the medial aspect of the hand remains in contact with the image receptor
- A radiolucent pad is placed under the lateral aspect of the hand as immobilisation and to keep the fingers extended and horizontal *or* the fingertips flex gently and rest upon the image receptor for support
- The fingers are separated

Beam direction and FFD
Vertical, at 90° to the image receptor
100 cm FFD

Centring point
Over the head of the 3rd metacarpal

Collimation
All phalanges, soft tissue outline of the hand, wrist joint

Previous descriptions of the DPO hand have shown the selection of a range of centring methods.[1,3] Originally, in the UK, centring for this projection was stated as over the head of the 5th metacarpal,[6,7] in order to utilise the effect of the oblique rays which 'opened out' the spaces between the metacarpal head. As the dose reduction culture in radiography gained influence, it became clear that this centring point required an unacceptably large field of radiation, almost half of which was not usefully employed. The result was to suggest that centring should remain the same, with the addition of angulation across the dorsum of the hand until the central ray lay over the head of the 3rd metacarpal. This would allow closer collimation around the hand, yet maintain the effects of the oblique rays afforded in the original centring point.

In principle, of course, this sounds a logical amendment. However, questions have arisen regarding this method.[3] Since the FFD for this projection lies at 100 cm and the distance between the heads of the 3rd to 5th metacarpals is generally around 3 cm, the oblique rays referred to will actually be around 2° and probably even less. How useful would such a small angle be? Can the human eye detect differences in images taken with or without this angle?

Why even consider 'opening up' the spaces between metacarpal heads when they are well-separated on the DP image? If it is really essential (and the authors question whether or not this would actually be essential) then why not utilise 2° less obliquity on the rotation of the hand? Could 2° even be assessed accurately by the human eye?

For these reasons the centring point is selected as the head of the 3rd metacarpal in this text.

Criteria for assessing image quality
- All phalanges, wrist joint and soft tissue outline of the hand are demonstrated
- Separation of the shafts of the metacarpals but with some overlap of metacarpal heads 3–5
- Separation of the soft tissues of the fingers and intermediate phalanges and distal phalanges
- Joint spaces will not be demonstrated as clear
- Sharp image demonstrating the soft tissue margins of the hand, bony cortex and trabeculae

Common error	Possible reason
Overlap of shafts of metacarpals	Excessive external rotation of the hand

■ Lateral hand (Fig. 5.13A,B)

The lateral projection is most useful for demonstration of direction of displacement in fractures of the metacarpals and is particularly useful to identify anterior displacement of distal bony fragment in the boxer's fracture.

If a cassette is used for the examination an 18 × 24 cm size is selected for most adults. Patients with large hands will require a 24 × 30 cm cassette.

Positioning
- The patient is seated with the affected side next to the table; lead rubber is applied to the waist
- From the DP position, the hand is externally rotated through 90° and its long axis placed obliquely across the available area if a cassette is used
- The fingers are extended and superimposed vertically, whilst the thumb is extended and abducted from the hand
- The thumb lies horizontally and supported on a radiolucent pad

Beam direction and FFD
Vertical, at 90° to the image receptor
100 cm FFD

Centring point
Over the medial aspect of the head of the 2nd metacarpal

Collimation
All phalanges, soft tissue outline of the hand, wrist joint

Criteria for assessing image quality
- All phalanges, the wrist joint and the soft tissue outline of the hand are demonstrated

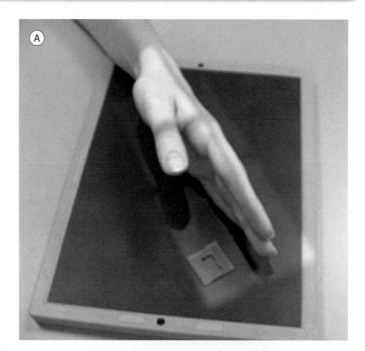

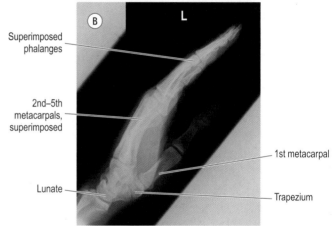

Superimposed phalanges

2nd–5th metacarpals, superimposed

Lunate

1st metacarpal

Trapezium

L

Figure 5.13   Lateral hand

- The fingers are superimposed, metacarpals 2–5 are superimposed and the thumb is cleared from other bones of the hand
- Sharp image demonstrating the soft tissue margins of the hand, bony cortex and trabeculae of the thumb phalanges and lunate. Outlines of superimposed bones are demonstrated but not showing trabecular detail. Penetration to demonstrate individual carpal bones

Common error	Possible reason
Poor superimposition of phalanges and poor superimposition of metacarpals	Over or under rotation of the hand; ensure dorsum of hand is at 90° to image receptor

Palmar dorsal oblique examination of both hands for rheumatoid arthritis assessment (ball catcher's)
(Fig. 5.14A,B)

Both hands are examined via the same, single exposure, image. Hands are palm upwards with relaxed fingers and slight medial rotation. The hands appear as though the patient is poised ready to catch a ball, hence the alternative name 'ball catcher's projection'.

If used, a 24 × 30 cm cassette is selected for this projection.

Positioning
- The patient is seated alongside the table but it may be necessary to turn the trunk slightly towards the image receptor
- The arms are abducted forwards towards the image receptor and externally rotated to bring the region of the dorsum of the hand overlying the 5th metacarpal in contact with the image receptor
- The dorsum of the hand lies at 30° to the image receptor and the hands are supported in this position by radiolucent pads. The fingers are slightly relaxed

Beam direction and FFD
Vertical, at 90° to the image receptor
100 cm FFD

Centring point
Midway between the medial borders of the hand, level with the heads of the 5th metacarpals

Collimation
Both hands and wrist joints

Criteria for assessing image quality
- Both hands and wrist joints are demonstrated
- Clear metacarpophalangeal joint spaces 2–5
- Sharp image demonstrating bony detail in contrast with the joint spaces

WRIST

The *Colles fracture* is a result of a fall onto an outstretched hand, resulting in fracture of the radius and possibly ulna. There is posterior displacement of the distal fragments, which most frequently requires manipulation to reduce this displacement. Less frequently, fracture of the distal radius and ulna may show anterior displacement of the distal fragments. These cases are categorised as *Smiths fractures*. The mechanism of injury is usually that of falling onto the back of the hand.

Wrist examinations are often undertaken with the wrist in plaster or other immobilisation medium, which will have implications for exposure factor selection, according to density of the fracture immobiliser. If a dense medium is used, as in plaster of Paris, both kVp and mAs will need to be increased, although more modern immobilisers are less dense and require less of an increase in exposure factors. Any increase results in a higher radiation dose for the area.

A popular method to counteract an increase in exposure factors is to select a standard speed cassette (if cassettes are used) for the examination, yet use the same or similar exposure factors as the examination would take with high definition screens and without plaster immobilisation. It could be suggested that this measure will result in loss of detail due to the selection of the faster screen.

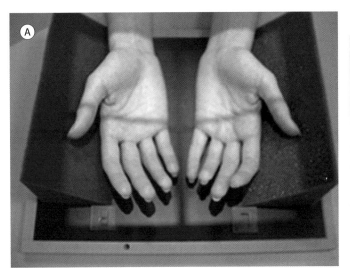
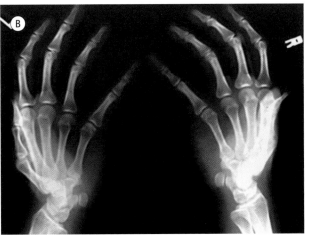

Figure 5.14   Ball catcher's. (b) Reproduced with permission from Ballinger PW, Frank ED. Merrill's atlas of radiographic positioning and radiologic procedures. 10th edn. St Louis: Mosby; 2003

However, when considering that the immobilisation medium will reduce image quality anyway, it becomes apparent that the fine detail strived for in initial radiographs is less achievable, especially when the increased area density will necessitate some increase in exposure factors and thus increase in scatter. The immobilisation medium will also overlie the area of interest and degrade the image detail. In addition, it should be remembered that the aim of examinations on body areas immobilised in this way is to demonstrate more gross features than in initial examination; e.g. progress of callus formation or evidence of fracture reduction.

If a cassette is used, two wrist projections can be undertaken on an 18 × 24 cm cassette divided transversely into two sections by the use of lead rubber. If three projections are undertaken as routine, use of a 24 × 30 cm cassette will facilitate inclusion of these.

▉ PA wrist (Fig. 5.15A,B)

Positioning
- The patient is seated with the affected side next to the table; lead rubber is applied to the waist
- The affected arm is flexed at the elbow and the wrist is internally rotated to pronate the hand
- The anterior aspect of the wrist is placed in contact with the image receptor; the fingers are relaxed to bring the forearm and wrist flat and in contact with the image receptor
- The radial and ulnar styloid processes are equidistant from the image receptor

Beam direction and FFD
Vertical, at 90° to the image receptor
100 cm FFD

Centring point
Midway between the radial and ulnar styloid processes

Collimation
Proximal third of metacarpals, carpals, distal third of radius and ulna, soft tissue outlines of wrist

Criteria for assessing image quality
- Proximal third of metacarpals, the carpals, distal third of radius and ulna, and soft tissue outlines of the wrist are demonstrated
- Clear demonstration of the distal radioulnar joint
- The radial and ulnar styloid processes seen on the lateral and medial margins of these bones

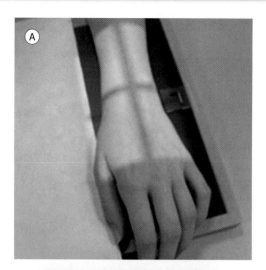

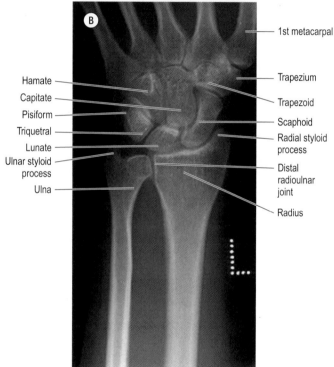

Figure 5.15   PA wrist

- Sharp image demonstrating the soft tissue margins of the area, bony cortex and trabeculae. Adequate penetration will demonstrate hook of hamate clearly

Good contrast is required over the soft tissue since there is evidence that changes in alignment and shape of the scaphoid fat pad, seen normally as a linear area of low density following the line of the medial edges of scaphoid and trapezium, can be an indicator of significant wrist injury. The fat pad sign alone cannot be considered unequivocal.[8] The fat pad is not usually noted in patients under 12 years of age.

Common error	Possible reason
Radial and ulnar styloid processes appear displaced from lateral and medial margins of these bones; superimposition of the radius and ulna over the distal radioulnar joint	Styloid processes are not equidistant from the image receptor

Lateral wrist (Fig. 5.16A,B)

Positioning
- The patient is seated with the affected side next to the table and a lead rubber sheet applied to the waist
- The arm is extended, abducted from the trunk and externally rotated 90°
- The medial aspect of the wrist is placed in contact with the image receptor
- The wrist is externally rotated approximately 5° further, in order to superimpose the radial and ulnar styloid processes

Beam direction and FFD
Vertical, at 90° to the image receptor
100 cm FFD

Centring point
Over the radial styloid process

Collimation
Proximal third of metacarpals, the carpals, distal third of radius and ulna, soft tissue outlines of wrist

Criteria for assessing image quality
- Proximal third of metacarpals, carpals, distal third of radius and ulna, soft tissue outlines of the wrist are demonstrated
- Superimposition of the distal radius and ulna; the lunate should have a crescent shaped appearance
- Sharp image demonstrating the soft tissue margins of the wrist, bony cortex and trabeculae. Penetration of carpus to demonstrate individual carpal bones

Common errors	Possible reasons
Radius appears posteriorly in relation to ulna	Excessive external rotation
Ulna appears posteriorly in relation to radius	Inadequate external rotation

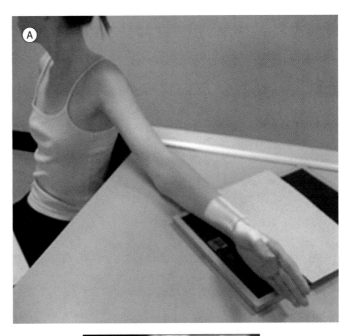

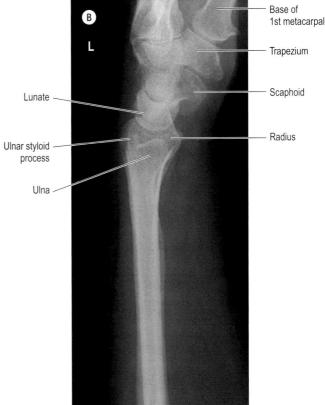

Base of 1st metacarpal
Trapezium
Lunate
Scaphoid
Ulnar styloid process
Radius
Ulna

Figure 5.16   Lateral wrist

PA oblique wrist (Fig. 5.17A,B)

Positioning
- The patient is seated with the affected side next to the table and a lead rubber sheet applied to the waist

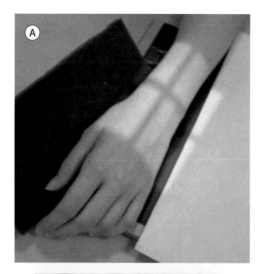

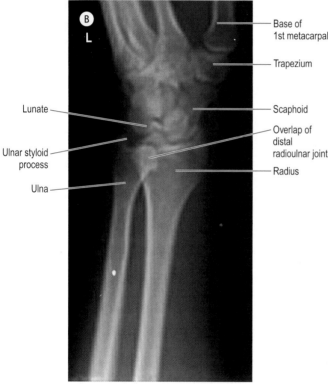

Labels on Figure 5.17:
- Base of 1st metacarpal
- Trapezium
- Scaphoid
- Overlap of distal radioulnar joint
- Radius
- Lunate
- Ulnar styloid process
- Ulna

Figure 5.17   PA oblique wrist

- From the PA position the wrist is externally rotated 45°
- The wrist is supported in this position with a radiolucent pad or by slight flexion of the fingers until their tips rest on the image receptor or table to support the obliquity; there should be no dorsiflexion or palmar flexion at the wrist

Beam direction and FFD
Vertical, at 90° to the image receptor
100 cm FFD

Centring point
Midway between the radial and ulnar styloid processes

Collimation
Proximal third of metacarpals, carpals, distal third of radius and ulna, and soft tissue outlines of wrist

Criteria for assessing image quality
- Proximal third of metacarpals, carpals, distal third of radius and ulna, and the soft tissue outlines of the wrist demonstrated
- Overlap of the distal radioulnar joint
- Scaphoid and trapezium are clearly demonstrated
- Sharp image demonstrating the soft tissue margins of the wrist, bony cortex and trabeculae. Adequate penetration to demonstrate differentiation between overlapped carpal bones

SCAPHOID

Scaphoid fractures are difficult to detect radiographically immediately after injury and are best demonstrated after 10–14 days when callus formation can be seen as increased bone density on radiographs. The scaphoid fat pad sign can be used to supplement bony information but the fat pad sign cannot be used as stand-alone evidence of injury.[8]

However, since fractures of the radius and ulna must also be excluded at the time of injury, wrist projections are undertaken initially. Disruption of the single blood supply to the proximal end of the scaphoid may result in bony necrosis and onset of bony degenerative changes if the fracture is not treated; as a result, even in the event of negative findings for radius and ulna at the initial stage, the wrist is treated conservatively, with the use of immobilisation. At the end of the 10–14 day callus formation period immobilisation is removed and well-collimated scaphoid projections are requested.

Many projections which will demonstrate the scaphoid have been described and it is necessary to use a minimum number which will provide the required information. Projections selected for description include ulnar deviation, to clear the scaphoid from adjacent carpal bones, and a 30° angle which has been shown to demonstrate fractures of the waist effectively. It may not be considered necessary to use all the projections described in one assessment of the scaphoid.

Descriptions include only those for the specifically centred, well-coned scaphoid assessment. In the PA wrist projection, where the centring point lies between the styloid processes, the scaphoid will be foreshortened due to its orientation within the carpus.[9] Centring over the scaphoid reduces this effect and the scaphoid is likely to be more clearly demonstrated, with minimum distortion. However, in an attempt to consider this concept realistically, it should be asked if this improved visualisation would be detected by the human eye since the obliquity of X-rays around the central ray at 100 cm FFD will only be approximately 2° over the fracture.

Initial assessment, which includes the wrist, should be positioned as described in the section on wrist examinations but with ulnar deviation applied. When employing this medial flexion on the wrist, care should be taken not to flex the joint anteriorly or posteriorly, as this can cause distortion of the image of the scaphoid itself.[9]

In this text, the term 'anatomical snuff box' is used in centring point descriptions. The position of the scaphoid can be identified as lying under this 'snuff box', a depression found on the lateral border of the carpus, between the base of the 1st metacarpal and radius. It is particularly evident when the thumb is in lateral abduction.

If part of an initial assessment of the wrist and scaphoid, projections can be undertaken using an 18 × 24 cm cassette, if used, split into two by the use of lead rubber.

If part of a specific scaphoid assessment, the cassette can be divided into up to five well-collimated sections. Similarly, a 24 × 30 cm cassette can be used.

■ PA with ulnar deviation (Fig. 5.18A,B,C)

Positioning
- The patient is positioned as for the PA projection of the wrist
- The 'snuff box' is placed in the centre of the available space if a cassette is used
- The hand is adducted towards the ulna; there should be no other flexion of the wrist. The thumb is in contact with the lateral aspect of the 2nd metacarpal

Beam direction and FFD
Vertical, at 90° to the image receptor
100 cm FFD

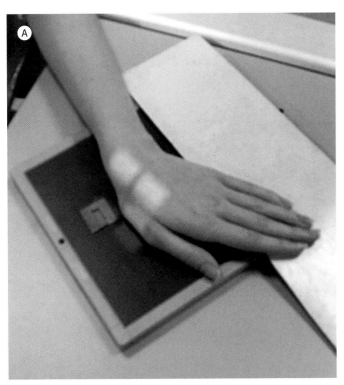

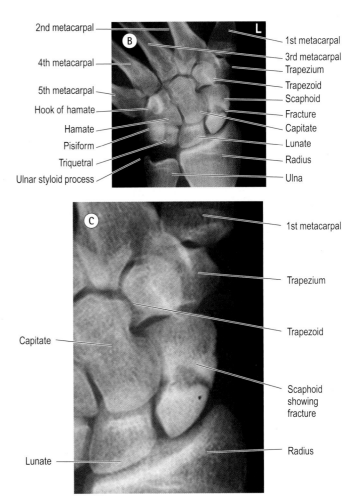

Figure 5.18 Scaphoid PA with **(A)** ulnar deviation, **(B)** showing fracture and **(C)** demonstrating close collimation

Centring point
Over the 'snuff box'

Collimation
Scaphoid, trapezium, trapezoid, lunate, 1st carpometacarpal joint, radiocarpal joint

Criteria for assessing image quality
- Demonstration of the scaphoid, trapezium, trapezoid, lunate, 1st carpometacarpal joint and radiocarpal joint
- Separation of the joint spaces around the scaphoid; adequate ulnar deviation will show long axis of the 1st metacarpal following that of the radius (if included in the image)
- Sharp image demonstrating bony cortex and trabeculae. Optimum penetration to demonstrate overlap of carpal bones and contrast to allow for demonstration of subtle scaphoid fat pat sign

Common error	Possible reason
Poor separation of joint space around scaphoid	Inadequate ulnar deviation

▇ Scaphoid: PA oblique with ulnar deviation
(Fig. 5.19A,B)

Positioning
- The patient is positioned as for the PA oblique projection of the wrist
- The 'snuff box' is placed in the centre of the available space if a cassette is used
- A radiolucent pad is used under the wrist to aid immobilisation
- The hand is adducted towards the ulna; there should be no flexion of the wrist

Beam direction and FFD
Vertical, at 90° to the image receptor
100 cm FFD

Centring point
Over the 'snuff box'

Collimation
Scaphoid, trapezium, trapezoid, lunate, 1st carpometacarpal joint, radiocarpal joint

Please note that Figure 5.19B shows less stringent collimation, to provide an example of the relationship of other carpal bones to the scaphoid.

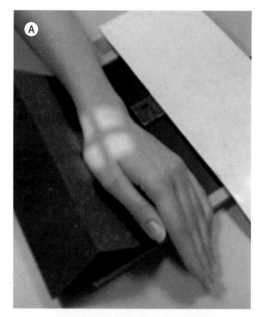

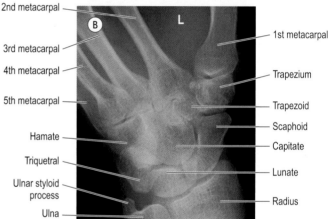

Figure 5.19 **(A)** Scaphoid PA oblique and **(B)** showing fracture

Criteria for assessing image quality
- Demonstration of the scaphoid, trapezium, trapezoid, lunate, 1st carpometacarpal joint and radiocarpal joint
- Separation of joint spaces around the scaphoid
- Sharp image demonstrating bony cortex and trabeculae. Adequate penetration to demonstrate differentiation between overlapped carpal bones

Common error	Possible reason
Poor separation of joint space around scaphoid	Inadequate ulnar deviation

▇ Scaphoid: AP oblique with ulnar deviation
(Fig. 5.20A,B)

Positioning
- The patient is positioned initially as for the lateral projection of the wrist

Please note that Figure 5.20B shows less stringent collimation, to provide an example of the relationship of other carpal bones to the scaphoid.

Criteria for assessing image quality
- Demonstration of the scaphoid, trapezium, trapezoid, lunate, 1st carpometacarpal joint and radiocarpal joint
- The scaphoid seen above the radius, partially overlapping the lunate but clear of the pisiform and triquetral
- Sharp image demonstrating bony cortex and trabeculae. Adequate penetration to demonstrate differentiation between overlapped carpal bones

▓ Lateral scaphoid (Fig. 5.21A,B)

Positioning
- The patient is positioned as for a lateral projection of the wrist; but since the projection is relevant to the scaphoid rather than the radius and ulna, the elbow may be flexed for external rotation at the wrist, rather than full abduction of the limb
- The 'snuff box' is placed in the centre of the available space if a cassette is used

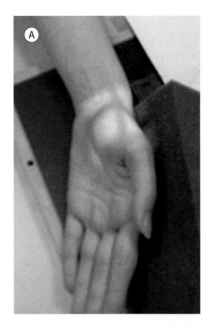

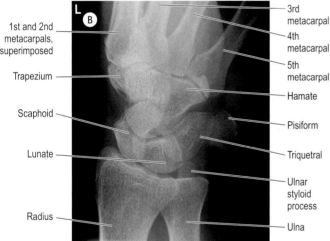

Figure 5.20   AP oblique scaphoid

Labels for Figure 5.20B:
- 1st and 2nd metacarpals, superimposed
- Trapezium
- Scaphoid
- Lunate
- Radius
- 3rd metacarpal
- 4th metacarpal
- 5th metacarpal
- Hamate
- Pisiform
- Triquetral
- Ulnar styloid process
- Ulna

- The wrist is externally rotated 45° and a radiolucent pad is placed under the wrist to aid immobilisation
- The 'snuff box' should be in the centre of the available space if a cassette is used
- The hand is adducted towards the ulna; there should be no flexion of the wrist

Beam direction and FFD
Vertical, at 90° to the image receptor
100 cm FFD

Centring point
Over the 'snuff box'

Collimation
Scaphoid, trapezium, trapezoid, lunate, 1st carpometacarpal joint, radiocarpal joint

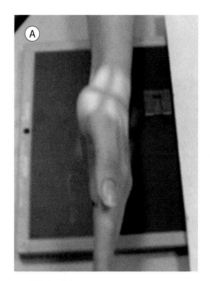

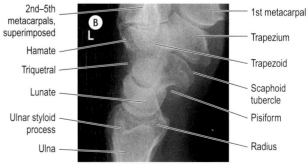

Labels for Figure 5.21B:
- 2nd–5th metacarpals, superimposed
- Hamate
- Triquetral
- Lunate
- Ulnar styloid process
- Ulna
- 1st metacarpal
- Trapezium
- Trapezoid
- Scaphoid tubercle
- Pisiform
- Radius

Figure 5.21   Scaphoid lateral

Beam direction and FFD

Vertical, at 90° to the image receptor
100 cm FFD

Centring point

Over the 'snuff box'

Collimation

Scaphoid, trapezium, lunate, 1st carpometacarpal joint, radiocarpal joint, radial and ulnar styloid processes

Please note that Figure 5.21B shows less stringent collimation, to provide an example of the relationship of other carpal bones to the scaphoid.

Criteria for assessing image quality

- Demonstration of the scaphoid, trapezium, lunate, 1st carpometacarpal joint, radiocarpal joint and radial and ulnar styloid processes
- The lunate projected as a crescent. The proximal end of the 3rd metacarpal, capitate, lunate and distal radius should be in alignment. The waist of the scaphoid should be superimposed over the pisiform, with the tubercle of scaphoid clear of the pisiform anteriorly on the palmar aspect of wrist
- Sharp image demonstrating bony cortex and trabeculae. Adequate penetration to demonstrate differentiation between overlapped carpal bones

■ Scaphoid: PA with 30° angulation and ulnar deviation

Positioning

- Position is as for the PA scaphoid with ulnar deviation (Fig. 5.18A)
- The 'snuff box' is positioned coincident with the centre of the available space if a cassette is used

Beam direction and FFD

Initially vertical, which is then directed 30° towards the elbow
100 cm FFD

Centring point

Over the trapezium

Collimation

Scaphoid and surrounding joints

This projection should be undertaken with the forearm positioned parallel to the median sagittal plain (MSP), in order that the central ray is not directed towards the trunk when angled towards the elbow. To achieve this, the patient's chair should be placed next to the longer dimension of the table rather than at the end, to allow easy and accurate angulation of the X-ray tube in the correct plane.

There are two alternative projections which will also place the scaphoid into a position where it will lie at 30° to the central ray, thus negating the need for angulation and these are with the wrist in dorsiflexion and the forearm raised 30° (see below).

■ Wrist in dorsiflexion (Fig. 5.22)

- An initial PA wrist position is modified by dorsiflexing the hand at the wrist until it makes an angle of 30° with the image receptor
- The hand is supported on a radiolucent pad and the wrist is placed in ulnar deviation. The anterior aspect of the wrist remains in contact with the image receptor

Beam direction and FFD

Vertical, at 90° to the image receptor
100 cm FFD

Centring point

Over the 'snuff box'

Collimation

Scaphoid and surrounding joints

■ Forearm raised 30° (Fig. 5.23)

- With the wrist in pronation, the forearm is raised 30° at the elbow
- The elbow remains in contact with the table
- The forearm and hand are supported on a radiolucent pad and the wrist is placed in ulnar deviation; the hand and forearm remain in the same plane

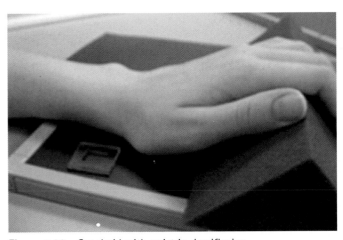

Figure 5.22   Scaphoid with wrist in dorsiflexion

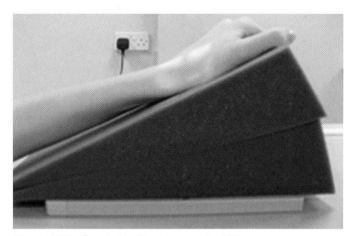

Figure 5.23   Scaphoid with forearm raised 30°

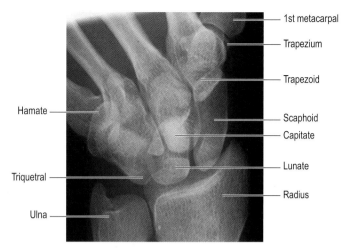

Figure 5.24   Scaphoid: PA 30° image

Beam direction and FFD
Vertical, at 90° to the image receptor

150 cm FFD, to reduce magnification caused by increased object film distance (OFD)

Centring point
Over the 'snuff box'

Collimation
Scaphoid and surrounding joints

Criteria for assessing image quality: all 30° projections
- The scaphoid and surrounding joints are demonstrated
- The scaphoid is cleared from other carpals due to ulnar deviation, with elongation due to 30° angle
- Sharp but elongated image demonstrating bony cortex and trabeculae of scaphoid. (See Fig. 5.24; *please note that this image shows less stringent collimation, to provide an example of the relationship of other carpal bones to the scaphoid*)

Common error	Possible reasons
Short appearance of scaphoid	Inadequate angle used or hand/forearm not raised enough

CARPAL TUNNEL

Compression of the median nerve in the carpal tunnel on the anterior aspect of the wrist results in pain and paraesthesia of the fingers; the collection of these symptoms is known as carpal tunnel syndrome.[10]

Whenever possible, magnetic resonance imaging (MRI) should be the imaging modality of choice for symptoms suggestive of this condition. However, bony spurs which emanate from the carpus, impinging upon innervation at the wrist, can be detected using plain film radiography. In addition, when there are valid reasons contraindicating the use of MRI (see Section 8, Ch. 41) it may still be necessary to undertake plain radiographic examination of the carpal tunnel.

Several methods for production of images of this region are available; implications of dose to radiosensitive organs, projectional principles and patient condition or capability should be considered when selecting the most appropriate method. Method 1 is given priority for description, since it is considered to show least magnification unsharpness and, with the trunk turned away from the primary beam, most effective in dose reduction to radiosensitive areas (thyroid, gonads, breast, eye lens). Unfortunately, carpal tunnel syndrome is highly likely to impair the patient's ability to forcibly dorsiflex the wrist and, in these cases method 3 should be selected.

If used, an 18 × 24 cm cassette is selected for all techniques.

▌ Method 1: superoinferior carpal tunnel – erect with patient facing away from the central ray
(Fig. 5.25A,B)

Positioning
- The image receptor is placed on the table, its edge coincident with the edge of the table-top
- A lead rubber apron is fastened to the back of the waist
- The patient stands with their back to the table, which should be adjusted so that its height lies just below the patient's waist level
- The affected arm is internally rotated until the palm faces posteriorly, towards the table and cassette

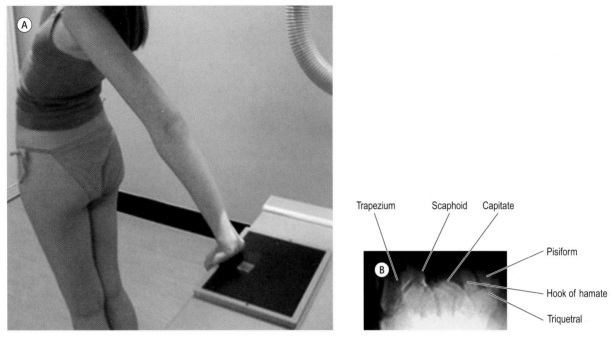

Figure 5.25   Superoinferior carpal tunnel (method 1) with **(A)** patient's back to X-ray beam; **(B)** carpal tunnel

- The proximal half of the palm is placed in contact with the image receptor and the fingers flexed around the edge of the receptor; the carpus should be as far away from the edge of the receptor as possible
- The patient effects dorsiflexion of the wrist in this position by leaning forward and exerting slight pressure on the forearm, which is extended at the elbow to allow maximum effect. The forearm is cleared from the wrist and carpus

Method 2: superoinferior carpal tunnel – erect with patient facing the central ray (Fig. 5.26)

Positioning
- The image receptor is placed on the table, its edge coincident with the edge of the table-top
- A lead rubber apron is fastened over the front of the waist
- The patient stands facing the table, which should be adjusted so that its height lies just below the patient's waist level
- The affected arm is externally rotated until the palm is in supination, facing anteriorly towards the table and cassette
- The proximal half of the palm is placed in contact with the image receptor and the fingers flexed around the edge of the receptor; the carpus should be as far from the edge of the receptor as possible
- The patient effects dorsiflexion of the wrist in this position by leaning back and exerting a slight pressure

on the forearm, which is extended at the elbow to allow maximum effect. The forearm is cleared from the wrist and carpus

Beam direction and FFD for methods 1 and 2
Vertical, at 90° to the cassette
100 cm FFD

Centring point
Over the midpoint of the anterior part of the wrist, within the depression caused by the tunnel arrangement of the carpus

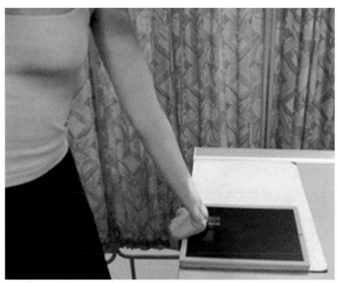

Figure 5.26   Superoinferior carpal tunnel (method 2) with patient facing X-ray beam

Collimation

Carpal bones, soft tissue of anterior aspect of wrist

■ Method 3: Inferosuperior carpal tunnel – patient seated facing the table (Fig. 5.27)

Positioning

- The patient is seated at the table and a lead rubber sheet is applied to the waist
- The image receptor is placed on the table-top, approximately 30–40 cm from the patient
- A 45° radiolucent pad is placed onto the image receptor. If a cassette is used, the pad should be placed over its middle
- The patient places the flexed elbow of the affected side onto the table, next to the image receptor
- Whilst maintaining some elbow flexion, the hand is pronated and the forearm rested on the pad
- The wrist should lie over, but not in contact with, the image receptor
- The hand is dorsiflexed at the wrist and a bandage passed around the fingers; pulling this bandage gently will facilitate the extent of dorsiflexion required to clear the forearm from the carpus
- The patient maintains the dorsiflexion by holding and pulling the ends of the bandage; the elbow remains in contact with the table-top
- The head is turned to the side, away from the primary beam

Beam direction and FFD for method 3

Vertical, at 90° to the image receptor
150 cm FFD

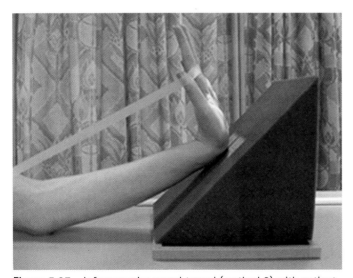

Figure 5.27   Inferosuperior carpal tunnel (method 3) with patient seated

Centring point

Over the midpoint of the anterior part of the proximal portion of the hand, within the depression caused by the tunnel arrangement of the carpus

Collimation

Carpal bones, soft tissue of anterior portion of distal hand

■ Criteria for assessing image quality (all methods)

- The carpal bones and soft tissue of the anterior portion of the wrist are demonstrated
- The carpal tunnel is seen as a curved, darker, soft tissue area anterior to the denser carpal bones
- The distal radius and ulna are cleared from the carpus to lie over the metacarpals
- The hook of hamate and pisiform are cleared from the rest of the carpus and on the medial aspect of the tunnel
- Sharp image demonstrating soft tissue of the carpal tunnel region, bony trabeculae of pisiform and hook of hamate. Optimum penetration to demonstrate these bones, whilst maintaining contrast with required soft tissue. Superimposed carpals will not be fully penetrated

Common errors	Possible reasons
Image overall appears pale with no distinguishable bony features	1. Inadequate penetration and exposure 2. Forearm may not have been cleared from carpus; improve dorsiflexion or consider examination using a method that may be more comfortable for the patient
Asymmetry of tunnel; 4th and 5th metacarpals are seen clear of forearm	Patient's arm is leaning towards radius; ensure forearm lies vertically over the hand and carpus
Asymmetry of tunnel; 1st and 2nd metacarpals are seen clear of forearm	Patient's arm is leaning towards ulna; ensure forearm lies vertically over the hand and carpus

References

1. Whitley AS, et al. Clark's positioning in radiography. 12th edn. London: Hodder Arnold; 2005
2. Richmond B. A comparative study of two radiographic techniques for obtaining an AP projection of the thumb. Radiography Today 1995; 61(696):11–15.
3. Unett EM, Royle AJ. Radiographic techniques and image evaluation. London: Chapman and Hall; 1997.

4. The Ionising Radiation (Medical Exposure) Regulations 2000. London: HMSO.
5. Lewis S. New angles on radiographic examination of the hand. Radiography Today 1988; 54(617):4–45, (618):20–30, (619):47–48.
6. Bell G, Finlay D. Basic radiographic positioning and anatomy. London: Baillière Tindall; 1986.
7. Clark KC. Clark's positioning in radiography. London: Heinemann; 1939.
8. Nicholson DA, Driscoll PA. ABC of emergency radiology. Cambridge: BMJ Publishing Group; 1995.
9. McQuillen Martensen K. Radiographic critique. Philadelphia: WB Saunders; 1995.
10. Helms CA. Fundamentals of skeletal radiology. 2nd edn. WB Saunders: Philadelphia; 1995.

CHAPTER 6

FOREARM, ELBOW AND HUMERUS

Elizabeth Carver

FOREARM (RADIUS AND ULNA)

This region of the upper limb is most usually affected by trauma. The Colles fracture is the most usual finding after trauma to radius and ulna and this is outlined in Chapter 5 (section on the wrist). Other fractures of these bones are much rarer. The *Galleazzi* fracture is more serious than the Colles fracture, being a fracture of the distal portion of the radius which is accompanied by subluxation or dislocation of the distal radioulnar joint. The *Monteggia* fracture, conversely, is a fracture of the ulna, accompanied by dislocation of the radius proximally.[1]

■ Anteroposterior (AP) forearm (Fig. 6.1A,B)

If used, the cassette size is selected for this examination according to patient size. Sizes suitable for adults include 15 × 40 cm, 30 × 40 cm split lengthwise for two projections or 35 × 43 cm similarly split lengthwise.

Positioning
- The patient is seated with the affected side next to the table; lead rubber is applied to the waist
- The arm is extended at the elbow, abducted away from the trunk and externally rotated until the hand lies in supination
- The posterior aspect of the forearm is placed in contact with the image receptor, to include elbow and wrist joints. The long axis of the forearm is coincident with the long axis of the cassette
- The joints must lie in the same plane

- The humeral epicondyles and radial and ulnar styloid processes are equidistant from the image receptor
- The head is turned away from the shoulder of the side under examination, aiming to reduce scattered radiation to the lenses of the eyes and thyroid

Beam direction and focus film distance (FFD)
Vertical, at 90° to the image receptor
100 cm FFD

Centring
Midway between the wrist and elbow joints

Collimation
Elbow, wrist, shafts of radius and ulna, soft tissue outlines of forearm

■ Criteria for assessing image quality
- Wrist and elbow joints, radius, ulna and soft tissue outline of the forearm are demonstrated
- Partial superimposition of the radius and ulna at proximal and distal ends, with separation of the shafts. Radial tubercle should overlap the cortex of the ulnar shaft, but no further
- Humeral epicondyles equidistant from coronoid and olecranon fossae
- Radial and ulnar styloid processes seen on the lateral aspects of these bones
- Sharp image demonstrating soft tissue margins of the forearm, bony cortex and trabeculae Adequate penetration to demonstrate overlap of olecranon over distal humerus whilst showing trabecular detail over shafts of radius and ulna

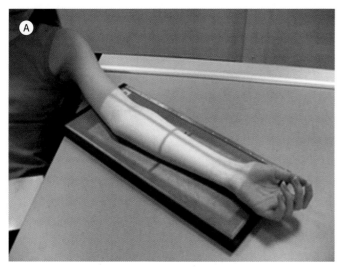

Figure 6.1   AP forearm

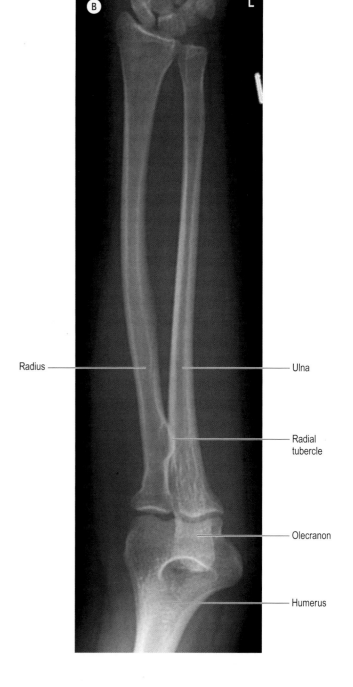

Common errors	Possible reasons
Radius cleared from ulna at the proximal end; radial head also shown clear	Externally rotated arm
Radial tubercle superimposed over shaft of ulna	Internally rotated arm
Shafts of radius and ulna show adequate contrast and density but elbow is 'thin' underpenetrated and shows poor contrast or bony detail	Inadequate kVp selected
Elbow joint shows adequate contrast and density but shafts of radius and ulna are dark, showing poor contrast and bony detail	Selected kVp too high

▇ Lateral forearm (Fig. 6.2A,B)

Positioning

- The patient is seated with the affected side next to the table; lead rubber is applied to the waist
- The arm is flexed at the elbow, abducted away from the trunk and internally rotated at the wrist
- The medial aspect of the forearm is placed in contact with the image receptor, to include elbow and wrist joints. The long axis of the forearm is coincident with the long axis of the cassette
- The joints must lie in the same plane
- The humeral epicondyles are superimposed, as are the radial and ulnar styloid processes Ensuring the shoulder lies in the same plane as the wrist and elbow will help facilitate this more easily
- The head is turned away from the shoulder of the side under examination, aiming to reduce scattered radiation to the lenses of the eyes and thyroid

Beam direction and FFD

Vertical, at 90° to the image receptor
100 cm FFD

Centring

Midway between the wrist and elbow joints, on the medial aspect of the forearm

Collimation

Elbow, wrist, shafts of radius and ulna, soft tissue outlines of forearm

▇ Criteria for assessing image quality

- The wrist and elbow joints, radius, ulna and soft tissue outline of the forearm are demonstrated
- Superimposition of posterior portion of radial head over coronoid process of ulna; superimposition of distal radius and ulna
- Shaft of the radius is seen anterior to that of the ulna
- There will be some superimposition of trochlea and capitulum of humerus. However, it may be unrealistic to expect to see full superimposition of these structures as the obliquity of the beam at its periphery is likely to pass through the elbow at around 3–4°
- Sharp image demonstrating soft tissue margins of the forearm, bony cortex and trabeculae. Adequate penetration to demonstrate overlap of radial head over the olecranon and distal radius over ulna, whilst showing trabecular detail over the shafts of the radius and ulna

Common errors	Possible reasons
Distal radius seen anteriorly in relationship to ulna	Wrist is medially rotated
Distal radius seen posteriorly in relationship to ulna; shafts of radius and ulna superimposed along most of their length	Wrist and elbow are externally rotated; this usually only occurs when the humerus does not lie in the same plane as the forearm and the shoulder lies above the table-top

ELBOW

Degenerative change and trauma are both major indicators for plain X-ray imaging. Dislocations at the elbow can be demonstrated radiographically and the head of the radius is the most likely part to be subluxed.

The *supracondylar fracture* of the humerus has many implications for the future of the patient's arm. Vasculature of the arm can be damaged, or existing damage can be exacerbated, by forced extension of the elbow joint; this can cause an ischaemic state for the lower arm, resulting in paralysis of the hand and forearm and, long term, in what is known as a *'Volkmann's ischaemic contracture'*. It is therefore essential that the radiographer undertakes modified projections of the elbow which cannot be extended; these are outlined in Chapter 27 on accident and emergency (A&E) radiography.

▇ AP elbow (Fig. 6.3A,B)

If used, two 18 × 24 cm cassettes are selected for AP and lateral projections. Alternatively, a 24 × 30 cm cassette can be split widthwise to include two projections on one cassette.

Positioning

- The patient is seated with the affected side next to the table; lead rubber is applied to the waist
- The arm is extended at the elbow, abducted away from the trunk and externally rotated until the hand lies in supination
- The posterior aspect of the elbow is placed in contact with the image receptor, the olecranon being positioned in the middle if a cassette is used

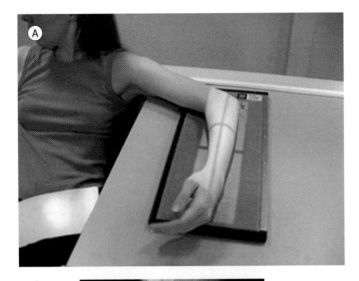

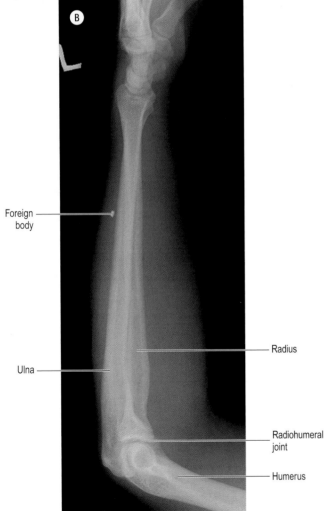

Figure 6.2   Lateral forearm

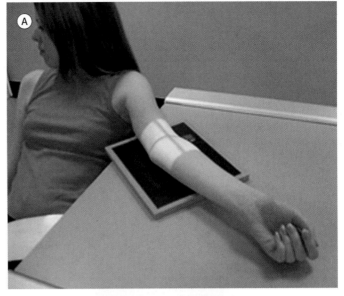

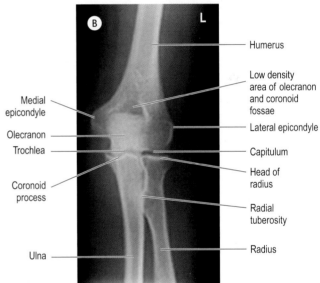

Figure 6.3   AP elbow

- The wrist, elbow and shoulder joints must lie in the same plane
- The humeral epicondyles are equidistant from the image receptor
- The head is turned away from the shoulder of the side under examination, aiming to reduce scattered radiation to the lenses of the eyes and thyroid

Beam direction and FFD

Vertical, at 90° to the image receptor

100 cm FFD

Centring

Midway between the humeral epicondyles

Collimation

Proximal radius and ulna, elbow joint, distal shaft of humerus, soft tissue outlines surrounding elbow joint

Criteria for assessing image quality

- The proximal radius and ulna, elbow joint, distal shaft of the humerus and soft tissue outlines surrounding the elbow joint demonstrated
- Partial superimposition of the radius and ulna at the proximal end. Radial tuberosity should overlap the cortex of the ulnar shaft, but no further
- Humeral epicondyles equidistant from the coronoid and olecranon fossae
- Sharp image demonstrating soft tissue margins around the elbow, bony cortex and trabeculae. Adequate penetration to demonstrate overlap of olecranon over distal humerus

Common errors	Possible reasons
Radius cleared from ulna; radial head also shown clear	Elbow is externally rotated
Radial tubercle superimposed over shaft of ulna	Internally rotated elbow
Radial head fully superimposed over ulna; distance between humeral epicondyles seems narrow	Hand may be in pronation rather than supination

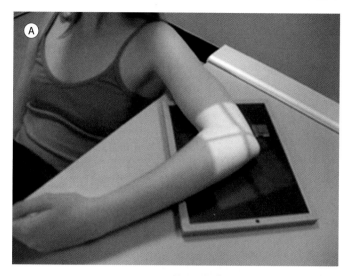

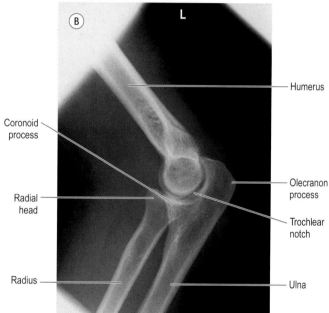

Figure 6.4   Lateral elbow

Lateral elbow (Fig. 6.4A,B)

Positioning

- The patient is seated with the affected side next to the table; lead rubber is applied to the waist
- The arm is abducted from the trunk, internally rotated and flexed 90° at the elbow
- The wrist is externally rotated until the radial and ulnar styloid processes are superimposed
- The medial aspect of the elbow is placed in contact with the image receptor; the medial humeral epicondyle is coincident with the middle if a cassette is used
- The shoulder, elbow and wrist joints must lie in the same plane
- The humeral epicondyles are superimposed. Ensuring the shoulder lies in the same plane as the wrist and elbow will help facilitate this more easily

- The head is turned away from the shoulder of the side under examination, aiming to reduce scattered radiation to the lenses of the eyes and thyroid

Beam direction and FFD

Vertical, at 90° to the image receptor
100 cm FFD

Centring

Over the lateral humeral epicondyle

Collimation

Proximal radius and ulna, elbow joint, distal shaft of humerus, soft tissue outlines surrounding elbow joint

Criteria for assessing image quality

- The proximal radius and ulna, elbow joint, distal shaft of the humerus and soft tissue outlines surrounding the elbow joint are demonstrated
- Superimposition of surfaces of trochlea and capitulum, with the posterior portion of the radial head shown over the coronoid process of ulna. Evidence of joint space of the elbow seen
- Shaft of the radius is seen anterior to that of the ulna
- Sharp image demonstrating soft tissue margins around the elbow, bony cortex and trabeculae. Adequate penetration to demonstrate overlap of radial head over the olecranon and superimposed epicondyles

The importance of optimum exposure factor selection cannot be emphasised enough, especially in the case of the elbow radiograph requested after trauma. Information on both bone and soft tissue becomes even more vital in trauma cases. This is because personnel assessing and/or reporting on the radiograph need to inspect the image for evidence of the 'fat pad sign', an indication of presence of abnormal fluid (usually blood) outside the elbow's joint capsule. This sign suggests bony damage, often supracondylar or radial head fractures, which may or may not be evident on the radiograph. On a normal lateral elbow radiograph, fat pads are not distinguishable from other soft tissues but when significant trauma causes displacement of the pads there will be an appearance similar to a downturned rose thorn (seen as more dark in contrast to surrounding soft tissue) anterior and/or posterior to the distal humerus, just above the epicondyles. The normal positions of the fat pads are along the anterior aspect of the humerus and within the olecranon fossa posteriorly.[1]

Flexion of the joint also affects fat pad appearance in the lateral elbow projection. Flexion which is less than 90° causes the olecranon to move towards the olecranon fossa, thus displacing the posterior pad superiorly to a position which may be visible on the lateral radiograph. This, potentially, may mimic appearances suggestive of trauma and thus impact upon radiological comment.[2]

The injured patient often finds it difficult or impossible to extend the elbow joint, making it impossible for the radiographer to undertake routine projections of the area. Modification in technique must be undertaken, especially if there is risk of Volkmann's ischaemic contracture after supracondylar fracture. These modifications are covered in Chapter 27 on A&E imaging.

HEAD OF RADIUS

A significant proportion of the radial head is superimposed over the proximal ulna in both the AP and lateral projections of the elbow joint. As a result small fractures of the radial head may fail to be demonstrated by more routine projections. Modifications of these are recommended in order to provide the required information. These modified projections are undertaken in addition to AP and lateral projections.

If used, two 18 × 24 cm cassettes are selected for individual projections. Alternatively, a 24 × 30 cm cassette can be split widthwise to include two projections on one cassette.

Oblique head of radius: external rotation
(Fig. 6.5A,B)

This projection will also demonstrate the proximal radio-ulnar joint.

Positioning
- The patient is positioned initially as for the AP elbow projection, with the centre of the cassette, if used, coincident with the radial head, rather than the middle of the elbow joint
- The arm is externally rotated through approximately 20° to clear the radial head from the ulna. Asking the patient to lean sideways, towards the table and cassette, will help facilitate this more easily
- A radiolucent pad placed under the medial aspect of the forearm will aid immobilisation
- The head is turned away from the shoulder of the side under examination, aiming to reduce scattered radiation to the lenses of the eyes and thyroid

Beam direction and FFD
Vertical, at 90° to the image receptor
100 cm FFD

Centring
Over the middle of the crease of the elbow

Collimation
Proximal radius and ulna, elbow joint, distal shaft of humerus, soft tissue outlines surrounding elbow joint

Criteria for assessing image quality

- The proximal radius and ulna, elbow joint, distal shaft of the humerus and soft tissue outlines surrounding the elbow joint are demonstrated

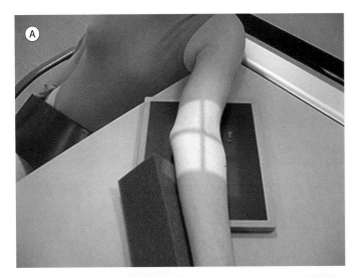

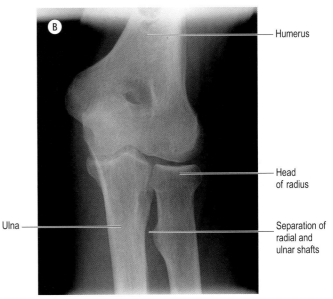

Humerus

Head
of radius

Ulna

Separation of
radial and
ulnar shafts

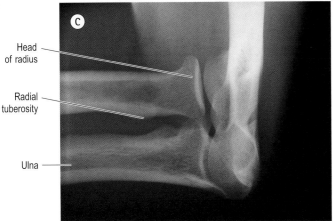

Head
of radius

Radial
tuberosity

Ulna

Figure 6.5 **(A,B)** Head of radius – oblique; **(C)** head of radius – lateral elbow with 45° lateromedial angulation to clear radial head from ulna. (C) Reproduced with permission from Ballinger PW, Frank ED. Merrill's atlas of radiographic positioning and radiologic procedures. 10th edn. St Louis: Mosby; 2003

- Radial head is cleared from the ulna, and the proximal radioulnar joint is clear
- Sharp image demonstrating soft tissue margins around the elbow, bony cortex and trabeculae

Common error	Possible reason
Radial head not cleared from ulna	Inadequate external rotation

Rotation which is as much as 45° has been suggested for demonstration of the radial head; this is significantly more than the 20° described here.[3] Since 20° adequately demonstrates clearance of the head it seems excessive to expect the injured patient to aim for further rotation.

An alternative projection for clearance of the radial head from the ulna has been described as a *lateral with 45° lateromedial angulation of the primary beam*.[4] This is acknowledged as a projection which will efficiently

clear the radial head but will cause some significant distortion of the image (Fig. 6.5C). Angulation of the beam towards the trunk also has implications of potential increase of radiation dose to more radiosensitive areas of the body. However, severe elbow trauma may render the patient incapable of adequate elbow extension for the oblique projection and the lateral with 45° angle may be the only suitable alternative. Clearly a situation when benefit versus risk assessment must be made by the radiographer.

Lateral head of the radius (Figs 6.6A,B, 6.7A,B)

Although the externally rotated oblique projection for the radial head will clear it from the ulna to show more of its medial aspect, and its anterior aspect is seen on the lateral elbow projection, other aspects of the head will not have been well demonstrated on any of the routine elbow images. As a result it is necessary to provide profile projections of the radial head. These are achieved with the elbow in a lateral position and as described below.

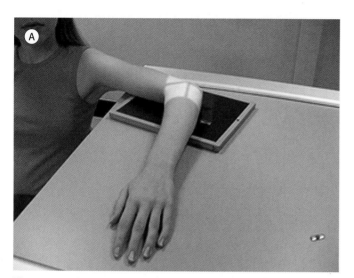

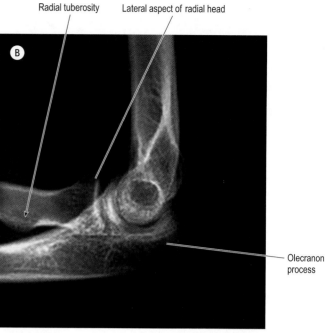

Figure 6.6   Lateral head of radius. Hand pronated. (B) Reproduced with permission from Ballinger PW, Frank ED. Merrill's atlas of radiographic positioning and radiologic procedures. 10th edn. St Louis: Mosby; 2003

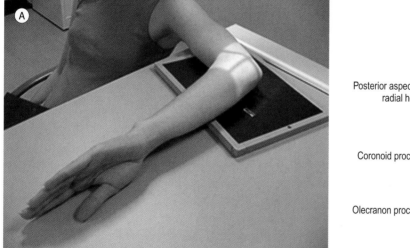

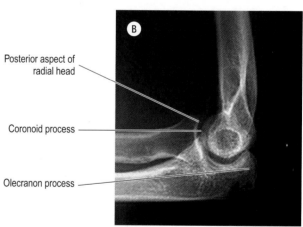

Figure 6.7   Lateral – head of radius. Hand medially rotated. (B) Reproduced with permission from Ballinger PW, Frank ED. Merrill's atlas of radiographic positioning and radiologic procedures. 10th edn. St Louis: Mosby; 2003

Positioning

- The patient is positioned initially as for the lateral elbow projection
- *1. To demonstrate the lateral aspect of the radial head:* Internally rotate the forearm until the hand is in pronation and in contact with the table-top

- *2. To demonstrate the posterior aspect of the radial head:* From the position described in 1, above, the forearm is rotated further until its medial aspect is in contact with the cassette and table-top
- A legend is applied to each image to identify the palm position used

- The head is turned away from the shoulder of the side under examination, aiming to reduce scattered radiation to the lenses of the eyes and thyroid

Beam direction and FFD

Vertical, at 90° to the image receptor
100 cm FFD

Centring

Over the lateral humeral epicondyle (both forearm positions)

Collimation

Proximal radius and ulna, elbow joint, distal shaft of humerus, soft tissue outlines surrounding elbow joint

▇ Criteria for assessing image quality

- As for the lateral elbow, plus demonstration of change of position of the radial tubercle as it moves with rotation at the elbow. With the hand pronated (position 1) it should be seen as a slight prominence on the radius, projecting into the space between the radius and ulna. With the hand further rotated medially (position 2) the tubercle appears more prominent and its outline will be nearer the outline of the ulna

▇ Olecranon and coronoid: AP oblique with internal rotation (Fig. 6.8A,B)

More detailed information of these areas on the ulna can be obtained by an internal oblique projection in cases where adequate AP and lateral projections cannot be undertaken due to patient condition.

If used, an 18 × 24 cm cassette is selected for this projection.

Positioning

- The patient is positioned initially as for the AP elbow projection
- The forearm is pronated by rotation of the wrist, to effect crossover of the radius and ulna
- The whole arm is medially rotated through 45° at the shoulder
- A radiolucent pad placed under the lateral aspect of the forearm will aid immobilisation
- The head is turned away from the shoulder of the side under examination, aiming to reduce scattered radiation to the lenses of the eyes and thyroid

Beam direction and FFD

Vertical, at 90° to the image receptor
100 cm FFD

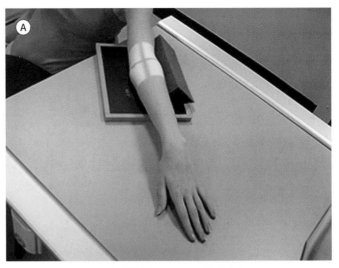

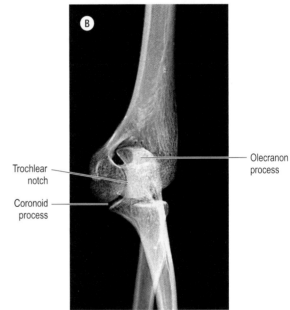

Figure 6.8   Olecranon and coronoid – AP internally rotated oblique. (B) Reproduced with permission from Ballinger PW, Frank ED. Merrill's atlas of radiographic positioning and radiologic procedures. 10th edn. St Louis: Mosby; 2003

Centring

Over the middle of the crease of the elbow

Collimation

Proximal radius and ulna, elbow joint, distal shaft of humerus, soft tissue outlines surrounding elbow joint

▇ Criteria for assessing image quality

- Proximal radius and ulna, elbow joint, distal shaft of the humerus and soft tissue outlines surrounding the elbow joint are demonstrated

- Proximal ulna appears as a 'spanner' with the olecranon process, trochlear notch and coronoid process shown in profile
- Olecranon process is superimposed over the olecranon fossa, the trochlear notch surrounds the outline of the trochlea and the coronoid process is shown clear of the radius
- Sharp image demonstrating soft tissue margins around the elbow, coronoid process in profile over soft tissue, bony cortex and trabeculae. Adequate penetration to demonstrate olecranon process overlying distal humerus

Common error	Possible reason
Coronoid process not cleared from radius	Inadequate medial rotation

Clearly this projection will not be possible in patients who cannot extend at the elbow joint, a common occurrence in cases of elbow trauma. An alternative has been suggested, where the partially flexed elbow is positioned with the posterior aspect of the forearm in contact with the cassette. A 45° central ray is then used and directed in a lateromedial direction, centred over the crease of the elbow. Appearance of the olecranon is similar to that in Figure 6.8b, in that the olecranon is seen as spanner shaped. This position can also be used to demonstrate the radial head, used in conjunction with a mediolateral central ray, which projects the radial head laterally from the ulna. For cases where supination is also not possible, the arm (which is flexed at the elbow, with the hand in pronation) is abducted with the humerus at 45° from the trunk, while the forearm is in contact with the table and the vertical central ray is centred over the lateral epicondyle;[5,6] this provides an image of the olecranon almost identical to that in Figure 6.8b but with less distortion since the central ray is not angled. The issue of benefit versus risk is certainly relevant regarding the projections described that have the hand in supination, since it appears that the patient's legs may come close to the primary beam and their trunk is leaning towards it.

ULNAR GROOVE

The ulnar groove lies between the medial humeral epicondyle and the trochlea. It acts as a channel along which the ulnar nerve passes, down to the forearm from the humerus. Ulnar nerve compression at this point can cause paraesthesia and neuralgia. Due to its excellent capacity for imaging soft tissue, magnetic resonance imaging (MRI) is most suited to investigation of possible ulnar nerve compression and should be the imaging method of choice, wherever possible

If used, an 18 × 24 cm cassette is selected for this projection.

Positioning (Fig. 6.9A)
- The patient is seated with the affected side next to the table; lead rubber is applied to the waist
- The arm is extended at the elbow, abducted away from the trunk and externally rotated until the hand lies in supination
- The posterior aspect of the elbow is placed in contact with the image receptor, the olecranon being positioned in the middle of the cassette, if used
- The elbow is fully flexed and the fist gently clenched. The wrist is also gently flexed, to bring the fingers and thumb in contact with the shoulder
- From a position when the humeral epicondyles are equidistant from the cassette, the upper arm is externally rotated 45°. This is best achieved by asking the patient to lean over towards the affected side before effecting

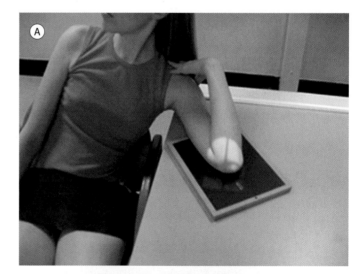

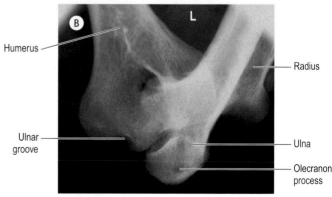

Figure 6.9   Ulnar groove

the external rotation. The fist remains in contact with the shoulder throughout

Beam direction and FFD
Vertical, at 90° to the image receptor
100 cm FFD

Centring
Over the medial epicondyle

Collimation
Olecranon process, distal humerus below shaft, soft tissue outlines around medial area of elbow

Criteria for assessing image quality

- Olecranon process, distal humerus below the shaft and soft tissue outlines around the medial area of the elbow are demonstrated
- Forearm is shown superimposed over the lateral portion of the distal humerus and clear of the medial epicondyle
- Olecranon process is seen distally in relationship to the humerus
- Ulnar groove is seen as a notch between the medial epicondyle and the trochlea
- Sharp image demonstrating soft tissue margins around the medial aspect of the elbow, bony cortex and trabeculae of the non-superimposed portion of the humerus (see Fig. 6.9B)

Common error	Possible reasons
Groove not seen as a distinct notch between trochlea and medial epicondyle	Inaccurate external rotation. If accompanied by superimposition of forearm over the midline of the humerus, this indicates inadequate external rotation. Superimposition of trochlea over the groove also indicates this.
	If the medial epicondyle appears flattened, there is over rotation of the arm

HUMERUS

AP humerus (Fig. 6.10A,B)

If used, cassettes should be selected according to the patient's humeral size. Most frequently, adults will require either a 30 × 40 cm or 35 × 43 cm cassette which is placed longitudinally in the erect cassette holder; this applies to both AP and lateral projections. If a patient presents supine,

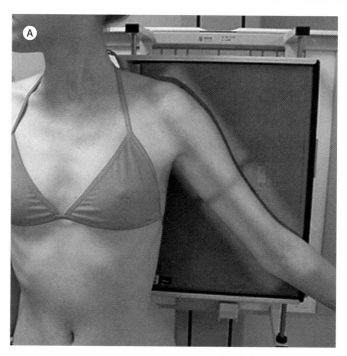

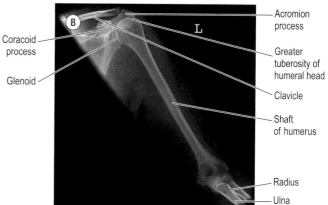

Figure 6.10   AP humerus

as on an A&E trolley, the cassette can be used under the humerus, on the trolley top.

Positioning
- If used, the cassette is placed in the erect cassette holder
- A lead rubber apron is applied to the patient's waist
- The patient stands erect facing the X-ray tube and the affected arm is extended and abducted from the trunk to avoid superimposition of the humerus and upper arm soft tissue over the soft tissue of the trunk
- The feet are slightly separated for stability
- The height of the image receptor is adjusted until its midpoint is coincident with the midshaft of the humerus
- Orientating the upper arm diagonally at 45° across the cassette or image receptor plate will maximise the available space for the area of interest which must include the shoulder and elbow joints on the image

- The palm faces forwards with the humeral epicondyles equidistant from the image receptor

Beam direction and FFD

Horizontal, at 90° to the image receptor
100 cm FFD

Centring

To the middle of the humerus, on the anterior aspect of the arm

Collimation

Shoulder joint, shaft of humerus, elbow joint, soft tissues surrounding the area

Aligning the light beam diaphragm housing along the long axis of the humerus before collimating will allow more effective collimation around the area of interest.

▮ Criteria for assessing image quality

- Shoulder joint, shaft of humerus, elbow joint and soft tissues are demonstrated
- Humerus is clear of the soft tissue of the trunk
- Greater tuberosity of humerus is in profile laterally on the head of humerus
- Humeral epicondyles are equidistant from coronoid and olecranon fossae
- Sharp image demonstrating soft tissue margins around the area of interest, bony cortex and trabeculae. Adequate penetration to demonstrate joints whilst maintaining trabecular detail over the humeral shaft

Common errors	Possible reasons
Pale shadow overlying medial aspect of the humerus and soft tissue of upper arm	Arm not abducted adequately from the trunk
Humeral epicondyles not shown as equidistant around coronoid and olecranon fossae; greater tuberosity projected over the humeral head	Arm is rotated. This is most frequently medial rotation, as this is a more comfortable position for the patient than with the rotation required for a true AP position of the humerus

▮ Lateral humerus (Fig. 6.11A,B)

Positioning

- If used, the cassette is placed in the erect cassette holder
- A lead rubber apron is applied to the posterior aspect of the patient's waist

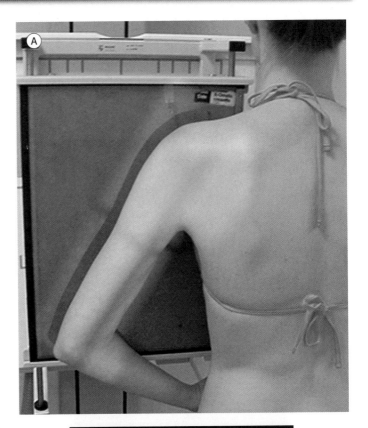

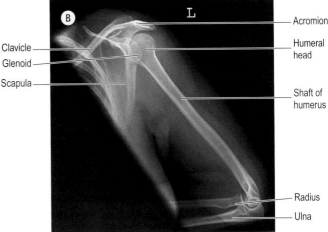

Figure 6.11   Lateral humerus

- The patient stands erect facing the image receptor and the affected arm is extended and abducted from the trunk to avoid superimposition of the humerus and upper arm soft tissue over the soft tissue of the trunk
- The feet are slightly separated for stability
- The height of the image receptor is adjusted until its midpoint is coincident with the midshaft of the humerus
- Orientating the upper arm at 45° across the image receptor will maximise the available space for the area of interest which must include the shoulder and elbow joints on the image

- The arm is medially rotated and the elbow flexed until the medial aspect of the hand comes into contact with the lower abdomen. The humeral epicondyles are superimposed
- The head is turned away from the side under examination
- A PA anatomical marker is usually used for this projection

The lateral humerus projection can also be undertaken with the patient facing the X-ray tube, in an AP position. The arm is flexed at the elbow and the limb medially rotated to bring the medial aspect of the humerus in contact with the image receptor. The hand is placed on the hip to immobilise the arm. Unfortunately this position is somewhat difficult, even for the non-injured patient, especially as the movement required at the shoulder results in the scapula being positioned almost perpendicular to the image receptor; this in itself is not disadvantageous but the position of the scapula does push the posterior aspect of the upper humerus away from the image receptor, making lateral representation of the image of the bone less accurate. The action of the hand resting on the hip also makes superimposition of the humeral epicondyles difficult.

Beam direction and FFD
Horizontal, at 90° to the image receptor
100 cm FFD

Centring
To the middle of the humerus, on the medial aspect of the arm

Collimation
Shoulder joint, shaft of humerus, elbow joint, soft tissues surrounding the area

Aligning the light beam diaphragm housing along the long axis of the humerus before collimating will allow more effective collimation around the area of interest.

Criteria for assessing image quality

- Shoulder joint, shaft of humerus, elbow joint and soft tissues are demonstrated
- Humerus is clear of soft tissue of trunk and humeral head is cleared from the image of the scapula
- Greater tuberosity of humerus is seen over the middle of humeral head
- Superimposition of the trochlea and capitulum (however, it must be remembered that oblique rays around the central ray are likely to impinge upon this area at around 5–8°, according to humeral length. This obliquity will almost certainly affect the superimposition of trochlea and capitulum. If this area of the humerus is of particular interest then elbow projections should be undertaken)
- Sharp image demonstrating soft tissue margins around the area of interest, bony cortex and trabeculae. Adequate penetration to demonstrate joints whilst maintaining trabecular detail over the humeral shaft

Common errors	Possible reasons
Pale shadow overlying the anterior aspect of the humerus (seen facing towards the thorax in this projection) and soft tissue of upper arm	Arm not abducted adequately from the trunk
Greater tuberosity appears towards or over the lateral margin of the humeral head	Arm is externally rotated. This can be avoided by ensuring that the entire length of the lateral aspect of the humerus is in contact with the image receptor; this encourages the patient to maintain the lateral position
Non-superimposition of trochlea and capitulum	Slight overlap, rather than full superimposition, can be explained by effects of obliquity of the beam around the central ray (see image quality criteria, above). However, when accompanied by incorrect appearance of the greater tuberosity (see above point) this may indicate external rotation of the humerus

INTERTUBEROUS SULCUS (BICIPITAL GROOVE)

The intertuberous sulcus lies on the anterior aspect of the humeral head, between the greater and lesser tuberosities; insertion of the long head of biceps lies here. Its position makes it difficult to image since it travels in a vertical direction and cannot be seen on an AP projection of the humerus or shoulder.

The projection aims to demonstrate the groove in profile, which is only possible in the superoinferior or inferosuperior direction. There are many problems associated with either of these approaches, the most obvious being implementation of either position with the bulky light beam housings commonly found in the 21st century. Other important considerations are dose implications when directing a beam in a caudal direction (for superoinferior projection) and immobilisation.

The option of the superoinferior method does cause serious concern for patient dose, since the caudal ray required would almost certainly irradiate anterior structures of the trunk in addition to the upper humerus, thus raising questions as to its suitability.

Therefore an inferosuperior approach may fit with the requirement for the radiographer to use a technique which reduces the risk of irradiating radiosensitive tissues. Older texts describe an inferosuperior method which involves the patient leaning over a tube head which is directed vertically, but in a cranial direction.[7] Use of the old long cones, which were replaced by modern collimators, meant that the patient could use the cone as an aid to immobilisation. The cassette was supported by use of a specialist holder. The method described in this text uses an adaptation of this, with the patient supine. In the absence of the long cone, the patient is immobilised by lying supine; a specialist cassette support is not always necessary but does prove useful.

Inferosuperior bicipital groove: method 1 (Fig. 6.12)

If used, an 18 × 24 cm cassette is used for this projection.

Positioning
- The patient lies supine on the examination table and a lead rubber apron is laid over the top of the trunk
- The cassette is supported vertically on the table with its tube side in contact with the superior aspect of the shoulder. Its centre is coincident with the humeral head
- The arm is abducted slightly from the trunk and externally rotated until the humeral epicondyles are approximately 45° to the table-top
- The greater and lesser tuberosities are palpated to ensure that the intertuberous sulcus is in profile superiorly
- The patient's head is turned away from the side under examination

Beam direction and FFD
Initially horizontal, with a 5° caudal angle

FFD may vary according to the size of the tube mounting but should be no less than 100 cm. A slightly longer FFD may be beneficial since there may be relatively long object film distance (OFD) in patients who have a significant amount of adipose or muscle tissue over the shoulder joint.

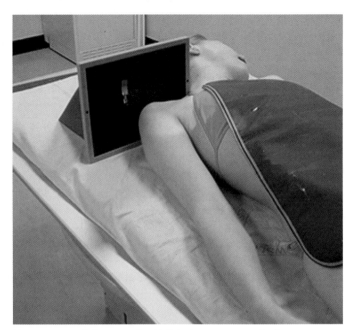

Figure 6.12   Inferosuperior bicipital groove – method 1

Inferosuperior bicipital groove: method 2 (Fig. 6.13)

If used, an 18 × 24 cm cassette is placed in the vertical holder.

Positioning
- The patient sits facing the X-ray tube, their back approximately 30 cm away from it
- The patient leans back, approximately 30° from vertical
- The arm is abducted slightly from the trunk and externally rotated until the humeral epicondyles are approximately 45° to the median sagittal plane (MSP)

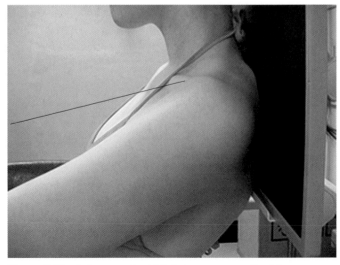

Figure 6.13   Inferosuperior bicipital groove – method 2

- The arm is elevated slightly to bring the long axis of the humerus to make an angle of approximately 30° with the floor (60° to cassette)
- The greater and lesser tuberosities are palpated to ensure that the intertuberous sulcus is in profile superiorly
- The patient's head is turned away from the side under examination

Beam direction and FFD

Initially horizontal, with a 15–20° cranial angle

As for method 1, FFD may vary according to the size of the tube mounting but should be no less than 100 cm.

Centring — both methods

Over the anterior aspect of the middle of the humeral head

Collimation

Anterior portion of humeral head, soft tissue overlying this area

Inclusion of the area within the cassette margins and collimation can be ensured by checking that the outline shadow of the area lies within the light beam representation and the cassette.

■ Criteria for assessing image quality

- Anterior portion of humeral head and the soft tissue overlying it are demonstrated

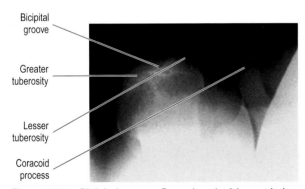

Bicipital groove

Greater tuberosity

Lesser tuberosity

Coracoid process

Figure 6.14 Bicipital groove. Reproduced with permission from Ballinger PW, Frank ED. Merrill's atlas of radiographic positioning and radiologic procedures. 10th edn. St Louis: Mosby; 2003

- Bicipital groove is seen in profile as a notch superiorly over the outline of the anterior aspect of humeral head, between the greater and lesser tuberosities
- Sharp image demonstrating soft tissue margins above the area of interest, bony cortex and its outline over the sulcus (see Fig. 6.14)

Common errors	Possible reasons
Humeral head seen but sulcus not in profile	1. Sulcus projected medially or laterally due to inaccurate rotation of the limb *or* 2. Extreme obliquity of the arm positions the sulcus obliquely, rather than perpendicular to cassette
Dense soft tissue shadow overlying area of interest	Tube position too low; the soft tissues of the arm may be superimposed over the area of interest

References

1. Scally P. Medical imaging. Oxford: Oxford University Press; 1999.
2. McQuillen Martensen K. Radiographic critique. Philadelphia: WB Saunders; 1995.
3. Bontrager K, Lampignano JP. Textbook of radiographic positioning and related anatomy. 6th edn. St Louis: Mosby; 2005.
4. Greenspan A, Norman A. The radial head capitellum view; a useful technique in elbow trauma. American Journal of Radiology 1982; 138:1186–1188.
5. Tomás FJ, Proubasta IR. Modified radial head-capitellum projection in elbow trauma. British Journal of Radiology 1998; 71:74–75.
6. Tomás FJ. Alternative radiographic projections of the ulnar coronoid process. British Journal of Radiology 2001; 74:756–758.
7. Clark KC. Clark's positioning in radiography. London: Heinemann; 1939.

THE SHOULDER GIRDLE

Linda Williams

The use of plain films is still an essential starting point when imaging the shoulder; basic diagnostic errors may occur if other imaging modalities are used alone, without the use of conventional plain radiography.[1] However, plain radiography of the shoulder is undertaken less frequently today as magnetic resonance imaging (MRI) is often the method of choice for imaging following initial assessment. It has become an increasingly important technique for evaluation of shoulder abnormalities, particularly rotator cuff disorders and joint instability.[12] The effectiveness of MRI is due to its high contrast sensitivity and multiplanar imaging capabilities; therefore diagnosis and appropriate management of the complex shoulder joint is established with greater confidence.[2]

Ultrasound is also used in imaging the shoulder joint and can be used to assess disorders such as defects in the long head of the biceps tendon.[1] Subacromial and acromioclavicular joint impingement are dynamic processes and these can be studied during ultrasound examination.

Computed tomography (CT) may be used in preoperative assessment of shoulder injuries, in order that fractures are not underestimated (as can be the case in some instances with plain image radiography). 3D reconstruction is often used to fully demonstrate complex fractures and assist in surgical planning.[2]

When imaging this region with plain radiography, radiation protection of the eyes and thyroid is an important consideration; the patient must always have their head turned away from the primary beam during exposure.

This area of high subject contrast has implications for overexposure of some structures involved in the joint. This is especially true of the acromioclavicular joint, which is often lacking in detail due to overexposure, whilst detail of denser structures of the region (e.g. the humeral head

or glenoid) are adequately demonstrated. Repeat examinations are often required as a result and can be avoided in the first instance by using a wedge filter placed between the image receptor and the upper shoulder. The most effective type of filter for this is rubberised and boomerang shaped and can therefore sit comfortably and safely around and behind the upper shoulder. Use of a relatively high kVp and lower mAs can offer a solution in the absence of a filter but the contrast of these images is somewhat reduced when compared with those produced with a filter. Patients with very dense muscle (e.g. body builders and rugby players) will certainly need effective beam penetration.

INDICATIONS

Arthropathy

Erosions are a relatively late feature in patients with rheumatoid arthritis and the shoulder should only be examined by plain film radiography if that joint is specifically affected. In patients with suspected osteoarthritis, X-ray is not indicated initially unless intervention is likely.

Fracture

This mostly affects the clavicle, humeral surgical neck, tuberosities of the humerus and scapula.

Fracture of the scapula is relatively uncommon, accounting for 3–5% of shoulder injuries.

Fractures of the surgical neck of the humerus and the tuberosities are sometimes classified using the Neer's method,[3] which considers the status and degree of displacement of the articular segment of the head of the humerus, the surgical neck of the humerus and the greater and lesser tuberosities.

Dislocation

This is of the shoulder joint and anterior dislocation is most common; only 2–4% occur posteriorly and an estimated 60–80% of these are missed on initial examination.

Subluxation of the acromioclavicular joint can also occur.

■ Anteroposterior (AP) shoulder (Fig. 7.1A,B)

This projection can be performed in the erect position, either standing or seated, depending on the patient's condition and ability. When examining a patient on a trolley, care should be taken to ensure the patient is either in the fully erect position or the beam is accurately angled to compensate for any tilt on the trolley back rest; this will ensure the central ray remains 90° to the image receptor.

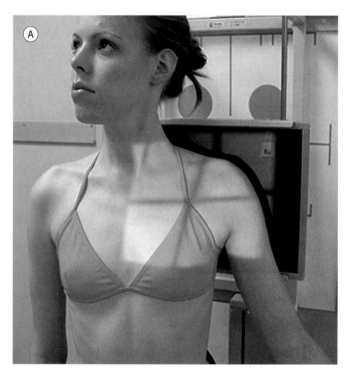

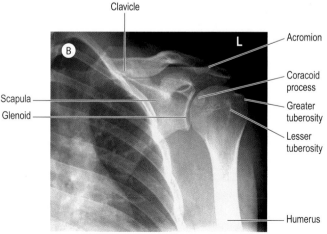

Figure 7.1   AP shoulder

If a cassette is used, 24 × 30 cm is selected and used transversely in the vertical holder (or supported behind the patient if on a trolley).

Positioning
- A lead·rubber apron is applied to the patient's waist for radiation protection
- The patient sits or stands erect, with the posterior aspect of the shoulder under examination in contact with the image receptor
- The arm is fully extended and slightly abducted with the palm of the hand facing forward to ensure the true anatomical position (with the greater tuberosity in profile on the lateral aspect of the humeral head)
- The patient's trunk is rotated approximately 20° towards the side under examination, to bring the scapula parallel to the image receptor
- The patient's head is turned away from the side under examination for radiation protection

Beam direction and focus film distance (FFD)
Horizontal at 90° to the image receptor
100 cm FFD

Centring point
To the coracoid process of the scapula, palpable anteriorly just below the lateral third of the clavicle and medial to the middle of the head of humerus

This centring point will bring the glenohumeral joint central to the image receptor but means that a large field of view is required to fulfil the image criteria for the area of interest. However, if the radiographic examination is for a general shoulder survey, the area of interest should be positioned to lie within the borders of the image receptor, with beam centring to the centre of the image receptor; this will ensure that the medial end of the clavicle, the whole of the scapula and upper third of the humerus can be included in one image with the minimum field of radiation.

Collimation
The head and proximal third of humerus, scapula, clavicle, lateral soft tissues of proximal humerus

Criteria for assessing image quality
- Head and proximal third of humerus, clavicle, acromioclavicular joint and the inferior end of the scapula are demonstrated
- Greater tuberosity is seen in profile on the lateral aspect of the head of humerus
- Glenohumeral joint is obscured by the head of humerus
- Acromion is demonstrated clear of the superior border of the humeral head

- Sharp image demonstrating the bony cortex and trabeculae of the head of the humerus in contrast with the shoulder joint and surrounding soft tissues; the acromioclavicular joint is seen clearly

The AP projection does not demonstrate the glenohumeral joint space clearly and orthopaedic departments may request either a 'True AP' or 'Grashey AP'[3] instead of, or to complement, the AP. This projection uses the same position and centring point as the AP described here but with an obliquity of the patient at 45° instead of 20°, to open the glenohumeral joint.

Common errors	Possible reasons
Inferior end of the scapula not included on the image	The image receptor is often positioned in the 'landscape' position; putting it in the 'portrait' position will usually prevent this
Foreshortening of the clavicle	The patient is rotated too much towards the side under examination
The acromioclavicular joint is over-penetrated	This is due to the difference in subject contrast in this area; the use of a wedge filter will prevent this

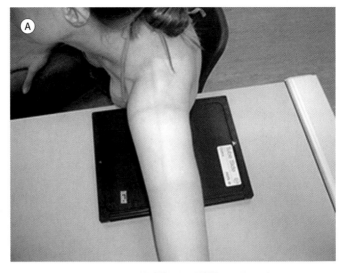

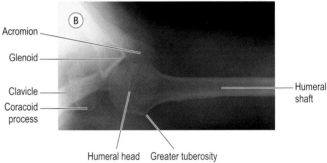

Figure 7.2 Superoinferior shoulder

AXILLARY/AXIAL PROJECTIONS OF THE SHOULDER

Evaluation of the shoulder joint, particularly for follow-up orthopaedic assessment, often requires an axillary projection to offer an image at 90° to the AP. Success of this projection will depend on the patient's condition and cooperation. Two methods are described here, method 1 is often difficult to implement or inappropriate, particularly in trauma, due to the extent to which the arm must be abducted. Method 2 is the method of choice for a patient with restricted movement of the humerus as there is more scope for adaptation to suit the patient's condition. Method 2 is sometimes referred to as the Lawrence axillary.[4]

If used, an 18 × 24 cm cassette is placed on the table-top, its short edge coincident with the table edge.

Method 1: superoinferior shoulder (Fig. 7.2A,B)

Positioning
- The patient sits with the side under examination next to and slightly away from the table

- For radiation protection purposes the legs are placed so they are not under the table and a lead rubber apron is worn around the waist
- The image receptor is placed on the table-top as described above
- The arm is abducted fully and the patient leans laterally over the image receptor; the hand is internally rotated and pronated. The axilla is positioned over the image receptor in a position which will ensure inclusion of the relevant anatomy, and with the axilla as close to it as possible
- The patient's head and neck are abducted away from the shoulder under examination as far as possible to clear them from the area of interest and reduce the radiation dose to these areas

Beam direction and FFD
Vertical at 90° to the image receptor
100 cm FFD

Centring point
To the superior aspect over the middle of the head of the humerus

Collimation

Head and proximal third of humerus, glenoid cavity, acromion, coracoid process, surrounding soft tissues

Criteria for assessing image quality

- Head and proximal end of humerus, glenoid fossa, lateral end of clavicle, acromion and coracoid process are demonstrated
- Greater tuberosity should be seen in profile anteriorly
- Acromion and lateral end of clavicle are superimposed on the superoposterior aspect of the head of humerus
- Coracoid process is demonstrated anterior to the head of humerus
- Sharp image demonstrating the soft tissue margins, bony cortex and trabeculae of the head of the humerus with adequate image density to demonstrate the bony detail of the humerus in contrast to the glenohumeral joint, acromion and clavicle

Common errors	Possible reasons
The glenohumeral joint is not demonstrated within the boundaries of the image receptor	The patient may not be stretching across the image receptor sufficiently. If the patient is capable of leaning further, try lowering the table top to enable the patient to flex more at the waist
Magnification and unsharpness of the resulting image, probably accompanied by foreshortening of humeral head	The axilla is not in close enough contact with image receptor and the humerus may not be fully abducted, causing its shaft to lie at an angle with the image receptor. Try using a pad to raise the image receptor or consider increasing the FFD to compensate for the large OFD

■ Method 2: inferosuperior shoulder (Fig. 7.3)

If used, an 18 × 24 cm cassette is selected.

Positioning

- The patient lies supine on the table
- A small radiolucent pad is placed beneath the shoulder to raise it slightly
- The head and neck are abducted as much as possible away from the side under examination to clear them from the area of interest and reduce radiation dose to these areas
- The image receptor is supported in the erect position, its tube side against the superior aspect of the head of the humerus and in contact with the neck

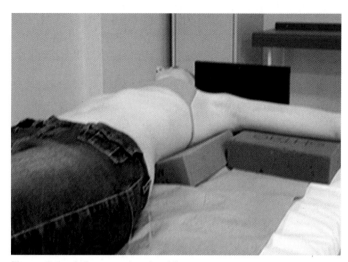

Figure 7.3   Inferosuperior shoulder

- The arm is abducted to 90° or as far as the patient's condition permits and the hand is supinated (although some internal rotation of the forearm is acceptable; supination acts mainly to help the patient maintain the correct relationship of the humerus to the cassette)
- A lead rubber apron is placed over the patient's chest and abdomen for radiation protection

Modern tube housings are usually too bulky to allow tube centring for this positioning. An alternative, *modified, inferosuperior* is suggested:

This technique can be achieved with as little as 30° arm abduction[3] but the tube needs to be brought in as close to the patient's body as possible. By lying the patient in a slightly diagonal position across the length of the table-top or trolley, access to the axilla is achievable (Fig. 7.4) Positioning the patient thus, diagonally across the table-top, requires consideration for the safety of the patient; this is directly related to table width and should only be considered in the relatively cooperative patient.

Beam direction and FFD (inferosuperior and modified inferosuperior projections)

Horizontal at 90° to the image receptor and coincident with the glenohumeral joint
100 cm FFD

The central ray must be at 90° to the image receptor and requires careful positioning to prevent a distorted image. To eliminate distortion, align the central ray with the patient first to ensure it is parallel to the glenohumeral joint, i.e. through the axilla, then position the image receptor until perpendicular to the central ray. This is suggested for both the inferosuperior and modified inferosuperior projections.

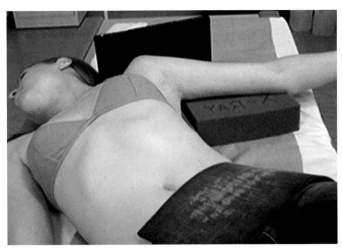

Figure 7.4 Modified inferosuperior shoulder

Common error	Possible reason
The glenohumeral joint is not demonstrated within the boundaries of the image receptor	The head and neck may not be sufficiently abducted away from the side under examination to enable the image receptor to be positioned correctly. Always ensure the image receptor is closely tucked into the neck

Centring point
Through the axilla

Collimation
Head and proximal third of humerus, glenoid cavity, acromion, coracoid process, surrounding soft tissues

The inferosuperior projections can be adapted to demonstrate the classic Hill Sachs compression fracture which results in patients who have recurrent anterior dislocation of the shoulder.[1] This adaptation involves maximum external rotation of the arm, with the patient aiming to press the thumb down towards the table or trolley top. Unfortunately this manoeuvre can be difficult for patients to achieve and the AP shoulder with maximum internal rotation can also demonstrate this lesion adequately.[1] In order to achieve the correct amount of rotation, the arm is medially rotated and flexed at the elbow; the dorsum of the hand is then rested on the waist.

Criteria for assessing image quality
- Head and proximal end of humerus, glenoid fossa, lateral end of clavicle, acromion and coracoid process should all be demonstrated
- Glenohumeral joint should be demonstrated
- Lesser tuberosity of humerus should be seen in profile
- Acromioclavicular joint will be superimposed on humerus
- Sharp image demonstrating the soft tissue margins, bony cortex and trabeculae of the head of humerus with adequate image density to demonstrate the bony detail of humerus in contrast to the glenohumeral joint

■ 30–45° modified superoinferior projection of the shoulder (Fig. 7.5A,B)

This projection is described by Unett and Royle[4] and a similar projection is described by Long and Rafert[3] but with more obliquity of the patient (i.e. the patient is rotated 45° onto the side under examination as opposed to bringing the scapula parallel to the image receptor; this is known as the 'Garth' Apical Oblique see Fig. 27.16). Unett and Royle describe this as 'modified Wallace and Hellier'[5] but the resulting image achieved with the 30–45° modified projection is much less magnified and distorted, which makes it easier to interpret. The Wallace and Hellier projection (see Fig. 27.17) (often called the 'Wallace' view) cannot be undertaken on the supine or semi-recumbent patient, since it requires the patient to sit with their back against the table, upon which the image receptor is placed horizontally. The air gap between the shoulder and image receptor will require some increase in exposure, thus increasing radiation dose in the Wallace and Hellier projection.

It is also easier to position the patient for the modified 30–45° view, since the patient position is identical to that for the AP shoulder, with the angle of central ray directed 30–45° caudally. The patient can satisfactorily be positioned supine or on a trolley or in a chair and this is therefore a very useful technique for trauma patients. Despite there being noticeable distortion caused by beam angulation, the humerus does still lie parallel to the image receptor, whereas the humerus lies at 90° to the image receptor in the Wallace and Hellier method, in addition to requiring 45° caudal tube angulation, which causes more distortion than with the 30–45° AP shoulder.

The projection demonstrates the glenohumeral joint in coronal profile and therefore an assessment of dislocation or intraarticular fractures can be made. The radiographer only needs to understand the basic radiographic principles involving effects of angulation on the image in order to assess direction of dislocation. Basically the structure lying closest to the image receptor will be less obviously displaced than structures further from it; therefore a posterior dislo-

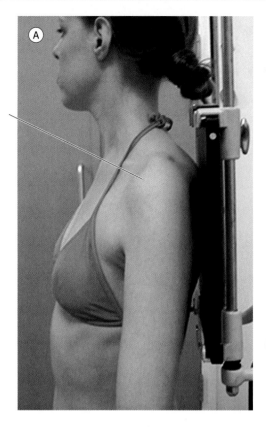

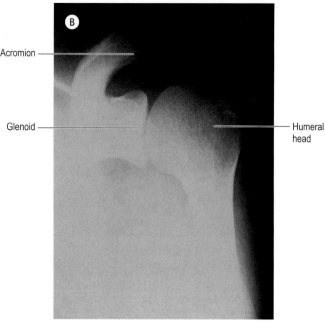

Acromion

Glenoid

Humeral head

Figure 7.5 30–45° modified superoinferior shoulder

cation will show the humeral head superimposed over the acromion, with anterior dislocation showing the humeral head well below the acromion and low when compared to the glenoid position. The Wallace and Hellier method does not appear to provide more useful information than the 30–45° modified projection and therefore its use should be questioned, considering it appears to have more disadvantages than the modified 30–45°.

If used, an 18 × 24 cm or 24 × 30 cm cassette is selected for this projection.

Positioning (as for AP shoulder)
- The image receptor is placed in the vertical holder or under/behind the patient's shoulder if supine or sitting on a trolley
- A lead rubber apron is applied to the patient's waist for radiation protection
- The patient can remain standing or be seated with the posterior aspect of the shoulder in contact with the image receptor
- The arm is fully extended and slightly abducted with the palm of the hand facing forward to ensure the true anatomical position
- The patient is rotated approximately 20° onto the side under examination to bring the scapula parallel to the image receptor

- The patient's head is turned away from the side under examination for radiation protection

Beam direction and FFD
Erect: Initially horizontal, directed caudally at 30–45° to the image receptor
Supine: Initially vertical, directed 30–45° caudally
If the patient is semirecumbent: The beam is initially positioned perpendicular to the image receptor and then directed a further 30–45° caudally from this angle
100 cm FFD

Centring point
Above the coracoid process and slightly superior to the head of the humerus

Collimation
Head and proximal third of humerus, glenoid cavity, acromion process, surrounding soft tissues

Criteria for assessing image quality
- Head and proximal shaft of humerus, glenoid fossa, lateral end of clavicle and acromion process should all be demonstrated
- Greater tuberosity is demonstrated on the lateral aspect of humerus

- Elongation of the head of humerus, the position of which will vary if the humeral head is dislocated
- The glenoid fossa and head of humerus are projected clear of the lateral margin of the rib cage
- Sharp image demonstrating the head of humerus in contrast to the shoulder joint and surrounding soft tissues

Lateral scapula/true lateral/'Y' view (Fig. 7.6A,B)

This projection may be used in cases of suspected gleno-humeral dislocation or fractures to the proximal humerus. It is similar to the basic lateral scapula projection but the humerus is not abducted in the same manner, to prevent the humerus overlying the body of the scapula; the humerus in this case is adducted alongside the patient's trunk. It is relatively simple to position and requires little cooperation from the patient. The resulting image allows an assessment of fractures or glenohumeral dislocation, as the shoulder girdle is demonstrated in the true lateral position. If the patient is presented on a trolley the technique can be performed in the AP position with the patient rotating approximately 25° towards the uninjured side.

This technique is considered to be superior to the modified axial (30–45° AP) described previously, as the modified axial can only help assess dislocations. This may then necessitate further radiographic examination. The 'Y' view is relatively simple to perform and can be achieved satisfactorily even if the patient presents supine on a trolley or in a chair, and is therefore a recommended technique for trauma patients.[6,7,8]

In the normal shoulder the humeral head will be demonstrated superimposed on the glenoid process as opposed to in the dislocated shoulder, where it will appear under the coracoid process in anterior dislocation and under the acromion in posterior dislocation.

If used, a 24 × 30 cm cassette is used longitudinally in the vertical holder.

Positioning
- A lead rubber apron is placed around the patient for radiation protection of the lower abdomen
- The patient stands or sits erect, facing the image receptor with their back to the X-ray tube.
- From an initial posteroanterior (PA) position, rotate the patient approximately 25° to bring the side under examination closer to, and bring the body of the scapula 90° to, the image receptor
- The arm on the side under examination is adducted from the trunk, with the elbow flexed and hand resting on the side of the waist. Alternatively, the elbow may be flexed with the forearm resting across the chest and the hand resting on the shoulder of the opposite side (this may be more comfortable for the injured patient)

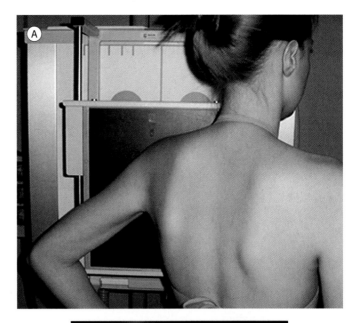

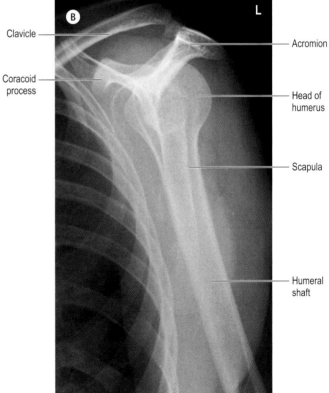

Figure 7.6   'Y' view

- The scapula is palpated to check the lateral and medial borders are superimposed
- The patient's head is turned as far as possible towards the unaffected side

If the patient is *supine*, this projection can be achieved by rotating their trunk 25° away from the side under examination, placing supporting radiolucent pads under the trunk for support. Although this will cause some magnification and have implications for scattered radiation exposure to the thyroid, eye lenses and female breasts, it is an acceptable alternative when a PA position is unsafe due to patient condition.

Beam direction and FFD
Horizontal at 90° to the image receptor
100 cm FFD

Centring point
To the upper end of the palpable medial border of the scapula to pass through the glenohumeral joint

Collimation
Scapula, the head and proximal third of the humerus, surrounding soft tissues

Criteria for assessing image quality
- Scapula and the head and proximal third of humerus are demonstrated
- Superimposition of the medial and lateral borders of the scapula
- Body of scapula is projected clear of the thorax
- Glenoid process is seen en face with the humeral head superimposed over it (in the normal shoulder)
- Sharp image demonstrating the bony cortex and trabeculae of the scapula and upper shaft of humerus in contrast with the surrounding soft tissue

The above technique can also be used with a *caudal angle of 10–15°* from the horizontal in cases of *suspected impingement syndrome*. The acromiohumeral space will appear more open than the true lateral scapula to show abnormalities of this area. The projection is sometimes referred to as the 'shoulder outlet'.[3]

Common error	Possible reason
Scapula not cleared from the ribs and thorax; not seen in profile	Inaccurate obliquity of position; there is often a temptation to turn the patient more than is required, since the correct trunk position does appear to be close to a PA projection

CLAVICLE

■ PA clavicle (Fig. 7.7A,B)

This projection is the method of choice, as opposed to an AP projection, because the object is in closer contact

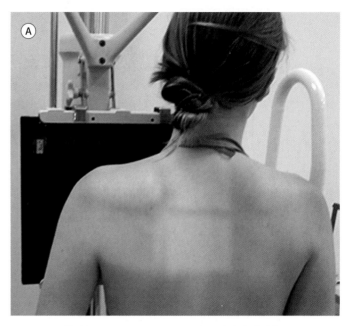

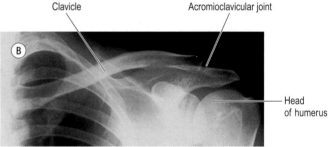

Clavicle   Acromioclavicular joint

Head of humerus

Figure 7.7   PA clavicle

to the image receptor, therefore reducing magnification and distortion of the clavicle. However, if the patient is injured or in a sling then positioning the patient for the AP clavicle may be more readily achievable and more comfortable.

If used, an 18 × 24 cm cassette is placed in the transverse position.

Positioning
- The image receptor is placed horizontally in the erect holder
- A lead rubber apron is applied to the patient's waist for radiation protection, ensuring the posterior aspect is protected
- The patient sits or stands erect with the anterior aspect of the shoulder under examination in contact with the image receptor
- The arm is made comfortable and may remain in a sling if presented this way
- The patient is rotated approximately 15° away from the side under examination to bring the plane of the clavicle closer and parallel to the image receptor

- The patient's head is turned away from the side under examination for radiation protection

Beam direction and FFD

Horizontal at 90° to the image receptor
100 cm FFD

Centring point

To the centre of the image receptor so that the central ray exits the mid shaft of the clavicle

Collimation

Clavicle, acromioclavicular joint, sternoclavicular joint

AP clavicle (Fig. 7.8)

The clavicle is demonstrated in the true AP position when both the shoulders are equidistant from the table or vertical cassette holder. Bontrager[9] and Ballinger & Frank[10] describe this positioning for the AP clavicle but Swallow et al[11] suggest a slight rotation towards the side under examination to ensure the medial end of the clavicle is not superimposed onto the vertebral column (although this will place the clavicle into a more oblique position than the other methods).

Positioning

- The image receptor is placed in the vertical holder
- A lead rubber apron is applied to the patient's waist for radiation protection

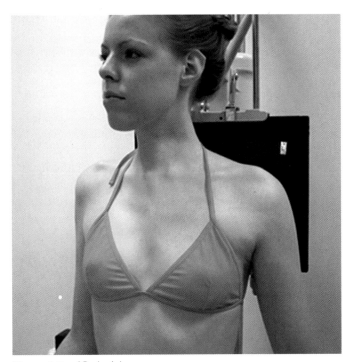

Figure 7.8 AP clavicle

- The patient sits or stands erect with the posterior aspect of the shoulder under examination in contact with the image receptor
- The arm is made comfortable and may remain in a sling if presented this way
- The patient stands with their median sagittal plane (MSP) perpendicular to the cassette or is rotated slightly towards the side under examination to bring the medial end of the clavicle away from the vertebral column
- The patient's head is turned away from the side under examination for radiation protection

Beam direction and FFD

Horizontal at 90° to the image receptor
100 cm FFD

Centring point

Over the mid point of the clavicle

Collimation

Clavicle, acromioclavicular joint, sternoclavicular joint

Criteria for assessing image quality: AP and PA projections

- Full length of the clavicle, including the acromioclavicular joint and the sternoclavicular joint, is demonstrated
- No or minimal distortion along the length of the clavicle
- Acromioclavicular joint should be demonstrated
- Sharp image demonstrating the soft tissue margins, bony cortex and trabeculae of the clavicle. The clavicle should be demonstrated with even contrast along the length and without overexposing the medial and lateral ends

Common error	Possible reason
High contrast on image which demonstrates the clavicle but the acromioclavicular joint appears blackened	kVp insufficient to reduce the subject contrast

Inferosuperior clavicle

There are two methods described here to provide an inferosuperior projection of the clavicle. Method 1 is the easiest to achieve and is normally used to assess fracture union; method 2 can be used on the supine patient, e.g. when presenting on a trolley. The AP is most frequently used alone, since fractures are rarely severely displaced; immobilisation with sling is usually quite effective as treatment. Occasionally the clavicular fracture may be so displaced that the fragments do not unify and these cases will almost certainly require an additional inferosuperior projection prior to making a decision on surgical intervention to pin the bone.

If used, an 18 × 24 cm cassette is used in the transverse position.

Method 1 (Fig. 7.9A)
Positioning
- The patient is seated and then positioned as for the AP clavicle projection
- The patient leans back by around 30°

Beam direction and FFD
Initially horizontal, angled cranially 30–45°; the maximum angle achievable will be governed by equipment variables
100 cm FFD

Centring point
Over the mid point of the clavicle

The image of the clavicle will be projected superiorly to the ribs and lung apices when compared to the AP or PA clavicle (Fig. 7.9B), due to the cranial angle used. Therefore the image receptor should be displaced cranially to compensate for this.

Collimation
Clavicle, acromioclavicular joint, sternoclavicular joint

Criteria for assessing image quality
- The full length of the clavicle, including the acromioclavicular joint and the sternoclavicular joint, is demonstrated
- Clavicle is projected above the apex of the lung
- Acromioclavicular joint should be demonstrated
- Sharp image demonstrating the soft tissue, bony cortex and trabeculae of the clavicle. The clavicle should be demonstrated with even contrast along the length and without overexposing the medial and lateral ends

Method 2 (Fig. 7.10A)
Positioning
- The patient lies supine with their arms resting at their side
- The image receptor is placed vertically and in contact with the superior aspect of the shoulder
- The head and neck are abducted for radiation protection of the eyes and thyroid
- A lead rubber apron is applied to the patient's waist for radiation protection

Beam direction and FFD
Initially vertical, angled at 45–60° towards the head, and 10–15° mediolaterally. *Again, the angle achieved will depend on equipment variables*
100 cm FFD

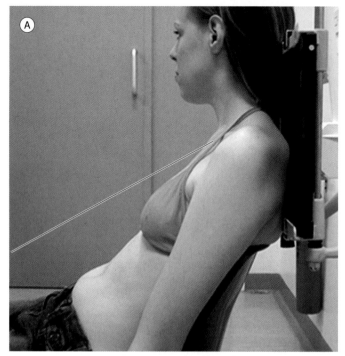

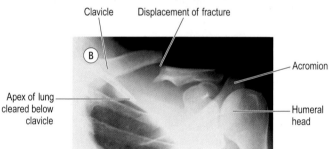

Figure 7.9 (A) Inferosuperior clavicle – method 1; (B) inferosuperior clavicle

Centring point
Over the mid point of the clavicle

For the supine inferosuperior projection, it is often not possible to position the X-ray tube low enough to achieve the required angulation (as is often the case with units which have large tube and light beam housing) and further modification may be necessary: The image receptor is placed in contact with the posterosuperior aspect of the shoulder and tilted backwards around 20° from vertical. The vertical central ray is then angled cranially until it is perpendicular to the image receptor, and an angle of approximately 10–15° mediolaterally away from the midline will clear the clavicle towards the centre of the image receptor. Centre over the middle of the clavicle. (Fig. 7.10B)

Collimation
Clavicle, acromioclavicular joint, sternoclavicular joint

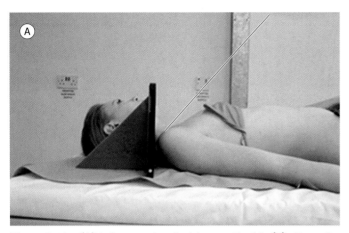
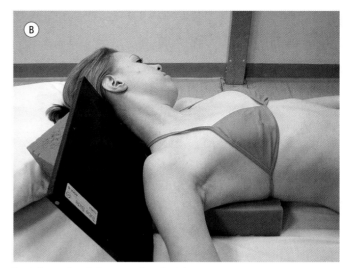

Figure 7.10   **(A)** Inferosuperior clavicle – method 2; **(B)** alternative method for supine inferosuperior clavicle

Criteria for assessing image quality
- Full length of the clavicle, including the acromioclavicular joint and the sternoclavicular joint, is demonstrated
- Clavicle is projected above the apex of the lung
- Acromioclavicular joint should be demonstrated
- Tubercle of the clavicle is visible on its under surface at the junction of the middle and lateral portions
- Medial end of the clavicle is slightly superior to the lateral end
- Sharp image demonstrating the soft tissue, bony cortex and trabeculae of the clavicle. The clavicle should be demonstrated with even contrast along the length and without overexposing the medial and lateral ends

Common errors	Possible reasons
Clavicle not cleared from lung apices	Inadequate cranial angle used (both methods) *or* Patient not leaning back enough (method 1)
Pale, soft tissue shadow overlying some or all the area of interest	Thorax or abdomen lying in the path of the primary beam; this may be due to a large abdomen, large female breasts or too much angulation (method 1)

SCAPULA

▄ AP scapula (Fig. 7.11A,B)

If used, a 24 × 30 cm cassette is used longitudinally in the vertical position.

Positioning
- The image receptor is placed in the vertical holder or supported behind the patient if on a trolley
- A lead rubber apron is applied to the patient's waist for radiation protection
- The patient sits or stands erect with the posterior aspect of the shoulder under examination in contact with the image receptor
- The arm is fully extended and slightly abducted with the palm of the hand facing forward to lie in the true anatomical position
- The patient is rotated approximately 20° towards the side under examination, to bring the scapula parallel to the image receptor
- The arm is flexed at the elbow and internally rotated, resting the dorsum of the hand on the patient's hip; this will move the scapula laterally away from the rib cage
- The patient's head is turned away from the side under examination for radiation protection

Beam direction and FFD
Horizontal at 90° to the image receptor
100 cm FFD

Centring point
To a point over the anterior chest (approximately 5 cm below the palpable coracoid process), to emerge over the mid scapular area

Collimation
Scapula, the head and proximal third of humerus, the surrounding soft tissues

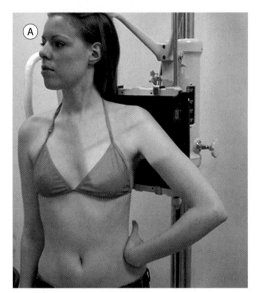

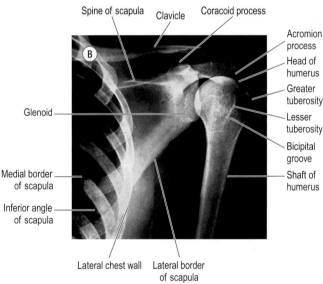

Figure 7.11   AP scapula. (B) Reproduced with permission from Ballinger PW, Frank ED. Merrill's atlas of radiographic positioning and radiologic procedures. 10th edn. St Louis: Mosby; 2003

Criteria for assessing image quality

- Head of humerus, the acromioclavicular joint and the superior and inferior angles of scapula are demonstrated
- Glenohumeral joint is obscured by the head of humerus
- Scapula projected laterally, clearing as much of the rib cage from the medial border of the body as possible
- Acromion is demonstrated clear of the superior border of the humeral head
- Sharp image demonstrating the bony cortex and trabeculae of the scapula through the air filled thorax. The bony detail of the scapula should be seen in contrast to the lungs, axilla and other soft tissue structures

◼ Lateral scapula (Fig. 7.12A,B)

If used, a 24 × 30 cm cassette is used longitudinally in the vertical holder.

Positioning

- A lead rubber apron is placed around the patient for radiation protection of the lower abdomen
- The patient stands or sits erect, facing the image receptor with their back to the X-ray tube.
- From an initial PA position, rotate the patient approximately 25° to bring the side under examination closer to, and bring the body of the scapula 90° to, the image receptor

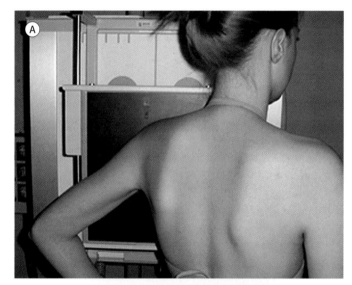

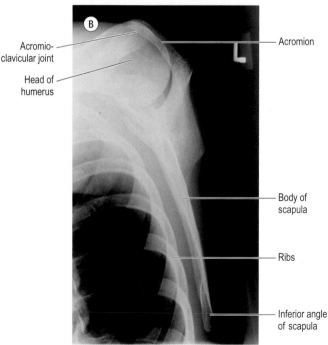

Figure 7.12   Lateral scapula

- The arm on the side under examination is flexed at the elbow, slightly abducted and the dorsum of the hand is placed on the hip, alternatively, the arm may rest across the chest with the hand resting on the shoulder of the opposite side (this may be more comfortable for the injured patient)
- The scapula is palpated to check the lateral and medial borders are superimposed

Beam direction and FFD
Horizontal at 90° to the image receptor
100 cm FFD

Centring point
To the middle of the palpable medial border of the scapula

Collimation
Scapula, the head and proximal third of humerus, the surrounding soft tissues

Criteria for assessing image quality
- Scapula, the head and proximal third of humerus are demonstrated
- Superimposition of the medial and lateral borders of the scapula
- Shaft of humerus should not overlie the body of the scapula
- The body of the scapula is projected clear of the thorax
- Sharp image demonstrating the bony cortex and trabeculae of the scapula in contrast with the surrounding soft tissue

Common errors	Possible reasons
Scapula not cleared from ribs and thorax; not seen in profile	Inaccurate obliquity of position; there is often a temptation to turn the patient more than is required, since the correct trunk position does appear to be close to a PA projection. Do not forget that the scapula will be moved into a position towards the lateral aspect of the thorax when the arm is placed in one of the required positions
Upper shaft of the humerus superimposed over the scapula	Arm not abducted or adducted sufficiently to clear the humerus from the body of scapula

ACROMIOCLAVICULAR JOINTS

These joints are normally examined to investigate subluxation of the joint following trauma. The radiographic examination should be requested following an orthopaedic assessment and not done routinely from A&E referrals, as clinical examination of the joint by an experienced orthopaedic surgeon often proves to be diagnostically accurate since severe disruption of the joint is palpable,[12] thus rendering radiographic examination unnecessary. Weight-bearing projections are often performed to assess the degree of subluxation although initial shoulder radiographs should be examined first to exclude fracture and because subluxation may be apparent without weights being given. However, research indicates that the weight-bearing examination offers little in the diagnosis of subluxation[13,14,15] and therefore the technique is not described in this text. A fourth article[16] supports this research but does suggest a rather extensive series of radiographs for acromioclavicular joints including:

AP projection with arm in internal rotation;
AP with 10–15° cranial central ray (Zanca projection);[17]
Axillary lateral (or lateral scapula or Wallace and Hellier projection if the axillary is unobtainable).

The full list of projections suggested by this article should not be routinely performed, particularly, as stated previously, clinical examination frequently offers sufficient diagnostic information and the axillary lateral shoulder is only helpful when assessing a possible posterior dislocation.[1] Comparative projections of both acromioclavicular joints should not be undertaken lightly, particularly in the light of the requirements of IR(ME)R 2000[18] and this practice should be discouraged.

■ **AP acromioclavicular joint** (Fig. 7.13A,B)

If used, an 18 × 24 cm cassette is placed transversely in the erect holder. (If both joints *must* be examined then careful collimation will allow them both to be included on one cassette, one on each side).

Positioning
- A lead rubber apron is applied to the patient's waist for radiation protection
- The patient sits or stands erect with the posterior aspect of the shoulder under examination in contact with the image receptor
- The arm is made comfortable and may remain in a sling if presented this way
- The patient is rotated approximately 10° towards the side under examination to bring the plane of the acromioclavicular joint perpendicular to the image receptor

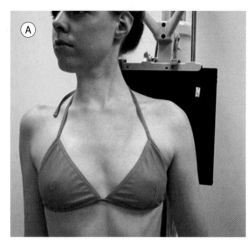

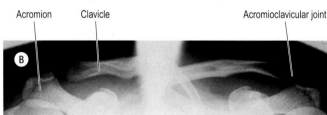

Acromion   Clavicle   Acromioclavicular joint

Figure 7.13   AP acromioclavicular joint

- The patient's head is turned away from the side under examination for radiation protection

Beam direction and FFD
Horizontal at 90° to the image receptor
100 cm FFD

Centring point
Over the acromioclavicular joint

Collimation
Acromioclavicular joint, acromion process, surrounding soft tissues

Criteria for assessing image quality
- Acromioclavicular joint, lateral end of the clavicle and soft tissue outlines are demonstrated
- If both joints are examined the images should be comparable in appearance
- Sharp image to demonstrate the bony trabeculae within the acromion and in contrast with the acromioclavicular joint and surrounding soft tissues

Common error	Possible reason
Dark image of joint with poor contrast between the joint and bones of the acromion and clavicle	Most obviously, exposure factors sets too high but poor collimation will allow scatter to overblacken the image or reduce contrast

References
1. Anderson JF, et al. Atlas of imaging in sports medicine. Sydney: The McGraw-Hill Companies; 1998.
2. Royal College of Radiologists working party. Making the best use of a department of clinical radiology: guidelines for doctors. 5th edn. London: Royal College Of Radiologists; 2003.
3. Long BW, Rafert JA. Orthopaedic radiography. Philadelphia: WB Saunders; 1995.
4. Unett EM, Royle AJ. Radiographic techniques and image evaluation. London: Nelson Thornes; 1997.
5. Wallace WA, Hellier M. Improving radiographs of the injured shoulder. Radiography 1983; 49(586):229–233.
6. Silverskoid JP, et al. Roentgenograph evaluation of suspected shoulder dislocation, a prospective study comparing the axillary and scapular Y view. Orthopaedics 1990; 13(1):63–69.
7. Wilson FC, Lin PP. General orthopaedics. New York: The McGraw-Hill Companies; 1997.
8. Grainger RG, Allison D. Diagnostic radiology. 3rd edn. Edinburgh: Churchill Livingstone; 1997.
9. Bontrager KL, Lampignano JP. Text book of radiographic positioning and related anatomy. 6th edn. St Louis: Mosby; 2005.
10. Ballinger PW, Frank ED. Merrill's atlas of radiographic positioning and radiologic procedures. 10th edn. St Louis: Mosby; 2003.
11. Swallow RA, et al. Clark's positioning in radiography. 11th edn. Oxford: Heinemann Medical Books; 1986.
12. Beim GM, Warner JJP. Clinical and radiographic evaluation of the acromioclavicular joint. Operative Techniques In Sports Medicine 1997; 5(2):65–71.
13. Varnarthos WJ, et al. Radiographic diagnosis of acromioclavicular joint separation without weight bearing, importance of internal rotation of the arm. American Journal of Roentgenology 1994; 162:120–122.
14. Bossart PJ, et al. Lack of efficacy of weighted radiographs in diagnosing acute acromioclavicular separation. Annals of Emergency Medicine 1998; 17(1):20–24.
15. Yap JJL, et al. The value of weighted views of the acromion clavicular joint. American Journal of Sports Medicine 1999; 27(6):806–809.
16. Reeves PJ. Radiography of the acromioclavicular joint: a review. Radiography 2003; 9:1–4.
17. Zanca P. Shoulder pain: involvement of the acromioclavicular joint (analysis of 1000 cases). American Journal of Roentgenology 1971; 112(3):493–506.
18. The Ionising Radiation (Medical Exposure) Regulations 2000. London: HMSO.

CHAPTER 8

FOOT, TOES, ANKLE, TIBIA AND FIBULA

Linda Williams

When imaging the foot and ankle all artefacts should be removed including socks, stockings and bandages. In cases of trauma this may not always be appropriate and extra care needs to be taken.

Gonad protection should always be used and particular care should be taken with the direction of the central beam as the gonads can easily be irradiated with the primary beam when examining the foot and ankle, particularly if a cranial angle is used. A lead rubber apron should always be applied when examining the lower limb extremities.

FOOT AND TOES

Indications

Examination of the foot for trauma should only be performed if there is true bony tenderness; the demonstration of a fracture rarely influences management.[1] Examination of the foot for hallux valgus is not indicated unless it is for preoperative assessment.

March fracture

March fractures are also known as fatigue or stress fracture to the metatarsals due to repetitive impact to this region; it is common for some new periosteal bone formation to be demonstrated on the images.

Lisfranc injuries

These are traumatic subluxations or dislocations at the base of the metatarsals at the tarsometatarsal joints, with or without fracture. This injury may involve some or all of the joints. The mechanism of injury can be from several incidents such as the foot hitting the floor of a car in a road traffic accident or missing the step of a kerb.[2]

Jones' fracture

This fracture is a transverse fracture of the proximal 5th metatarsal, usually as a result of an inversion injury to the foot, the same mechanism that causes an ankle sprain.[2]

If used, a 24 × 30 cm cassette can be divided into two for the examination of the foot, with lead rubber being used to cover the side not in use.

Dorsiplantar (DP) foot (Fig. 8.1A,B)

In both the DP and DP oblique position, in order to enable the joint spaces between the tarsal bones to be demonstrated more clearly, a 15° cranial angle may be used as described in *Clark's Positioning in Radiography*.[3] When using this projection the tarsometatarsal articulations are demonstrated without as much bony overlap as when a perpendicular central ray is used. However, careful consideration must be given when directing the tube towards the gonads and adequate radiation protection must be used. The same image can be produced by using a 15° foam wedge under the image receptor, the thickest end being placed at the toe end; this removes the necessity for angulation of the central ray directly towards the gonads but magnification of the image of metatarsals and phalanges will occur if used in this way, as the object to film distance will vary along the length of the foot.

Exposure for a foot requires the toes and the tarsal bones to be demonstrated on the one image and a suitable

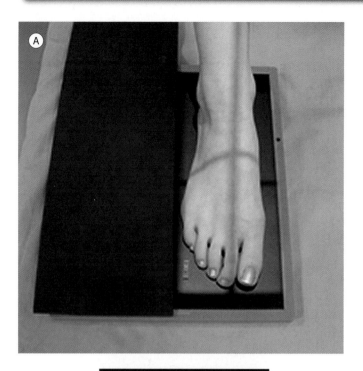

kVp should be selected, high enough to reduce subject contrast without over-penetrating the thinner end of the area. The use of a slim wedge filter, the thickest part of the filter being placed at the toes, will have the effect of reducing subject contrast. The wedge can be used under the foot but some magnification of the metatarsals and phalanges will occur in a similar way to that mentioned in the last paragraph.

Positioning
- The patient is seated on the table with their legs extended and their hands are used to support themselves
- The patient's knee on the side under examination is flexed and the plantar aspect of the foot is placed in contact with the image receptor
- The opposite leg is abducted and a lead rubber sheet is placed over the abdomen and pelvis for radiation protection

Beam direction and focus film distance FFD
Vertical central ray, at 90° to the cassette
100 cm FFD

Centring point
Over the base of 2nd metatarsal

Collimation
All phalanges, metatarsals, tarsals, soft tissues

Criteria for assessing image quality
- Demonstration of the phalanges, metatarsals, navicular, cuboid and cuneiform bones and soft tissue shadowing of the outline of the foot
- Adjacent phalanges should be demonstrated separately with exception of the bases of metatarsals 2–5 which will be slightly overlapped. Toes of patients with toe deformities are unlikely to all be separated
- Shafts of the metatarsals separated
- Tarsal bones should appear overlapped
- Talus and calcaneum should be superimposed over the tibia and fibula
- Sharp image demonstrating the soft tissue margins, bony cortex and trabeculae of the phalanges, metatarsals and tarsus. The proximal calcaneum and talus will not be penetrated sufficiently to be demonstrated

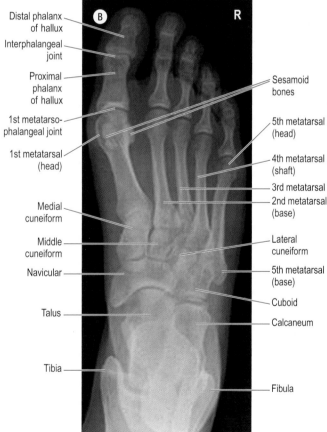

Figure 8.1   DP foot

Common error	Possible reason
Superimposition of the lower leg over the tarsal bones	Knee may be flexed too much, encouraging too much ankle flexion

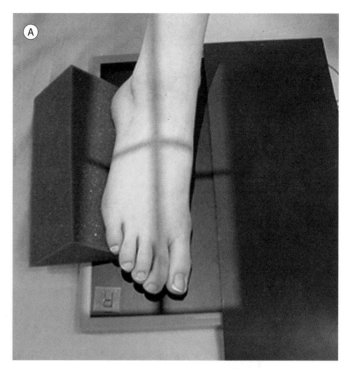

Dorsiplantar oblique (DPO) foot (Fig. 8.2A,B)

Positioning
- The plantar aspect of the foot is placed on the unexposed side of the cassette, if used, and lead rubber is placed over the exposed half
- From the DP position the patient's foot is internally rotated to bring the plane of the dorsum of the foot parallel to the image receptor
- A radiolucent pad is placed under the plantar aspect of the foot for immobilisation
- The opposite leg is abducted and a lead rubber sheet is placed over the abdomen and pelvis for radiation protection

Beam direction and FFD
Vertical central ray, at 90° to the image receptor
100 cm FFD

Centring point
Over the base of 3rd metatarsal

Collimation
All phalanges, metatarsals and tarsal bones, surrounding soft tissues

Criteria for assessing image quality
- Demonstration of the phalanges, metatarsals, navicular, cuboid and cuneiform bones and soft tissue shadowing of the outline of the foot
- Adjacent phalanges are not likely to all be separated, due to obliquity, especially in the case of patients with toe deformities (i.e. 'hammer toe')
- Shafts of metatarsals 2–4 separated
- Overlap of the bases of the 1st and 2nd metatarsals
- Separation of the tarsal bones, although the medial and middle cuneiforms will appear superimposed, with some overlap of middle and lateral cuneiforms
- Talus and calcaneum are clear of the tibia and fibula
- Sharp image demonstrating the soft tissue margins of the foot, bony cortex and trabeculae of the phalanges, metatarsals and tarsus

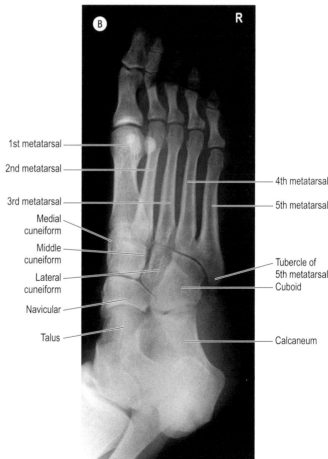

Figure 8.2 DPO foot

Common errors	Possible reasons
Superimposition of the lower leg over the tarsal bones	Knee may be flexed too much, or the foot may be under-rotated
Overlapping of metatarsals	Over-rotation of foot

■ Lateral foot (Fig. 8.3A,B)

Positioning

- With the leg extended, it is externally rotated until the lateral aspect of the foot is in contact with the image receptor. This may be more comfortable if the knee is slightly relaxed and not fully extended. The plantar aspect of the foot is 90° to the image receptor
- Radiolucent foam pads may be placed under the lower leg and foot for support in this position
- A lead rubber apron is placed over the abdomen for radiation protection

Beam direction and FFD

Vertical central ray, at 90° to the cassette
100 cm FFD

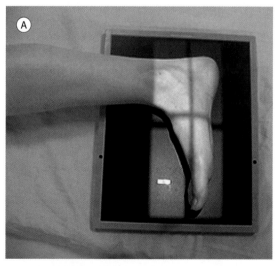

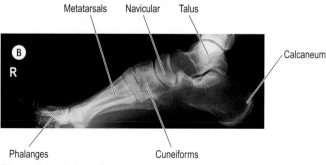

Metatarsals   Navicular   Talus

Calcaneum

Phalanges   Cuneiforms

Figure 8.3 Lateral foot

Centring point
Over the navicular cuneiform region

Collimation
All phalanges, metatarsals, tarsals, soft tissues

The lateral foot projection can be achieved by external rotation from the DP position but the position with the leg extended draws the area of the primary beam further from the trunk.

Criteria for assessing image quality
- Demonstration of the phalanges, metatarsals, navicular, cuboid and cuneiform bones and soft tissue shadowing of the outline of the foot
- Phalanges should be superimposed; the distal phalanges of the longest toe (hallux or 2nd toe) will lie clear
- Metatarsals should be overlapped, with the 1st metatarsal lying most superiorly and the 5th inferiorly
- Sharp image demonstrating the superimposition of the phalanges and metatarsals and the bony trabeculae of the tarsal bones, navicular, talus and calcaneum

■ Weight-bearing lateral foot (Fig. 8.4A,B)

This projection is usually performed as part of an orthopaedic assessment. It is important to include the whole length of foot on the image as the relationship of the joints of the tarsal bones and the metatarsals is an important indication of the degree of surgical intervention required following trauma. This is particularly important in Lisfranc injuries where fracture dislocations are involved and a complete radiographic evaluation of the foot is required.[2]

A suitably designed platform is required for good radiography of this area. The platform should be made of radiolucent material, with a groove in the centre for positioning the film vertically and to allow the image receptor to be placed at a level below the soft tissues of the plantar aspect of the foot to enable the soft tissues to be included on the image. The platform should be of a dimension to allow both feet to be placed comfortably on either side of the groove (Fig. 8.5).

A 24 × 30 cm cassette is placed vertically in the groove of the support.

Positioning
- Stand the patient on the specially designed platform
- Ensure the patient is stable and suitable support is provided to allow even distribution of the weight of both feet
- Support the image receptor in the erect, transverse position in the groove of the platform on the medial aspect of the foot

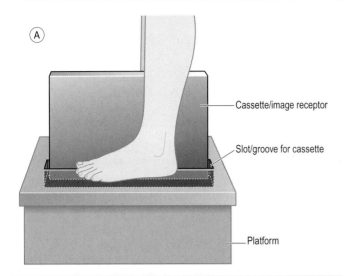

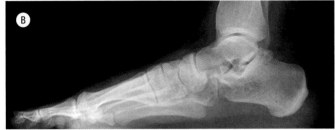

Figure 8.4   Weight-bearing lateral foot

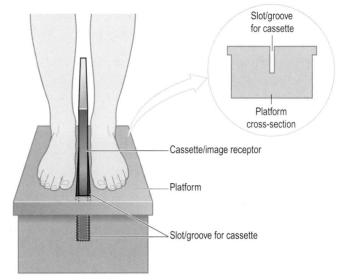

Figure 8.5   Cross-section of platform used for weight-bearing lateral foot

- Use a sheet of lead rubber between the back of the film and the foot that is not under examination, for radiation protection
- The long axis of the foot should be parallel to the long axis of the image receptor
- A lead rubber apron is placed over the abdomen for radiation protection

Beam direction and FFD
Horizontal central ray, at 90° to the cassette
100 cm FFD

Centring point
Over the tubercle of the fifth metatarsal

Collimation
The phalanges, metatarsals, tarsal bones, surrounding soft tissues

Criteria for assessing image quality
- Distal phalanges, calcaneum, ankle joint and soft tissue outlines of the foot should all be demonstrated
- Phalanges should be superimposed, with the longest toe cleared as for non-weight-bearing lateral
- Metatarsals should be overlapped as for the lateral foot
- Medial and lateral articular surfaces of the talus should be superimposed

- Sharp image demonstrating superimposition of the phalanges and metatarsals, bony trabeculae of the tarsal bones, navicular, talus and calcaneum. The soft tissue of the heel pad should not be over-blackened. kVp should be sufficient to reduce the subject contrast along the length of the foot

TOES

DP and DPO toes

It is often a requirement to examine all the toes, but most often toes 2–5, in one projection. Therefore the description that follows gives the option to do this or to examine the toes individually. The practice of including other toes on an image is often employed to establish which phalanx is being examined (see also the section on fingers in Ch. 5), however this involves irradiating areas that are not required for examination and it could be argued that this contravenes IR(ME)R 2000.[4] Collimation to include just part of the adjacent toe either side may be sufficient for identification purposes.[5]

Single toe examination
If used, an 18 × 24 cm cassette is orientated vertically, divided in two using a sheet of lead rubber.

Multiple toes examination
If used, an 18 × 24 cm cassette is placed in the transverse position, divided in two using a sheet of lead rubber. Patients with wide feet may require a 24 × 30 cm cassette.

▪ DP toe/toes (Figs 8.6A,B, 8.7A,B)

Positioning

- The patient is seated on the table with their legs extended and their hands are used to support themselves

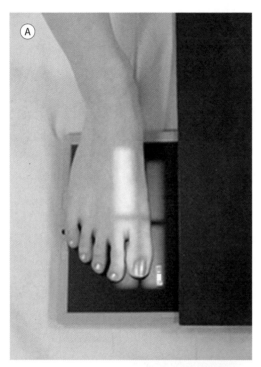

- The patient's knee on the side under examination is flexed and the plantar aspect of the toes is placed in contact with the image receptor
- The opposite leg is abducted and a lead rubber sheet is placed over the abdomen and pelvis for radiation protection

Beam direction and FFD

Horizontal central ray, at 90° to the cassette
100 cm FFD

Centring point

To the individual toe under examination at the metatarsophalangeal joint (Fig. 8.6A) or to the 3rd metatarsophalangeal joint if all the toes are to be included (Fig. 8.7A)

Collimation

Distal half of metatarsals and phalanges of the relevant toe/toes

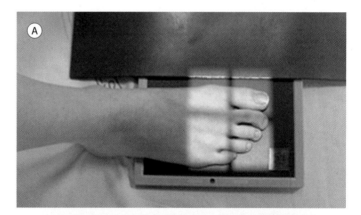

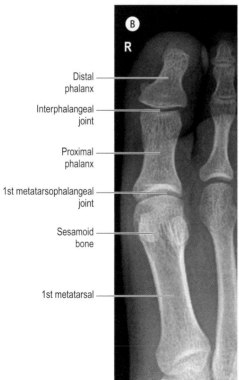

Figure 8.6   DP individual toe – hallux

R

Distal phalanx
Interphalangeal joint
Proximal phalanx
1st metatarsophalangeal joint
Sesamoid bone
1st metatarsal

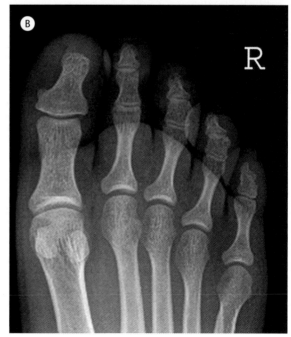

Figure 8.7   DP for all toes

Criteria for assessing image quality

- All the phalanges and the distal half of the metatarsals should be included
- Symmetry of the phalangeal condyles
- Joint spaces of the interphalangeal joint spaces are demonstrated clearly. Separation of the toe or toes from the adjacent toes. Neither of these may be possible with patients with toe deformity
- Separation of adjacent metatarsal heads
- Sharp image demonstrating the soft tissue margins of the toe/toes, bony cortex and trabeculae of the phalange/s

▇ DPO toes (Fig. 8.8A,B)

Positioning

- The patient is seated on the table with their legs extended and their hands are used to support themselves
- If a cassette is used, the plantar aspect of the toes is placed on the unexposed half and lead rubber is placed over the exposed half
- From the DP position the patient's foot is internally rotated to approximately 30° to the image receptor
- A radiolucent pad is placed under the plantar aspect of the foot for immobilisation
- The opposite leg is abducted and a lead rubber sheet is placed over the abdomen and pelvis for radiation protection

Beam direction and FFD

Horizontal central ray, at 90° to the cassette
100 cm FFD

Centring point

To the individual toe under examination at the metatarsophalangeal joint or to the 3rd metatarsophalangeal joint if all the toes are to be included

Collimation

Distal half of metatarsals and phalanges of relevant toe/toes

Criteria for assessing image quality

- All the phalanges and distal half of the metatarsals should be included on the image
- As much separation of the phalanges as possible
- Sharp image demonstrating the soft tissue margins of the toe/toes, bony cortex and trabeculae of the phalange/s

▇ Lateral hallux (Fig. 8.9A)

Positioning

- The patient is seated on the table with their legs extended and their hands used to support themselves

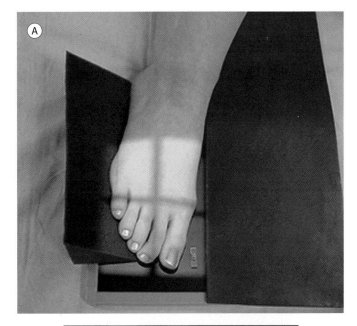

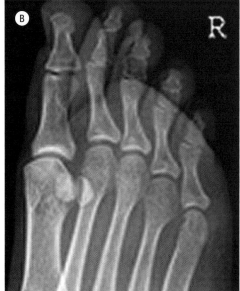

Figure 8.8   DPO toes

- The plantar aspect of the toes are placed on the image receptor
- From the DP position the patient's leg is internally rotated so that the medial aspect comes in contact with the table
- The patient is asked to assist with use of a crepe bandage to pull the toes that are not being examined away from the toe under examination either in (1) a plantar direction or (2) a dorsal direction (Fig. 8.9B) depending on the patient and how their toes most easily flex
- The opposite leg is abducted and a lead rubber sheet is placed over the abdomen and pelvis for radiation protection

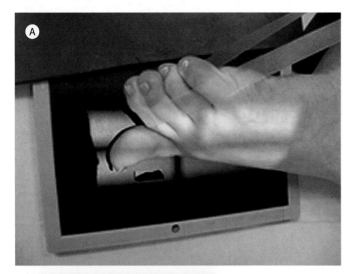

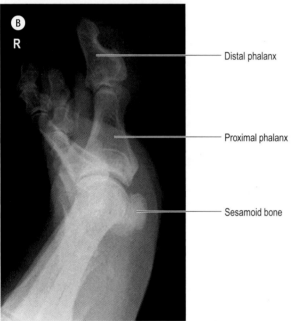

Figure 8.9 Lateral toe – hallux. Note that in (B) flexion of toes is opposite to (A)

The crepe bandage may be replaced with a piece of gauze between the toes. The radiographer examining the patient should assess which is the most suitable method for the individual patient depending on the flexibility of the patient's toes. It has been suggested that the use of a tongue depressor/spatula can be used to separate the toes, but if the patient has suffered trauma to the region then this is not advisable. In any case, use of the relatively short spatula will bring the patient's fingers closer to the primary beam. Also consider the use of dental film placed between the toes with the tube side of the film in contact with the medial aspect of the toe under examination.

Beam direction and FFD
Horizontal central ray, at 90° to the cassette
100 cm FFD

Centring point
To the individual toe under examination at the proximal interphalangeal joint

Collimation
Distal half of metatarsals and phalanges of the relevant toe

Criteria for assessing image quality
- Relevant phalanges and the metatarsophalangeal joint demonstrated on the image
- Clear interphalangeal and metatarsophalangeal joints demonstrated with the phalangeal condyles superimposed
- Sharp image demonstrating the soft tissue margins of the toe and the bony cortex and trabeculae of the phalanges

Common error	Possible reason
Poor joint spaces with non-superimposition of the phalangeal condyles	Long axis of the toe may not lie parallel to the cassette; the leg may not be rotated sufficiently medially

ANKLE

The ankle is a ring structure consisting of the tibia, talus and fibula, linked by the medial and lateral collateral ligaments and the interosseous ligament. A break in the ring is commonly associated with a second break in the ring elsewhere which could be either ligamentous or bony.[1]

Most ankle fractures are a result of inversion or eversion injuries occurring with a combination of adduction, abduction, lateral rotation, or axial forces. Inversion injuries with supination and lateral rotation account for over half of ankle fractures.[2]

Fractured ankles can be complex and many attempts have been made to separate them into several classifications depending on the degree of injury. There is also an increasing element of dislocation with each degree of fracture. Pott's fractures are one such method of classification.

Pott's classifications

Abduction, external rotation type
Pott's I   A fracture of the lateral malleolus of the fibula
Pott's II   The fibular fracture, with also a transverse fracture of the medial malleolus and lateral subluxation of the talus
Pott's III In addition to the fibular fracture, the posterior part of the medial malleolus is displaced upwards and the talus subluxed backwards

The above description of the Pott's classifications are those most commonly found, however several more classifications are described for the more unusual adduction injury.

Adduction type

Pott's I   Vertical fracture of the medial malleolus

Pott's II   The fractured medial malleolus is accompanied by a transverse fracture of the lateral malleolus and medial subluxation of the talus

Pott's III   The talus is dislocated backwards. There is a fracture of the posterior part of the medial malleolus and a transverse fracture of the lateral malleolus

▮ Ankle trauma in children and adolescents

It is much more likely for a child to suffer from an epiphyseal injury than a fracture or ligament tear due to the ligaments in children being stronger than the physis. The distal tibial epiphysis is only second to the radius in the number of bony injuries occurring in children for the entire skeleton. The Salter Harris classifications are used to describe these injuries; these are explained in the introductory section for skeletal radiography in Chapter 4.

The ankle joint may be examined for demonstration of the joint alone but is often examined for suspected fracture and therefore the image usually requires inclusion of the lower third of tibia and fibula. To achieve this, collimation is required to be extended further up the tibia and fibula, while the centring point should remain the same as for the joint (midway between the malleoli). This will result in there being an excessive field of primary radiation below the plantar aspect of the foot and beyond the image receptor; to reduce the patient dose and prevent unnecessary scattered radiation reaching the image receptor (and thus improve image quality) place a sheet of lead rubber below the image receptor. Follow-up examinations need only include the affected area.

If used, a 24 × 30 cm cassette is split with a piece of lead rubber. This will enable the anteroposterior (AP) and the lateral projections to be included on one film. When the ankle is examined specifically for the joint itself it can be demonstrated on an 18 × 24 cm cassette, split into two by use of lead rubber.

▮ AP ankle (Fig. 8.10A,B)

The AP ankle is described in this text with the malleoli being equidistant from the image receptor. When positioning the ankle in this way there will be superimposition of distal tibia by the fibula, and the distal tibiofibular joint

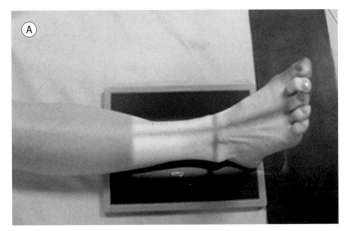

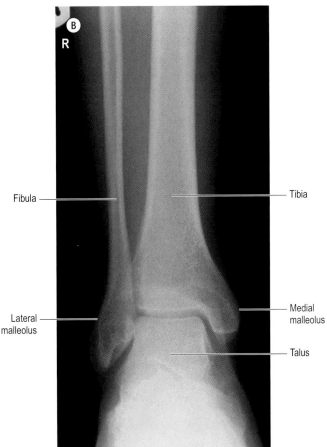

Figure 8.10   AP ankle

will be obscured. The lateral aspect of the mortice, i.e. the fibiotalar joint, will be demonstrated ('mortice', or 'mortise', refers to the appearance of the joint space around the upper talus, in the AP ankle projection, as it fits between the distal tibia and both malleoli; this is likened to the mortice joint used in carpentry). Some texts[5,6,7] describe this position as an oblique ankle and suggest, for the AP, the inter malleoli line forms an angle of approximately 15–20° with the image receptor (with the lateral malleolus being closer to the image receptor). However, this positioning will obscure the lateral mortice and demonstration of the distal fibula will be incomplete. Other texts[3,8,9] are concurrent with that described in this text, i.e. that the malleoli should be equidistant to the image receptor.

If used, a 24 × 30 cm cassette is selected. Lead rubber can be used to mask off half of the cassette in order to perform both AP and lateral projections on one image.

Positioning

- The patient is seated on the table with their legs extended
- The leg under examination is adducted away from the opposite leg to offer protection from the main beam
- A lead rubber apron is worn to protect the gonads
- The posterior aspect of the lower leg is placed in contact with the image receptor with the heel 2 cm above its lower edge
- The ankle joint is flexed to 90° (this is achieved by asking the patient to pull their toes towards their knee)
- The ankle is internally rotated to bring the medial and lateral malleoli equidistant to the image receptor
- The patient is immobilised in this position by using a 45° foam pad placed on the dorsal aspect of the foot with a sandbag resting on it

Beam direction and FFD

Vertical central beam, at 90° to the image receptor
100 cm FFD

Centring point

Midway between the malleoli

Collimation

Lower third of tibia and fibula, ankle joint, lateral and medial malleoli, talus, surrounding soft tissues

Criteria for assessing image quality

- Demonstration of the lower third of tibia and fibula, lateral and medial malleoli with soft tissue outlines
- Tibiotalar joint is well demonstrated with equal space surrounding the superior aspect of the talus
- Talus and its articulation with the malleoli should be clearly demonstrated and free of superimposition
- Distal tibiofibular joint will be obscured
- Sharp image demonstrating the soft tissue margins, bony cortex and trabeculae of the distal tibia and fibula with the cortical margins of the superior aspect of the talus demonstrated

Common errors	Possible reasons
Joint space not demonstrated between the talus and fibula	The leg is not sufficiently internally rotated; make sure the malleoli are equidistant to the table-top
The tibiotalar joint is not clearly demonstrated	There is insufficient dorsiflexion of the foot

■ Lateral ankle (Fig. 8.11A,B)

To most easily achieve the best position for a lateral ankle, ask the patient to keep their leg extended and dorsiflexed at the ankle, and then roll over onto the side under examination. A common problem when performing the lateral ankle projection is that the patient tends to invert the foot and it is difficult to rectify this once in the lateral position.

Positioning

- From the AP position the leg is externally rotated onto the side under examination until the malleoli are superimposed vertically
- The foot is dorsiflexed to bring the foot and tibia into an angle of 90°
- A small foam pad can be placed under the lateral border of the forefoot to support the patient in this position, as the lateral aspect of the forefoot will not be in contact with the table-top when the malleoli are superimposed

Beam direction and FFD

Vertical central ray at 90° to the image receptor
100 cm FFD

Centring point

Over the medial malleolus

Collimation

Lower third of tibia and fibula, talus, calcaneum, navicular, surrounding soft tissues

Criteria for assessing image quality

- Lower third of tibia and fibula, talus, calcaneum, navicular and the surrounding soft tissues are demonstrated
- Medial and lateral borders of the talus are superimposed to give a clear joint space
- Extreme distal aspect of the fibula is superimposed centrally over the distal tibia, although the shaft becomes more posterior proximally
- Single line representing superior articulatory surface of the talus, with clear tibiotalar joint space

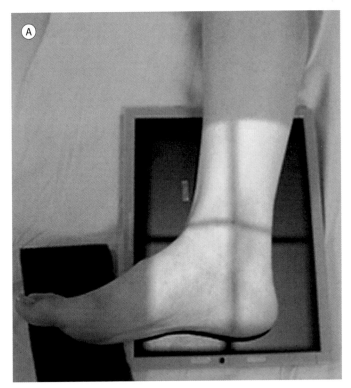

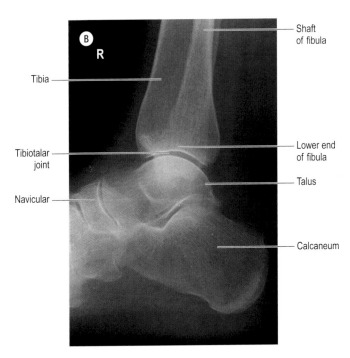

Figure 8.11   Lateral ankle

- Sharp image demonstrating the soft tissue, bony cortex and trabeculae of tibia, fibula and talus

Common errors	Possible reasons
Distal fibula projected posterior to the tibia	The leg is over-rotated laterally, make sure the malleoli are superimposed
Shaft of the fibula projected over the tibia	The leg is under-rotated
Loss of joint space and/or double edge to line representing superior articulatory surface of talus	Over- or under-rotation of the leg and/or inversion of the foot

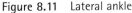 Ankle obliques

Obliques can be performed to further clarify or demonstrate any disruption to the joint, or to help in diagnosing a fractured malleolus. (a) Lateral/external and (b) medial/ internal obliques with 45° rotation are usually required. In order to assess distal tibiofibular joint, distal fibula, talus and its articulation with the lateral malleolus and tibia, then the medial oblique has a reduced rotation of 30°(c). The 30° oblique projection is sometimes referred to as a *mortice*

projection and it has been noted that some referring clinicians erroneously refer to the routine AP projection as 'mortice', thinking that the slight obliquity required to bring the malleoli into the correct position constitutes an oblique projection.

It must be mentioned, however, that magnetic resonance imaging (MRI) is the method of choice when provision of a visual account of the biomechanics of the ankle joint is required, although it is noted that some imaging centres advocate ultrasound as the imaging method of choice.

If used, an 18 × 24 cm cassette is selected.

Positioning
(a) 45° lateral/external oblique (Fig. 8.12A,B)
- From the AP position the ankle is rotated 45° externally and a radiolucent foam pad is used to support the ankle in this position

(b) 45° medial/internal oblique (Fig. 8.13A,B)
- From the AP position the ankle is rotated 45° internally and a radiolucent foam pad is used to support the ankle in this position

(c) 30° medial/internal oblique (Fig. 8.14A,B)
- From the AP position the ankle is rotated 30° internally and a radiolucent foam pad is used to support the ankle in this position

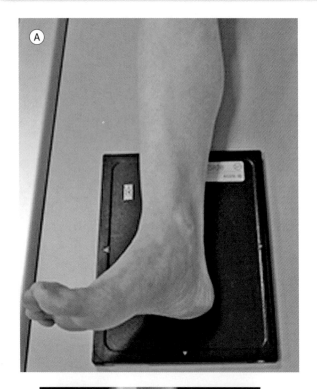

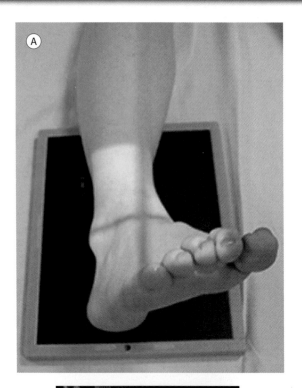

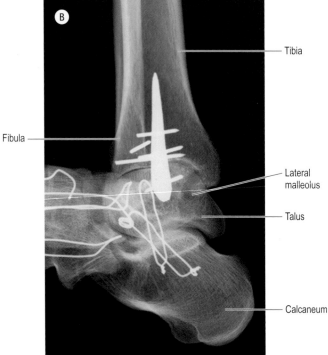

Fibula

Tibia

Lateral
malleolus

Talus

Calcaneum

Figure 8.12   45° external oblique ankle

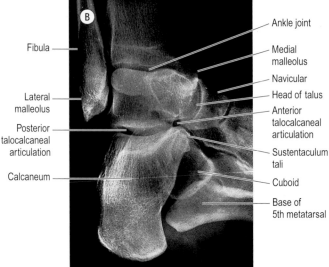

Fibula

Lateral
malleolus

Posterior
talocalcaneal
articulation

Calcaneum

Ankle joint

Medial
malleolus

Navicular

Head of talus

Anterior
talocalcaneal
articulation

Sustentaculum
tali

Cuboid

Base of
5th metatarsal

Figure 8.13   45° internal oblique ankle. (B) Reproduced with permission from Bryan GJ. Skeletal anatomy. 3rd edn. Edinburgh: Churchill Livingstone; 1996

Beam direction and FFD

Vertical central ray at 90° to the image receptor, although a 15° cranial angle will clear the distal fibula more efficiently 100 cm FFD

Centring point

For all projections, midway between the malleoli

Collimation

Medial and lateral malleoli, distal tibia and fibula, talus, surrounding soft tissues

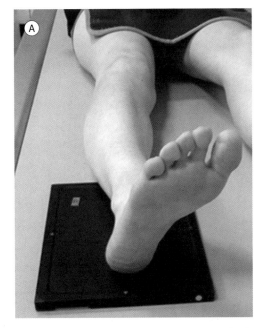

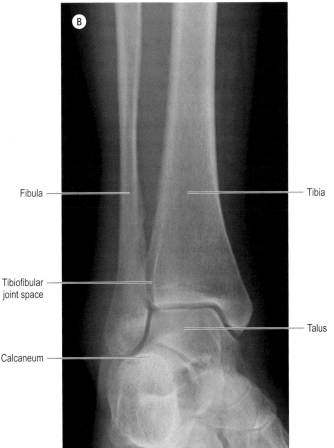

Figure 8.14   30° internal oblique ankle

Criteria for assessing image quality

- *(a) 45° external rotation:* The malleoli should be superimposed on the talus. The lower end of fibula should be obscured by the anterior aspect of the distal tibia
- *(b) 45° internal rotation:* The lateral malleolus, lateral aspect of mortice and distal tibiofibular articulation should be well demonstrated. The medial aspect of the mortice will appear closed
- *(c) 30° internal rotation/mortice projection:* The talo-tibial joint should be well visualised and the medial and lateral aspects of the mortice should be open. The medial and lateral malleoli should be well demonstrated

SUBTALAR JOINT/TALOCALCANEAL JOINTS

The following projections are described here for completeness, however it is now unusual to find them requested, as MRI will provide high contrast sensitivity and has multi-planar capabilities. It therefore facilitates superior demonstration of these articular surfaces.

◼ Medial obliques, subtalar joint

If used, an 18 × 24 cm cassette is selected.

Positioning
- As for 45° medial oblique (Fig. 8.13A)

Beam direction and FFD
1. *40° cranial angle* to show the anterior portion of the posterior talocalcaneal articulation
2. *30° cranial angle* to show the articulation between the talus and sustenaculum
3. *10° cranial angle* to show the posterior portion of the posterior talocalcaneal articulation
100 cm FFD

Centring point
All angulations – to a point beneath the lateral malleolus

Collimation
Distal end of the tibia and fibula, calcaneum, tarsal bones

Criteria for assessing image quality
- Distal end of tibia and fibula, calcaneum and tarsal bones are demonstrated

- (1) should demonstrate the anterior part of the posterior talocalcaneal articulation
- (2) should demonstrate the articulation between the talus and sustenaculum
- (3) should demonstrate the posterior part of the posterior talocalcaneal articulation. The sinus tarsi should be demonstrated as open on this projection
- Sharp image with adequate penetration to demonstrate the subtalar joint with visualisation of the bony cortex and trabeculae of the talus in contrast to the surrounding soft tissue margins

Lateral oblique subtalar joint

If used, an 18 × 24 cm cassette is selected.
This demonstrates the posterior subtalar joint and will also confirm a fracture involving the joint surface[2] and disclose DP compression.

Positioning
- As for 45° external oblique projection (Fig. 8.12a)

Beam direction and FFD
15° cranial angle
100 cm FFD

Centring point
To a point just below and anterior to the medial malleolus

Collimation
Distal end of tibia and fibula, calcaneum, tarsal bones

Criteria for assessing image quality
- Distal end of tibia and fibula, calcaneum and tarsal bones are demonstrated
- Posterior subtalar joint should be well demonstrated with the middle and anterior subtalar joint obscured by the inferior aspects of the talar neck and head
- Sharp image with adequate penetration to demonstrate the posterior subtalar joint with visualisation of the bony cortex and trabeculae of the talus in contrast to the surrounding soft tissue margins

CALCANEUM

The calcaneum is often examined when a patient presents after falling feet first from height but fractures of this area can result from a twisting injury. Some fractures will only become apparent when the Bohler's Angle[1] is assessed; this angle is normally found to be between 30° and 40° and is reduced to below 30° when a fracture is present (see

Fig. 8.15). CT is useful for assessment of the extent and involvement of fragments in the fractured calcaneum.

If used, an 18 × 24 cm cassette is selected. Lead rubber may be used to mask off half of the cassette in order to perform two projections on one image.

Lateral calcaneum (Fig. 8.16A,B)

For assessment of the calcaneal spur, the lateral projection only should be undertaken.

Positioning
- The patient is seated on the table, and the ankle of the side under examination is rotated externally
- The lateral aspect of the foot is brought into contact with the image receptor
- The ankle is dorsiflexed to 90° and the rotation of the leg adjusted until the malleoli are superimposed
- A lead rubber apron is worn to protect the gonads

Beam direction and FFD
Vertical central ray, at 90° to the image receptor
100 cm FFD

Centring point
To the middle of the calcaneum below the medial malleolus

Collimation
Calcaneum, ankle joint, navicular, surrounding soft tissues

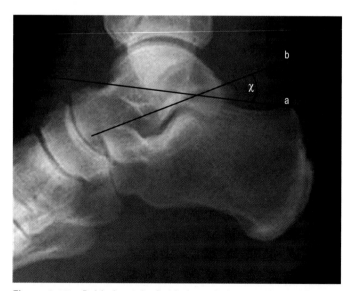

Figure 8.15 Bohler's angle. Bohler's angle is assessed by drawing 2 intersecting lines (a) from the highest point on the posterior aspect of the calcaneum to its highest midpoint and (b) from the highest midpoint to the highest anterior point. The lines are extended here to demonstrate the angle more accurately. If the angle x is less than 30° this suggests calcaneum fracture with compression

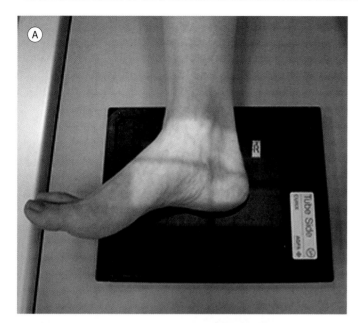

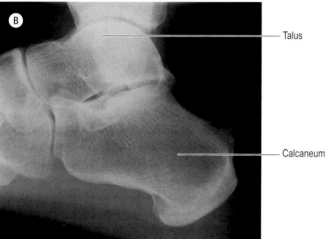

Figure 8.16   Lateral calcaneum

Criteria for assessing image quality
- Calcaneum, talocalcaneal and cubocalcaneal joints and soft tissue outlines are demonstrated
- Distal fibula should be superimposed over the tibial malleolus
- Sharp image demonstrating the soft tissue margins, bony cortex and trabeculae of the calcaneum

Axial calcaneum

This projection can be achieved by several methods. It is commonly described with the patient seated on the table and the central ray directed 40° cranially towards the extended leg (method 4) but this method has the X-ray beam directed towards the trunk and should only be performed if the other methods described cannot be achieved due to the patient's condition.

Method 1 is easily achieved by the ambulant patient and methods 2 and 3 can be achieved in the less ambulant patient and most trolley patients. Methods 1–3 position the long axis of the calcaneum parallel to the image receptor, producing an image with minimal distortion. Method 4 positions the long axis of the calcaneum at 90° to the image receptor and produces maximum distortion to the image. All four techniques can be used to examine both calcanei simultaneously, with the X-ray beam centred between the heels, at the levels stated for the individual calcaneum. This method will cause a degree of image distortion but will reduce the exposures made to one; two separate exposures will increase radiation dose but will provide less distortion due to accurate centring over each heel in turn.

Method 1: patient erect (Fig. 8.17A,B)
Positioning
- The patient stands in the erect position with their back to the X-ray tube and the plantar aspect of the heel under examination is placed directly on the image receptor

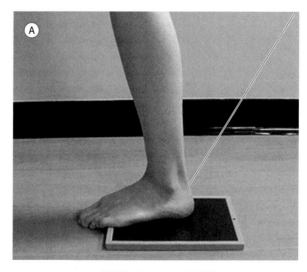

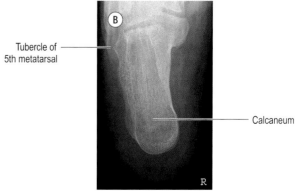

Figure 8.17   (A) Erect axial calcaneum; (B) axial calcaneum

- The other leg is abducted to clear it from the radiation field
- A lead rubber apron is placed around the patient's waist to protect the gonads
- With the patient's knees slightly flexed the hands can be placed onto a table or chair in front for support. A vertical bucky stand can also be used
- The malleoli are checked until equidistant from the image receptor

Beam direction and FFD
Initially vertical, the beam is directed 30° towards the toes, i.e. 60° to the image receptor
100 cm FFD

Method 2: patient prone (Fig. 8.18)
An erect cassette holder is required for this method, with a cassette supported vertically. Some digital plate image receptors may not be suitable for this method.

Positioning
- The patient lies prone on the table with the toes projecting over the end of the table
- The cassette in the holder is placed at the end of the table with the tube side of the image receptor facing the plantar aspect of the patient's feet
- Both legs are extended and the unaffected leg is abducted to clear it from the radiation field
- A lead rubber sheet is placed over the pelvis to protect the gonads
- The plantar aspect of the foot under examination is placed in contact with the image receptor
- The malleoli are equidistant from the image receptor

Beam direction and FFD
Initially horizontal, the X-ray tube is directed caudally towards the toes at approximately 30°, to create an angle of 60° with the image receptor
100 cm FFD

Method 3: patient lying on side (Fig. 8.19)
Positioning
- The patient lies in the lateral position on the side under examination
- The unaffected leg is abducted posteriorly and placed behind the side under examination
- The leg of the side under examination is supported above the table-top using foam pads and the image receptor is supported vertically, its tube side in contact with the plantar aspect of the heel
- The malleoli are equidistant from the image receptor
- A lead rubber sheet is placed over the hips for gonad protection

Beam direction and FFD
1. Initially the beam is horizontal, directed towards the posterior aspect of the heel and coincident with the long axis of the calcaneum *and then*
2. The angle is approximately 30° caudally towards the toes to form an angle of 60° with the image receptor
100 cm FFD

Centring point for methods 1, 2 and 3
At the level of the malleoli, in the middle of the posterior aspect of the heel

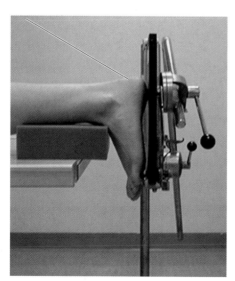

Figure 8.18   Prone axial calcaneum

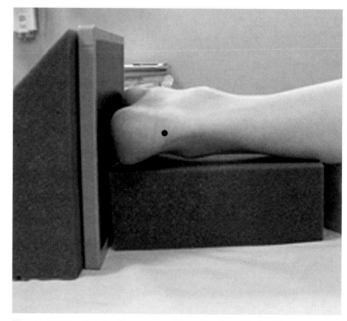

Figure 8.19   Axial calcaneum with patient on their side

Method 4: patient seated (Fig. 8.20)

Positioning

- The patient is seated on the table with their legs extended and separated
- The posterior aspect of the heel under examination is placed on the image receptor with the inferior border of the heel pad at the lower edge
- A lead rubber sheet is placed over the pelvis to protect the gonads
- The foot is dorsiflexed; this position can be assisted and maintained by providing the patient with a bandage looped around the forefoot and pulled on towards the trunk. This is held by the patient
- The malleoli are equidistant from the image receptor

Beam direction and FFD

A vertical central ray is directed 40° cranially
100 cm FFD

Centring point

At a point midway on the plantar aspect of the heel, to pass through the malleoli

Collimation

Calcaneum, talocalcaneal and cubocalcaneal joints, the soft tissue outline

Criteria for assessing image quality

- Calcaneum, talocalcaneal and cubocalcaneal joints and the soft tissue outlines demonstrated
- Cubocalcaneal joint space clearly visualised without the metatarsals superimposed
- Lateral malleolus demonstrated on the lateral aspect of the calcaneum
- Calcaneum demonstrated without rotation and distortion

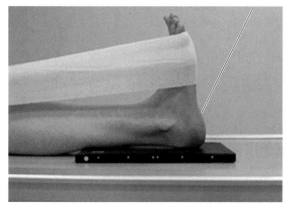

Figure 8.20 Axial calcaneum with patient seated

- Sharp image demonstrating the soft tissue margins and bony cortex and trabeculae of the calcaneum, cubocalcaneal joint shown adequately without over-penetration of the distal aspect of calcaneum

Common errors – all methods	Possible reasons
Elongated long axis of the calcaneum	Over-angulation of X-ray beam
Foreshortening of long axis of the calcaneum	Not enough angulation on X-ray beam
Cubocalcaneal joint not demonstrated	Not enough dorsiflexion of the foot

TIBIA AND FIBULA

When examining the tibia and fibula both the knee and the ankle joint must be demonstrated. This is particularly important in the case of gross injuries in order to show general alignment and to be certain that a contra-coup injury has not occurred. The fibula acts as a support for the tibia and a fracture at one end of one bone often results in a fracture at the opposite of the other. The ankle joint is often described as a bony ring and the ring may be considered to extend into the knee. An external rotation injury of the ankle joint, resulting in a seemingly isolated fracture of the medial malleolus, may result in a fracture of the proximal fibula, this is called a Maissoneuve fracture.[1] In the case of spiral fracture the full length of the fracture may not be demonstrated if the full length of the tibia and fibula is not shown.

The image receptor size selected should either be two 18 × 43 cm (usually cassette sizes rather than digital receptors) or in the case of most male patients 35 × 43 cm (or, in the case of some digital receptors, 43 cm²) used diagonally, to ensure the full lengths of the tibia and fibula are included; indeed, it may be necessary to use two image receptors per projection to ensure both joints are included.

▉ AP tibia and fibula (Fig. 8.21A,B)

Positioning

- The patient is seated on the table and may support themselves by leaning on their hands
- Both legs are extended and the leg that is not under examination is abducted to clear it from the radiation field
- A lead rubber sheet is placed over the pelvis to protect the gonads

Beam direction and FFD

A vertical central ray, at 90° to the image receptor
100 cm FFD

Centring point

Midway between the ankle and knee joint on the anterior aspect of the lower leg or, if both joints cannot be included on one image, in the middle of the area being exposed

Collimation

Tibia and fibula, ankle and knee joints, surrounding soft tissues

Criteria for assessing image quality

- Tibia and fibula, ankle and knee joints and surrounding soft tissues are demonstrated
- Separation of the tibial and fibular shafts
- Proximal tibiofibular joint should show slight superimposition of tibia and fibula
- The distal tibiofibular joint should have slight superimposition of tibia and fibula
- Demonstration of the joint space between the medial and lateral borders of the talus and the medial and lateral malleoli respectively
- Sharp image demonstrating the soft tissue margins, bony cortex and trabeculae of tibia and fibula with adequate penetration to demonstrate both the ankle joint and knee joint

▪ Lateral tibia and fibula (Fig. 8.22A,B)

Positioning

- From the AP position the leg externally rotated onto the side under examination
- The opposite leg is abducted to clear from the main beam
- A lead rubber apron is applied to the lower abdomen for gonad protection
- The lateral aspect of the leg is in contact with the image receptor which is positioned to include the ankle and knee joint
- The long axis of the tibia and fibula should be parallel to surface of the image receptor
- The ankle is flexed and the malleoli are superimposed
- A small foam pad can be placed under the lateral border of the forefoot to support the patient in this position

Beam direction and FFD

Vertical central ray at 90° to the image receptor
100 cm FFD

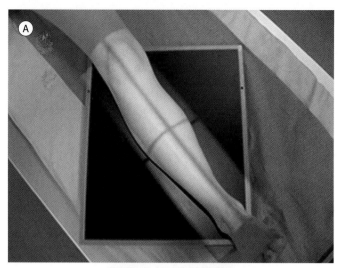

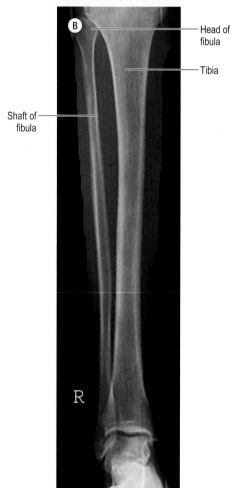

Head of fibula

Tibia

Shaft of fibula

R

Figure 8.21   AP tibia and fibula

- The leg under examination is placed with its posterior aspect in contact with the image receptor
- The malleoli are positioned equidistant to the image receptor and the ankle is dorsiflexed; this position may be supported with use of a radiolucent pad and sandbag at the plantar aspect of the foot

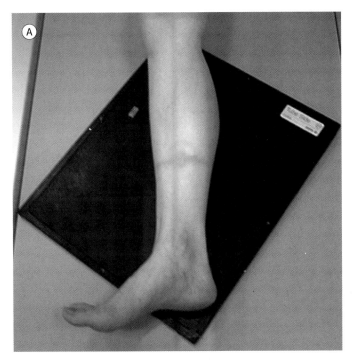

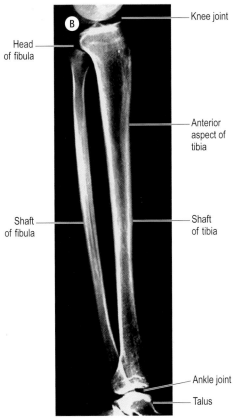

Head of fibula

Knee joint

Anterior aspect of tibia

Shaft of fibula

Shaft of tibia

Ankle joint

Talus

Figure 8.22   Lateral tibia and fibula. (B) Reproduced with permission from Bryan GJ. Skeletal anatomy. 3rd edn. Edinburgh: Churchill Livingstone; 1996 and Gunn (2002)

Centring point

Midway between the ankle and knee joint on the medial aspect of the lower leg or if both joints cannot be included on one image, in the middle of the area being exposed

Collimation

Tibia and fibula, ankle and knee joints, soft tissues

Criteria for assessing image quality

- Ankle, knee joints and soft tissue demonstrated
- Mid-shaft of fibula should project slightly posterior to tibia
- Proximal end of fibula should be slightly posterior to tibia with partial superimposition
- The distal end of fibula should be superimposed over the middle of the distal tibia
- Sharp image demonstrating the soft tissue margins, bony cortex and trabeculae of tibia and fibula with adequate penetration to visualise the ankle and knee joints. The kVp should be sufficient to reduce the high subject contrast along the length of the tibia and fibula

References

1. Raby N, et al. Accident and emergency radiology, a survival guide. 2nd edn. London: Saunders; 2005.
2. Long BW, Rafert JA. Orthopaedic radiography. Philadelphia: WB Saunders; 1995.
3. Whitley AS, et al. Clark's positioning in radiography. 12th edn. London: Hodder Arnold; 2005.
4. The Ionising Radiation (Medical Exposure) Regulations 2000, London (HMSO).
5. Bontrager KL. Textbook of radiographic positioning and related anatomy. 5th edn. St Louis: Mosby; 2001.
6. McQuillen-Martensen K. Radiographic critique. Philadelphia: WB Saunders; 1996.
7. Eisenberg RL, et al. Radiographic positioning. 2nd edn. Boston: Little Brown and Company; 1995.
8. Unett EM, Royle AJ. Radiographic techniques and image evaluation. London: Nelson Thornes; 1997.
9. Bell GA, Finlay DBL. Basic radiographic positioning. Eastbourne: Baillière Tindall; 1986.

KNEE AND FEMUR

Linda Williams

The knee joint has a complex arrangement of ligaments, tendons and muscles which together provide stability to the joint. Because of the anatomical location and the complex biomechanics of the knee, it is susceptible to a variety of injuries.[1] The knee and femur are often investigated in the event of trauma, however this should only be the case if there is a suspected fracture as ligamentous and menisceal injuries may appear as normal on plain films.[2] The knee should not be investigated for knee pain unless there is locking and restricted movement or suspected loose body. Osteoarthritic changes are commonly found in the knee and radiographic examination should only be undertaken when considering surgery.[3]

Plain radiography of the knee is undertaken less frequently in the 21st century as magnetic resonance imaging (MRI) is often the method of choice for imaging the joint. This is due to its high contrast sensitivity and multiplanar imaging capabilities. It is particularly effective in investigating the effects of trauma to the anterior and posterior cruciate ligaments and menisci.[4] The images gained by this modality, of non-bony parts of the joint, are far superior to, and carry more information than, plain radiographic images and diagnosis and appropriate management of this complex joint is established with greater confidence after MRI examination.[3]

Ultrasound is also used as a method of imaging some lesions of the knee joint, e.g. Bakers cyst; these can show as a vague mass behind the knee on plain films but ultrasound will give a clear account of the full extent of the cyst.[4]

However, there is still an important role for plain radiography of the knee for initial diagnosis in trauma and follow-up orthopaedic assessment.

FRACTURES AND INJURIES AFFECTING THE REGION OF THE KNEE AND FEMUR

Shaft of femur

The shaft is usually fractured as a result of considerable force to the femur, commonly in road traffic accidents.

Supracondylar

These are fractures superior to the femoral condyles; the gastrocnemius muscle may pull the distal fragments posteriorly.

Tibial plateau

These fractures are often associated with considerable damage to the medial collateral or cruciate ligaments. The most common finding is depressed lateral tibial plateau due to a car bumper injury; this is seen in 80% of cases.[1]

Patellar

Patellar comminuted fractures are usually the result of a direct blow. Muscle spasm (quadriceps), if severe enough, can cause transverse fractures. The bipartite patella (unfused secondary ossification centre) can be confused with a fracture but these have well-defined margins. The patella may also be *dislocated* medially or laterally, and can be recurrent due to a shallow intercondylar groove. Dislocations usually occur following a twisting force, typically as in sports injuries.

▉ Anteroposterior (AP) knee (Fig. 9.1A,B,C)

If used, an 18 × 24 cm cassette is selected, its long axis coincident with the long axis of the leg.

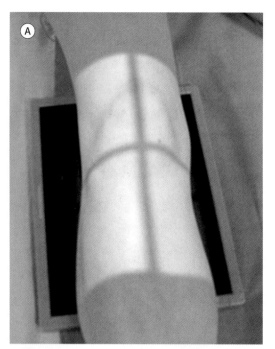

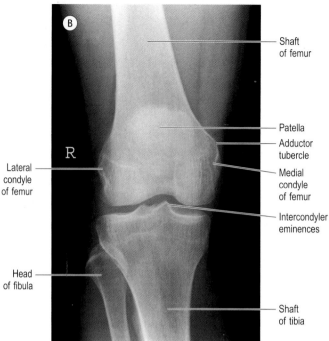

Shaft
of femur

Patella

Adductor
tubercle

Lateral
condyle
of femur

R

Medial
condyle
of femur

Intercondyler
eminences

Head
of fibula

Shaft
of tibia

Figure 9.1   **(A,B)** AP knee **(C)** Patella not centralised but joint space shown
adequately

Positioning

- The patient is seated on the table with their legs extended
- The posterior aspect of the knee under examination is in contact with the image receptor
- The unaffected leg is abducted from the leg under examination to clear it from the field of radiation
- A lead rubber apron is worn for radiation protection of the lower abdomen
- The leg is rotated to align the patella midway between the femoral condyles

Orthopaedic requests may require this projection to be undertaken with the patient erect. This allows for assessment of the joint space and alignment of the joint whilst weight bearing, prior to surgery.[1] Positioning for the erect AP remains the same as for the seated version, except for the first step. In the case of the erect AP the patient stands erect in front of an erect image receptor holder, facing the horizontal X-ray tube. The stability of the patient should also be considered in the erect position and there should be provision of a support for the patient to hold. The patient must be asked to distribute their weight evenly on both feet.

Beam direction and focus film distance (FFD)

Patient seated: Vertical central beam, at 90° to the image receptor *or* 90° to the long axis of the tibia (which will improve joint space demonstration if the patient cannot fully extend the knee)

Patient erect: Horizontal beam, at 90° to the image receptor *or* long axis of the tibia

100 cm FFD

Centring point

In the middle of the joint space, midway between the tibial condyles

A centring point of 2.5 cm below the apex of the patella is often cited as the centring point for AP of this joint but this specific measurement does not allow for variation in patient build.

Collimation

Lower third of femur, knee joint, proximal third of tibia, head of fibula, surrounding soft tissues

Criteria for assessing image quality

- Distal third of femur, proximal third of tibia, head of fibula, patella and soft tissue outlines are demonstrated
- Medial and lateral epicondyles of the femur are demonstrated in profile
- Head of fibula should appear partially obscured by the tibia
- Shafts of tibia and fibula should be separated
- Joint space should appear clear and the upper margin of the tibial plateau should be shown in profile
- Sharp image demonstrating the soft tissue margins, bony cortex and trabeculae of tibia, fibula, femur and patella, with sufficient penetration to visualise the bony trabeculae and cortical outline of the patella over the femur. Demonstration of the knee joint space in contrast with bony areas

Common errors	Possible reasons
The patella appears medially in relation to the femur and the proximal tibiofibular joint is demonstrated. The joint space may appear narrowed or obscured, unilaterally or bilaterally. Part, or all, of the tibial plateau does not appear to be seen in profile	The leg is excessively internally rotated; ensure the femoral condyles are equidistant from the image receptor and the patella is centralised. However, take care to note if the patient has a naturally medially positioned patella or knock knees before attempting repeat projection. *If the tibiofibular joint appears to be demonstrated correctly, and joint space shown clear, then it is likely that the patient's patella does not naturally lie centrally positioned; an example of this is shown in Figure 9.1C*
The patella is projected laterally in relation to the femur and the proximal tibiofibular joint is obscured by the tibia. The joint space may appear narrowed or obscured, unilaterally or bilaterally. Part or all of the tibial plateau does not appear to be seen in profile	There is excessive external rotation of the leg. Patellae are less likely to naturally lie on the more lateral aspect over the femur than medially, as above, but note should still be made to check if this is the case
There is no bony detail of the patella demonstrated – pale image of patella but femur may show trabecular detail outside the periphery of the patella	The radiograph is under-penetrated; increase kVp

▨ Lateral knee (Fig. 9.2A,B)

If used, an 18 × 24 cm cassette is selected, its long axis coincident with the long axis of the table-top.

Positioning

- The patient is seated on the table with their legs extended
- The patient is rotated laterally onto the side under examination and the hip and knee is flexed; the lateral aspect of the knee is in contact with the image receptor. Flexion of the knee should be at least 45°, to a maximum of 80°. Generally flexion through 60° (making an angle of 120° between the femoral and tibial shafts) is most commonly adopted

- The unaffected leg is abducted away from the knee under examination to clear it from the field of radiation; this may be posterior or anterior to the knee under examination. If cleared posteriorly, it is more comfortable if the unaffected leg remains extended, if cleared anteriorly it is more comfortable for the knee and hip to be flexed
- The ankle of the affected leg is supported with a sandbag to bring the long axis of the tibia parallel to the table-top
- The condyles of the femur are superimposed; this may be achieved by placing the middle finger on the lateral condyle and the thumb on the medial condyle, rotating the patient's femur until they are superimposed. Rotation at the pelvis may help with this adjustment

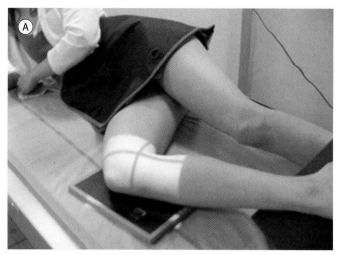

Figure 9.2 Lateral knee

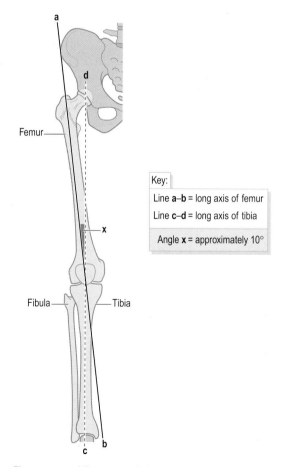

- The transverse plane of the patella is at 90° to the table-top
- A lead rubber apron is placed over the lower abdomen for radiation protection

Comments on superimposing the femoral condyles

Criteria for assessing the lateral knee radiograph require the knee joint to be demonstrated with the condyles of the femur superimposed. However there is often difficulty in producing this as the femur and tibia do not follow a straight line. The femoral shaft angles medially through approximately 10° from hip to knee yet the plane of the articular surface of the knee joint is at right angles to the long axis of the tibia (Fig. 9.3); this means that there is an angle of approximately 170° made between the femur and tibia at the lateral aspect of the knee joint. Therefore, when the patient is placed on their side in a recumbent position for the lateral knee position, it is unlikely that a vertical central ray would travel through the joint at 90° or superimpose the femoral condyles. To correct this the lower leg needs to be raised from the table-top, with pads or sandbags, to ensure the tibia lies parallel to, and the tibial plateau is perpendicular to, the image receptor.[5] Padding at the ankle end of the limb is likely to be most effective.

Without padding at the ankle, the condylar surfaces will not lie in the same plane and, if padding is not used, some texts claim the solution is to apply a cranial angle of approximately 7° as compensation.[6,7] If this method is used the main beam will be directed towards the gonads and therefore this technique is not recommended. It has been noted that some radiographers will adapt the above technique by centring lower, in conjunction with a vertical central ray, to achieve the same effect as applying a cranial

angle but this will necessitate a larger collimated field of radiation and this is also not recommended. Indeed, this practice must be actively discouraged and is in contradiction to the requirements of IR(ME)R 2000.

Figure 9.3 Alignment of shafts of femur and tibia

Beam direction and FFD

Vertical at 90° to the image receptor and coincident with the transverse axis of the joint

100 cm FFD

In cases of trauma, horizontal beam laterals must be performed; this method will demonstrate any joint effusion displacing the suprapatellar bursa, which may contain fat released from the bone marrow following fracture.[2] A fat-blood effusion may be seen (lipohaemarthrosis), indicating a fracture even if not seen on the resulting radiograph. Use of a horizontal beam will also ensure that the unstable joint is not disrupted further, or fracture fragments further displaced. This is especially a risk in the case of transverse patellar fracture or fractures of the femoral shaft.

Centring point

Over the middle of the medial tibial condyle, through the middle of the knee joint

2.5 cm below and behind the apex of the patella has been described for the centring point for this projection but, as discussed in the AP knee projection description, this does not consider variation in patient build.

Collimation

Lower third of femur, knee joint, proximal third of tibia, head of fibula, surrounding soft tissues

Criteria for assessing image quality

- Distal third of femur, proximal third of tibia, head of fibula and soft tissues should all be demonstrated
- Knee joint is demonstrated as clear, with the condyles of femur superimposed
- Patellofemoral joint space is demonstrated. However, if the patella is not naturally positioned centrally over the femur, the patellofemoral space will not be seen despite good superimposition of the femoral condyles. This is seen in Figure 9.2b
- Head of fibula is partly superimposed over tibia (approximately one-third to one-half of the head should be overlapped)
- Head of fibula is seen posteriorly in relation to tibia
- Sharp image demonstrating the soft tissue margins, bony cortex and trabeculae of femur, tibia, fibula and patella. Joint space is shown in contrast to denser bone

Common errors	Possible reasons
The condyles of the femur are not superimposed anteriorly and posteriorly and the patellofemoral joint space is not clear	Incorrect rotation but is the leg over-rotated or under-rotated? The *head of fibula* is a good indication of the direction to correct rotation: 1. If the *head of fibula* is excessively or completely superimposed over the tibia then there is insufficient rotation – further external rotation is required 2. If the proximal tibiofibular joint is shown clearly then there is excessive rotation – less rotation is therefore required The *adductor tubercle*, found on the posterior, upper aspect of the medial femoral condyle, can also be used as an indicator when assessing knee rotation. In the correct position the tubercle is hardly discernible but in cases of incorrect rotation it becomes more apparent and can be used as follows: 1. If the tubercle lies anteriorly in relationship to the other condyle, the knee is over-rotated 2. If the tubercle lies posteriorly, the knee is under-rotated The *patellofemoral* joint space will clear once the rotation is corrected but it must be remembered that the patella may not be centralised naturally and this may result in unavoidable loss of joint space. If the condyles are superimposed and the patellofemoral space is not evident, this may be due to a naturally occurring non centralised patella (this will also have been apparent when positioning for the AP projection) Another method for assessing direction of rotation is to estimate the relative *size of each condyle*; it is assumed that the outline of the apparently larger condyle will be that most remote from the image receptor (the medial condyle) since it will be more magnified than the lateral condyle. Unfortunately it is difficult to make this assessment when only part of the condyle lies clear of the other. Some patients also have one slightly flattened condyle (usually on its anterior aspect), which will never appear superimposed over the other, more normally curved, condyle
Femoral condyles not superimposed along the knee joint surface, i.e. nearest the upper surface of the tibial plateau	The tibia is not parallel to the table-top; usually this is due to a lack of attention to adequate padding of the lower leg. It is more difficult to assess correction requirements in this situation but estimation of size of condyles (as described above) may help. It is more likely that the lower leg is inadequately raised rather than excessively raised

INTERCONDYLAR NOTCH

Projections for this area are sometimes referred to as 'tunnel' projections as the appearances are similar to that of a railway tunnel. It is commonly performed to investigate knee pain if there is locking, restricted movement and a suspected loose body. Three methods will be described here to achieve this projection; methods 1 and 2 are the methods of choice as the primary beam is not directly pointing towards the gonads. Method 3 will also provide a more distorted, magnified image. The third method should only be attempted in patients who are unable to achieve the positions required for method 1 or 2.

Method 1 (Fig. 9.4A,B,C)

If used, an 18 × 24 cm cassette is selected for this projection, its long axis coincident with the long axis of the leg.

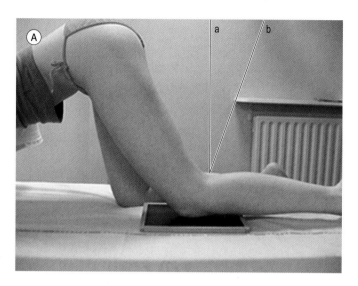

a - 90° to long axis of tibia
b - 70° to long axis of tibia

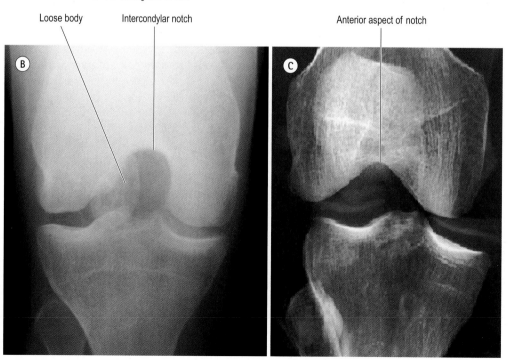

Figure 9.4 **(A)** Intercondylar notch – method 1, **(B)** with beam 90° to tibia and **(C)** with beam 70° to tibia

Positioning

- The patient kneels on the table with the knee of the leg under examination on the image receptor, their hands placed on the table for support
- The unaffected leg is separated from that under examination, to clear it from the radiation field
- The angle between the tibia and femur should be 120°
- The femoral condyles should be equidistant to the table-top and the patella centralised between them
- A lead rubber apron is worn for radiation protection to the lower abdomen, on its posterior aspect

Beam direction and FFD

1. Vertical central beam, at 90° to the long axis of the tibia. This will demonstrate the posterior aspect of the notch
   This is the only projection necessary to demonstrate loose bodies as the whole of the notch can be visualised, with the exception of its anterior aspect.
2. Cranial angle at 70° to the tibia. This will demonstrate the anterior aspect of the notch

100 cm FFD

Centring point

In the middle of the crease of the knee

▌ Method 2 (Fig. 9.5)

Positioning

- The patient lies prone on the table with the knee under examination in contact with the image receptor
- The unaffected leg is separated from that under examination, to clear it from the radiation field
- The knee is flexed until the tibia is at angle of 45° to the table-top and is supported in this position
- The femoral condyles are adjusted to centralise the patella
- A lead rubber apron is worn for radiation protection to the lower abdomen

Beam direction and FFD

1. Caudal central beam, at 45° to the image receptor and femur. This will demonstrate the whole of the notch, with the exception of the anterior aspect
2. Caudal angle at 65° to the femur. This will demonstrate the anterior aspect of the notch

100 cm FFD

Centring point

In the middle of the crease of the knee

▌ Method 3 (Fig. 9.6)

- The patient is seated on the table with the leg under examination flexed through 60° until the angle between the tibia and femur is 120°
- The unaffected leg is separated from that under examination, to clear it from the radiation field
- The image receptor is supported on a pad under the flexed knee so that it is elevated high enough to ensure the upper and lower leg are in contact with it
- The femoral condyles should be equidistant to the image receptor to centralise the patella
- A lead rubber apron is worn to protect the lower abdomen. This should be adjusted to lie between the thighs to ensure adequate protection to the gonads

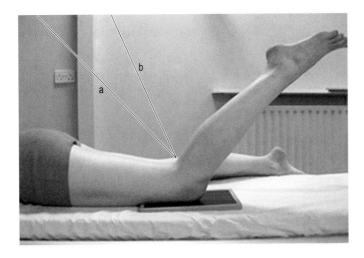

a - Beam 45° to femur
b - Beam 65° to femur

Figure 9.5 Intercondylar notch – method 2

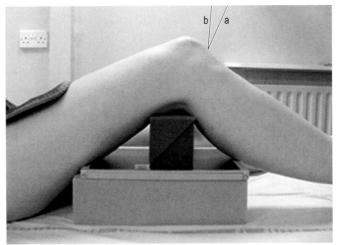

a - Beam 90° to tibia
b - Beam 110° to tibia

Figure 9.6 Intercondylar notch – method 3

Beam direction and FFD

1. Initially vertical, the central beam is angled cranially until at 90° to the long axis of tibia. This will demonstrate the whole of the notch, with the exception of the anterior aspect

2. Initially vertical, the central beam is angled until at 110° to the long axis of the tibia. This will demonstrate the anterior aspect of the notch

100 cm FFD

Accurate estimation of angulation can be achieved by initially positioning the tube housing or light beam housing parallel to the long axis of the tibia, then checking the angulation indicator on the unit before adding the required angulation to this reading.

Centring point

Immediately below the apex of the patella

Collimation

Femoral and tibial condyles

Criteria for assessing image quality

- Femoral and tibial condyles are included in the image
- Patella is cleared above the intercondylar notch
- Patella is central between the femoral condyles
- Tubercles of the intercondylar eminences of tibia are visualised
- Tibiofemoral joint space should be clear
- *For the whole notch:* the notch should be seen as tunnel or 'n' shaped, with almost vertical lateral margins and an arched roof
- *For the anterior aspect of the notch:* the notch is shallower than required for the full notch, rather like an inverted 'v' with sloped lateral margins and narrow roof
- Sharp image demonstrating the soft tissue in the notch in contrast with the adjacent bone, intercondylar eminences and any loose bodies

Common error	Possible reason
Patella superimposed over notch	Beam angle not correctly set in relation to tibia (too much cranial angle in PA projections, methods 1 and 2; not enough cranial angulation in method 3, AP projection) Incorrect flexion can also cause this

PATELLA

Posteroanterior (PA) patella (Fig. 9.7A,B)

Although the PA is the preferred method for the patella projection, as it is in close contact with the image receptor, the patient may not be able to achieve the PA position (due to injury or patient condition). In these cases a satisfactory image can be obtained by positioning the patient as for an AP knee projection, with a 10 kVp increase on exposure factors. Consideration to increasing the FFD must be given to compensate for the relatively large object image receptor distance.

Positioning

If used, an 18 × 24 cm cassette is placed on the table-top.

- The patient lies prone on the table with their legs extended and the affected patella in contact with the image receptor
- The affected patella is placed centrally on the cassette, if one is used
- The unaffected leg is separated from that under examination to clear it from the radiation field
- A lead rubber apron is worn to protect the abdomen and pelvis
- The leg is rotated to align the patella between the femoral condyles and a small pad is placed under the tibia to prevent rotation of the leg

Beam direction and FFD

Vertical central beam, at 90° to the image receptor
100 cm FFD

Centring point

In the middle of the of the crease of the knee

Collimation

Femoral and tibial condyles, knee joint, surrounding soft tissues

Criteria for assessing image quality

- Distal third of femur, proximal third of tibia, head of fibula, patella and soft tissue outlines should all be demonstrated
- Patella is centralised over the femur
- Head of fibula should appear slightly obscured by tibia
- Shafts of tibia and fibula should be separated
- Sharp image demonstrating the bony cortex and trabeculae of patella in contrast with the femur

a suspected fracture of the patella, as in the case of a transverse fracture, because the fragments can be further separated and thus exacerbate the effects of injury. However, if the patient presents with some flexion of the knee, method 3 may be considered.

There are several methods for achieving this projection and three will be described here. Method 1 is the preferred method since the central ray is not directed directly towards the gonads. In method 2, although the main beam is not directly towards the patient's abdomen, it is still aimed in the direction of the trunk. Method 3 is commonly described with the patient seated and supporting the image receptor themselves.[1,5,7,8] However, where the patient is supine[9] and a portable cassette holder is used, not only will greater radiation protection be achieved for the patient, i.e. the main beam will not be directed at the patient's torso and towards the patient's fingers, but the risk of movement unsharpness from the patient holding the image receptor will be removed. In all cases the patient should wear a lead rubber apron for radiation protection.

To demonstrate the lateral movement of the patella if subluxation is suspected the projection can be performed with the knee at varying angles of flexion, e.g. 30°, 60° and 90°.[10]

If used, an 18 × 24 cm cassette is selected.

Positioning

Method 1 (Fig. 9.8A,B)

- The patient lies in the prone position with the image receptor placed under the knee of the leg to be examined
- The unaffected leg is separated from the leg under examination, to clear it from the radiation field
- The knee is flexed through 60° and immobilised with the use of a bandage around the ankle; this is held by the patient. Alternatively, radiolucent pads and sandbags may be placed under the lower leg for support (although a significant depth of pad would be required for this)
- The patella is centralised over the femur

Method 2 (Fig. 9.9)

- The patient lies on the side under examination with knee flexed through approximately 75°
- The unaffected leg is cleared backwards, away from the leg under examination, to clear it from the radiation field
- The patient's arms are used as support
- Using a portable cassette holder, place the image receptor in the vertical position on the table, tube side in contact with the lower end of the femur and at 90° to the long axis of the patella, or support using pads and sandbags

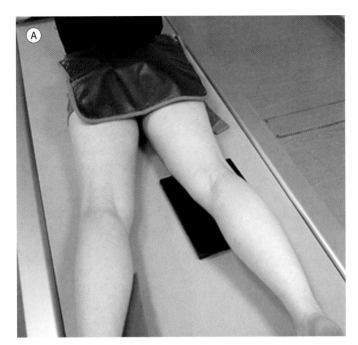

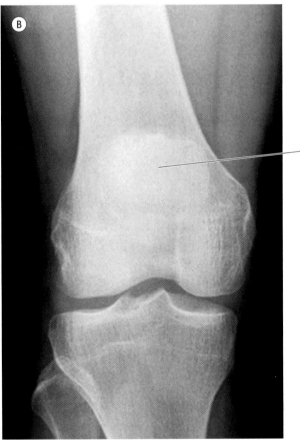

Patella

Figure 9.7   PA patella

Inferosuperior patella

This projection is often undertaken to evaluate the patellofemoral joint in an orthopaedic assessment prior to and post knee surgery. It must not be attempted if there is

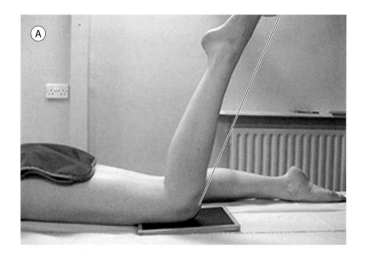

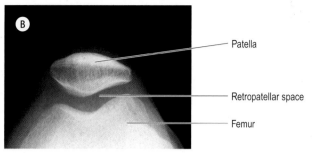

Figure 9.8 **(A)** Inferosuperior patella – method 1;
(B) inferosuperior patella

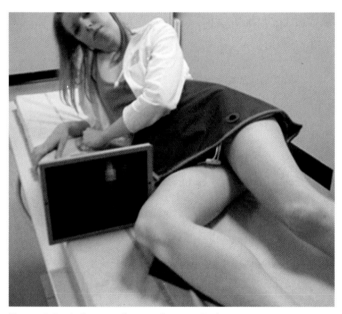

Figure 9.9   Inferosuperior patella – method 2

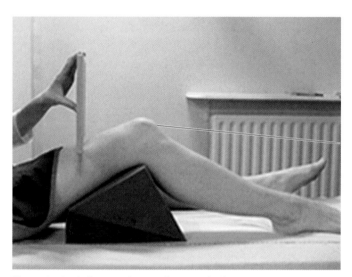

Figure 9.10   Inferosuperior patella – method 3

Method 3 (Fig. 9.10)

• The patient lies supine on the table with the affected knee flexed through 60°
• The unaffected leg is separated from the leg under examination, to clear it from the radiation field
• The image receptor is supported vertically in the portable holder, its lower edge in contact with the lower end of the femur and at 90° to the long axis of the patella (the tube side of the image receptor is towards the knee and feet)
• If no holder is available the image receptor must be supported by the patient but this presents with increased radiation dose, especially to the trunk and hands. There is also increased potential for movement unsharpness and distortion of image if the patient does not maintain the correct relationship of the image receptor to patella

Beam direction and FFD

Method 1: Vertical, directed cranially (approximately 15°) to coincide with the long axis of the patella
100 cm FFD
Method 2: Horizontal, at 90° to the image receptor and to coincide with the long axis of the patella
Method 3: Horizontal, directed cranially up to approximately 15° and to coincide with the long axis of the patella

Centring point: all methods

Immediately below (behind) the apex of the patella

Collimation

Patellofemoral joint space, articular surfaces of the femur, anterior surface of the patella, surrounding soft tissues

Criteria for assessing image quality

• Patella is projected clear from the femoral condyles for a clear view of the patellofemoral joint space

- Sharp image demonstrating the joint space and surrounding soft tissues, in contrast with the bony cortex and trabeculae of patella

FEMUR

The femur has a wide variation in subject contrast from the hip joint, through the shaft and down to the knee joint; therefore, to reduce this wide subject contrast it is advisable to use a kVp of at least 75.

The increasing size of the population, particularly in the western world,[11] has not been reflected in the availability of significantly larger image receptor sizes and, unfortunately, average limb length has been seen to have increased even more than trunk length. This has implications for radiographic examination of the femur, which ideally should have only one exposure per projection, with the entire femur from hip to knee included. In reality, limitations of image receptor space very often requires the radiographer to provide images of the upper and lower femur on two, overlapping images of the same projection.

Cassettes remain at a maximum 35 × 43 cm in size but some digital image receptors do now have an increased maximum size, to 43 cm². Despite there being no increase in size beyond the 43 cm dimension, there will be increased space for the femoral length on the 43 cm² receptor if it is positioned across the diagonal, compared to the space available across the diagonal of the 34 × 43 cm cassette. Simple mathematical calculation of the length of the diagonal in the 43 cm² receptor shows it to be 60.8 cm, compared to 55 cm in the case of the 35 × 43 cm cassette, although it must be noted that this only relates to the extreme measurement from corner to corner. Until more digital plates of larger dimensions are in more regular use, it is likely that making two exposures of the same projection (one of the upper femur and one of the lower femur) will remain as the norm.

If the femur is too long for inclusion on one image, it must be noted that the leg should remain in the same position for both images used for the same projection, to assess the rotation of any fracture, and there should be overlap of the mid shaft of the femur on each image. Follow-up images taken for orthopaedic assessment only require demonstration of the fracture site and associated or nearest joint (unless there is a surgical prosthesis or pin present), thus reducing the radiation exposure to one projection for these assessments.

Radiation protection is an essential consideration and the 28-day rule should be applied when the whole femur is to be demonstrated. Gonad protection is also essential and careful positioning of this, to avoid covering the hip joint or upper femoral shaft, will prevent unnecessary repeats.

If it is considered that the gonad protection available may exclude part of the required information on the lateral projection then it may be excluded for the upper end of the femur but should always be used for the lower end of the femur.

If used, an 18 × 43 cm cassette is used lengthwise to coincide with the length of the femur for the AP and lateral positions

or

a 35 × 43 cm cassette or 43 cm² digital receptor is used, with the femur positioned across the diagonal for the AP and lateral positions. This will allow the maximum amount of leg length to be demonstrated

AP femur (Fig. 9.11A,B,C)

Positioning

- The patient lies supine on the table with their legs extended
- The posterior aspect of the femur under examination is placed in contact with the image receptor and positioned to include the hip and knee joint if possible. If this is not possible, ensure that the knee is included if the lower two-thirds of the femur is required (Fig. 9.11A). If the upper third is required, the hip joint should be included
- The unaffected leg is separated from the leg under examination, to clear it from the radiation field
- The leg is internally rotated approximately 15° to bring the femur into the true AP position and the neck of the femur parallel to the image receptor
- A lead rubber apron is applied to the lower abdomen for radiation protection

Beam direction and FFD
Vertical at 90° to the image receptor
100 cm FFD

Centring point
Mid shaft, on the anterior aspect of the femur*

Collimation
Knee and hip joints, surrounding soft tissues*
*Note that the asterisked sections will require consideration for amendment if two images of the projection are required, when femoral length dictates this. Realistically, the *central ray* can be considered to be in the middle of the area covered by the image receptor space.

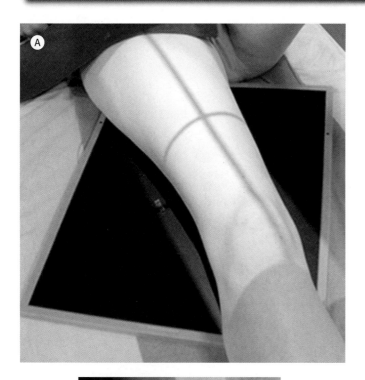

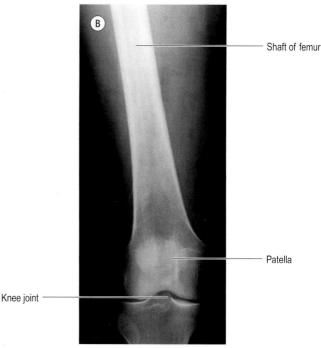

Shaft of femur

Patella

Knee joint

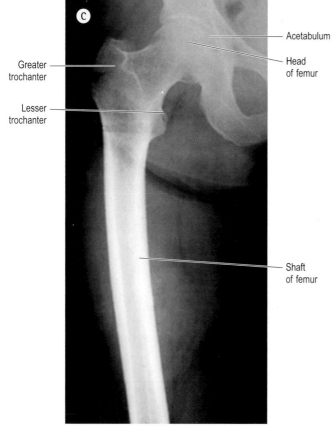

Acetabulum

Head of femur

Greater trochanter

Lesser trochanter

Shaft of femur

Figure 9.11 **(A)** AP lower femur; **(B)** AP lower femur **(C)** AP upper femur. (B) and (C) Reproduced with permission from Bryan GJ. Skeletal anatomy. 3rd edn. Edinburgh: Churchill Livingstone; 1996 and Gunn C. Bones and joints. 4th edn. Edinburgh: Churchill Livingstone; 2002

Criteria for assessing image quality

- Knee and hip joints, patella and all the soft tissue outlines should be demonstrated (or the area intended for inclusion if the whole femur cannot be included on the image receptor)

- Greater trochanter should be seen in profile on the lateral aspect of the upper femur and cleared from the neck
- Lesser trochanter, if included, should be seen on the medial aspect of the femur

- Sharp image demonstrating the soft tissue margins, bony cortex and trabeculae of femur, care should be taken in kVp selection to reduce the inherent contrast in the femur

Common errors	Possible reasons
Both joints not demonstrated	Inaccurate assessment of adequacy of receptor size *or* Image receptor not positioned accurately
Greater trochanter overlaps neck of femur	Inadequate internal rotation of leg

Lateral femur (Fig. 9.12A,B,C)

Positioning

- From the AP position the patient is rotated onto the side under examination with the opposite leg placed behind them, on the table-top

- With the knee and hip slightly flexed, the image receptor is placed under the lateral aspect of the femur and is positioned to include the hip and knee joint if possible. If this is not possible, ensure that the knee is included if the lower two-thirds of the femur is required (Fig. 9.12A). If the upper third is required, the hip joint should be included
- The femoral condyles are superimposed and a sandbag is placed under the ankle joint to help facilitate this. The more the hip is flexed, the easier it becomes to rotate the patient into a lateral position
- Foam pads may also be used to aid positioning and immobilisation, as for the lateral knee projection
- A lead rubber apron is place over the lower abdomen for radiation protection

Beam direction and FFD
Vertical at 90° to the image receptor
100 cm FFD

Centring point
Mid shaft, on the medial aspect of femur*

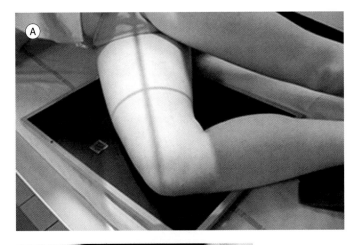

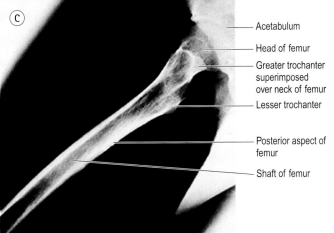

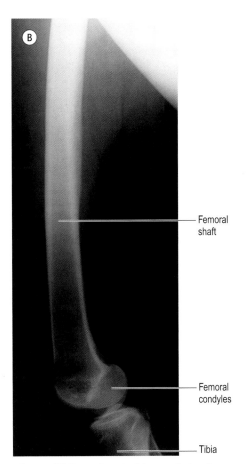

Acetabulum

Head of femur

Greater trochanter superimposed over neck of femur

Lesser trochanter

Posterior aspect of femur

Shaft of femur

Femoral shaft

Femoral condyles

Tibia

Figure 9.12 **(A)** Lateral femur; **(B)** lateral lower femur **(C)** lateral upper femur. (C) Reproduced with permission from Bryan GJ. Skeletal anatomy. 3rd edn. Edinburgh: Churchill Livingstone; 1996 and Gunn (2002).

Collimation

Hip and knee joints, surrounding soft tissues*

*As for the AP femur, these will vary according to the amount of femur that can be included on the image receptor.

Following *trauma or surgery* it may be necessary to undertake *horizontal beam lateral* projections. In either of these cases consider undertaking a horizontal beam lateral neck of the femur as described in Chapter 10 and horizontal beam lateral of the knee and lower two-thirds of the femur. To take this mediolateral approach, the opposite leg must be uninjured so that it can be raised. If this is not possible a lateromedial approach should be used for the lower two-thirds of the femur, with appropriate protection for the other leg, and a mediolateral oblique used as for the femoral neck lateral. This is described in Chapter 27 and in Figure 27.22.

Criteria for assessing image quality

- Hip, knee joint, patella and surrounding soft tissues are demonstrated, or the area intended for inclusion if the whole of the femur cannot be included on the image receptor
- Patellofemoral joint space is visualised (unless the patella is not naturally centralised on the individual patient)
- Greater trochanter is superimposed on the shaft of femur
- Lesser trochanter is seen in profile on the posterior aspect of the femur

- Sharp image demonstrating the soft tissue margins, bony cortex and trabeculae of femur; care should be taken in kVp selection to reduce the inherent contrast in the femur

References

1. Long BW, Rafert JA. Orthopaedic radiography. Philadelphia: WB Saunders; 1995.
2. Raby N, et al. Accident and emergency radiology, a survival guide. London: Saunders; 2001.
3. Radiation protection 118 Referral guidelines for imaging. European Commission Directorate-General for the Environment 2000.
4. Burnett S, et al. A–Z orthopaedic radiology. London: WB Saunders; 2000.
5. Whitley AS, et al. Clark's positioning in radiography. 12th edn. Oxford: Hodder Arnold; 2005.
6. McQuillen-Martensen K. Radiographic critique. Philadelphia: WB Saunders; 1996.
7. Eisenberg RL, et al. Radiographic positioning, 2nd edn. Boston: Little Brown and Company; 1995.
8. Bontrager KL. Textbook of radiographic positioning and related anatomy, 5th edn. St Louis: Mosby; 2001.
9. Bontrager KL, Lampignano JP. Textbook of radiographic positioning and related anatomy. 6th edn. St Louis: Mosby; 2005.
10. Unett EM, Royle AJ. Radiographic techniques and image evaluation. London: Nelson Thornes; 1997.
11. Cole TJ. Secular trends in growth. Nutrition Sociology 2000; 59(2):317–324.

CHAPTER 10

PELVIS AND HIPS

Linda Williams

Radiographic examination of the pelvis and hips must be undertaken with care as the region surrounds the radiosensitive reproductive organs. Gonad protection should be used in all cases and should be correctly positioned (Figs 10.1A,B); an exception is made when examining the female pelvis in trauma, for an initial examination of a child, or when there is a non-specific region of pain in the first examination. The 28-day rule should always be used in females of reproductive capacity, when examining this area.

INDICATIONS

The pelvis and hips may be examined for the following reasons:

Multiple myeloma
Osteolytic lesions may occur in the pelvis and the pelvis may be examined as part of a skeletal survey, although radionuclide imaging plays a greater role in this instance.

Osteoarthritis
The hip joints may degenerate due to this condition but radiographic examination should only be performed if the patient is likely to require hip replacement.[1]

Trauma
The pelvis and hips are commonly examined in the event of trauma; this is most likely to establish if a fracture or dislocation has occurred.

Since the pelvis consists of three bony rings, the main pelvic ring and the two secondary rings formed from the pubic and ischial bones, it is important to remember that a fracture of such a bony ring is usually associated with a fracture elsewhere in the ring (contra coup fracture).

Perthes
A disorder of the upper femoral epiphysis, this manifests as osteonecrosis of the capital femoral epiphysis.[2] This is where the growing epiphysis shows ischaemic changes. It presents most commonly in children aged 4–9 years and boys are four times more likely to be affected than girls.[3]

Slipped upper femoral epiphysis (SUFE)
The epiphysis is displaced, usually medially and posteriorly. The patient often presents with spontaneous pain in the groin. Thirty percent of patients suffering from this are obese and the condition is possibly related to hormonal imbalance.[3]

Anteroposterior (AP) pelvis and hips (Fig. 10.2A,B,C)

There are two methods for producing the AP pelvis, the first demonstrates the full pelvis and hip joints, whilst the second is required for hips only. This second projection is usually requested for follow up following hip replacement surgery and is often referred to as a 'low centred' pelvis. However it is a recognised projection and has been described in texts for many years.[4,5] Radiographers should not, therefore, assume that this is simply a 'mis-centred pelvis' and consider it to be a suboptimal procedure. Suggested image receptor size is as for the pelvis and hips AP, as it is often necessary to include a longer section of the femur to ensure the whole length of hip prosthesis is demonstrated (if relevant).

Both examinations are performed using a 43 cm^2 or 35 × 43 cm image receptor placed in the bucky transversely.

Positioning
- The patient lies supine on the table with their legs extended and their head resting on a pillow
- The median sagittal plane (MSP) is at 90° to the table-top and the anterior superior iliac spines (ASISs) should be equal distance from the table-top

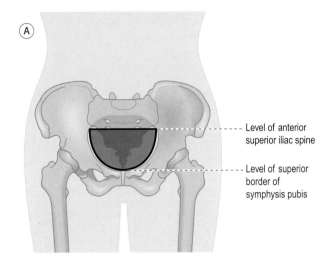

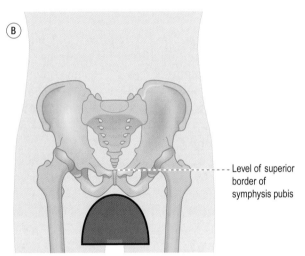

Figure 10.1   Position for gonad protection for **(A)** female patient and for **(B)** male patient

- The arms are raised onto the pillow
- The legs are slightly internally rotated to bring the necks of femora parallel to the table-top
- Gonad protection is applied if appropriate. Exceptions are when examining the female pelvis in trauma, for a first examination of a child, or when there is a non-specific region of pain in the first examination

For this projection both feet are internally rotated slightly during positioning to bring them into the true anatomical position and allow the neck of femur (NOF) to lie parallel to the image receptor.[4] This facilitates demonstration of the femoral neck with minimal foreshortening, and also clears the greater trochanter from the femoral neck. The lesser trochanter appears in profile medially. If the feet are excessively internally rotated the lesser trochanter will be obscured and if they are externally rotated, or even if the toes point in an upwards and vertical direction, the NOF will appear foreshortened on the resulting image, with the greater trochanter superimposed over the neck.[4]

In the case of trauma, foot position can provide an indication of a fractured NOF. The patient will present with the affected leg in noticeable external rotation, often with the lateral aspect of the foot in contact with the trolley top and apparent shortening of the leg. No attempt must be made to move this leg.[2]

A line known as Shenton's Line (Fig. 10.3) follows the curve of the upper border of the obturator foramen and continues to travel inferiorly down the medial border of the femoral neck. This line can be used as a guide to compare both sides when checking for injury, as a disruption in the normally smooth, curved line indicates subluxation, dislocation or change in femoral neck position as a result of fracture.

Overexposure of the greater trochanters can be a problem in this projection, particularly in thin patients who have little soft tissue in this region. This can be resolved by careful consideration of exposure factors; a reduction in mAs will reduce the degree of film blackening, and to cater for this a kVp of at least 70 will reduce the level of subject contrast.[4] It is suggested that a minimum of 70 kVp is used in all AP pelvis examinations.

Some patients will present with a body shape which is relatively slim over the legs and hip joint but is larger over the pelvis and abdomen. This shape appears to most frequently occur in the elderly female patient group and can pose a problem for production of an image with a useful range of densities. Selection of kVp even higher than 70 may be useful in these cases, as the central region of the pelvis may appear underexposed when the hips appear correctly exposed (and vice versa) on the image when insufficient kVp is used.

Beam direction and focus film distance (FFD)

Vertical at 90° to the image receptor

115 cm FFD

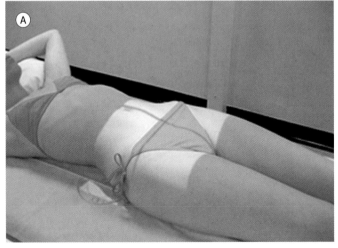

Figure 10.2   **(A)** AP position – pelvis and hips

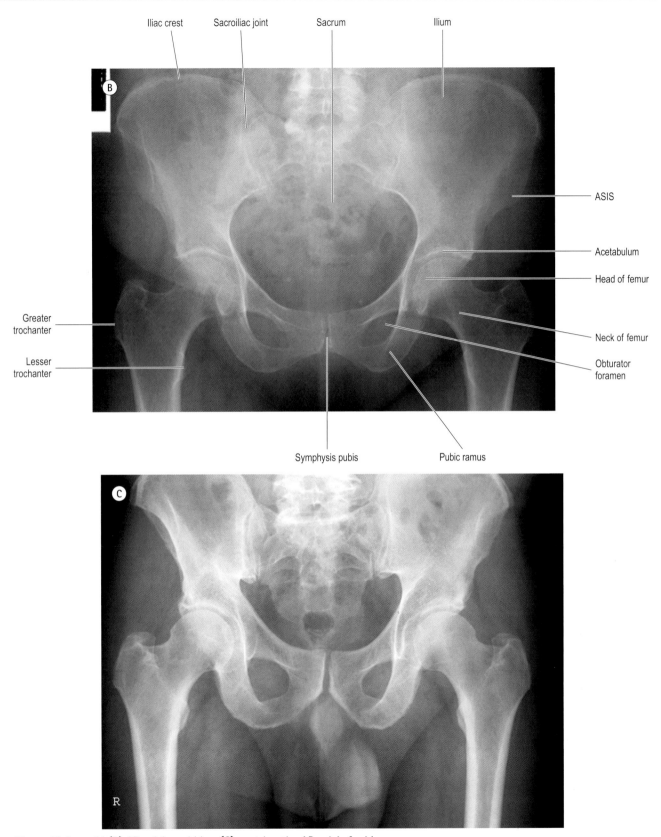

Figure 10.2 cont'd (B) AP pelvis and hips; (C) centring the AP pelvis for hips

Figure 10.3 Shenton's line

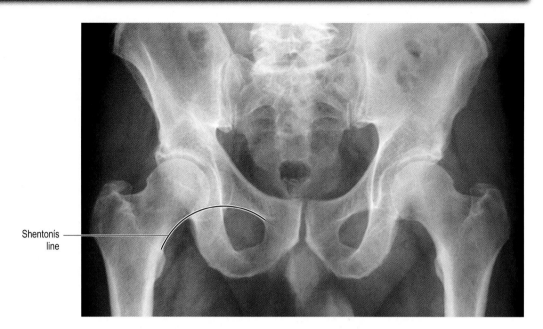

Shentonís
line

Note that the FFD suggested is longer than the traditional 100 cm used for the majority of radiographic projections. The buttocks elevate the pelvis, which is a relatively large structure, thus increasing OFD and magnification of the pelvis. Potentially the larger pelvis will be less likely to be included within the perimeter of the image receptor; to overcome this, increasing the FFD reduces this magnification and improves on image sharpness.

Those patients with a noticeably larger amount of adipose tissue will, in effect, find their pelvis raised even higher above the image receptor than slimmer patients. Therefore consideration should be given to raising the FFD even higher than the 115 cm suggested.

Centring point

For the pelvis and hips: in the midline, midway between the ASIS and the upper border of the symphysis pubis

It is wise to check, while centring, that the top of the iliac crests lie within the upper border of the image receptor; this will ensure that the maximum amount of anatomy distal to the iliac crests is demonstrated on the image.

For the hips: in the midline, 2.5 cm above the superior border of the symphysis pubis (the upper border of the symphysis pubis is located level with the greater trochanters)

Collimation

For the pelvis and hips: iliac crests, proximal portion of femora, greater and lesser trochanters

The image receptor may be aligned with the X-ray beam before examining the patient and, as suggested by Unett and Royle, collimation can be adjusted at this point. This avoids the temptation to open the collimators wider than necessary when X-raying a larger than average patient.[4]

For the hips: acetabulae, greater and lesser trochanters, upper third of femur or full length of the prosthesis (if present)

If previous images are available it is recommended that they are viewed to establish the length of any surgical device that may be present in the hip/s to ensure the image receptor is positioned correctly for their inclusion.

Criteria for assessing image quality

- Iliac crests and greater and lesser trochanters are demonstrated for full pelvis, acetabulae, trochanters and appropriate amount of femur for the hips only
- Iliac bones, heads and necks of femora and the greater and lesser trochanters and obturator foramina should be symmetrical
- Sharp image demonstrating the range of densities of the bony cortex and trabeculae of the pelvis and its soft tissues, hips and trochanters

Common errors	Possible reasons
Asymmetry of structures	MSP not 90° to table-top (rotated patient) This could be due to muscular atrophy or simply the patient lying awkwardly. Use of radiolucent pads may help correct this in the case of muscular atrophy
Greater trochanters obscured and overlying the NOF	Feet are not internally rotated (this is unavoidable on patients with fractured NOF)

Common errors (*cont'd*)	Possible reasons (*cont'd*)
Overexposed image (see section after positioning, for overexposure of the greater trochanters and uneven exposure of hips and pelvis)	If an automatic exposure device has been used for a patient with hip prostheses the exposure will continue for longer than necessary to try and expose the hips. Setting a manual exposure will prevent this

AP single hip (Fig. 10.4A,B)

If used, a 24 × 30 cm cassette is placed longitudinally in the table bucky.

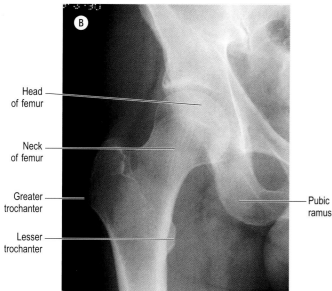

Figure 10.4   AP single hip

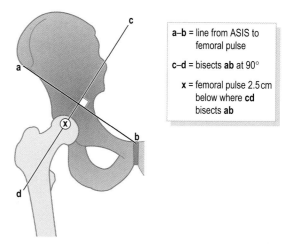

a–b = line from ASIS to femoral pulse

c–d = bisects **ab** at 90°

x = femoral pulse 2.5 cm below where **cd** bisects **ab**

Figure 10.5   Location of femoral pulse

Positioning

- Initial positioning is as for the AP pelvis
- The leg of the side under examination is slightly internally rotated to bring it into the true anatomical position
- The unaffected leg is abducted to clear it from the radiation field
- Gonad protection is applied and should be clear from the hip joint

Beam direction and FFD

Vertical at 90° to image receptor
100 cm FFD

Centring point

Over the femoral pulse

The femoral pulse (and therefore the centre of the head of femur) is located thus: draw an imaginary line from the ASIS to the upper border of the symphysis pubis; bisect this line perpendicularly, and then locate a point 2.5 cm distally along this bisecting line (Fig. 10.5).

Collimation

ASIS, greater and lesser trochanters, proximal third of femur

Criteria for assessing image quality

- ASIS, proximal third of the femur and trochanters are demonstrated
- Greater trochanter is seen cleared from and laterally to the NOF, and slightly in profile
- Lesser trochanter is visible on the medial aspect of the femur
- Obturator foramen is seen 'open' and not obscured by the ischium
- Sharp image demonstrating the soft tissue margins, bony cortex and trabeculae of the distal ilium, ischium and proximal femora whilst demonstrating the greater trochanter

Common errors	Possible reasons
Length of hip prosthesis not fully demonstrated	Inaccurate centring or presence of prosthesis not known or considered. Ensure previous images are available to view and if necessary, use a larger image receptor or field
Greater trochanter obscured and overlying the NOF	Lack of internal rotation
Overexposed image	See relevant italicised section under AP pelvis above, for overexposure of the greater trochanters and use of automatic exposure chambers (AECs) for patients with hip replacement

Lateral oblique for both hips ('frog lateral')
(Fig. 10.6A,B)

This projection is usually undertaken on children when investigating both hips for conditions such as Perthes' disease or SUFE and must not be used in the case of trauma. If cassettes are used, size selected will depend on the size of the child but it is placed transversely in the table bucky (if child size dictates), as for adult AP hips. The use of a grid is not necessary for children under the age of about 9 years (clearly depending on their size and weight) and the exposure factors can be reduced significantly from those given for the adult pelvis, hence reducing the radiation dose to the child. This projection is usually undertaken in conjunction with an AP pelvis, therefore gonad protection should be applied for at least one of the images, even if it is a first examination (usually the AP pelvis for ease of positioning).

Positioning
- Initial positioning is as for the AP pelvis projection
- The knees and hips are flexed and knees and hips are externally rotated
- The plantar aspects of the feet are placed together and rotation of the legs continued until through approximately 60° (femoral shafts at 30° to the table-top)
- The legs are supported with radiolucent pads under their lateral aspects
- Gonad protection is applied

Beam direction and FFD
Vertical at 90° to the image receptor
100 cm FFD

Centring point
1–2.5 cm above the middle of the upper border of the symphysis pubis (varying according to child size) or position a cassette with its upper border level with the ASIS and centre to the middle of the cassette

Collimation
ASISs, greater and lesser trochanters

Criteria for assessing image quality
- ASISs, proximal thirds of femora and trochanters are demonstrated
- Iliac bones, heads and necks of femora and obturator foramina should appear symmetrical
- Greater trochanters are superimposed over the necks of femora
- Lesser trochanters are in profile on the medial aspects of the shafts of femora
- Sharp image demonstrating bony cortex and trabeculae of the head and neck of femur and surrounding soft tissues

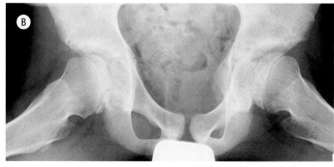

Figure 10.6 (A) Frog lateral position; (B) frog lateral hips

Common errors	Possible reasons
Asymmetry of structures	Rotation – note that the pelvis is not stable when in this position. Care should be taken in the initial stages to ensure stability with radiolucent foam pads to support the legs
Hyperdense area over the hip/s, increasing distally over the femoral shaft/s. Foreshortened femoral neck/s; the greater trochanter not superimposed over the neck of femur	Inadequate external rotation of the legs. This is often caused by inadequate flexion of the knees; good knee flexion facilitates more comfortable external rotation

Lateral oblique single hip (Fig. 10.7A,B)

This projection must not be used in the case of trauma and is usually performed to supplement an AP pelvis when examining patients with non-specific hip pain. However, its use is rarely justified since information gained is not significantly greater than that found on the AP hip projection.

If used, a 24 × 30 cm cassette is placed longitudinally in the table bucky.

Positioning
- Initial positioning is as for the AP pelvis projection
- The MSP is 90° to the table; from this position the patient is rotated laterally through 45° onto the side under examination and supported in this position with foam pads
- The knee and hip are flexed and externally rotated to bring the lateral aspect of the thigh in contact with the table-top; the more flexion to the knee the easier the patient finds this positioning
- The arms are rested on the pillow
- Gonad protection is applied (due to patient position, care should be taken to prevent the gonad shield from slipping and therefore obscuring essential anatomical structures)

Beam direction and FFD
Vertical at 90° to the image receptor
100 cm FFD

Centring point
Over the femoral pulse (see centring for AP single hip)

Collimation
ASIS, greater and lesser trochanters, anterior and posterior soft tissue outline of the femur

If, after positioning, the long axis of the femur lies obliquely across the table-top, consider rotating the light beam diaphragm to coincide with the long axis of the femur, to enable closer collimation.

Criteria for assessing image quality
- ASIS and proximal third of femur are demonstrated
- Greater trochanter is superimposed over the NOF
- Lesser trochanter is seen in profile on the medial aspect of the upper femur
- Ischium and pubic ramus will be superimposed
- Sharp image demonstrating the bony cortex and trabeculae of the proximal femora with sufficient penetration to demonstrate the acetabulum

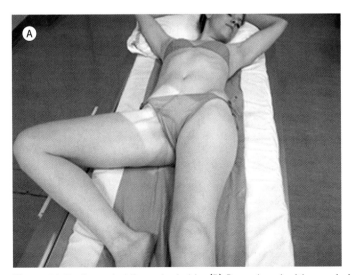
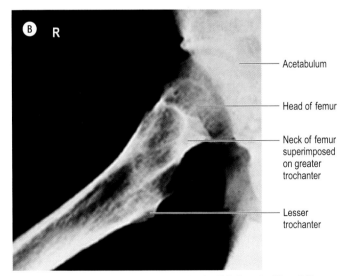

Figure 10.7   Lateral oblique single hip. (B) Reproduced with permission from Bryan GJ. Skeletal anatomy. 3rd edn. Edinburgh: Churchill Livingstone; 1996 and Gunn (2002).

Common error	Possible reason
Hyperdense area over the hip, increasing distally over the femoral shaft. Foreshortened femoral neck; the greater trochanter not superimposed over the NOF	Inadequate external rotation of the leg. This is often caused by inadequate flexion of the knee; good knee flexion facilitates more comfortable external rotation

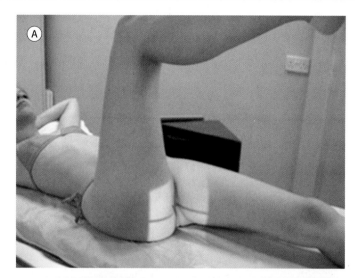

▇ Horizontal beam lateral for NOF (Fig. 10.8A,B)

This projection must always be used in cases of hip or pelvic trauma and following surgery to the hip. In these cases it is inadvisable to move the patient but a projection at 90° to the AP projection is still required. It is the most frequent lateral performed on the hip, despite being described as an adaptation to technique in most texts.

The NOF lies at 45° to the MSP and correct positioning of the image receptor, at 45° to the MSP and parallel to the NOF, will produce an image of the femoral neck at 90° to the AP hip. Positioning of the image receptor is best achieved with the use of a 45° radiolucent pad which is placed next to the patient's thigh (see positioning section).

Since the projection requires the use of a medial approach to the hip, with horizontal beam, the unaffected leg must be cleared from the primary beam. This is achieved by the use of a leg support. This support should be of a design that is radiolucent with a comfortable lower leg and foot rest. One example of this is the 'Poole' leg support (Fig. 10.9). Great consideration for the maintenance of patient dignity and comfort are essential when positioning the leg on the support, as the position can be difficult to achieve and revealing of this somewhat private area most often proves to be embarrassing for patients.

Care should be taken when selecting exposure factors, as the inherent contrast of this area is high, from the dense hip joint down to the shaft of femur. kVp chosen should be high enough to reduce this and it is suggested that the range of 75–90 kVp is used.

A 24 × 30 cm image receptor is used with a stationary grid.

Positioning
Method 1 (Fig. 10.8A,B)

- The patient is supine on the A&E trolley, with the MSP perpendicular to the trolley top. The long axis of the trolley should be parallel to the ceiling track of the X-ray tube
- The MSP should also be coincident with the long axis of the trolley or parallel to the ceiling track of the X-ray tube if the patient is lying obliquely on the trolley

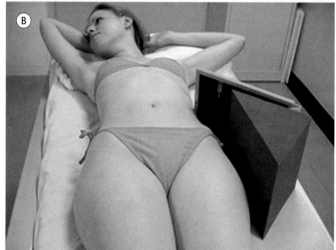

Figure 10.8   **(A)** Horizontal beam lateral for NOF – method 1; **(B)** cassette position for horizontal beam lateral hip

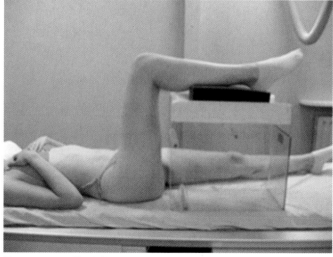

Figure 10.9   'Poole' leg support

Method 2 (Fig. 10.10A,B)

- The X-ray tube is positioned next to the unaffected side, its light beam housing directed horizontally towards the patient
- The trolley is rotated to bring the leg on the patient's unaffected side nearer to the X-ray tube, until the patient's MSP is at 45° to the beam

Both methods

- The image receptor is placed horizontally in a lateral holder. The upper edge of the image receptor is adjacent to, and gently pushed into, the soft tissues immediately above the iliac crest on the affected side; it is then positioned at 45° to the MSP and parallel with the NOF
- The use of a 45° foam pad next to the patient aids in correct assessment of receptor angle for this positioning
- The holder is then adjusted to ensure the image receptor and grid are pressed firmly down onto the mattress; this prevents the ischial tuberosity being omitted from the image

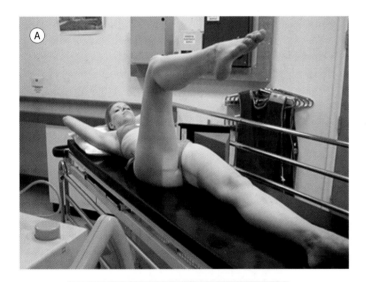

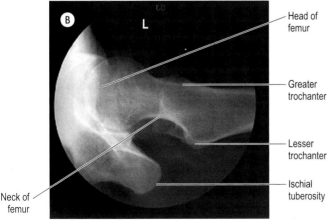

Neck of femur — Head of femur — Greater trochanter — Lesser trochanter — Ischial tuberosity

Figure 10.10 **(A)** Horizontal beam lateral for NOF – method 2; **(B)** horizontal beam lateral. (B) Reproduced with permission from Ballinger & Frank (2003)

- A leg support is placed on the table-top and the unaffected leg is flexed at the knee and hip to bring the anterior aspect of the femur as close to the trunk as possible (and at least into the vertical position to prevent super-imposition of the thigh on the image)
- The ankle and foot are placed on the leg support. The greater the knee flexion, the more effective the clearance of the thigh from the hip under examination. If the patient's condition permits slight external rotation of the opposite limb, this will clear the soft tissues of this thigh even more efficiently

Beam direction and FFD
Horizontal at 90° to the image receptor (the tube will require 45° rotational adjustment to achieve this in method 1)
100 cm FFD

Centring point
To the middle of crease of the internal and medial aspect of the groin of the affected leg

Collimation
Acetabulum, proximal femur, trochanters, anterior and posterior soft tissue outlines

Criteria for assessing image quality
- Head of femur and acetabulum clearly demonstrated
- Greater trochanter superimposed on neck of femur
- Lesser trochanter superimposed inferiorly on greater trochanter
- Soft tissue shadowing of raised thigh cleared from head and neck of femur
- Ischial tuberosity demonstrated posteriorly
- Sharp image demonstrating the soft tissue margins of the thigh, bony cortex and trabeculae of the head neck and proximal femur. The kVp chosen should be sufficient to demonstrate the acetabulum and head of femur but the femoral neck should not be overpenetrated.

Common errors	Possible reasons
The acetabulum and joint space not clearly demonstrated (dense soft tissue shadow overlying area)	The soft tissues of the opposite leg have obscured the area of interest and the exposure used was insufficient to penetrate them. Flex the knee and hip of the opposite leg to a greater degree
Part of the image has grid cut off	The grid is either not in a vertical position or the central ray is not at 90° to the grid

Common errors (cont'd)	Possible reasons (cont'd)
The acetabulum and joint space are clearly demonstrated but the NOF is overexposed	Incorrect exposure factors have been chosen, consider using a higher kVp and reducing the mAs or using a filter
The image appears very grey and it is difficult to distinguish features	The collimation is insufficient and too much scattered radiation has reached the film or receptor. Collimate more closely and consider the use of lead rubber sheets over the patient's anterior aspect of the thigh

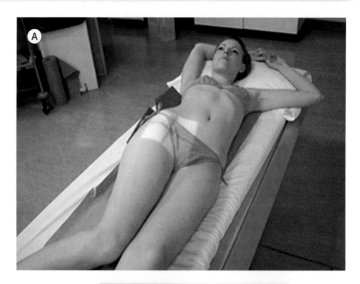

ACETABULUM

Acetabular fractures carry significant clinical sequelae but are difficult to assess in some cases, for example when the femoral head has pushed through the acetabulum but sprung back by the time the radiograph is taken, leaving only subtle soft tissue signs.[6] Reports show that as much as 57% of acetabular fractures are missed on plain film radiography and it is advisable to use computed tomography (CT) to accurately assess existence, nature and extent of an injury to the acetabulum.[7] To some degree the extent of the injury can be established if the appropriate plain radiographic obliques of the acetabulum are undertaken.

The techniques described here are sometimes referred to as Judet obliques, first described by the brothers Judet in 1964;[2] they are also referred to as 'acetabulum en-face' and 'profile' in Unett and Royle.[4] The projections, if taken in conjunction with an AP pelvis, allow for a more complete assessment of the acetabulum. Both obliques are necessary for a complete examination.

If used, 24 × 30 cm cassettes are placed longitudinally in the table bucky.

Acetabulum posterior rim/obturator oblique position (Fig. 10.11A,B)

Positioning
- The patient lies supine on the table with their legs extended and their head resting on a pillow
- Initially the MSP is 90° to the table; from this position the patient's trunk is rotated through 45°, away from the side under examination
- The raised side is supported in this position with radiolucent pads
- Gonad protection is carefully applied, avoiding the area of interest

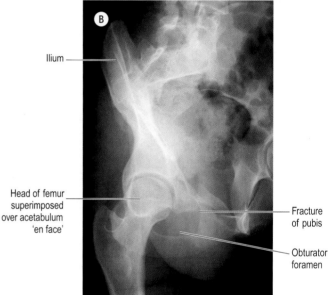

Figure 10.11   Acetabulum posterior rim/obturator oblique

Acetabulum anterior rim/iliac oblique position (Fig. 10.12A,B)

Positioning
- The patient lies supine on the table with their legs extended and their head resting on a pillow
- Initially the MSP is 90° to the table; from this position the patient's trunk is rotated through 45° towards the side under examination
- The raised side is supported in this position with radiolucent pads
- Gonad protection is carefully applied

Beam direction and FFD
Vertical at 90° to the image receptor
100 cm FFD

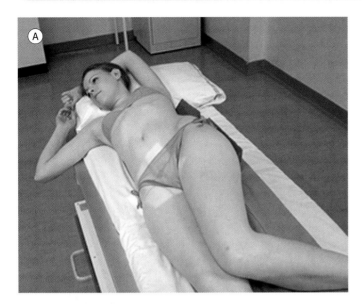

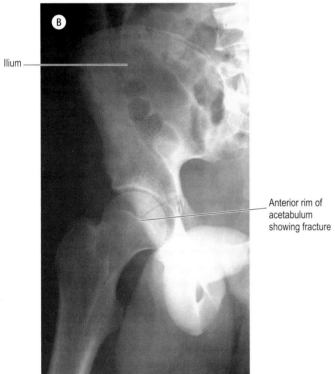

Figure 10.12   Acetabulum anterior rim/iliac oblique position

Centring point

Over the femoral pulse (Fig. 10.5)

Collimation

ASIS, ischium, pubic ramus

The obliques described should be undertaken when a complete orthopaedic assessment of the patient's pelvis has been carried out and it has been established that the pelvis is stable enough for movement. If not, and it is possible to lower the unaffected side of the pelvis, the projection for acetabulum en face can be undertaken as normal. For acetabulum in profile the patient remains in this position and the image receptor is supported vertically behind the raised side, using a horizontal central ray. Centre over the raised hip.

If injury is suspected to both acetabulae, two 35 × 43 cm image receptors may be used to examine one acetabulum in the en face position whist the opposite one is in the lateral position and vice versa. This will cut the number of exposures from four to two but, by centring in the midline, the accuracy of the resulting radiograph of each acetabulum will not be as great as performing separate, well centred projections. The central portion of the pelvis will also be irradiated when it is likely that this area would not be irradiated if four well-coned exposures were made.

If there is access to a fluoroscopy suite with transverse C-arm rotational function, the injured patient can, using a suitable patient handling aid, be moved across onto the table and be examined using this equipment. The C-arm is rotated through 45° towards either side and this will achieve the same images as described above. This technique can be used with an ordinary X-ray tube and table but problems with cross gridding arise unless the bucky can be adjusted to bring the grid slats 90° to the long axis of the table-top. Using a stationary grid will allow the grid slats to be placed in the correct direction but this method does require placement of the image receptor in a tray under the table or trolley.

Criteria for assessing image quality

Acetabulum posterior rim/obturator oblique position

- The head and neck of femur are demonstrated with the acetabulum rim outlined as a circle ('en-face')
- The posterior rim of the acetabulum is particularly well demonstrated
- The ilium is demonstrated in profile with the obturator foramen seen open
- Sharp image demonstrating the bony cortex and trabeculae of the head of femur and cortical outline of the acetabular rim

Acetabulum anterior rim/iliac oblique position

- The anterior acetabular rim is superimposed across the head of femur
- The iliac wing is seen 'en-face' and without foreshortening
- The ischial spine is demonstrated in profile medial to the acetabulum
- Sharp image demonstrating the bony cortex and trabeculae of the head of femur and cortical outline of the acetabular rim

Lateral ilium

Positioning

- As for the acetabulum posterior rim/obturator oblique position (Fig. 10.11A)

AP ilium

Positioning

- As for the acetabulum anterior rim/iliac oblique position (Fig. 10.12A)

Beam direction and FFD for both projections of the ilium

Vertical at 90° to the image receptor
100 cm FFD

Centring point

For the AP ilium: midway between the midline and the ASIS of the raised side
For the lateral ilium: over the ASIS of the raised side

Collimation

Sacroiliac joint, iliac crest, ischium, pubic ramus

Criteria for assessing image quality

AP ilium
- Iliac crest, symphysis pubis, sacroiliac joints and ASIS are demonstrated
- Ilium demonstrated 'en face' with the iliac fossa seen without foreshortening
- Obturator foramen will appear closed
- Sharp image demonstrating the bony cortex and trabecular patterns of the ilium, acetabulum and femoral head

Lateral ilium
- Iliac crest, symphysis pubis, sacroiliac joint and ASIS are demonstrated
- Ilium is demonstrated in profile
- Opening of the obturator foramen as compared to the AP pelvis
- Sharp image demonstrating the bony cortex and trabecular patterns of the ilium, pubis, acetabulum and femoral head

PELVIMETRY

The imaging examination of the maternal pelvis is known as pelvimetry. In circumstances when obstetricians need to decide if a caesarean section is required, accurate measurements of the pelvic inlet and outlet are taken and compared with the biparietal diameter of the baby's skull, which has been measured during ultrasound examination. Any cephalopelvic disproportion can then be established. The examination is usually performed around the 38th week of pregnancy when the radiation risk to the viable fetus has been reduced. In some circumstances the examination is taken after a caesarean section to establish the mother's measurements for future pregnancy and delivery.

In the last decade of the 20th century, accurate CT became the method of choice for this assessment, superseding the traditional method of plain film pelvimetry.[4] Although CT is seen as a high dose examination, CT pelvimetry involves a relatively low dose, yet accurate, technique when compared to plain film pelvimetry. One method uses AP and lateral scanogram/scout scans to identify the fovea over the femoral heads and a single axial CT slice to take the pelvimetric measurement. Alternatively a single lateral scanogram from iliac crests down to include symphysis pubis may be used.

Use of MRI has also evolved as a pelvimetric method and has been suggested to be the method of choice for this assessment, since its use avoids exposing patient and fetus to ionising radiation.

It is clear that plain radiographic pelvimetry need not and should not be undertaken. Indeed, description of plain film pelvimetry has been purposely discontinued by some authors.[8] However, in the absence of CT or MRI, the technique described below may be used but it must be recognised that this must only be when no other measurement technique is available. No antiscatter device is required, since the method described uses an air-gap to eliminate its use; this, at least, reduces the radiation dose from plain pelvimetric techniques which use a grid. Special equipment is required for this method, to cater for support of the patient in the erect position 25 cm away from the erect image receptor.

Two methods of measurement are advocated: (1) a radioopaque ruler placed between the buttocks to coincide with the midline, allowing for actual measurements to be taken as both the ruler and the bony structures will be magnified proportionally; (2) The object to film distance is recorded on the resulting radiograph and used in conjunction with a pelvimetry chart to calculate the actual measurements.

If used, a 35 × 35 cm cassette is placed in the erect cassette holder.

Positioning

- The patient stands erect with their side against a perspex screen which is supported 25 cm from the image receptor
- The feet are separated for comfort and stability and the toes placed in alignment on the floor; equal weight is applied to each leg
- The arms are folded across the chest

- The MSP is parallel to the image receptor and the pelvis is adjusted to align the greater trochanters in the horizontal plane

Beam direction and FFD
Horizontal at 90° to the image receptor
180 cm FFD

Centring point
2.5 cm above the greater trochanter

Collimation
Iliac crest, upper femora, symphysis pubis, coccyx

The light beam diaphragm housing should be rotated through 45° to reproduce a diamond shape; this allows close collimation while still including the bony landmarks required for measurement.

Criteria for assessing image quality
- Sacral promontory, greater trochanters, symphysis pubis and sacral coccygeal junction are demonstrated
- Femoral heads should be completely superimposed
- Sharp image demonstrating the bony cortex and trabeculae of the femoral heads, the whole of the symphysis pubis in contrast with the pubic rami and the sacral promontory, and the sacrococcygeal junction in contrast with the soft tissues of the abdomen and any overlying fetal tissue

Common error	Possible reason
The femoral heads are not superimposed vertically	The patient may have one leg slightly shorter than the other, (a small wooden block placed under the shorter leg during positioning will remedy this) or the patient may be leaning sideways

References
1. Radiation protection 118 Referral guidelines for imaging. European Commission Directorate-General for the Environment 2000.
2. Long BW, Rafert JA. Orthopaedic radiography. Philadelphia: WB Saunders; 1995.
3. Burnett S, et al. A–Z of orthopaedic radiology. London: WB Saunders; 2000.
4. Unett EM, Royle AJ. Radiographic techniques and image evaluation. London: Nelson Thornes; 1997.
5. Kreel L, Paris A. Clark's positioning in radiography. 10th edn. London: Heinemann Medical Books; 1979.
6. Nicholson DA, Driscoll PA. ABC of emergency radiology. London: BMJ Publishing Group; 1995.
7. Heller M. Radiology of trauma. Berlin: Springer; 2000.
8. Bontrager K. Textbook of radiographic positioning and related anatomy. 5th edn. St Louis: Mosby; 2001.

CERVICAL SPINE

Barry Carver

REASONS FOR EXAMINATION

Trauma

Cervical spine injury is relatively common and is typically seen in association with road traffic accidents, falls from a height and sporting injuries. Most neck injuries are caused by transmission of force to the neck from force applied to the head. Consequently evidence of head or facial trauma, particularly in the comatose patient, requires 'clearing the cervical spine'.[1] The overriding concern is of damage to the spinal cord, as this may result in varying degrees of paralysis or even fatality.

The tendency in the past has been to order plain film radiography on all patients who have undergone trauma which may have involved the cervical spine, however minor. The positive yield of such examinations is extremely low, believed to be only 2.4% of almost 34 000 examinations in a recent study in Alabama.[2] Much work has been done, particularly in Canada and the USA (National Emergency X radiography Utilization Study - NEXUS:) to establish criteria for imaging referral.[3,4,5,6,7]

The clinical criteria have been reported to have the potential to reduce requests for cervical spine radiography by 12.6%.[8] This represents one in eight requests, so significant savings could be made in staff and patient time, leading to financial savings, as well as reduction in patient dose.

Between 2 and 3% of all victims of blunt trauma suffer injury to the spinal column, many of whom are young adults under the age of 40 years.[9] Damage to the spinal cord, secondary to spinal trauma and due to squeezing or shearing forces caused by displaced bone, herniated disc material, or buckling of ligaments, is an important consideration in this group of patients. Despite the fact that at least three times as many spinal column injuries occur without neurological deficit as with neurological deficit,

care must be taken and immobilisation of the cervical spine utilised until its requirement is eliminated.[10] This caution must be observed since spinal cord injury without radiographic abnormality is a well-known phenomenon, most commonly described in children.[11] In addition, hyperextension injuries of the cervical spine may injure the spinal cord without apparent damage to the spine seen on radiographs.

Another cause of spinal cord injury is the 'whiplash' injury which involves extremes of flexion and extension of the neck. This is most frequently the result of a road traffic accident. As the driver or passenger in a vehicle, and restrained by seatbelts, the patient's head might be whipped backwards if the vehicle is struck from behind. Alternatively, the vehicle may stop abruptly causing sudden forward flexion of the neck followed by forced extension. Most commonly, muscular injury is seen but in extreme circumstances quadriplegia may result from such a violent whiplash injury.[10]

As stated above, all patients whose mechanism of injury is such that injury to the spinal column is suspected should be immobilised by application of a spinal collar or similar device, until such time as the presence or absence of such injury is proven. Initial imaging must be obtained with minimal patient movement to avoid aggravation of potentially unstable injuries.

The mechanism of injury is an important consideration as symptoms of spinal injury may be masked by other distracting injuries,[12] or difficult to determine due to cranial or facial trauma.[13,14] Reliance on the mechanism of injury for referral criteria is controversial but there are specific mechanisms associated with high risk of injury, and work is ongoing in this field.[15]

Spinal clearance should, however, be achieved as promptly as possible as there is significant morbidity associated with the prolonged use of spinal immobilisation in those who have undergone significant trauma.[16]

In the cervical spine, a careful evaluation of the soft tissues may provide significant information regarding the location and extent of an injury. Even this can be the subject of debate. In adult patients it is said that the normal distance between the posterior aspect of the pharyngeal air column and the anterior vertebral margin measured at the body of C3 should be less than 7 mm,[17] however in their study Herr et al[18] quote less than 4/5 mm. The distance from the posterior aspect of the trachea to the anterior vertebral margin measured at the inferior aspect of C6 is more uniformly referred to as, 'should be less than 21 mm'.[17] An increase in these measurements is strongly indicative of the presence of a haematoma.

Such prevertebral soft-tissue haematomas are common in patients with injury to the anterior spinal column, commonly avulsion fracture or hyperextension injury.[18] Ligament damage can occur without fracture; visualisation of the prevertebral haematoma will help demonstrate the presence of such an injury, but is insensitive as a predictor of fracture or injury site.

Vertebral alignment can be demonstrated on the lateral cervical spine radiograph and is commonly assessed using examination of continuous convex lines as described below and shown in Figure 11.1.

Lines 1 and 2: The anterior and posterior spinal lines join the respective portions of the vertebral bodies.

Line 3: The spinolaminar line joins the anterior margins of the junction of the lamina and spinous processes.

Line 4: The fourth line joins the tip of the spinous processes.

Disruption of one or more of these lines can be indicative of injury. For example, if an upper vertebral body is anterior to the one below, this may be an indication of disruption of the posterior ligaments.

The cervical spine is normally lordotic in curvature; loss of lordosis has been said to be an indication of severe muscular spasm and is taken as a sign of cervical spine injury,[10] commonly seen in 'whiplash' type injuries. However, such loss of lordosis can be accentuated by neck position and may be a normal finding if the 'stiff neck' is held in a slightly flexed position during imaging. Hence it is not a reliable sign of definite injury.

Neck pain

Radiographic examination of the cervical spine is not recommended for the routine investigation of neck pain. However, cervical spine radiography may be useful where there is a history of trauma, or worsening/unresolved neurological symptoms, and in children where such pain is uncommon without a cause.[19]

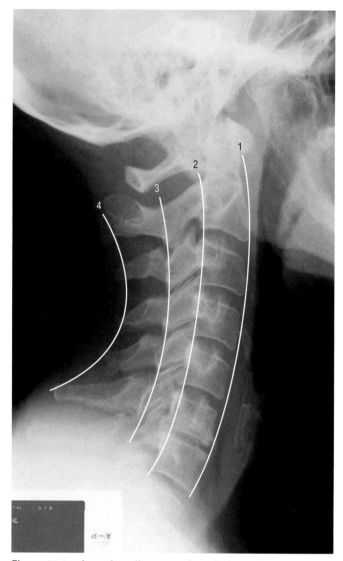

Figure 11.1   Assessing alignment of cervical vertebrae

Torticollis

This causes the neck to lie in abnormal lateral flexion with the head and neck rotated to the same side. This is usually caused following trauma by spasm in the sternocleidomastoid and trapezius muscles, and in isolation is not an indication for radiographic examination.

Degenerative disease processes

Symptoms of degenerative disease are commonly due to disk or ligamentous changes not demonstrated by plain film radiography.[19]

Rheumatoid arthritis

This can cause instability of the atlantoaxial joint. Subluxation may be demonstrated by a lateral view in flexion.[19]

Osteoarthritis

Osteoarthritis is not normally an indicator for radiography unless osteophytic impingement requires demonstration.

Neoplasia

See the 'Commonly Encountered Pathologies that affect the Skeleton' section in Chapter 4.

Congenital processes

Klippel-Feil syndrome – short neck and fused cervical vertebrae. This is not an indicator for cervical spine radiography but is seen as an incidental finding.

Cervical rib

This rib is an extra rib arising from C7. It varies in size and shape and clinical symptoms may bear little relationship to the size of the rib. Its position relative to adjacent anatomy is the determining factor for severity of symptoms. It might cause compression of the subclavian artery or the brachial plexus.

RECOMMENDED PROJECTIONS

Imaging of the cervical spine, particularly in cases of trauma, has been the subject of worldwide debate for some considerable time. Whilst the cervical spine radiograph has long been the routine method for imaging this anatomical region, imaging department protocols vary widely as to the required 'routine' series to be undertaken. More recently, computed tomography (CT) has been an additional examination for equivocal findings. The use of CT itself has been the subject of considerable debate as to its efficacy, but this has changed relatively recently due to the proliferation of helical CT equipment, and latterly with the introduction of multi-slice CT acquisition. The increased capabilities of CT allow for better image detail and hence enables the detection of injuries not seen on plain film.

However the cervical spine is still most rapidly and most commonly initially assessed with plain film examination. The NEXUS study has looked at its appropriateness for imaging and has proposed that there is no risk of cervical spine injury if their 'low risk' criteria are met, these are:

1. 'no posterior midline tenderness;
2. are not intoxicated;
3. have normal level of alertness;
4. exhibit no focal neurological deficit;
5. have no painful distracting injuries.'[4]

As previously stated, imaging department protocols vary widely. Many centres perform a three-view series: lateral C1–C7 plus AP C3–C7 and AP C1–C2 ('odontoid process or peg'/'open mouth' view); others use a two-view series, not utilising the 'open mouth' view routinely.

Unfortunately there is no consensus in the literature as to what should be used; Harris et al[20] reported that, whilst 81% of Orthopaedic Trauma Association members responding to his survey utilised the three-view series, only 31% of the National Association of Spinal Surgeons respondents did so.

Studies such as West et al[21] in 1997 compared single-view to three-view screening, finding an increase in sensitivity from 81.8% to 83.3% in a comparatively small sample. A similar study in paediatrics by Baker et al[22] found that a lateral view had a sensitivity of 79% for cervical spine injury, compared to 94% for the three-view series. MacDonald et al[23] had similar findings to West and concluded that the three-view series alone was not always sufficient for adequate diagnosis.

There are other suggestions within the literature. Holliman et al[24] suggest that the AP C3–C7 view adds little to the diagnostic ability of the series; Turetsky et al[25] suggest its replacement by 30° trauma obliques. Doris & Wilson[26] advocate the use of the AP and obliques in a routine five-view series.

A problem with inclusion of oblique views as a five-view series is the question of 'which obliques?'. Thirty degrees, as above, 60° as advocated by Abel[27], or something in between such as 45°, is a familiar suggestion in radiographic positioning texts.[28]

Daffner goes further and discusses a routine six-view series – the five-view series as discussed above (with again no mention as to the angle of obliquity) with the addition of a swimmer's view.[29] It is interesting, from the perspective of a UK radiographer, to look at his results for plain film radiography: examinations taking up to 46 minutes, with 13 radiographs being taken in one case, and 77% of patients requiring at least one repeated radiograph – standards related to radiation dose and patient care which would be unacceptable in the UK.

Following performance and evaluation of the lateral and such accessory views as may be required, the 'cervical spine series' including anteroposterior (AP), open mouth, and oblique views can then be completed, if no significant instability has been previously demonstrated.[30]

Some studies advocate the inclusion of flexion and extension radiographs in the 'routine cervical spine series' (seven-view?) but care must be taken depending on the degree of suspicion of instability. Where a small subluxation is demonstrated, significant ligamentous injuries may be revealed by flexion and extension views. However, Pollack et al[31] found that flexion and extension images failed to demonstrate any injuries not already demonstrated by other images; hence their usefulness has to be questioned.

The cost and clinical efficacy of such protocols has also been called into question by Mirvis et al.[32] They query the use of 'routine' CT for clarifying areas of uncertainty, or non-visualised areas in asymptomatic patients, finding a less than 1% positive yield and that finding was said to be a clinically unimportant injury. Careful clinical assessment of the patient is held to be more effective.

Also, information gained from the initial lateral film can be readily, if not necessarily fully, interpreted by the attending casualty doctor. This is less likely with CT examination which would require radiological interpretation. Additionally, Kaneriya et al[33] in their 1998 study, calculated that the five-view series was more cost effective in the exclusion of C7/T1 injury than CT, and that the use of CT in this area should be limited to those cases where the five-view series had failed to adequately demonstrate all required anatomy.

Nunez et al[34] found that 35% of fractures detected by CT were not seen on initial plain film radiography in the most seriously ill group of patients and that a third of these were unstable fractures, mostly located at C1/2 or C7/T1, again stressing the importance of adequate visualisation of C7. Suboptimal examinations were often found to be due to patient condition and the suggestion is that CT be included for this most seriously injured patient group.

For patients with significant cranial trauma, screening of the craniocervical junction or the entire cervical spine with helical CT scanning has also been advocated.[13] This is due to the correlation between major head injury and cervical spine injury, especially in the comatose patient.

Facial trauma, especially when sustained in road traffic accidents, has also been shown to have a correlation with cervical spine injury, and proper evaluation of the cervical spine is also required in this group.[14]

Both the groups mentioned above show the importance of distracting injuries and stress the point that, if the mechanism of injury makes a cervical spine injury likely, it must be assumed that there is an injury until proven otherwise, in order to avoid potential catastrophic effects upon the patient.

◼ Lateral cervical spine

The image receptor should be used vertically. If used, an 18 × 24 cm cassette is placed longitudinally in the erect holder. A 24 × 30 cm cassette may be used but is only necessary for *very* tall patients.

Positioning
Method 1: patient standing/sitting erect (Fig. 11.2A,B)
- The patient should be seated/standing with the lateral aspect of their shoulder resting against the image receptor
- If used, the cassette is positioned with its upper border level with the upper part of the pinna of the ear and to enable inclusion of the anterior and posterior soft tissue outlines of the neck

- The median sagittal plane (MSP) is parallel to the image receptor, with the neck extended to raise the jaw and prevent the angles of the mandible being superimposed over the vertebral bodies
- The shoulders should be relaxed and depressed as much as possible as they may obscure the lower cervical vertebrae and the cervicothoracic junction. It has been suggested that patients with broad muscular shoulders should be given a weight to hold in each hand to assist in projecting the shoulder masses below the level of C7.[28] However this is often counter-productive, as patients frequently hunch their shoulders in an attempt to hold the weights firmly whilst keeping still. This is especially likely if careful explanation of what is being attempted is not given to the patient. Exposing the radiograph on arrested expiration may help

Method 2: patient supine (Fig. 11.3)
This is a modification of method 1 to account for the change in patient position. This position is the one typically used in trauma, hence movement of the patient for the performance of this projection is contraindicated. Before attempting the examination, it is always worth checking for necklaces beneath cervical collars that should have been, but often are not, removed at initial examination of the patient.

Superimposition of the shoulders can be more problematic in this position and several methods of applying shoulder traction have been described.[35,36] The key to success is again careful explanation to the patient to achieve their cooperation; traction should be applied above the elbow joints, and slowly to prevent the patient working against the application of traction.

A 24 × 30 cm cassette is suggested for this position, to ensure that its posterior border can be positioned low enough to include the spinous processes of the cervical vertebrae.

- The trolley is positioned to ensure that the long axis of the cervical vertebrae is parallel to the wall or ceiling track of the X-ray tube
- 2 m focus film distance (FFD) is selected and the tube is centred approximately to the middle of the lateral aspect of the neck; approximate collimation to the neck should also take place at this point
- The cassette/image receptor is placed vertically at the side of the neck remote from the tube, its long axis parallel to the patient's MSP. Support for the image receptor may be via independent cassette support designed for A&E examinations, erect cassette holder as used for chest radiography, or sponge pads and sandbags
- The midpoint of the cassette, if used, should be level with the thyroid eminence

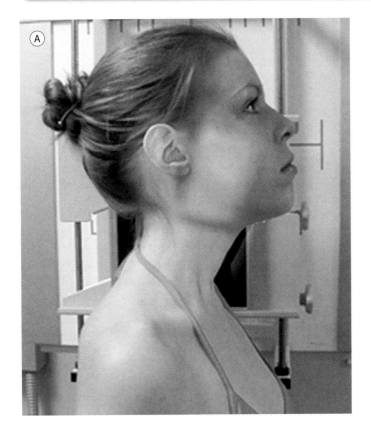

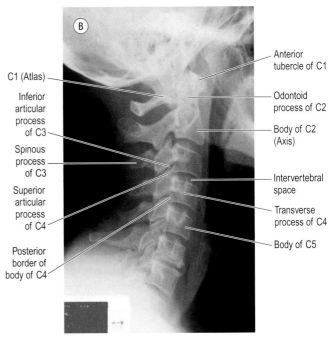

Figure 11.2   Lateral cervical vertebrae

The following labels appear on Figure 11.2:

- C1 (Atlas)
- Inferior articular process of C3
- Spinous process of C3
- Superior articular process of C4
- Posterior border of body of C4
- Anterior tubercle of C1
- Odontoid process of C2
- Body of C2 (Axis)
- Intervertebral space
- Transverse process of C4
- Body of C5

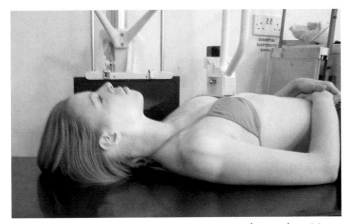

Figure 11.3   Lateral cervical vertebrae – supine (trauma) position

Beam direction and FFD: both methods

Horizontal, at 90° to the cassette

200 cm FFD – to minimise magnification caused by object film distance (OFD), which does however provide an air gap that reduces scatter reaching the image receptor

Centring point

In the middle of the neck at the level of the thyroid eminence

There are a range of centring points quoted for this examination. Fixed centring points such as '2.5 cm posterior and inferior to the angle of mandible'[37] take no account of patient size or shape and in a larger than average person would lead to the beam being centred at soft tissues anterior to C2/3.

Collimation

Atlantooccipital articulations, body of T1, cervical spinous processes, soft tissue structures of the pharynx

Soft tissues must be included, particularly in cases of trauma, where as previously discussed, changes in appearance of the soft tissues can be a strong indicator of the presence of bony injury.[17,18]

Criteria for assessing image quality

- Atlantooccipital articulations, body of T1, cervical spinous processes and soft tissue structures of the pharynx are included on the image
- Mandible should be cleared from the vertebral bodies, and the angles of the mandible in close approximation
- Left and right posterior borders of the vertebral bodies are superimposed to show no rotation
- There should be clear intervertebral joint spaces with no overlap of superior and inferior borders of vertebral bodies, to show no tilt of the cervical column
- Sharp image demonstrating soft tissue structures of the pharynx in contrast to bone and air in the trachea, detail of the bony cortex and trabeculae, the joint space between C7 and T1 and spinous processes of the cervical vertebrae

Common errors	Possible reasons
Posterior borders of the vertebral bodies not superimposed	Rotation of neck; MSP not parallel to image receptor (Accuracy in positioning may be affected if the patient is supine and immobilised)
Superior borders of the vertebral bodies not superimposed; joint spaces may be obscured	Tilt of the neck in relationship to image receptor; MSP not parallel. (Accuracy in positioning may be affected if patient is supine and immobilised)
Superimposition of the mandible over vertebral bodies	Failure to raise the chin adequately – again may be difficult in the immobilised patient
Failure to demonstrate the body of T1	Usually due to superimposition of the shoulders over the field or insufficient kVp may have been used

Bony injury can manifest in many ways; fractures of the vertebrae may be obvious or very subtle, a typical example being the 'fat C2' sign, where the body of C2 appears wider than the body of C3 on a lateral radiograph.[38] This suggests the possibility of an oblique fracture of the body of C2, which may or may not be readily apparent on the lateral radiograph.

It has been estimated that, in acute cervical spine injury, up to 33% of fractures and dislocations have been missed,[10] hence the requirement for high quality, appropriate imaging. Given this figure it is not surprising that there exists the culture of ordering radiography on all possibly neck injured patients.

The American College of Surgery and the American College of Radiology (ACR) currently recommend routine performance of lateral cervical radiographs of C1–C7 for all patients admitted following major blunt trauma.[30] Inclusion of C7 is vital, although not always easy! Unfortunately, incidence of injuries at this level has been reported as up to 30% of patients with cervical spine injury, whilst C7 is not demonstrated in some studies in up to 40% of patients on 'cross table' (horizontal beam) lateral radiographs.[10]

■ Modified projections to supplement the lateral

As previously mentioned, the cervicothoracic junction is often inadequately demonstrated on lateral projections of the cervical spine due to superimposition of the shoulders. Where it is suspected that this may be the case, traction should be applied whenever possible to assist prevention of superimposition; failure to do so inevitably results in a substandard and useless/unnecessary radiograph.

Should the body of T1 still not be demonstrated, alternatives such as the use of beam shaping filters or CT of the area should be considered. If neither are available the 'swimmers' view may be considered as a last resort. Other alternatives to this include trauma oblique projections of the cervical vertebrae, which are described later in this chapter (see Fig. 11.12A,B).

■ 'Swimmers' view of C7–T1 junction
(Fig. 11.4A,B,C)

Consideration should be given to the suitability of this projection for trauma patients due to the movements required. Visualisation of the required anatomy is poor due to the overlying structures; this is exacerbated in patients of larger build due to the significant increase in exposure factors required by the projection and their size. Scatter is also considerable. Consequently, other alternatives should be considered, such as utilisation of obliques,[25,26,27,33] or methods for moving the shoulders down and clear from the C7–T1 junction.[35,36]

The image receptor should be placed in a vertical stand, either in the bucky or used with a stationary grid as required. If used, an 18 × 24 cm cassette is placed longitudinally in the erect holder (if the patient position is erect) with an antiscatter device.

Positioning
- The patient should be seated/standing, or may be supine, with the lateral aspect of the shoulder resting against the image receptor; MSP is parallel to it
- The centre of the image receptor is level with the heads of the humeri
- Without altering the relationship of the MSP to the image receptor, the arm nearest the image receptor is raised and flexed at the elbow with the forearm resting across the top of the head
- The shoulder nearest the X-ray tube is lowered as far as possible

Beam direction and FFD
Horizontal at 90° to the cassette
100 cm FFD

Centring point
Over the superior aspect of the head of humerus on the side nearest the tube

Collimation
C6, T2, the anterior aspect of the vertebral bodies, the spinous processes

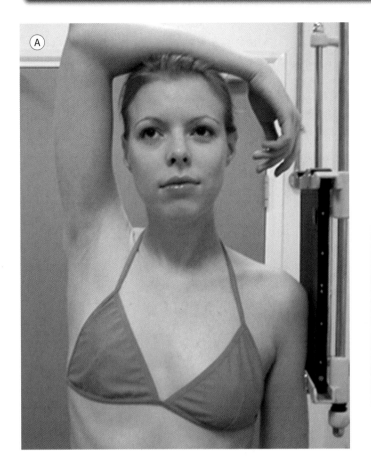

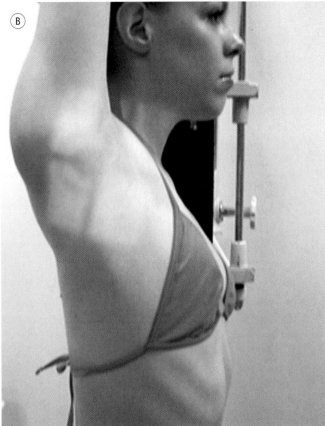

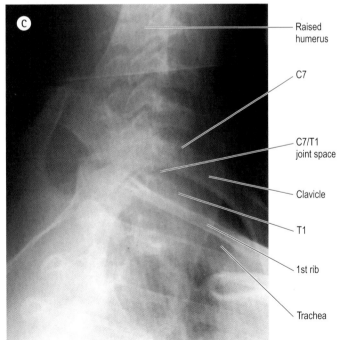

Raised humerus

C7

C7/T1 joint space

Clavicle

T1

1st rib

Trachea

Figure 11.4   (A) 'Swimmers' projection of C7/T1; (B) centring and collimation for swimmer's view; (C) swimmer's view

Criteria for assessing image quality

- C6, T2, the vertebral bodies and spinous processes are included on the image
- Right and left posterior, superior and inferior borders of the vertebral bodies are superimposed to show no rotation, or tilt
- There should be vertical separation of the right and left shoulder masses enabling visualisation of the cervicothoracic junction
- Sharp image demonstrating detail of the bony cortex and trabeculae within the vertebral bodies of C6–T2, joint space between C7 and T1 and spinous process of 7th cervical vertebra

Common errors	Possible reasons
Failure to demonstrate the cervicothoracic junction – due to under/ overexposed image	Exposure factors and their effect on image detail are the main problems in producing diagnostic radiographs of the cervicothoracic junction. This may be overcome with the use of an automatic exposure device with the centre chamber selected. Good collimation must be used to ensure correct exposure
Failure to demonstrate cervicothoracic junction – due to the humeri overlying vertebrae	The shoulders not adequately displaced – if due to patient condition – consider other investigations to demonstrate the area (commonly CT)
Low contrast 'grey' image	Strict collimation will significantly improve the quality of the image through a reduction in scatter

■ **Lateral in flexion and extension** (Fig. 11.5A,B, Fig. 11.6A,B)

This projection is used to demonstrate abnormal movements or deformities such as atlantoaxial instability, and in cases of suspected ligamentous injury when initial radiographic examination is normal, use of fluoroscopy is an alternative to the projections described below.[19]

Positioning

Principles of the technique are the same as described for the lateral projection above. The centre of the image receptor is coincident with the middle of the neck, with the long axis of the cassette parallel to the long axis of the

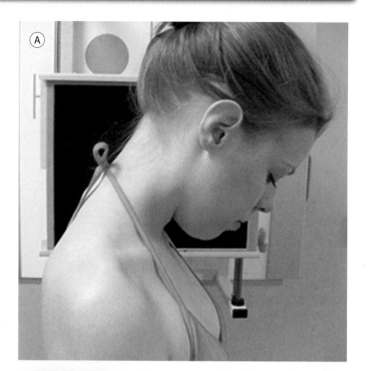

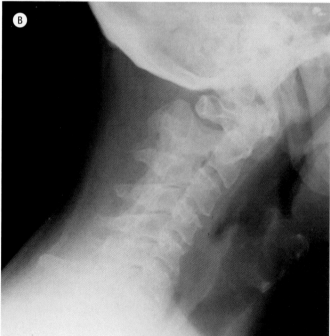

Figure 11.5   (A) Neck in flexion; (B) C-spine in flexion

neck. For flexion the image receptor is most suitably orientated horizontally in the holder and extension with it vertically.

Two exposures are made, one with the neck in full flexion and one with the neck in full extension; the degree of movement will be determined by patient condition and clinical indications and should take place under medical

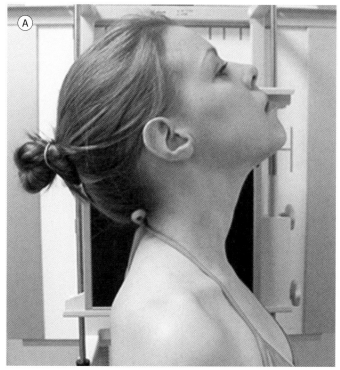

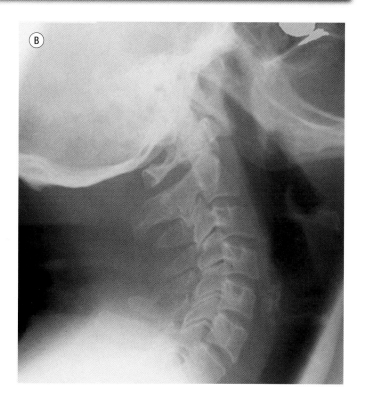

Figure 11.6 **(A)** Neck in extension; **(B)** C-spine in extension

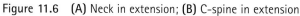

supervision as required. The movements should not be forced and will be limited by the patient. This may be uncomfortable for the patient so the position should be maintained for as short a time as possible.

Beam direction and FFD
Horizontal, at 90° to the cassette
200 cm FFD

Centring point
To the middle of the neck at the level of the thyroid eminence

Collimation
Atlantooccipital articulations, the body of T1, the anterior and posterior soft tissues

Criteria for assessing image quality
- Atlantooccipital articulations, body of T1, anterior soft tissue structures of neck and spinous processes demonstrated
- Superimposition of right and left posterior, superior and inferior borders of vertebral bodies
- Sharp image demonstrating soft tissue structures of the pharynx in contrast to bone and air in the trachea, detail of bony cortex and trabeculae, joint space between C7 and T1 and spinous processes of cervical vertebrae

■ AP cervical spine: C3–C7 (Figs 11.7A,B, 11.8A,B)

Positioning
Method 1: patient standing or sitting erect (Fig. 11.7A)
The image receptor should be placed in a vertical stand. If used, an 18 × 24 cm cassette is placed longitudinally in the erect holder.

- The patient is sitting or standing with the back of their neck resting on the image receptor
- The MSP is 90° to the image receptor, if a cassette is used the upper border should be placed level with the external auditory meati (EAMs)
- The chin is slightly raised to superimpose the symphysis menti and the base of occiput to provide clear visualisation of C3

Method 2: patient supine (Fig. 11.8A,B)
This is as for the lateral cervical spine in method 1, and is usual for trauma where the patient will typically present on a trolley.

- The image receptor is placed beneath the neck or supported beneath the trolley on a cassette tray. If placed beneath the neck then the lateral view must have been inspected prior to patient movement. If supported beneath the trolley in a tray the effects of the increased OFD must be taken into account
- The MSP should be perpendicular to the image receptor wherever safely possible

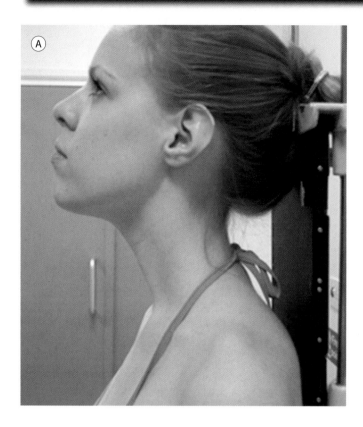

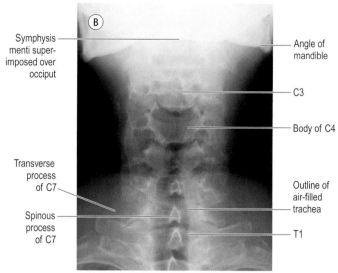

Figure 11.7 **(A)** AP C3–C7 with patient erect; **(B)** AP C3–C7

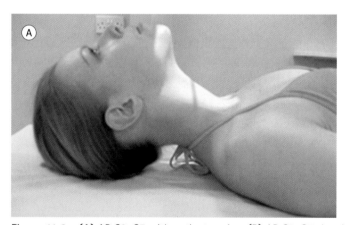

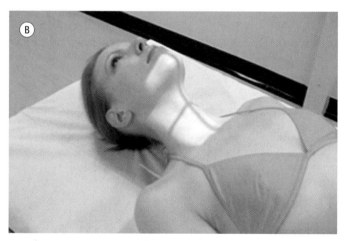

Figure 11.8 **(A)** AP C3–C7 with patient supine; **(B)** AP C3–C7 showing centring

- Superimposition of the symphysis menti and occiput are as for method 1, but this may not be possible with the patient who is immobilised

Beam direction and FFD: both methods
90° to the cassette

100 cm FFD

Consider the effect of increased OFD if the patient is supine – a grid is not usually required but consideration needs to be given to patient size; a large patient may necessitate the use of a grid.

If the patient has undergone trauma and/or is in a cervical collar, or even has neck stiffness, it may not be possible to raise the chin, in which case a cranial angle should be applied to the X-ray beam sufficient to superimpose the lower mandible over the base of the occiput. The angle selected should equate to the line joining the symphysis menti to occiput. Some neck immobilisation collars actually keep the chin elevated and superimpose the occiput over C3; in these cases a caudal angle should be employed. If angulation is used, it may be necessary to displace the image receptor to ensure the image falls within its boundaries.

Centring point
Over the MSP at the level of the thyroid eminence

Collimation
C2/3, T1, the transverse processes on each side

Criteria for assessing image quality
- C2/3 joint space, T1, and transverse processes are demonstrated
- Lower border of the mandible is superimposed on the base of occiput
- There is no rotation – the spinous processes are equidistant to the pedicles on each side
- Sharp image demonstrating air in the pharynx/trachea in contrast to the detail of the bony cortex and trabeculae; intervertebral disc spaces clearly seen

Common errors	Possible reasons
Failure to visualise C3 – obscured by the mandible	The chin not raised sufficiently to superimpose the mandible over the base of occiput
Failure to visualise C3 – obscured by the occiput	Chin raised too much

■ Cervical rib

If it is suspected that a patient has a cervical rib, the AP cervical spine projection is modified. If required, a 24 × 30 cm cassette is used longitudinally and the patient is positioned as described above. The vertical central ray is directed over the sternal notch and collimation includes C3 to T5 and the lateral soft tissues of the neck.

■ AP projection for C1–C2 (Fig. 11.9A,B)

If used, an 18 × 24 cm cassette is placed in the cassette holder or bucky if the patient is large.

Positioning
- The patient initially is positioned as for the basic AP cervical spine position, erect or supine
- If used, the cassette is positioned with its middle level with the upper incisors
- The patient opens their mouth as much as possible; if moving the head is an option it should be adjusted to bring the hard palate perpendicular to the image receptor. This may be achieved using the alatragal line, which lies parallel to the hard palate, as a guide. Positioning of the hard palate in this way superimposes the lower border

of the upper incisors over the base of the occiput, thus clearing these structures from the odontoid process and C1–C2 joints
- The mouth is checked to ensure it is open far enough to adequately clear the teeth and mandible from the C2–C3 joint spaces

Beam direction and FFD
Parallel to the alatragal line

This is especially useful as a guide for beam angulation in trauma cases where head movement is contraindicated. 100 cm FFD

Centring point
Through the open mouth at the level of the lower border of the upper incisors

Collimation
Atlantooccipital joints, C2/3 joint space, the transverse processes on each side

Criteria for assessing image quality
- Odontoid process, atlas, axis, and atlantoaxial articulations are demonstrated and visualised symmetrically
- Upper teeth and base of the skull are superimposed
- Lower teeth are superimposed over the body of C3 but cleared from the C7–C3 joint space
- No rotation – the spinous processes are demonstrated centrally to the vertebral bodies
- Sharp image demonstrating the bony cortex and trabeculae, in contrast to adjacent soft tissues

Common errors	Possible reasons
The odontoid process obscured by upper teeth	The chin not raised sufficiently or caudal beam angle is too much
The odontoid process obscured by the occiput	The chin raised too much or cranial beam angle is too much
C1 and C2 not symmetrical and/or the lower teeth on one side obscure the C2/3 joint space on one side	Rotation of the head
Lower teeth obscuring C2/3 joint space bilaterally	The mouth not open sufficiently

The difficulty of obtaining the AP C1/2 view in unconscious patients is emphasised by Blacksin & Lee who suggest CT of the craniocervical region in these patients.[39]

For other (non-trauma) patients, for whom it is difficult to obtain an image of the odontoid process, and when the

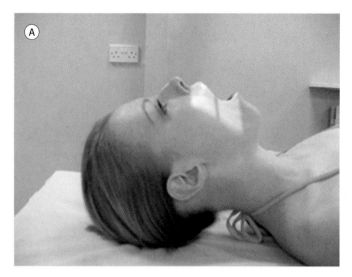

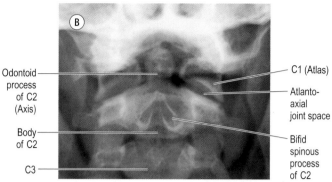

Figure 11.9   (A) AP C1–C2 (odontoid process); (B) AP C1–C2; (C) axial odontoid process. (C) Reproduced with permission from Ballinger PW, Frank ED. Merrill's atlas of radiographic positions & radiologic procedures. Missouri: Mosby; 2003

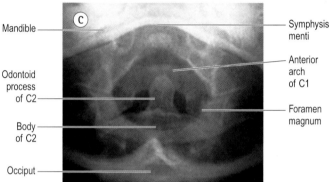

C2/C3 joint space has been adequately demonstrated, an axial odontoid peg projection can be undertaken. It is easier to undertake supine, as the chin is raised as much as possible and requires the patient to maintain this position. The central ray is then angled 25° cranially and directed midway between the angles of the mandible. The image produced shows the odontoid process through the foramen magnum (Fig. 11.9C).

OBLIQUE PROJECTIONS OF THE CERVICAL SPINE

For neurological referrals, magnetic resonance imaging (MRI) examination of the neck is preferable to oblique projections of the cervical spine, which were used in the past to demonstrate the shape of the intervertebral foramina. The main use for obliques of the cervical spine is in trauma cases; obliques used are a modification of the 'routine' erect obliques and are described at the end of the obliques section.

It must be noted that a wide variety of oblique projections have been described, the main variation being the tube angulation applied.[25,27,28,40] Which of the alternatives is used should be dependent upon the pathology to be demonstrated, but those used are all too often selected due to habit or protocol. For the sake of clarity and uniformity of approach, 45° neck obliquity (or 45° lateromedial tube angulation to produce appearances equivalent to 45° neck obliquity in the injured patient) is used throughout the next section of this chapter, but this does not indicate that this is necessarily the 'recommended technique'; reference needs to be made to the individual circumstances and the texts mentioned above before selecting the appropriate obliquity.

Whatever obliquity is ultimately selected, the technique is broadly the same; to change from one to another simply insert the number of degrees required (not forgetting to displace the image receptor appropriately if using lateromedial angulation!).

Where practicable, posteroanterior (PA) obliques should be used in preference to AP obliques due to the potentially lower absorbed dose to the thyroid.

■ Anterior obliques of the cervical spine (Fig. 11.10A,B)

The right anterior oblique (RAO) demonstrates the *right* intervertebral foramina.

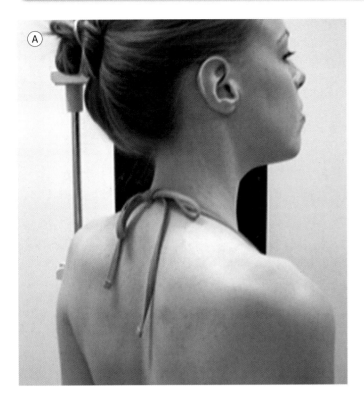

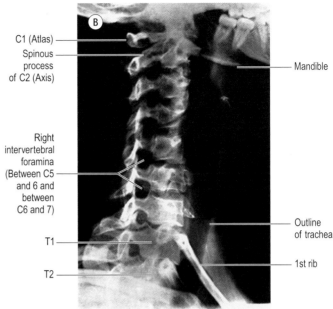

Figure 11.10 Anterior oblique cervical vertebrae

The left anterior oblique (LAO) demonstrates the *left* intervertebral foramina.

The image receptor should be placed in a vertical stand. If used, an 18 × 24 cm cassette is placed longitudinally in the erect holder. A 24 × 30 cm cassette may be used but is only necessary for *very* tall patients.

Positioning
- The patient is erect, facing the *image* receptor
- If used, the upper border of the cassette is placed level with the top of the pinna of the ear
- The patient is rotated away from the side under examination, until the MSP is at 45° to the image receptor. The head is turned a further 45° until the MSP of the head is parallel to the image receptor
- The chin is raised sufficiently to clear the mandibular rami from the upper vertebrae

Beam direction and FFD
Horizontal central ray
200 cm FFD

A 15° caudal angulation may be applied to better demonstrate the intervertebral foramina.

Centring point
To a point in the middle of the neck, at the level of the thyroid eminence

Collimation
Atlantooccipital joints, T1, lateral soft tissue outlines

Criteria for assessing image quality
- Base of the occiput, the body of T1, and soft tissue outlines of the neck are demonstrated
- Mandible is cleared from the upper vertebrae
- Intervertebral foramina is demonstrated on the opposite side of the spine to the mandible – should be symmetrical ovoids
- Pedicles of the opposite side are projected centrally at the superior border of the vertebral bodies
- Spinous processes are demonstrated posterior to the intervertebral foramina
- Soft tissue structures of the neck are demonstrated anterior to the vertebral bodies
- Sharp image demonstrating detail of the bony cortex and trabeculae in contrast to the intervertebral foramina and adjacent soft tissue structures

Posterior obliques of the cervical spine
(Fig. 11.11)

This projection may be used as an alternative to the anterior oblique, however, it should be noted that this position will lead to increased absorbed dose in the thyroid gland.

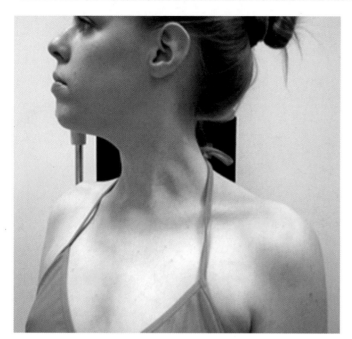

Figure 11.11   Posterior oblique cervical vertebrae

This projection may be achieved in trauma cases with the patient supine, however the modified technique for trauma must be used – not the routine projection which requires patient movement, which would be contraindicated for the trauma setting.

The **right posterior oblique (RPO)** demonstrates the *left* intervertebral foramina.

The **left posterior oblique (LPO)** demonstrates the *right* intervertebral foramina.

The image receptor should be placed in a vertical stand. If used, an 18 × 24 cm cassette is placed longitudinally in the erect holder. A 24 × 30 cm cassette may be used but is only necessary for *very* tall patients.

Positioning
- The patient is erect, facing the X-ray tube and with their back against the image receptor
- If a cassette is used, its upper border is placed level with the top of the pinna of the ear
- The patient is rotated away from the side under examination, until the MSP is at 45° to the image receptor. The head is turned a further 45° until the MSP of the head is parallel to the image receptor
- The chin is raised sufficiently to clear the mandibular rami from the upper vertebrae

Beam direction and FFD
Horizontal central ray
200 cm FFD

A 15° cranial angulation may be applied to better demonstrate the intervertebral foramina.

Centring point
To a point in the middle of the neck at the level of the thyroid eminence

Collimation
Atlantooccipital joints, T1, lateral soft tissue outlines

Criteria for assessing image quality
This is the same as for the anterior obliques.

■ Modified technique for trauma (Fig. 11.12A,B)

Oblique projections of the cervical spine may be required as a supplementary examination in trauma cases where there is concern over the integrity of the facet joints.

AP oblique projections can be undertaken without moving the patient, using lateromedial angulation to provide an apparently oblique neck image.

The **RPO** demonstrates the *left* facet joints and intervertebral foramina.

The **LPO** demonstrates the *right* facet joints and intervertebral foramina.

Positioning
- The patient is supine and the image receptor is supported beneath the trolley top
- The patient position is as close as possible to that for the AP cervical spine projection
- If a cassette is used, the upper border is placed level with the top of the pinna of the ear and displaced after centring, as described under 'beam direction and FFD'

Beam direction and FFD
The beam is angled 45° lateromedially across the patient from either side in turn. The image receptor should be displaced from the centre sufficiently to ensure that its centre is coincident with central ray, allowing for the applied beam angulation

100 cm FFD, which may need to be increased if there is a long OFD (neck to cassette tray)

If a 15° cranial angulation is required, this may be obtained by rotating the X-ray tube 15° around its horizontal axis after the initial lateromedial angulation.

Centring point
To a point in the middle of the neck, at the level of the thyroid eminence, on the side nearest the X-ray tube

Collimation
Atlantooccipital joints, T1, lateral soft tissue outlines

Criteria for assessing image quality
This is the same as for the erect obliques.

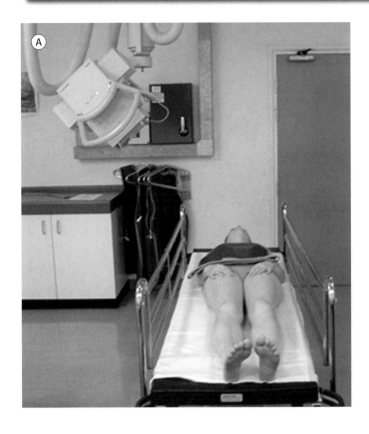

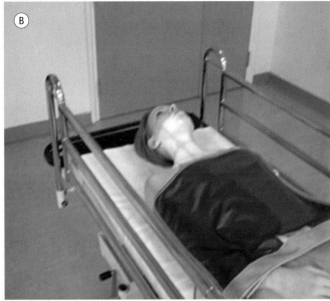

Figure 11.12 **(A)** Trauma cervical oblique; **(B)** trauma oblique – showing collimation

Common errors – all methods	Possible reasons
Narrowed foramina	Under-rotation of the neck
Foreshortening of the pedicles	Over-rotation of the neck
The foramina distorted/disc space not demonstrated	Insufficient cranial/caudal tube angulation

Note that if lateromedial angulation is used, as for modified projections in trauma, this will cause more image distortion than projections using neck rotation

OTHER IMAGING MODALITIES AND THE CERVICAL SPINE

Even though CT scanning provides the most detailed evaluation of bony injuries, MRI has some clear advantages, being the most sensitive modality for the detection of intrinsic spinal cord pathology, and also providing the most detailed evaluation of the soft tissues. An added advantage is that there is no loss of resolution in areas such as the lower cervical spine where the shoulders may interfere with visualization, even with the use of CT.

It has been suggested that MRI should be available within the emergency department setting to be used as routinely as plain film radiography is currently,[41] however even MRI is not without its disadvantages particularly with the group of patients under consideration. Artefact can be a problem, either from the posterior fat pat in adults, or the pulsatile flow of cerebrospinal fluid (CSF) in children.[42]

There are other suggestions as to how imaging may be used in this group of patients. Brookes & Willett, researching in Oxford, have proposed a protocol for spinal clearance involving dynamic screening of the cervical spine in unconscious trauma patients to enable rapid, safe discontinuation of spinal precautions.[16]

As with all debates in the field of medical imaging, it is not practicable to provide a concrete 'once and for all answer' to the question as to which of the above imaging methods is 'best'; the practice of medical imaging has changed dramatically in the latter decade of the 20th and into the 21st century, with a constant stream of new technologies that shows no sign of slowing down. CT could become unrecognisable in the next few years from the slice-by-slice technology of 10 years ago with the introduction of flat plate digital detector systems.

These advances in medical imaging technology are being driven by the rapid advances in computing and associated technologies. Already we can look to the image registration of various cross-sectional studies; for example, the registration of CT and MRI images may enable bony and soft tissue structures and their relationships to be better demonstrated than is possible with each individual modality.[43] As we are in such a state of flux we can only offer a snapshot and consider how to best use what is available today, but have a system with the flexibility to adapt to the changes tomorrow may bring.

References

1. Zimmerman R. Head injury. In: Taveras J, Ferrucci J, eds. Radiology on CD-ROM. June 2001; 3, Ch. 37.
2. Lowery DW, et al. Epidemiology of cervical spine injury patients. Academic Emergency Medicine 2000; 7(5):591.
3. Hoffman JR, et al. Selective cervical spine radiography in blunt trauma. Annals of Emergency Medicine 1998; 32(4):461–469.
4. Mower WR, et al. Selective cervical spine radiography of blunt trauma victims. Academic Emergency Medicine 1999; 6(5):451.
5. Stiell IG, et al. Obtaining consensus for a definition of 'clinically important cervical spine injury' in the CCC study. Academic Emergency Medicine 1999; 6(5):435.
6. Stolberg HO. The development of radiology guidelines in Canada. Canadian Association of Radiologists Journal 1999; 50:83–88,152–155.
7. Stiell IG, et al. Application of the NEXUS low-risk criteria for cervical spine radiography in Canadian Emergency Departments. Academic Emergency Medicine 2000; 7(5):566.
8. Hoffman JR, et al. Validity of a set of clinical criteria to rule out injury to the cervical spine in patients with blunt trauma. New England Journal of Medicine 2000; 343(2):94–99.
9. Hills MW, Dean SA. Head injury and facial injury: Is there an increased risk of cervical spine injury? Journal of Trauma 1993; 34:549–554.
10. Melville GE, Taveras JM. Traumatic injuries of the spinal cord and nerve roots. In: Taveras J, Ferrucci J, eds. Radiology on CD-ROM. Lippincott. June 2001.
11. Pang D, Pollack I. Spinal cord injury without radiographic abnormality in children – the SCIWORA syndrome. Journal of Trauma 1989; 29:654–663.
12. Ullrich A, et al. Distracting painful injuries associated with cervical spinal injuries in blunt trauma. Academic Emergency Medicine 2001; 8(1):25–29.
13. Link TM, et al. Substantial head trauma: value of routine CT examination of the cervicocranium. Radiology 1995; 196:741–745.
14. Hackl W, et al. Prevalence of cervical spine injuries in patients with facial trauma. Oral Surgery Oral Medicine Oral Pathology Oral Radiology & Endodontics 2001; 92(4):370–376.
15. Stiell IG, et al. How important is mechanism of injury in predicting the risk of cervical spine injury? American Emergency Medicine 2001; 8(5):456–457.
16. Brookes RA, Willett KM. Evaluation of the Oxford protocol for total spinal clearance in the unconscious trauma patient. Journal of Trauma 2001; 50(5):862–867.
17. Matar LD, Doyle AJ. Prevertebral soft-tissue measurements in cervical spine injury. Australasian Radiology 1997; 41:229–237.
18. Herr CH, et al. Sensitivity of prevertebral soft tissue measurement of C3 for detection of cervical spine fractures and dislocations. American Journal of Emergency Medicine 1998; 16(40):346–349.
19. European Commission Directorate-General for the Environment 2000. Referral guidelines for imaging. Radiation protection 118.
20. Harris MB, et al. Evaluation of the cervical spine in the polytrauma patient. Spine 2000; 15;25(22):2884-2891.
21. West OC, et al. Acute cervical spine trauma: diagnostic performance of single view versus three view radiographic screening. Radiology 1997; 204:819–823.
22. Baker C, et al. Evaluation of paediatric cervical spine injuries. American Journal of Emergency Medicine 1999; 17:230–234.
23. MacDonald RL, et al. Diagnosis of cervical spine injury in motor vehicle crash victims: how many x-rays are enough? Journal of Trauma 1990; 30(4):392–397.
24. Holliman CJ, et al. Is the anteroposterior cervical spine radiograph necessary in initial trauma screening? American Journal of Emergency Medicine 1991; 9(5):421–425.
25. Turetsky DB, et al. Technique and use of supine oblique views in acute cervical spine trauma. Annals of Emergency Medicine 1993; 22(4):685–689.
26. Doris PE, Wilson RA. The next logical step in the emergency radiographic evaluation of cervical spine trauma: The five view trauma series. Journal of Emergency Medicine 1985; 3:371–375.
27. Abel MS. The exaggerated supine oblique view of the cervical spine. Skeletal Radiology 1982; 8:213–219.
28. Unett EM, Royle AJ. Radiographic techniques and image evaluation. London: Chapman and Hall; 1997.
29. Daffner RH. Cervical radiography for trauma patients: A time-effective technique? American Journal of Roentgenology 2000; 175:1309–1311.
30. American College of Radiology. ACR standard for the performance of radiography of the cervical spine in children and adults. 1999. Online. Available: http://www.acr.org/departments/stand_accred/standards/dl_list.html
31. Pollack CV, et al. The utility of flexion-extension radiographs of the cervical spine in blunt trauma. Academic Emergency Medicine 2001; 8(5):488.
32. Mirvis SE, et al. Protocol-driven radiologic evaluation of suspected cervical spine injury: efficacy study. Radiology 1989; 170:831–834.
33. Kaneriya PP, et al. The cost-effectiveness of oblique radiography in the exclusion of C7–T1 injury in trauma patients. American Journal of Roentgenology 1998; 171:959–962.
34. Nunez DB, et al. Cervical spine trauma: how much do we learn by routinely using helical CT? RadioGraphics 1996; 16:1307–1318.
35. Ballinger P. Merrill's atlas of radiographic positions and radiologic procedures. 8th edn. St Louis: Mosby; 1995.

36. Carver BJ, Roche D. An alternative technique for visualisation of the C7/T1 junction in trauma. Supplement to British Journal of Radiology 2000; 73:73.

37. Swallow R, et al. Clark's positioning in radiography. 11th edn. London: Heinemann; 1986.

38. Pellei DD. The fat C2 sign. Radiology 2000; 217:359–360.

39. Blacksin MF, Lee HJ. Frequency and significance of fractures of the upper cervical spine detected by CT in patients with severe neck trauma. American Journal of Roentgenology 1995; 165(5):751-754.

40. Woodford MJ. Radiography of the acute cervical spine. Radiography 1987; 53(607):3–8.

41. Rogers LF. To see or not to see, that is the question. American Journal of Roentgenology 2001; 176:1.

42. Westbrook C. Handbook of MRI technique. Oxford: Blackwell Science; 1994.

43. Panigrahy A, et al. Registration of three-dimensional MR and CT studies of the cervical spine. American Journal of Neuroradiology 2000; 21:282–289.

THORACIC SPINE

Linda Williams

The thoracic spine should not be routinely examined by X-ray for pain without trauma, unless in the elderly when osteoporosis may cause sudden collapse of vertebrae. Magnetic resonance imaging (MRI) may be indicated if local pain continues.[1]

Clinical significance of wedge fractures should not be overlooked as, occasionally, there may be fragments displaced within the spinal canal that could cause spinal cord compression.[2]

The 28-day rule should be applied when examining the thoracic spine in patients of reproductive capacity.

INDICATIONS

Fracture

The most common reason for examining this area radiographically is due to major or minor trauma involving the region. Fractures of the upper and middle sections of the thoracic spine do not occur as frequently as those of the cervical vertebrae and thoracolumbar region. However with thoracic spine fractures there is a higher incidence of spinal cord injury.[3]

Osteomyeloma

The thoracic spine may be examined as part of a skeletal survey to stage the condition and assess which lesions may benefit from radiotherapy.[1]

Osteomyelitis

A 2–3 phase skeletal scintinogram is more sensitive than an X-ray examination[1] so it is not routinely indicated but in the later stages an area of porosis may be seen; the diagnosis at this stage can usually be made by blood cultures.[4]

▮ Anteroposterior (AP) thoracic spine (Fig. 12.1A,B)

Much research has been undertaken on the advantages and disadvantages of the posteroanterior (PA) versus the AP projection of the lumbar spine, particularly with relation to dose reduction. Brennan[5] in his article analysing the PA projection of the lumbar spine recommends the employment of this procedure to facilitate dose reduction without loss of image quality. However, with regard to the principle of undertaking a PA projection of the thoracic spine, it must be remembered that, due to its natural kyphotic curvature, oblique rays from the X-ray beam will be angled in the opposite direction to the intervertebral joint spaces. The resulting PA image is therefore not likely to demonstrate the intervertebral joint spaces as adequately as with the AP projection. This is somewhat unfortunate, as the PA projection may reduce radiation dose to the breast, eyes and thyroid, all radiosensitive areas. However, breast shields may be used and with good collimation this can significantly reduce the dose. Levy et al, have studied the use of the PA projection in examining the whole spine for scoliosis in adolescents;[6] their work suggests that a PA study of the spine will effect a reduction in dose to the patient without any loss of image quality and although the assessment for scoliosis using plain films has reduced significantly with the increased use of other imaging methods, their work indicates that PA thoracic spine examination may be a possibility in some cases.

A consideration when examining the thoracic spine is the variation in densities along the length of this section of the vertebral column, the upper end being superimposed by the air filled trachea and vertebrae 5–12 being superimposed by the heart and great vessels. Abdominal contents are usually superimposed over T11 and T12 and size of individual vertebrae increase gradually, with T1 being significantly smaller than T12.

Clearly this range of densities has implications for selection of exposure factors that will provide adequate contrast and density along the entire length of the region under examination. To achieve even density, certain techniques may be employed as follows:

1. A high enough kVp can be used to reduce the subject contrast along the length of the spine.
2. A wedge filter can be used with the thicker end at the upper region of the thoracic spine.
3. A flour filter can be used. The filter consists of flour inside a radiolucent bag (usually plastic which is covered by a cotton bag that can be washed). The contents of the bag can be shaken to distribute the flour into a thicker layer at one end; this thicker end of the bag is then placed over the upper end of the sternum and the flour is patted by the radiographer until the thickness decreases towards the lower end of the thoracic vertebrae. The filter is therefore adaptable to any patient size, unlike set size aluminium filters. The filter can be made extremely cheaply and requires no specialist attachment feature on the light beam mounting, although manufacture of such a filter should only be attempted after consultation with health and safety and cross-infection specialists from the hospital where the filter is to be used.
4. Graduated intensifying screen: this technique is rarely used as these screens are expensive and therefore not readily available in most imaging departments.

Some texts suggest the use of the anode heel effect to help reduce the subject contrast along the length of the spine.[7,8] However, anode targets in modern X-ray tubes are set at such an angle that this effect will have little or no difference on the resultant image.

When using an automatic exposure device (AED) for the thoracic spine, accurate centring and good collimation is essential. If the beam is not collimated sufficiently then the AED will end the exposure before the required radiographic density of the image is achieved. This is due to the effect of additional scatter from the excess irradiated tissue lateral to the spine.

The AP thoracic spine is exposed on arrested inspiration to ensure the diaphragm is lowered and a maximum number of thoracic vertebrae are demonstrated. However it has been suggested that the use of arrested expiration to reduce the amount of air in the thorax will provide a more uniform density over the thoracic spine by helping to reduce the subject contrast.[8,9]

If cassettes are used, AP and lateral projections of the thoracic spine should be carried out on 18 × 43 cm or 30 × 40 cm cassettes, placed in the table bucky.

Positioning

- The patient is supine with their arms at their sides and legs extended
- A low radiolucent pillow or pad may be used to support the head, and the knees may be supported slightly with a pad for patient comfort
- A lead rubber apron is applied to the lower abdomen for gonad protection
- The median sagittal plane (MSP) is 90° to the table-top and the coronal plane is parallel to the table-top

Note that this technique may be performed erect, either standing or seated; the positioning is the same but a vertical

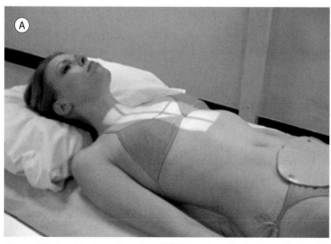
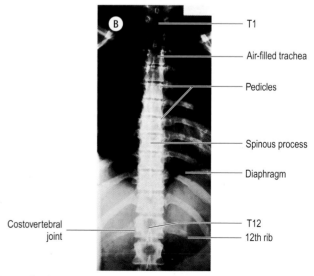

Figure 12.1 AP thoracic spine. (B) Reproduced with permission from Bryan GJ. Skeletal anatomy. 3rd edn. Edinburgh: Churchill Livingstone; 1996 and Gunn (2002)

image receptor and antiscatter device is used. Central ray direction is adjusted accordingly.

Beam direction and focus film distance (FFD)

Vertical central ray, at 90° to the image receptor
100 cm FFD

Centring point

In the midline approximately two-thirds of the distance between the sternal angle and the xiphoid sternum, nearest the xiphoid end

Many texts quote the centring point for this projection as between the sternal notch and the xiphoid sternum.[10,11] This point locates the central ray over T6, i.e. numerically at the middle of the thoracic vertebrae. Unfortunately vertebrae T1–T6 are shorter in length than T7–T12 and a centring point over T6 will therefore not lie over the midpoint of the thoracic section of the vertebral column. Indeed it will be in a relatively high position in relation to the actual midpoint of the area. Other texts quote a centring point as either between the sternal angle and the xiphoid sternum, or 3–5 cm below the sternal angle to a point over T7[8,9,12] which is still not low enough to coincide with the actual midpoint of the thoracic vertebrae. It has therefore been thought necessary to reassess the situation. Several radiographs have been studied by the author and it has been noted that the actual half way point between T1 and T12 lies, in fact, approximately over T7/8 junction. Since anterior surface markings need to be used for assessing this point it has been identified, from skeletons and radiographs, that T7/8 junction lies three-quarters of the way down the sternum itself – hence the centring point quoted (Fig. 12.2).

Collimation

C7–L1, all transverse processes

> Expose on arrested respiration

Criteria for assessing image quality

- C7 down to L1 and all their transverse processes are demonstrated
- The thoracic vertebrae are in the centre of the film
- Spinous processes are centralised over the midline of the vertebral bodies
- Paraspinal line[2] should be clearly demonstrated
- Intervertebral joint spaces are demonstrated
- Sharp image demonstrating the bony cortex and trabeculae of the vertebral bodies of C7 down to L1, adequately

Common errors	Possible reasons
Overexposure of the upper region or underexposure of the lower region	Failure to employ any of the techniques described above for even image density throughout
Superimposition of the vertebral bodies vertically	The long axis of the spine is not near parallel to the table-top. Reducing the size of the head support and giving the patient a small pad beneath the knees for support can rectify this. (However, severely kyphotic patients may require two exposures with beam angled in each direction of the kyphosis)

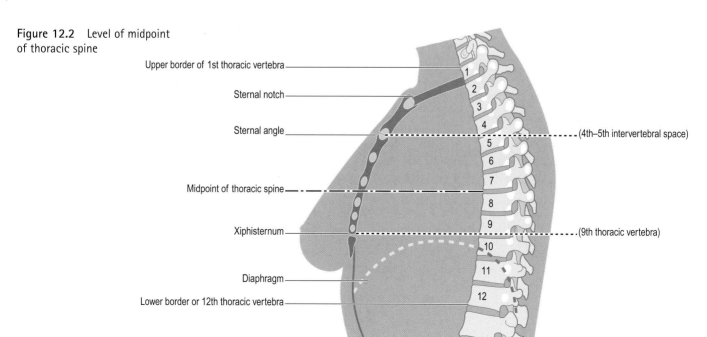

Figure 12.2 Level of midpoint of thoracic spine

Upper border of 1st thoracic vertebra
Sternal notch
Sternal angle ------- (4th–5th intervertebral space)
Midpoint of thoracic spine
Xiphisternum ------- (9th thoracic vertebra)
Diaphragm
Lower border or 12th thoracic vertebra

penetrated through the denser mediastinal and upper abdominal structures without overblackening of the upper vertebrae

■ Lateral thoracic spine (Fig. 12.3A,B)

As in the case of the AP projection, there also exists a range of densities along the area covered by the lateral thoracic spine projection. The more dense area in this case is the upper end of the thoracic region, since the average person is wider at the shoulders than they are lower down the thoracic region. The use of the filter described earlier in this chapter is used with the thicker end orientated in the opposite direction to that used for the AP, i.e. the thicker end at the shoulder end. This will even out the densities encountered along the length of the spine.

There are two schools of thought when choosing exposure factors for the lateral projection. One that is commonly used is the breathing technique, accompanied by the use of a low mA and long exposure time (2 seconds plus) to provide the required mAs. This technique is designed to blur rib shadows and lung markings which lie over the vertebrae, thus enabling the viewer to see the vertebral bodies more clearly.[8,9,12,13] The other suggests that, as the ribs are actually attached to the vertebrae, in using the breathing technique, the rib shadow cannot be blurred without blurring the vertebrae also; in other words, what is actually happening is that whilst breathing, the vertebral bodies are moving but to a lesser extent than the ribs move. This gives an apparent sharpness of the vertebral bodies due to the differential sharpness between the ribs and the bodies.[14]

There is sometimes difficulty in demonstrating the intervertebral joint space of all the thoracic vertebrae on one image and this can be overcome by the use of a greater FFD (150 cm). This relatively long distance means there is less divergence of the beam around the central ray when it reaches the thoracic spine and there is more chance of the joint spaces being demonstrated on the image, especially those at the extreme ends of the thoracic spine. Although this method has been used by many radiographers for many years a recent study[15] has provided evidence to support this practice, while also showing that magnification and unsharpness is reduced. This technique requires adjustment of exposure factors, with due attention to the inverse square law, unless an AED is used.

A lead rubber sheet placed behind the patient, next to the skin surface, will absorb some of the scattered radiation produced during exposure and enhance the image. Some research disputes the necessity to place lead rubber

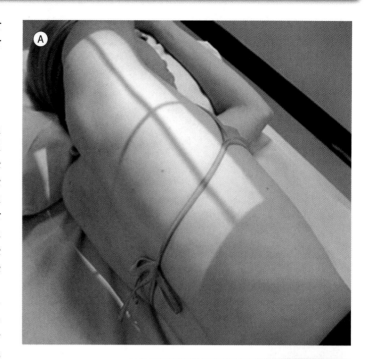

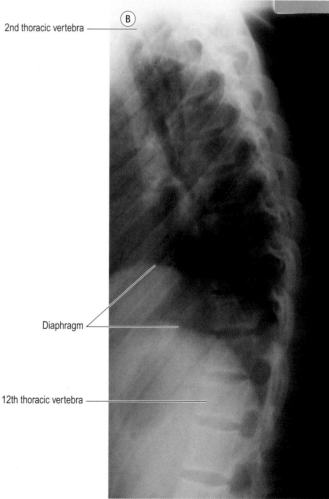

2nd thoracic vertebra

Diaphragm

12th thoracic vertebra

Figure 12.3   Lateral thoracic spine

behind the patient for the lateral spine projection,[16] arguing that the resulting radiograph is not enhanced by this practice. It also claims that the action is not necessary with the use of the accurate collimators available today, which prevent any scatter reaching the film. However, a more recent study[15] actually supports the use of lead rubber in this way, claiming that the resulting radiographic contrast is improved due to less scatter reaching the film.

Positioning
- From the AP position the patient is turned 90° onto their side to bring the coronal plane 90° to the table-top and the MSP parallel to it, with their back to the radiographer for ease of positioning
- The patient's head is rested on a low radiolucent pad and the knees and hips are flexed for stability
- The patient's upper arm is placed stretched above their head to help bring the spine parallel to the table-top and clear the humerus and soft tissue of the arm from the field. The lower arm is raised onto the pad to clear it from the field
- A lead rubber apron is placed across the lower abdomen and pelvis for radiation protection
- The spinous processes are palpated and assessed to ensure that the long axis of the spine and the MSP are parallel to the table-top; this may require the use of a radiolucent pad under the lower end of the thoracic spine, but comments after the beam angulation section for this projection should also be noted before considering this. If the spine has a lateral curvature when the patient is lying on their side, with the curve appearing as a slight 'u' shape, it is usually not necessary to make adjustments in central ray or to use pads. This is because the oblique rays around the central ray are likely to correspond with the obliquity of the intervertebral joint spaces. If a curvature appears as a slight 'n' shape, it will be more advantageous to turn the patient onto their opposite side for this projection. In any case, lateral curvature is often best assessed by viewing the AP projection before attempting the lateral position
- A sheet of lead rubber is placed behind the patient to absorb some scattered radiation and improve image quality

Beam direction and FFD
Vertical at 90° to the long axis of the thoracic spine

Reference has already been made to the use of radiolucent pads to help the spine lie parallel to the image receptor but it must be remembered that the effectiveness of this will vary, according to the weight of the patient (heavier patients will squash the pad more than slimmer patients, thus reducing the effect of the pad). Variation in anatomy of individual patients will require varying compensation to allow the thoracic column to lie parallel to the image receptor. Insertion of pads can also be somewhat difficult when a patient is elderly, obese, suffering from back pain and lying in the lateral position. Angulation of the beam in a direction that will ensure the central ray strikes the long axis of the thoracic vertebrae at 90° can also be employed as an alternative strategy. It is easier to use this, rather than the pad method and beam angulation will more accurately facilitate the correct 90° beam/vertebral column relationship.

115–150 cm FFD

Note the range of FFDs offered; this is after consideration of the comments made in the introductory notes for this projection.

Centring point
At the level of T8 approximately 2–3 cm behind the mid-axillary line, and 7–9 cm anterior to the spinous process of T7

Note that the spinous process of T7 lies level with body of T8. T8 can also be located from the posterior aspect of the patient by palpation of the inferior angle of scapula, which lies level with T8, even when the arm is raised. Approximations in given measurements are due to the vast difference in the sizes and shapes of all patients.

Collimation
C7 to L1, anterior vertebral bodies, spinous processes

Criteria for assessing image quality
- T2 should be demonstrated and not obscured by the upper arms and shoulders; the body of L1 should be included inferiorly (it is not usually possible to demonstrate T1 on the lateral projection because of the shoulder thickness; it may be necessary to take a supplementary projection of this area if the clinical history indicates need for this)
- All anterior bodies and spinous processes are demonstrated
- There is superimposition of the posterior ribs and superimposition of the anterior and posterior borders of the vertebral bodies
- Superimposition of the inferior and superior borders of the vertebral bodies and intervertebral disc spaces is demonstrated
- There is blurring of the ribs and lung markings if the breathing technique used
- Correct image density to demonstrate the bony cortex and trabeculae of all the vertebrae with sufficient penetration of the shoulder region to visualise the upper vertebrae, without overblackening of the lower vertebrae

Common errors	Possible reasons
Collimation may result in some of the vertebral column being excluded from the image	The curvature of the spine due to kyphosis has not been taken into consideration; if a large kyphosis is suspected on visual examination of the patient, view the AP image first and adjust collimation accordingly
The anterior and posterior borders of the bodies are not superimposed	The patient is either rotated too far forward or too far back; ensure the coronal plane is 90° to the table-top
The intervertebral joint spaces are not demonstrated; upper and lower borders of the vertebral bodies are not superimposed	The long axis of the spine is not parallel to the table-top. Care should be taken to ensure the spinous processes are all parallel to the table-top, with use of radiolucent pads if necessary, or the beam should be angled to strike the spine at 90° to its long axis

References

1. RCR Working Party. Making the best use of a Department of radiology: guidelines for doctors. 5th edn. London: The Royal College of Radiologists; 2003.
2. Raby N, et al. Accident and emergency radiology, a survival guide. London: Saunders; 2001.
3. Long BW, Rafert JA. Orthopaedic radiography. Philadelphia: WB Saunders; 1995.
4. Duckworth T. Lecture notes on orthopaedics and fractures. UK: Blackwell Science; 1995.
5. Brennan PC, Madigan E. Lumbar spine radiology; analysis of the posteroanterior projection. European Radiology 2000; 10:1197–1201.
6. Levy AR, et al. Reducing the lifetime risks of cancer from spinal radiographs amongst people with adolescent idiopathic scoliosis. Spine 1996; 21(13):1500–1507.
7. Eisenberg RL, et al. Radiographic positioning. 2nd edn. Boston: Little Brown and Company; 1995.
8. Bontrager KL. Textbook of radiographic positioning and related anatomy. 5th edn. St Louis: Mosby; 2001.
9. McQuillen-Martensen K. Radiographic critique. Philadelphia: WB Saunders; 1996.
10. Unett EM, Royle AJ. Radiographic techniques and image evaluation. London: Nelson Thornes;1997.
11. Bell GA, Finlay DBL. Basic radiographic positioning. Baillière Tindall; 1986.
12. Ballinger PW, Frank ED. Merrill's atlas of radiographic positioning and radiologic procedures, 10th edn. St Louis: Mosby; 2003.
13. Swallow RA, et al. Clark's positioning in radiography, 11th edn. Oxford: Heinemann Medical Books; 1986.
14. Oldnall NJ. Thoracic spine technique. Online. Available http://www.xray2000.co.uk
15. Thomas A. Imaging the lateral thoracic spine. Synergy 2003; April:10–13.
16. Mitchell FE. Scattered radiation and the lumbar spine. Part 1; initial research. Radiography Today 1991; 57(644):18–20.

CHAPTER 13

LUMBAR SPINE

Barry Carver, Margot McBride, Elizabeth Carver

CONDITIONS AFFECTING THE REGION

Trauma

Wedge fractures can occur when the anterior border of a vertebral body is crushed due to flexion or vertical pressure, i.e. a high fall landing on the feet or head. More serious bony injury can occur, including fracture and dislocation of vertebrae, which can cause misalignment of the vertebral column. Below the first lumbar vertebra (L1) the cauda equina is more resistant to injury than the spinal cord. Plain radiography is most likely to be undertaken in the acute setting when injury has been sustained.

Pars interarticularis fractures are shown on oblique lumbar spine projections; this type of injury can result in a spondylolisthesis (forward slippage of one vertebra in relationship to the vertebra below), although plain radiography may not be the most appropriate investigative method. L5 slippage on the first sacral segment (S1) is most frequently found. They are often an incidental finding on images and are not usually directly related to specific traumatic incidents.

Back pain

Lumbago
Low back pain; often no radiological cause is found.

Sciatica
Pain radiating to the leg due to the compression of the lumbar nerve roots. May be associated with a lumbar disc prolapse or spondylosis.

Back pain, whether acute or chronic, is not on its own an indicator for plain film radiography (except in the case of possible osteoporotic collapse),[1] however back pain may be associated with more serious features in which case magnetic resonance imaging (MRI) is the investigation of choice.[2]

Degenerative disease processes

Degenerative change is part of the normal ageing process. Amongst those affecting the lumbar region are spondylosis, spondylitis, spondylolisthesis, intervertebral disc collapse and osteoarthritis. In order to justify imaging, the potential for affecting patient management must be considered.

Studies have shown that only a very small percentage of requests for plain film radiography change patient management,[3] and are not cost effective.[4] The high radiation dose associated with lumbar spine radiography should not be used for patient reassurance, or indeed reassurance for the referrer.[5]

Metastatic disease

Metastatic disease is characterised by secondary deposits seen as lytic, and in some cases sclerotic lesions; pathological fractures may be present. Early detection via radionuclide imaging (RNI) or MRI are generally the most appropriate examinations.[2]

Congenital processes

Spina bifida
This is a congenital defect usually occurring in the lumbosacral region. The laminae do not fuse, causing the vertebral arch to be incomplete posteriorly. Spina bifida has varying degrees of severity as it may or may not be associated with protrusion of the meninges and spinal cord. Today, plain radiography is unlikely to be required as an initial investigation, since awareness of the existence of the abnormality is usually raised after routine prenatal ultrasound scanning. In spina bifida occulta the defect

does not involve the meninges or spinal cord and is usually an incidental finding on an anteroposterior (AP) radiograph of the area.

■ Challenges of the lumbar spine examination

There are a number of challenges the radiographer will encounter when positioning a patient, not only due to the patient's physical shape and size but in the judgement of radiographic planes of the body in relation to the patient and X-ray table. The following tips may be helpful in overcoming difficulties which may be encountered.

Positioning tips

Prior knowledge of the patient's clinical history, when initially studying a patient's X-ray request form, assists in the problem-solving and decision-making processes crucial for the optimum choice of positioning technique required, in order to achieve a high quality diagnostic image. Initial clinical evaluation of the spinal shape will assist in any positioning adjustment requirements when the patient is placed on the X-ray couch. This is particularly important for patients with abnormal configurations of the spine.

The patient should be made to feel comfortable and relaxed; tension can cause difficulty when attempting to move a patient into position. The examination gown should be adjusted if necessary to ensure that no creases will interfere with their movement into the required position and that the anatomical landmarks are easily palpated. If the gown design includes a split, this must be at the back of the patient, to allow for visualisation of the spinal column whilst palpating its surface markings.

Palpation of the prime anatomical landmarks is important when adjusting the patient into the correct position for each projection. Clinical palpation is a skill, which if practised with reservations could lead to mistakes. Physical contact involving the lower trunk, as required by lumbar spine examination, requires a degree of tact and diplomacy whilst employing precision and gentleness but firmness.

A key requisite for accurate positioning of the lateral lumbar projections is to assess the position of the long axis of the vertebral column in relationship to the image receptor. The column should be palpated *and* visually assessed along the lumbar section, with the *eyes level with the vertebrae*. Radiographers often assess visually from a point that is higher than the spine; this does not give a true impression of the vertebral position. Palpation of the spinous processes is also essential and must be implemented in addition to visual assessment, since the muscles on the posterior aspect of the patient can sag (especially in the middle-aged and elderly patient), giving an inaccurate impression if visual assessment only is used.

For lumbar spine X-ray examinations, the anatomical landmarks chosen during positioning set-up techniques are considered as reasonably standard although their position relative to the surrounding anatomical structures can vary due to osteological changes. Excessive fatty tissue can also cause difficulty in palpation techniques. There is a large variation in total body fat in individuals of varying age and between populations. Therefore, standardisation of the anatomical sites used for positioning and palpation is important.

■ AP lumbar spine (Fig. 13.1A,B)

If used, a 30 × 40 cm cassette is selected and placed longitudinally in the table bucky.

Positioning
- The patient is supine with their arms placed on the pillow and legs extended
- The knees may be supported slightly with a pad for patient comfort; this is also said to reduce the lumbar lordosis enabling better visualisation of the intervertebral joint spaces. However, there is some dispute regarding the effectiveness of this (please see relevant discussion at the end of this section)
- The median sagittal plane (MSP) is 90° to the table-top and the coronal plane is parallel to the table-top
- Gonad protection should be applied to all patients – if it is correctly positioned it will not obscure any relevant detail, and is essential to reduce the dose to the gonad

Beam direction and focus film distance (FFD)
Vertical central ray, 90° to the image receptor
100 cm FFD

Centring
In the midline, at the level of the lower costal margin (level of L3)

Collimation
Psoas muscles, transverse processes of LV1–LV5, T12–L1 joint space, sacroiliac joints

Note that this technique may be performed erect, either standing or seated; the positioning is the same but a vertical image receptor and antiscatter device is used.[6] The central ray direction is adjusted accordingly.

Criteria for assessing image quality
- Psoas muscles, transverse processes of LV1–LV5, T12–L1 joint space, sacroiliac joints are demonstrated
- Spinous processes are in the centre of vertebral bodies, demonstrating no rotation

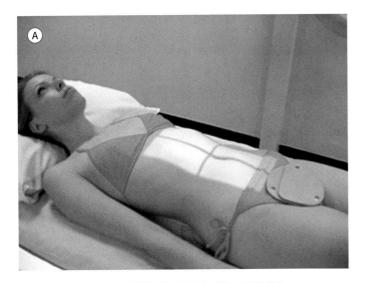

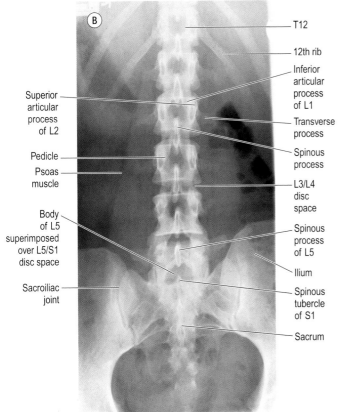

Figure 13.1   AP lumbar spine

Labels on Figure 13.1:
- T12
- 12th rib
- Inferior articular process of L1
- Transverse process
- Spinous process
- L3/L4 disc space
- Spinous process of L5
- Ilium
- Spinous tubercle of S1
- Sacrum
- Superior articular process of L2
- Pedicle
- Psoas muscle
- Body of L5 superimposed over L5/S1 disc space
- Sacroiliac joint

Common errors	Possible reasons
Spinous processes not in the midline of vertebral bodies	1. Rotation of the spine – MSP not perpendicular to the image receptor. Adjust the patient position so that the pelvis and shoulders are not rotated 2. Scoliosis may cause this appearance and may not be improved upon. This is distinguishable from rotation due to position error by the distinct lateral curve of the column and potential variation of rotation down its length[7]
Intervertebral disc spaces not clearly demonstrated	Excessive lordosis – the direction of the primary beam can be adjusted so that the beam is directed through the required joint spaces *(see comments below)*

Expose on arrested respiration

Exposure is made on arrested respiration, to prevent blurring of abdominal contents. The respiratory phase is unimportant as the diaphragms will not move over the body of L1 in either phase. It is likely though, that selection of exposure factors will be affected by opposite phases of respiration, since extreme inspiration will increase the volume and density of abdominal tissue overlying the lumbar area. This will be likely to necessitate an increase in exposure factors, which will result in an increase in radiation dose to the patient and decrease in image contrast due to increased scatter from the greater tissue volume and density.

An alternative to demonstrate the transverse processes free from overlying gas shadows is to use a long exposure with the patient gently panting, using the effect of autotomography to prevent the gas obscuring bony detail.

- L2–L3 and L3–L4 joint spaces are demonstrated; other intervertebral spaces will be projected obliquely due to lumbar curvature
- Sharp image demonstrating soft tissue of abdominal viscera in contrast to bone and air in the gastro-intestinal tract (GIT); detail of bony cortex and trabeculae; spinous processes visualised through vertebral bodies

It is commonly believed that the curvature of the lumbar spine can be reduced by an angled pad being placed under the knees, enabling better visualisation of the inter-vertebral joint spaces by associated flattening of the lumbar lordotic curve.[8] If this is not sufficient to enable demonstration of the disc spaces then this effect can be increased by flexing the knees and hips further and bringing the plantar surface of the feet in contact with the table-top.

The effect has been disputed by Murrie et al,[9] but the effectiveness of the knee flexion is traditionally claimed to be felt by a simple experiment: if one lies supine with legs extended and a flat hand placed under the lumbar curve, the hand slides easily under the arch made by the lumbar curve. When the knees and hips are flexed, the hand feels the lumbar area press down onto its palmar aspect, suggesting reduction in lumbar curve. The more the hips and knees are flexed, the more the curve appears to reduce. Is the movement felt by the hand merely muscular movement rather than reduction of lordosis? Would an increase in knee/hip flexion actually show a more significant lumbar curve reduction?

A repeat of the process described in the experiment by Murrie et al was undertaken by the authors and has resulted in the MRI images in Figure 13.2. The knees and hips were placed into maximum possible flexion (which was noticeably restricted in the scanner bore available). The images show minimal (and probably non-detectable on an AP X-ray image) reduction in the curve, although some intervertebral joint space angles did appear to change more than with the first experiment. The repeat experiment was undertaken only on one person. However, even the initial research was only undertaken on a very small sample of 5 examinations.[9]

It was also noted that Murrie et al flexed the knees over a 45° pad, which may not offer adequate hip flexion for lumbar curve reduction anyway. When repeating the experiment the authors noted that the bore of the MRI scanner did not allow a particularly effective flexion of the hips and knees, and it was felt that further flexion might have given different results. It is suggested that the experiment be repeated with a larger sample using a wide bore or open-sided MRI scanner and the authors recommend that this research be repeated in this way. Use of an open-sided MRI scanner would allow the sample to achieve hip and knee flexion which is more comparable to that used in AP lumbar spine radiography.

Therefore we can see, without more scientific evidence to support knee flexion as a means to reduce lordosis, that the only reason for flexing the patient's knee may be for patient comfort. However, the question must be asked 'Do we require all joint spaces to be visualised on an AP?' – information regarding intervertebral disc spaces is more readily available on the lateral view, and on MRI, which after all is the investigation of choice for most lumbar pathologies.

Posteroanterior (PA) or AP?

Due to the anterior curvature of the lumbar spine it would seem reasonable that the PA projection could be preferable

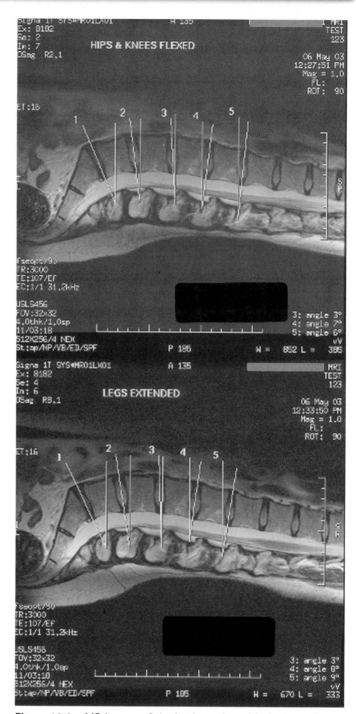

Figure 13.2 MR images of the lumbar spine with the knees in flexion and extension

to AP, as in this position the diverging X-ray beam coincides more closely with the intervertebral joint spaces, enabling better demonstration.

This is not, however, a commonly adopted practice, reasons being the magnification and consequent unsharpness due to increased object film distance (OFD). This could be compensated by an increase in FFD and exposure factors.

Colleran[10] has shown that the magnification produced does not cause significant reduction in image quality and indeed recommends its adoption because of the superior demonstration of the sacrum, sacroiliac (SI) joints and intervertebral joint spaces. Her work has resulted in the adoption of the PA projection in a small number of imaging departments.

Lateral lumbar spine (Fig. 13.3A,B)

If used, a 30 × 40 cm cassette is selected and placed longitudinally in the table bucky. Erect weight-bearing horizontal beam technique may be employed for this projection.[6]

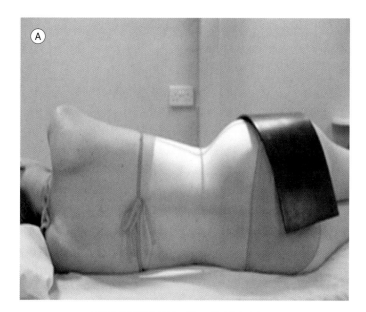

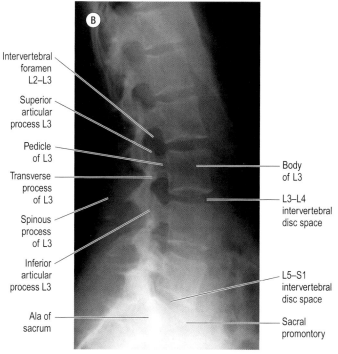

Intervertebral foramen L2–L3

Superior articular process L3

Pedicle of L3

Transverse process of L3

Spinous process of L3

Inferior articular process L3

Ala of sacrum

Body of L3

L3–L4 intervertebral disc space

L5–S1 intervertebral disc space

Sacral promontory

Figure 13.3   Lateral lumbar spine

Positioning

- From the AP position the patient is turned 90° onto their *left* side (see the end of the positioning section for the justification for this) to bring the coronal plane 90° to the table-top and the MSP parallel to it, with their back to the radiographer for ease of positioning
- The knees and hips are flexed for stability and comfort and the arms are rested on the pillow in front of the patient's head; this clears the patient's arms from the required area. A pad may be inserted between the knees to aid patient comfort and stability. Note that the choice of size of the pad is important and should be large enough to ensure that the raised knee enables the pelvis to be adjusted into the lateral position relative to the X-ray couch
- A lead rubber apron is placed across the lower anterior aspect of the abdomen and pelvis for radiation protection, without obscuring the lower lumbar vertebrae and first sacral segment. A thin sheet of lead rubber may not be sufficient to absorb primary beam if this impinges upon any aspect of the sheet, and should not be used
- The spinous processes are palpated and assessed to ensure that the long axis of the spine and the MSP are parallel to the table-top; if not it will be necessary to angle the beam in a direction which will ensure the central ray strikes the long axis of the lumbar vertebrae at 90°. Very often, the female pelvis causes the spine to tilt upwards towards the pelvic end of the vertebral column, whereas the male shoulders can cause the opposite effect (although this has more effect on the lateral thoracic spine projection). Use of radiolucent pads, placed under the lateral aspect of the lower end of the tilted vertebral column, can be used to address this problem. However, the authors question the accuracy and effectiveness of this (see Ch. 12 on the lateral thoracic spine). Assessment of the alignment of the spinous processes must be made with the eyes level with the spine to ensure accuracy (also see 'Positioning Tips' earlier in the chapter). Palpation of the posterior superior iliac spines (PSIS) to check their vertical superimposition will assure accurate lateral position of the pelvic end of the lumbar vertebrae. The shoulder end of the column should also be assessed so that the posterior aspect of the patient's shoulders is vertical
- If the spine has a lateral curvature when the patient is lying on their side, with L1 and L5 higher than the middle vertebrae, it is not usually necessary to make adjustments in the central ray or to use pads. This is because the oblique rays around the central ray are likely to correspond with the obliquity of the intervertebral joint spaces. If a slight curvature appears with L1 and L5 higher than the middle vertebrae (not commonly encountered), it will be more advantageous to turn the patient

onto their opposite side for this projection. In any case, lateral curvature is often best assessed by viewing the AP projection before attempting the lateral position

- If the patient has scoliosis, it is recommended that the side to which the largest curvature is more prominently demonstrated is placed nearest the X-ray couch. The central ray is then directed towards the lowest point of the convex shape of the curvature. This ensures that the oblique rays which penetrate each of the vertebral bodies produce an image which assists in reducing the superimposition of the vertebral bodies over intervertebral joint spaces, demonstrating the joint spaces as efficiently as is possible under the circumstances

- A sheet of lead rubber is placed on the table-top behind the patient to prevent scatter reaching the film, thus improving image quality. There has been some discussion as to the efficacy of use of lead rubber in this circumstance,[11] however its use should be mandatory and has been shown to be effective[12]

Unless otherwise indicated, e.g. by scoliosis, the left lateral should be routinely performed as this results in up to 38% less effective patient dose.[13,14] However, there is some evidence that the right lateral may be preferable in paediatric patients due to the greater radiosensitivity of the liver in children.[15,16]

Beam direction and FFD
Vertical central ray 90° to the long axis of the lumbar spine
100–150 cm FFD

Consider using the longer FFD (e.g. 150 cm) to compensate for large OFD. This will also enable better visualisation of the intervertebral joint spaces as shown in Figure 13.4.

Centring point
At the level of the lower costal margin, which is coincident with L3

The beam is required to be directed through the vertebral body of L3; this can be located 7.5 cm to 10 cm anterior to the spinous process of L3, the distance varying with patient build.

Collimation
T12 to S1, anterior aspects of the vertebral bodies, spinous processes

It may be useful to include the aorta anteriorly in patients where calcification may indicate the presence of atheromatous degeneration within the aorta. Localised deviation (apparent bulge) of the calcified outline of the aorta is indicative of abdominal aortic aneurysm.

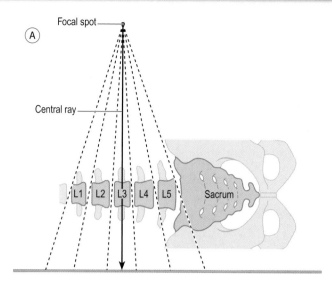

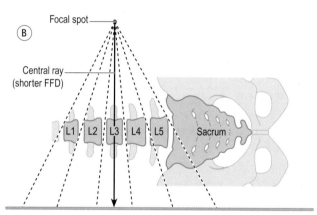

Figure 13.4 Effects of varying FFDs on joint space demonstration. This is a diagrammatic representation of the lumbar vertebrae in the lateral position. **(A)** shows the position which uses a longer FFD than in **(B)**. Notice how the obliquity of the rays at the periphery (L5/S1 and T12/L1) increase with the shorter FFD and increase the chances of vertebral overlap on the image. L3 is unaffected as it lies below the central ray

---

Expose on arrested respiration

The exposure is made on expiration, to ensure the posterolateral aspects of the diaphragms do not overlie L1.

Exposure factors
A kVp high enough to allow penetration and visualisation of the L5/S1 joint space, as well as to demonstrate the lumbar vertebrae, should be used. 80–95 kVp is suggested in EU guidelines.[17]

Criteria for assessing image quality
- T12 to S1, spinous processes and soft tissues anterior to vertebral bodies are demonstrated on the image

- Posterior, superior, and inferior borders of each vertebral body should be superimposed
- Posterior ribs and superior surfaces of the sacral ala should be superimposed
- Joint spaces between each vertebra should be clearly demonstrated *(see discussion below on L5/S1 joint space)*
- Sharp image demonstrating soft tissue structures anterior to the vertebral bodies in contrast to detail of bony cortex and trabeculae; bone seen in contrast with intervertebral joint spaces between T12/L1 down to L5/S1. Spinous processes of lumbar vertebrae visualised

Common errors	Possible reasons
The posterior condyles of the vertebral bodies do not appear superimposed	Rotation of the patient – MSP not parallel to the table-top. Adjust the hips and/or shoulders so that they are superimposed
Disc spaces are not clearly demonstrated – the superior and inferior surfaces of the vertebral bodies are not superimposed	The long axis of the vertebral column is not parallel to the table-top (tilt). See notes in positioning section for methods which may be utilised to correct or compensate. Is there a degree of scoliosis which may be affecting joint space demonstration?
Pale (low density) over L5/S1 region, rest of lumbar spine well demonstrated	Inadequate kVp selected

Modification of technique for trauma

Clearly it is important not to move the patient if trauma is indicated; consequently it is necessary for the lateral view to be obtained using a horizontal beam.

◼ Lateral lumbosacral junction (LSJ)
(Figs 13.5, 13.6A,B)

The LSJ or L5/S1 projection is normally only required if the joint space is not adequately demonstrated on the lateral projection (i.e. if there is overlap of the vertebral body of L5 onto S1 or if there is insufficient penetration to demonstrate the joint space or bony detail of S1), to enable assessment of the intervertebral height. Realistically it is probably unnecessary for the joint space to be 'perfectly' demonstrated, allowing some superimposition of the superior surfaces of S1 and the inferior surfaces of L5. A clear disc

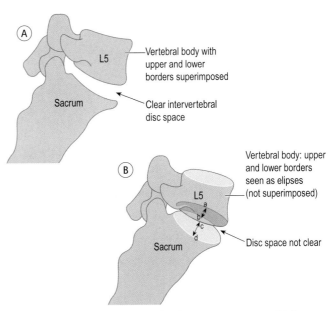

Figure 13.5 'Tilted' lateral lumbar image: assessment of joint space. **(A)** 'Perfect' – L5/S1 showing disc space as seen in (b); **(B)** acceptable – because disc height can be assessed as indicated, by measuring a–b and c–d

space with no superimposition of the vertebral bodies over the space is the ideal result and is what we should be looking to achieve; however, the radiation dose burden of this examination needs to be considered. In order to avoid undertaking a lateral L5/S1 projection in addition to the lateral lumbar, assessment of disc space height can often be made on a less than perfect image as shown in Figure 13.5B, which shows the lower end of the lumbar vertebrae as they might appear on a lateral lumbar spine image. As long as the four surface edges can be identified then an assessment of joint space is possible. These measurements can only be made when the lateral lumbar spine image shows adequate penetration and exposure which provides good detail of the bony trabeculae of the first sacral segment.

If used, an 18 × 24 cm cassette is placed longitudinally in the table bucky.

Erect weight-bearing horizontal beam technique may be employed.[6]

Positioning

- The patient is placed on to their side as for the lateral projection position, i.e. with the MSP parallel to the X-ray table and the vertebral bodies parallel with the table
- An imaginary line adjoining the PSISs will demonstrate the plane of the L5/S1 joint space. If not superimposed, the beam should be angled to coincide with this line

Beam direction and FFD

A vertical central ray, coincident with the L5/S1 joint space (vertical alignment of PSISs). Beam angulation may

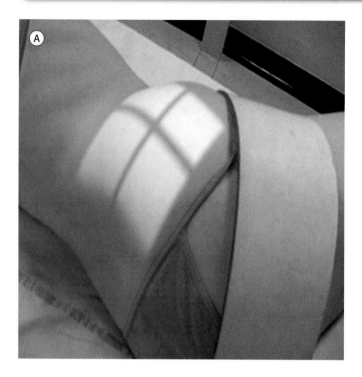

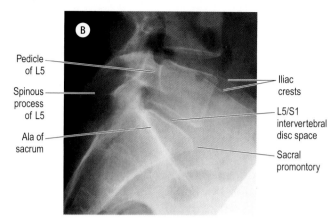

Pedicle of L5

Spinous process of L5

Ala of sacrum

Iliac crests

L5/S1 intervertebral disc space

Sacral promontory

Figure 13.6　Lateral lumbosacral junction

be required to ensure the central ray is directed through the joint space, which should be assessed by viewing:

1. The AP projection to see if there is a lateral tilt of the lower lumbar spine and/or the joint space at the LSJ. The AP projection *must* be available for assessment before attempting the lateral L5/S1 projection
2. The position of the PSISs when lying in the lateral position. They should be vertically aligned in order to justify use of a vertical central ray. Deviation from this position will mean that the central ray must be angled to coincide with the angle made by the PSISs
3. The lateral lumbar spine image. The radiographer may have used a vertical, caudally or cranially angled central ray for the lateral lumbar projection and the appearance of the lateral L5/S1 area on the lateral lumbar spine can be used as a reference point for assessment of the central ray. Modification of the central ray for this projection can be summarised thus:
   - If the lateral lumbar image undertaken with a vertical central ray shows a good L5/S1 joint space (but is underexposed or under-penetrated), angle approximately 5–7° caudally when the beam is centred over the LSJ
   - If the lateral lumbar image undertaken with a caudally angled central ray shows a good L5/S1 joint space (but is underexposed or under-penetrated), add more

caudal angulation before centring the beam over the LSJ
   - If the lateral lumbar image undertaken with a cranially angled central ray shows a good L5/S1 joint space (but is underexposed or under-penetrated), use a vertical beam centred over the LSJ
   - If the lateral lumbar image undertaken with a vertical central ray shows a poor L5/S1 joint space it is most likely that a vertical central ray will be required for the lateral L5/S1 projection unless the AP projection and the PSISs show the opposite is required

100–150 cm FFD

Again, consider using the longer FFD to compensate for long OFD.

Centring point

Through the lumbar sacral junction which lies anterior to the spinous process of L5

This is most readily located as shown in Figure 13.7. An imaginary triangle is drawn between the readily palpable anterior superior iliac spine (ASIS), PSIS and apex of the iliac crest. The L5/S1 junction lies in the centre of this triangle.

Collimation

Body of L5, 1st sacral segment, spinous processes

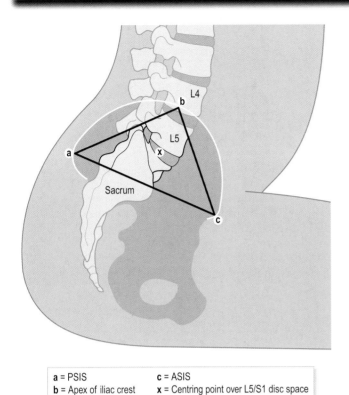

a = PSIS   c = ASIS
b = Apex of iliac crest   x = Centring point over L5/S1 disc space

Figure 13.7 Location of centring point for lateral L5/S1 projection. 'a', 'b' and 'c' show the landmarks which make the triangle around the centring point. The triangle is not necessarily equilateral or isosceles but this is still an effective way to centre accurately

Common errors	Possible reasons
Both sides of ala of sacrum not superimposed; posterior parts of L5 do not appear superimposed	Rotation of the patient. MSP not parallel to the table-top (rotated) – adjust the hips and shoulders so that they are superimposed
Disc spaces are not clearly demonstrated – the superior and inferior surfaces of the vertebral bodies are not superimposed	Incorrect choice of beam angulation *or* The long axis of the vertebral column is not parallel to the table-top

Criteria for assessing image quality
- Bodies of L5 and S1, spinous processes and soft tissues anterior to vertebral bodies are demonstrated on the image
- Posterior, superior, and inferior borders of L5 and S1 should be superimposed
- L5/S1 joint space should be clearly demonstrated *(but see Fig. 13.5)*
- Ala of sacrum superimposed*
- Sharp image demonstrating soft tissue structures anterior to the vertebral bodies in contrast to detail of bony cortex and trabeculae, joint space and spinous process of L5

*Use of the term 'ala' refers to the oblique white lines noted on the lateral projection, which have previously been described as ileopectineal lines, basis ossis sacri or pelvic lines.[18] The lines, whatever their correct name, do lie coincident with the sloped and expanding ala of the sacrum as they join with the pelvis at the sacroiliac joints. The author therefore feels that the use of the name 'ala' is simple and less confusing.

■ AP L5/S1 junction (Fig. 13.8A,B)

Due to the orientation of the lumbar curve, L5 tilts in opposition to the oblique rays of the X-ray beam; thus the L5/S1 joint is not well demonstrated on the standard AP projection. The AP L5/S1 projection is rarely used but may be utilised for additional evaluation in relevant clinical circumstances,[19] which is most commonly requested for specialist orthopaedic assessment.

If used, an 18 × 24 cm cassette is placed in the table bucky.

Positioning
The patient is positioned as for an AP lumbar spine projection

Beam direction and FFD
Initially vertical, with a cranial angle of 10–20°, according to the patient's lumbar lordosis, which tends to be more extreme in the female adult.[20] The lateral projection should be viewed before assessing the angulation required

Centring point
In the midline, level with the ASISs; this may vary slightly, according to cranial angle used

Collimation
L4/L5 junction, L5, transverse processes, L5/S1 junction

Criteria for assessing image quality
- L4/L5 junction, L5, transverse processes, and L5/S1 junction are demonstrated
- L4/L5 and L5/S1 joint space shown clearly
- Spinous process of L5 centralised over vertebral body
- Sharp image showing contrast between bony trabeculae of vertebral bodies and the joint spaces between

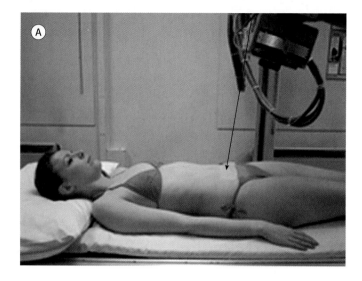

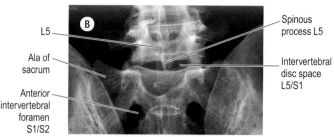

Figure 13.8 AP LSJ. **(B)** Notice how the appearances of L5 and its spinous process and L5/S1 joint space change from the AP lumbar spine image (Fig. 13.1b) to this, the AP L5/S1 image. This is because: (1) the oblique rays in the AP lumbar image are caudal and the lumbar curve tilts the body of L5 forwards over the joint space; (2) the beam is angled opposite to this (cranially) for the AP L5/S1 projection, coinciding with the disc space

Common error	Possible reason
Poor joint space visualisation	Inaccurate angle selection

OBLIQUE LUMBAR SPINE

Oblique projections may be undertaken with the patient prone or supine. Posterior oblique projections are used and demonstrate the side closest to the image receptor. Anterior obliques could be used and would demonstrate the side furthest from the receptor, raising the side under examination and centring over the 3rd lumbar vertebra. Oblique projections demonstrate the apophyseal joints, laminae, pedicles and pars interarticularis. They are used in particular to demonstrate defects in the pars inter-articularis which may result in spondylolisthesis. Both obliques are undertaken, for comparison.

Traditionally, posterior obliques have been used most extensively, in order to reduce the OFD and therefore minimise magnification unsharpness. Unfortunately the lumbar curve lies in opposition to the oblique rays, which gradually increase in obliquity towards each end of the lumbar vertebrae, increasing the longitudinal obliquity of all but L3 on the image. Use of the anterior oblique approach would bring the lumbar curve into a position which more closely follows the pattern of central and oblique rays, reducing the longitudinal obliquity of L1, L2, L4 and L5. Although OFD would be increased for this projection, anterior abdominal tissue is compressed; this allows for reduction in scatter and a reduction in exposure factors may be considered if tissue compression is significant. However, patients with back pain or limited movement are likely to find the semi-prone position difficult and for this reason the posterior obliques are described in more detail.

MRI is the investigation of choice in the symptomatic patient, however non-specific abnormalities are commonly detected even in asymptomatic patients, so careful thought must be given to the appropriateness of imaging.[21]

If used, a 24 × 30 cm cassette is placed longitudinally in the table bucky for posterior or anterior obliques (30 × 40 cm may be used for taller patients).

■ Posterior obliques (Fig. 13.9A,B)

Positioning
- The patient lies supine, their MSP coincident with and perpendicular to the midline of the table
- The arm on the side under examination is raised onto the pillow, for comfort and ease of positioning
- The patient is rotated 45° *towards* the side under examination
- Radiolucent pads are placed under the trunk and raised shoulder for support. The arm on the unaffected side must be clear of the area under examination

Beam direction and FFD
Vertical

or – the beam is angled with a cranial or caudal tilt of between 10°–15° *if the patient presents with a marked lordosis*. The degree of angle used is dependent upon the degree of lordosis and the direction of angle employed relates to which vertebrae are under examination (e.g. caudal angle for L1 and L2, cranial for L4 and L5)
100 cm FFD

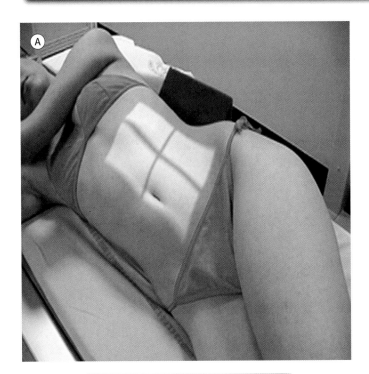

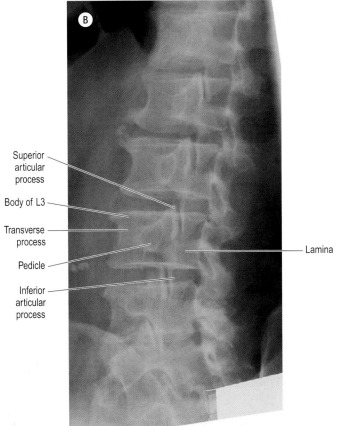

Superior articular process

Body of L3

Transverse process

Pedicle

Inferior articular process

Lamina

Figure 13.9 Posterior oblique lumbar spine

Centring point

Over the raised side of the trunk at the level of the lower costal margin (level of L3), in the mid-clavicular line

Collimation

T12/L1 junction, L5/S1 junction, bodies and transverse processes of lumbar vertebrae

Criteria for assessing image quality

- T12/L1 junction, L5/S1 junction, bodies and transverse processes of lumbar vertebrae are demonstrated
- 'Scottie dog' appearance seen within the associated vertebral body, with a dog's nose seen touching the edge of the vertebral body and the back of the dog's front leg coincident with the middle of the vertebral body. Structures correspond to the dog as follows:
  - Nose = transverse process
  - Eye = pedicle
  - Ear = superior articular process
  - Body = lamina
  - Neck = pars interarticularis
  - Front leg = inferior articular process
  - Please note that the position of the dog in relationship to its associated vertebral body will vary slightly in a longitudinal direction, according to the relationship of the vertebral body and its distance from the central ray. It is suggested that L3 is used to assess positional accuracy, since it lies most perpendicular to the central ray
- Sharp image showing soft tissue in contrast with bone and 'scottie dog' in contrast with the bony trabeculae of the associated vertebral body

Common errors	Possible reasons
Dog's nose is elongated and most of it lies outside the vertebral body outline	Inadequate rotation
Dog's nose squashed and lies well within vertebral body outline	Excessive rotation

◼ Posterior oblique L5 (Fig. 13.10A,B)

For this projection, positioning is as for the posterior oblique lumbar vertebrae, with the following adjustments due to the position of the vertebral body and its extreme tilt at the end of the lumbar lordosis: Anterior obliques may also be considered, with the direction of beam angulation in opposition to that used for posterior obliques and the centring point adapted to lie over the PSIS of the raised side.

Beam direction and FFD

Initially vertical, angled 10–20° cranially. The image receptor is displaced until coincident with the primary beam
100 cm FFD

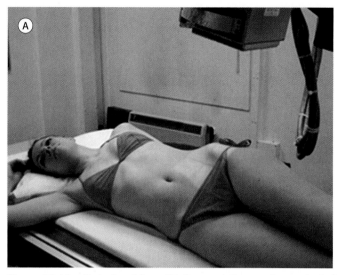

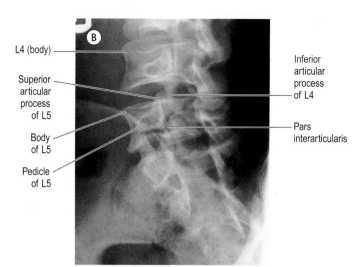

L4 (body)

Superior articular process of L5

Body of L5

Pedicle of L5

Inferior articular process of L4

Pars interarticularis

Figure 13.10   Posterior oblique L5. Compare the pars interarticularis on this image to that of L3 on Figure 13.9B. The neck of the Scottie dog in Figure 13.9B is intact whereas here there appears to be a dark line or collar, which is suggestive of spondylolisthesis

Centring point
Level with the ASIS in the midclavicular line

Collimation
L4/L5 junction, L5, S1

Criteria for assessing image quality
- L4/L5 junction, L5 and S1 are demonstrated
- 'Scottie dog' appearance seen within L5 as explained for oblique lumbar vertebrae
- Clear joint space between L4 and 5, and L5 and S1
- Sharp image showing soft tissue in contrast with bone and 'scottie dog' in contrast with the bony trabeculae of L5. Bone seen in contrast with joint spaces

■ Erect laterals in flexion and extension

Flexion and extension views may be used to demonstrate the range of movement within the lumbar spine. With the development of erect scanning by FONAR, it is now possible to perform this examination by MRI.[22,23]

If used, a 30 × 40 cm cassette is placed longitudinally in the erect bucky.

Positioning
- The patient is in the erect lateral position – the patient can be seated or standing. The MSP is parallel to the erect bucky, usually with the left side in contact with it
- For the flexion projection the patient bends forward, flexing the spine as far forward as possible, arms extended forward, holding a fixed support or their legs to aid immobilisation

- For the extension projection the patient leans backwards, extending the spine as far as possible; again immobilisation devices can be provided

Central ray, FFD, centring point
Central ray horizontal, at 90° to the long axis of the spine. The rest of the technique is as for the lateral projection

SACROILIAC JOINTS

The sacroiliac joints are difficult to assess on AP projections of the lumbar spine or pelvis, due to the oblique nature of the joints. The sacral angle, which lies in opposition to the oblique rays at the periphery of the X-ray beam, causes foreshortening of the joints on the AP lumbar projection. On the AP pelvis projection, the sacral and sacroiliac joint angle is far greater than the obliquity of X-rays around the central ray. The joints travel from the back of the sacrum and pelvis in an anterolateral direction (approximately 15°), again crossing the oblique rays in any AP position, rather than lying coincidentally with them. Therefore it is necessary to use a technique that considers the effects normal anatomy has on the demonstration of these joints.

Many years ago it was believed that the joints were demonstrated with a prone patient position and very short FFD; the short FFD was suggested in order to provide maximum angulation of oblique rays around the central ray and pass more accurately through the joints. This was combined with the prone position, which placed the sacral angle in a more suitable orientation. Unfortunately, although a prone position is often recommended for dose reduction to gonads, this method increases skin dose significantly and is not likely to provide noticeable improvement of joint visualisation; it has been estimated that an unobtainable and unfeasible FFD of 18 cm would be required in order to provide obliquity of rays which will coincide with the 15° angles of the joints.[24] A prone projection at 100 cm FFD, with the caudal angle selected to pass through the sacral angle at 90°, is therefore recommended if a single projection is required. Alternatively, individual posterior oblique projections of each joint will demonstrate the joints most effectively but will require the patient to be exposed to ionising radiation twice (although close collimation will reduce the associated risks of exposure to ionising radiation).

▪ Prone sacroiliac joints (SIJs) (Fig. 13.11A,B)

If used, a 24 × 30 cm cassette is placed crosswise in the table bucky.

Positioning
- The patient lies prone, arms placed on the pillow and head turned to the side for comfort
- The MSP is perpendicular to the table-top and positioned to lie coincident with the long axis of the table

Beam direction and FFD
A vertical central ray is angled caudally until at 90° to the long axis of the sacrum
100 cm FFD

Centring
Midway between the PSIS

Collimation
SIJs, L5/S1 joint

Criteria for assessing image quality
- SIJs and L5/S1 joint are demonstrated
- Symmetry of sacrum and sacroiliac joints
- Sharp image demonstrating the trabecular pattern of sacrum and ilium and lower density of the SIJs in contrast with the sacrum and ilium

▪ Posterior oblique SIJs (Fig. 13.12A,B)

Both joints are examined for comparison.
If used, an 18 × 24 cm cassette is placed longitudinally in the table bucky.

Positioning
- The patient lies supine, with the MSP initially coincident with the long axis of the table
- The side under examination is raised 15° and a radiolucent pad placed under the raised side for immobilisation
- The arm on the lowered side is placed on the pillow for comfort and the leg on the same side flexed at the knee to aid stability
- A sheet of lead rubber is applied to the lower pelvis region, below the level of the SIJs

Beam direction and FFD
1. Vertical *or*
2. Angled 10–15° cranially, to compensate for the sacral angle
   The second option can, in some cases, project the image of the ischium over the inferior aspect of the SIJ. This is more likely in males, due to the shallower pelvis.

Centring
1. 2.5 cm medial to the ASIS on the raised side
2. 2.5 cm medial to and below the ASIS on the raised side

Collimation
SIJ on the raised side

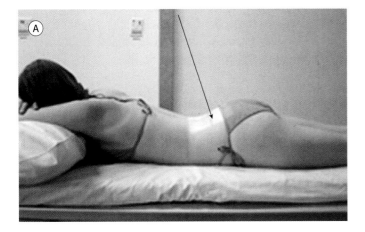

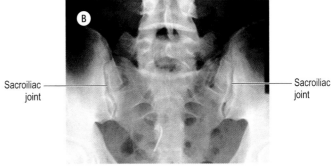

Figure 13.11   Prone SIJs

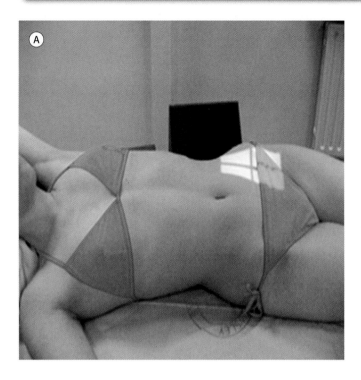

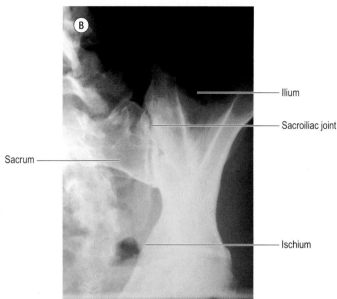

Figure 13.12 Posterior oblique sacroiliac joints

Criteria for assessing image quality
- SIJ is demonstrated
- SIJ is shown clear of iliac crest and ASIS
- Joint space seen clearly
- Sharp image showing bony trabeculae of sacrum and ilium and the lower density joint in contrast with sacrum and ilium

Common errors	Possible reasons
Joint space overlaps	Since the joint surfaces are not flat, some irregularity of the joint will be noted. Total loss of joint space is due to inaccurate obliquity. There may be indistinct or lost joint space in cases of degenerative diseases, such as ankylosing spondylitis
Ilium superimposed over joint	Too much obliquity

OTHER IMAGING MODALITIES AND THE LUMBAR SPINE

As previously stated, MRI is generally recognised as the most appropriate modality for lumbar spine imaging in many circumstances.[1,4,21] Cost and availability are factors which will still predispose some departments to the continued use of plain film radiography; the significant radiation dose burden must, however, always be considered for justification of this procedure.[14] New techniques are in development such as erect MRI scanning, enabling a wide variety of examinations to be performed.[23]

Computed tomography (CT) has been advocated for demonstration of pars interarticularis abnormalities which lead to spondylolisthesis,[25] but its role in imaging the intervertebral disc should now be limited to patients unable to undergo MRI. CT also has a role in significant trauma where modern multislice scanners can utilise multiplanar and 3D bony reconstruction techniques.

References
1. van den Bosch M, et al. Evidence against the use of lumbar spine radiography for low back pain. Clinical Radiology 2004; 59(1):69–76.
2. Royal College of Radiologists working party. Making the best use of a department of clinical radiology: guidelines for doctors. 5th edn. London: Royal College of Radiologists; 2003.
3. Kendrick D, et al. Radiography of the lumbar spine in primary care patients with low back pain: randomised controlled trial. British Medical Journal 2001; 322:400–405.
4. Miller P, et al. Cost-effectiveness of lumbar spine radiography in primary care patients with low back pain. Spine 2002; 27(20):2291–2297.
5. Editor's choice. Challenges to orthodoxy? British Medical Journal 2001; 322(7283):0.
6. Wood A. Imaging the spine: Why take it lying down? Synergy 2003; Dec:16–19.

7. McQuillen Martensen K. Radiographic critique. Philadelphia: WB Saunders; 1995.

8. Whitley A, et al. Special procedures in diagnostic imaging. Oxford: Butterworth Heinemann; 1991.

9. Murrie VL, et al. Supportive cushions produce no practical reduction in lumbar lordosis. British Journal of Radiology 2002; 75:536–538.

10. Colleran C. PA lumbar spines; a future concept. Radiography Today 1994; 60(681):17–20.

11. Mitchell F, et al. Scattered radiation and the lumbar spine. Radiography Today 1991; 57(645):12–14.

12. Thomas A. Imaging the lateral thoracic spine. Synergy 2003; Apr:10–13.

13. Hart D, et al. Estimation of effective dose in radiology from entrance surface dose and dose area product measurements. NRPB 262 Chilton 1994.

14. Nicholson R, et al. Awareness by radiology staff of the difference in radiation risk from two opposing lateral lumbar spine examinations. British Journal of Radiology 1999; 72:221.

15. Hart D, et al. Coefficients for estimating effective doses from paediatric x-ray examinations. NRPB 279 Chilton 1996.

16. Chapple C, et al. Awareness by radiology staff of the difference in radiation risk from two opposing lateral lumbar spine examinations. British Journal of Radiology 2000; 73:568.

17. European Guidelines on Quality Criteria for Diagnostic Radiographic Images. EUR 16260 Luxembourg Office for Official Publications of the European Communities; 1997.

18. Wong-Chung J, et al. Two parallel linear densities on lateral radiographs of the lumbosacral spine: neither ileopectineal lines nor basis ossis sacri. British Journal of Radiology 1997; 70:58–61.

19. ACR Practice guideline for the performance of spine radiography in children and adults. ACR; 2002.

20. Murrie VL, et al. Lumbar lordosis measurement: a study in patients with and without low back pain. Clinical Anatomy 2001; 14:298.

21. ACR Appropriateness criteria. Acute low back pain – radiculopathy. ACR; 1996.

22. Jinkins J, et al. Upright, weight-bearing, dynamic-kinetic magnetic resonance imaging of the spine – review of the first clinical results. Journal of Hong Kong College of Radiology 2003; 6:55–74.

23. www.fonar.com

24. Unett EM, Royle AJ. Radiographic techniques and image evaluation. London: Chapman and Hall; 1997.

25. Mayor P. Invited review: spondylolysis: current imaging and management. Proceedings of UK Radiological Congress 2003. British Journal of Radiology 2003; 76(Supp):35.

SACRUM AND COCCYX

Elizabeth Carver

SACRUM

Trauma relating to the sacrum may well be associated with other injury to the pelvic ring and imaging of the pelvis is likely to be required in addition to examination of the sacrum. In cases of severe trauma it is inadvisable to undertake a lateral projection of the sacral area in the position described in this section; a horizontal beam approach would be the method of choice. However, since serious pelvis trauma will probably be assessed by initial pelvis images which will be supplemented by CT examination, a lateral sacrum image is unlikely to be required.

The sacrum may be a site for metastatic spread of malignancy and plain images of the region will demonstrate such lesions. The appearance of sacral foraminae should not be confused with areas of loss of bone density caused by metastases.

The lumbar curve varies with each individual patient and causes variation in the angles created between the sacrum and lumbar vertebrae. As a result it is suggested that the cranial angulation required to strike the sacrum at 90° in the anteroposterior (AP) position will vary from 10–25°, according to the individual patient's build. The most efficient strategy for making a decision on appropriate angulation is to undertake the lateral projection initially and use it to assess the required angle before proceeding with the AP projection. This also applies to the coccyx.

If the examination request outlines that information on the coccyx is required, the lateral projection of the coccyx can be included on the lateral sacrum projection, to reduce the number of exposures made. For this reason, the coccyx is also referred to in the description of the lateral projection.

If used, a 24 × 30 cm cassette is placed longitudinally in the table bucky for both lateral and AP projections of the sacrum.

Lateral sacrum (Fig. 14.1A,B)

Positioning
- The patient lies on their side, with hips and knees flexed to maintain stability and the feet placed together to prevent the patient from rolling forwards or backwards. The arms are flexed at the elbow and raised to rest on the pillows for comfort and to clear them from the area of interest
- Lead rubber is applied over the raised side, diagonally from anterior superior iliac spine (ASIS) to the femoral head, to cover the anterior portion of the pelvis and to protect the gonads
- The palm of the radiographer's hand is used to palpate the posterior aspect of the sacrum and ensure that its transverse axis is perpendicular to the table-top
- The long axis of the sacrum is parallel to the table-top; this should be checked with the area at the radiographer's eye level for accuracy. If patient build affects the relationship of the sacrum to the table-top, a compensating cranial or caudal central ray can be used (see beam direction, below)

Beam direction and FFD
Vertical, directed at 90° to the long axis of the sacrum once this has been assessed
100 cm FFD

Centring
Midway between the posterior superior iliac spines (PSISs) and sacrococcygeal junction

As the coccyx is more difficult to palpate than the sacrum, the level of its first segment may be difficult to locate. An alternative method to palpation uses the relationship of sacrococcygeal junction which lies approximately level with the midpoint of the upper border of the

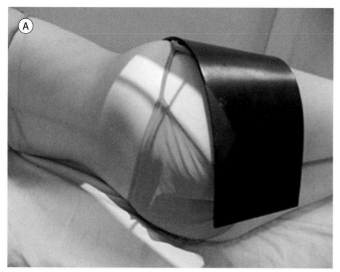

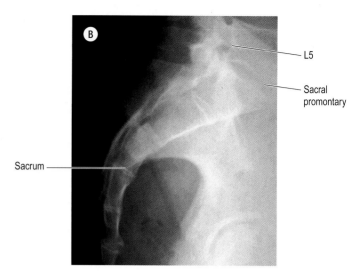

Figure 14.1 Lateral sacrum

symphysis pubis; palpation of the symphysis pubis anteriorly will allow the radiographer to estimate the level of the first coccygeal segment posteriorly.

Collimation

Lumbosacral junction, sacral promontory, soft tissues overlying the sacrum posteriorly, coccyx

Criteria for assessing image quality

- Lumbosacral junction, sacral promontory, soft tissues overlying the sacrum posteriorly and coccyx are demonstrated. Omission of the coccyx from the field may be acceptable if demonstration of the coccyx is not required specifically for the examination
- Joint space at the lumbosacral junction is demonstrated

Common errors	Possible reasons
Non-superimposition of ala	Rotation
Sacrum demonstrated but detail of coccyx less so, or not seen *If information relating to the coccyx is not required for the examination, repeat examination should not be attempted*	1. kVp may not be correct to demonstrate the range of densities encountered over sacrum and coccyx 2. A combination of the higher exposure factors and increased scatter associated with larger patients may have affected image contrast and quality. This is not necessarily considered a radiographer error; close collimation will reduce scatter but will not eliminate it

- Ala of sacrum superimposed*
- Sharp image demonstrating bony trabeculae. Adequate penetration to demonstrate detail of sacrum and less dense coccyx on the one image

*Use of the term 'ala' refers to the oblique white lines noted on the lateral projection, which have previously been called ileopectineal lines, basis ossis sacri or pelvic lines.[1] The lines, whatever their correct name, do lie coincidentally with the sloped and expanding ala of the sacrum as they join with the pelvis at the sacroiliac joints. The author therefore feels that use of the name 'ala' is simple and less confusing.

■ AP sacrum (Fig. 14.2A,B)

Positioning

- The patient is supine with arms slightly abducted from the trunk
- The median sagittal plane (MSP) is coincident with the long axis of the table
- For male patients, lead rubber or lead gonad protection is applied below the symphysis pubis
- ASISs are equidistant from the table-top

Beam direction and focus film distance (FFD)

The lateral sacrum projection is examined to assess the angle of the sacrum

Initially, the central ray is vertical, angled 10–25° cranially until 90° to the long axis of the sacrum

Centring

In the midline, midway between the level of the ASISs and the upper border of symphysis pubis

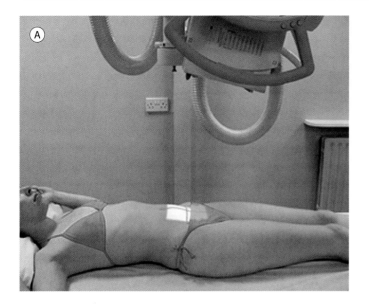

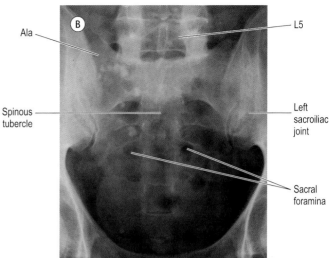

Figure 14.2   AP sacrum

The centre of the cassette, if used, is displaced to coincide with the emerging central ray. A digital plate receptor should include the field of radiation

Collimation
Lumbosacral joint space, sacrococcygeal junction, sacroiliac joints

Criteria for assessing image quality
- Lumbosacral joint space, sacrococcygeal junction and sacroiliac joints are demonstrated
- Symphysis pubis is superimposed over coccyx
- Symmetry of sacral foraminae
- Sharp image demonstrating bony detail of spinous tubercles in contrast with the body of the sacrum and all bony detail of the sacrum in contrast with the soft tissues of the pelvic cavity

Common errors	Possible reasons
Asymmetry of sacral foraminae	Rotation about the MSP
Symphysis pubis superimposed over lower sacral segments	Angle of beam is too great
Foreshortened sacrum	Inadequate angle used
Ala of sacrum seen but sacral segments 2–4 superimposed; 5th segment seen	Angle selected is in wrong direction (caudal)

COCCYX

Under EU 118 and RCR guidelines, trauma to the coccyx and coccydinia are not routine indicators for radiographic examination of the coccyx since confirmation of effects on the coccyx does not alter patient management.[2,3] The range of 'normal' appearances of the human coccyx can make radiological assessment a difficult task.

However, although guidelines rule out these, the most frequently encountered problems associated with the coccyx, as routine indicators it must be assumed that cases of extreme pain or trauma may necessitate radiographic examination of the area.

If used, 18 × 24 cm cassettes are selected for lateral and AP projections of the coccyx, placed longitudinally in the bucky.

Lateral coccyx (Fig. 14.3A,B)
Positioning
- The patient lies on their side and is positioned as for the lateral sacrum and coccyx projection
- A lead rubber sheet is applied diagonally from ASIS to the femoral head

Beam direction and FFD
Vertical, directed at 90° to the long axis of the sacrum and coccyx
100 cm FFD

Centring
At the base of the sacrum, level with the midpoint of the symphysis pubis

Collimation
Coccyx, sacrococcygeal junction

Criteria for assessing image quality
- Coccyx and sacrococcygeal junction are demonstrated

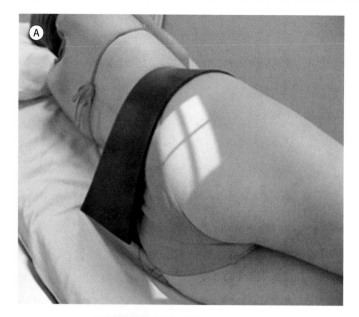

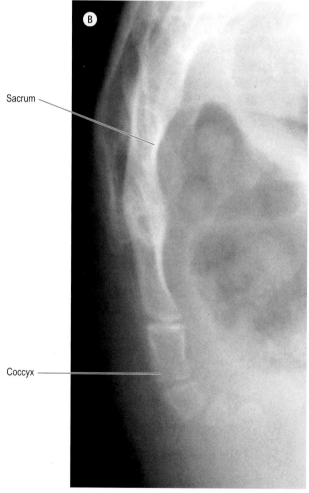

Sacrum

Coccyx

Figure 14.3   Lateral coccyx

- Sharp image demonstrating separate coccygeal segments in contrast to the surrounding soft tissues

Common error	Possible reason
Inadequate contrast to distinctly demonstrate coccyx in contrast to soft tissues of buttocks	Usually due to patient build and implications of associated scatter (see errors section under AP coccyx)

AP coccyx (Fig. 14.4A,B)

Positioning
- The patient is supine as for the AP sacrum projection
- For male patients, lead rubber or lead gonad protection is applied below the symphysis pubis, to protect the gonads

Beam direction and FFD
The lateral coccyx or sacrum and coccyx projection is examined to assess the angle of the coccyx

Initially the central ray is vertical, angled approximately 15° caudally until 90° to the long axis of the coccygeal segments
100 cm FFD

Centring
In the midline, midway between the level of the ASISs and the upper border of symphysis pubis

The centre of the cassette, if used, is displaced to coincide with the emerging central ray. A digital plate receptor should include the field of radiation.

Collimation
Sacrococcygeal junction, all coccygeal segments

Criteria for assessing image quality
- Sacrococcygeal junction and all coccygeal segments are demonstrated
- Symphysis pubis is cleared from the coccyx
- Foreshortened sacrum
- Sharp image demonstrating coccygeal segments in contrast with the soft tissues of the pelvic cavity

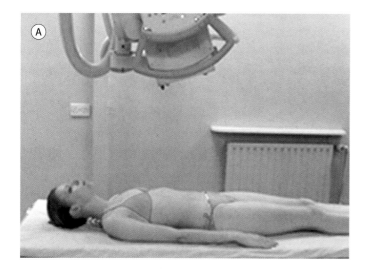

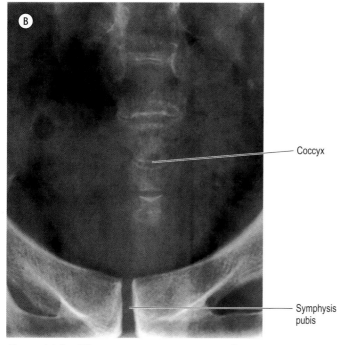

Figure 14.4 AP coccyx

Common errors	Possible reasons
Poor contrast between coccyx and soft tissues or coccyx not demonstrated	1. Although the coccyx itself is not particularly dense, the pelvic area in the larger patient is an area of relatively large body thickness. Increased scatter associated with larger patients may thus have affected image contrast and quality. This is not necessarily considered a radiographer error and may be unavoidable in some cases 2. Faecal matter and bowel gas may also overlie the area and mask the low density structure of the coccyx
Coccygeal segments superimposed over the sacrum	Excessive angle used
Sacrum not foreshortened; coccygeal segments foreshortened or superimposed	Angle selected is in wrong direction (cranial)

References

1. Wong-Chung J, et al. Two parallel linear densities on lateral radiographs of the lumbosacral spine: neither ileopectineal lines nor basis ossis sacri. British Journal of Radiology 1997; 70:58–61.
2. Radiation Protection 118. Referral Guidelines for Imaging. 2000. European Commission. Luxembourg.
3. Royal College of Radiologists working party. Making the best use of a department of clinical radiology: guidelines for doctors. 5th edn. London: Royal College Of Radiologists; 2003.

THORACIC SKELETON

Elizabeth Carver

The bones of the thorax comprise the ribs and sternum but radiographic examination of the area also involves demonstration of the sternoclavicular joints. Referrals for radiography of the ribs have declined, especially in cases of trauma. Although painful, rib fractures are treated conservatively unless displacement causes fracture fragments to penetrate the soft issue of the thorax and induce pneumothorax or haemothorax. Evidence of these conditions is definitely required via radiographic examination but the posteroanterior (PA) chest projection is considered to be the most appropriate means for demonstration of these appearances since the most important aspect of diagnosis is that of assessing the effect injury may have had on thoracic contents.[1] The PA chest film is also very likely to demonstrate the fractured rib and fragments causing a pneumothorax, haemothorax or evidence of visceral damage.[2,3] Ribs positioned below the diaphragm on the PA image are those that are less likely to penetrate the pleura. The PA chest image also shows ribs 1–6 reasonably well, but not ribs 7–12.

There may be, however, a case for demonstration of pathological fractures, for example those caused by metastatic deposits. This is often due to the need for diagnosis of the presence of metastatic spread itself rather than specific evidence of its effects on the rib. For this reason oblique projections of the ribs are included in this chapter. In addition to fractures and metastasis, other rib lesions seen on plain radiography include fibrous dysplasia, aneurysmal bone cysts, myeloma and granuloma.[1]

OBLIQUE RIBS

The oblique projection is designed to turn the lateral portions of the ribs away from their profiled position as seen on the PA chest radiograph. Of course, this means that other aspects of the ribs will not be well demonstrated on the oblique projection. For this reason oblique rib examinations should always be undertaken in addition to a PA chest radiograph.

It is more than obvious that exposures should be made on arrested respiration but the phase varies according to ribs under examination, due to diaphragmatic position in relationship to individual rib height. Since the diaphragm effectively splits the area covered by ribs into two density thicknesses, this has implications for adequate demonstration of ribs on the radiograph. As a result, exposure for oblique projections of the upper ribs (1–6) is made on arrested inspiration to facilitate their demonstration over the air-filled lung tissue, and ribs 7–12 on expiration to demonstrate them over abdominal tissue below the diaphragm.

In addition to the phase of respiration, angulation can be used to maximise the number of ribs shown above or below the diaphragm. Caudal angulation will project the image of the diaphragm lower in the case of the upper ribs, as can cranial angulation to project it higher and maximise the number of lower ribs shown below the diaphragm.

◼ Posterior oblique for upper ribs (Fig. 15.1A,B)

If used, a 30 × 40 cm cassette is selected and placed longitudinally in the erect cassette holder (or bucky for large patients).

Positioning
- A lead rubber apron is applied to the patient's waist
- The patient stands with their back to the image receptor and faces the X-ray tube; the side under examination is positioned with the lateral borders of ribs 1–6 well within

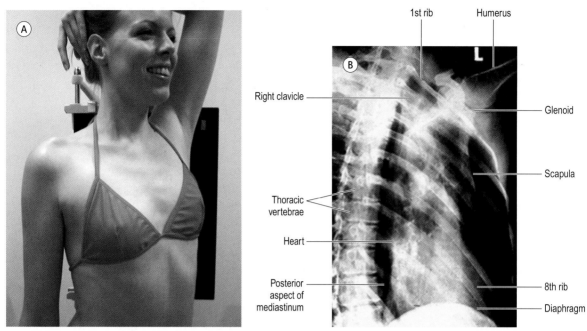

Figure 15.1   Posterior oblique – upper ribs. (B) Reproduced with permission from Bryan GJ. Skeletal anatomy. 3rd edn. Edinburgh: Churchill Livingstone; 1996 and Gunn (2002)

the cassette border, if used. *Or* collimate to the size of the area of interest if using a digital system
- The arm on the side under investigation is raised and the forearm rested on the head; this will clear the arm from the area of interest
- The patient is rotated 30–45° towards the side under examination; the thorax on the side of interest rests against the image receptor

Beam direction and focus film distance (FFD)
100 cm FFD
If a cassette is used: the upper edge of the cassette is positioned level with C7 and a horizontal beam is centred over the middle of the upper border of the cassette. The beam is then directed caudally until coincident with the centre of the cassette
For a digital system: initially horizontal, with 12° caudal angulation to the centre of the image receptor

Centring
If a cassette is used: to the middle of the cassette, as outlined above
For a digital system: midway between the sternal notch and xiphisternum

Collimation
C7 to T12, lateral margins of ribs on affected side, mid-clavicular line on the opposite side

It is not necessary for this projection to be undertaken erect but it is described thus as it is simpler for the radi-

ographer to adjust the cassette height using an erect cassette holder and is more comfortable for the patient who has painful ribs, since their weight does not lie on their injured thoracic rib cage. Traditionally the upper rib oblique projection has been described using a moving grid (bucky)[4,5] but, since ribs 1–6 lie superior to the diaphragm in a low density area, direct exposure is possible without an anti-scatter device. This allows reduction in exposure factors and therefore affords less radiation dose to the patient. Supine oblique positioning can still be adopted on patients who cannot sit or stand erect.

In the case of larger patients it is possible that provision of adequate contrast may be compromised by an increase in tissue density. This, coupled with the higher density over the mediastinum, may require the use of a grid or bucky.

> Expose on arrested inspiration

Criteria for assessing image quality
- The entire length of ribs 1–6 are demonstrated above diaphragm
- Arm is cleared from thorax
- Heart shadow may overlie medial aspect of 6th rib in the case of right-sided ribs, or most of the 6th rib in the case of the left
- Oblique appearance of thoracic vertebrae
- Image of anterior ribs moved laterally in comparison to their position as seen on the PA chest image
- Sharp image demonstrating ribs in contrast to air-filled lung tissue and viscera of the mediastinum and heart

Common errors	Possible reasons
High contrast image which does not demonstrate ribs in contrast to viscera and heart	kVp selected is too low. It will be necessary to compensate for kVp increase by decreasing mAs proportionally to avoid over-blackening over the lung area
Over-blackened image generally	If AEC used, the central ray and chamber selected may be lying over the dense mediastinum
Pale shadow overlying lateral ribs	Arm not cleared from area
Lower ribs (4–6) pale and shown below diaphragm	Exposed on expiration

▨ Posterior oblique for lower ribs (Fig. 15.2A,B)

If used, a 30 × 40 cm cassette is selected and placed longitudinally in the erect bucky.

Positioning

- A lead rubber apron is applied to the patient's waist
- The patient stands with their back to the image receptor and faces the X-ray tube; the side under examination is positioned with the lateral borders of ribs 7–12 well within the cassette border *or* collimate to the size of the area of interest if using a digital system
- The arm on the side under investigation is raised and the forearm rested on the head; this will clear the arm from the area of interest
- The patient is rotated 30–45° towards the side under examination; the thorax on the side of interest rests against the image receptor

Beam direction and FFD

100 cm FFD

If a cassette is used: the lower edge of the cassette is positioned level with the lower costal margin and a horizontal beam is centred over the middle of the lower border of the cassette. The beam is then directed cranially until coincident with the centre of the cassette

For a digital system: initially horizontal, with 12° cranial angulation to the centre of the image receptor

Centring

If a cassette is used: to the middle of the cassette, as outlined above

For a digital system: midway between the lower costal margin and xiphisternum

Collimation

2.5 cm below lower costal margin to midway between the sternal notch and xiphisternum, lateral margins of ribs on the affected side, midclavicular line on the opposite side

> **Expose on arrested expiration**

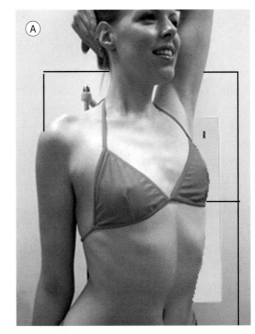

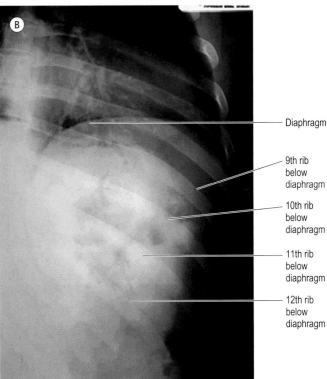

Diaphragm

9th rib below diaphragm

10th rib below diaphragm

11th rib below diaphragm

12th rib below diaphragm

Figure 15.2 Posterior oblique – lower ribs

Note that the oblique for lower ribs has been described, as for the upper ribs, with the patient erect. This is in contrast with other texts,[5] which suggest this projection be undertaken with the patient in a supine oblique position. The erect position has been used here simply for reasons of patient comfort.

Criteria for assessing image quality
- The entire length of ribs 7–12 demonstrated below the diaphragm; ribs 7 and 8 are frequently shown above the diaphragm but, since the heart shadow tends to overlie these ribs in the oblique position, contrast over these ribs is usually similar to those seen below the diaphragm
- Arm cleared from thorax
- Oblique appearance of thoracic vertebrae
- Ribs appear less curved than in a PA or anteroposterior (AP) image
- Sharp image demonstrating ribs in contrast to abdominal and heart tissue

Common errors	Possible reasons
Pale shadow overlying lateral ribs	Arm not cleared from area
Ribs 7–8 dark and shown above diaphragm	Exposed on inspiration; more likely to affect the right side than the left due to there being less heart tissue superimposed over the ribs on this side

STERNUM

Mechanism for injury to the sternum is most likely to be that of a crush injury as in road traffic accidents when the steering wheel impacts upon the driver's chest. The lateral projection is recommended for patients with sternal injury[2] and can be undertaken with the patient seated or supine on a trolley.

■ Lateral sternum (Fig. 15.3A,B)

If used, a 24 × 30 cm cassette is selected for this examination and placed in an erect holder. A grid or erect bucky may be required for larger patients.

Positioning
- A lead rubber apron is applied to the patient's waist
- The patient stands or sits erect with the lateral aspect of their chest placed in contact with the image receptor. If standing, their feet are separated for stability

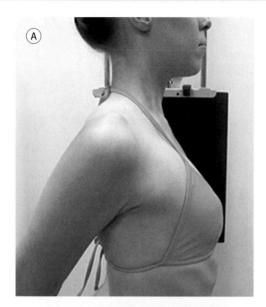

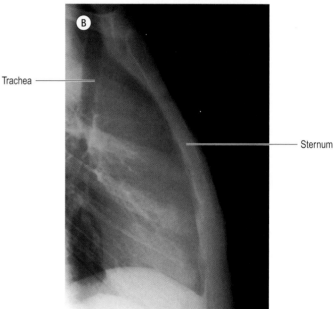

Trachea

Sternum

Figure 15.3 Lateral sternum

- The height of the cassette, if used, is adjusted until its middle is coincident with a point midway between the sternal notch and xiphisternum
- The anterior aspect of the sternum is placed coincident with the longitudinal midline of the cassette, if used
- The median sagittal plane (MSP) is parallel to the image receptor
- The arms are raised above the head to clear from the area of interest as for the chest lateral *or* the shoulders are pulled back (this may be difficult for some patients)

Beam direction and FFD
Horizontal, at 90° to the image receptor
100 cm FFD

Centring
Midway between the sternal notch and xiphisternum

Collimation
Sternoclavicular joints, manubrium, sternal body and xiphisternum, soft tissues of anterior sternal area, retrosternal lung tissue

Rotation of the light beam diaphragm housing to coincide with the long axis of the sternum will maximise efficiency of collimation to the field.

> **Expose on arrested respiration**
> Arrested respiration avoids movement unsharpness on the image, which is the primary function of the manoeuvre. However, arrested inspiration will serve to press the sternum further forward, which is especially beneficial when the arms are pulled backwards rather than raised.

Criteria for assessing image quality
- Sternoclavicular joints, manubrium, sternal body and xiphisternum, soft tissues of anterior sternal area, retrosternal lung tissue are demonstrated
- Arms are cleared from the area of interest
- Sternoclavicular joints are superimposed
- Sharp image demonstrating bony trabeculae in contrast with anterior soft tissues and retrosternal lung tissue

Common errors	Possible reasons
Pale density over upper sternum and sternoclavicular joints	Arms not cleared from field
White sternum with no bony detail evident	kVp too low
Lower aspect of sternum not included on image	During inspiration the patient may lean back or elevate the lower chest during the manoeuvre, moving the lower sternum outside the field of collimation or off the receptor completely. Care should be taken to observe the patient during the manoeuvre

▇ Anterior oblique sternum (Fig. 15.4A,B)

This projection is not recommended for trauma cases since it involves a prone position if the patient cannot stand

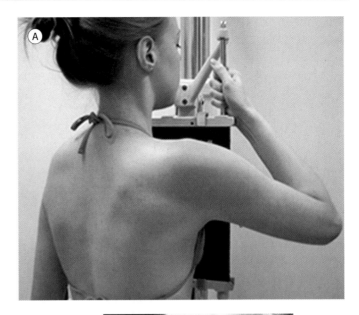

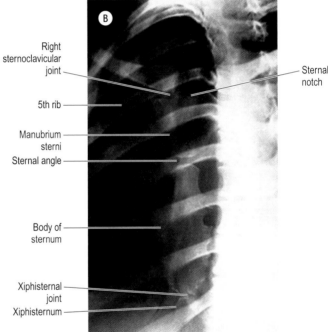

Figure 15.4 **(A)** Anterior oblique sternum; **(B)** oblique sternum. (B) Reproduced with permission from Bryan GJ. Skeletal anatomy. 3rd edn. Edinburgh: Churchill Livingstone; 1996 and Gunn (2002)

and, in any case, does not provide valuable additional information to the lateral.[2] However, it has been recommended for demonstration of inflammatory conditions.[4]

The oblique position clears the sternum from the vertebral column; some texts describe a right anterior oblique[4,6] but consideration must be given to the fact that the majority of the heart shadow lies over to the left. For this reason, the left anterior oblique is described here, where the right side is moved away from the image receptor to position the sternum over the right lung. The right atrium of the heart will also move to the right but this forms a significantly lower proportion of heart tissue than that which would be projected if a right anterior oblique were performed.

The projection can be undertaken erect or prone. If used, a 24 × 30 cm cassette is placed longitudinally in the bucky. A cassette with a stationary grid can also be utilised.

Positioning
- A lead rubber apron is applied to the back of the patient's waist
- The patient lies prone *or* stands facing the image receptor
- The middle of the cassette, if used, is level with a point midway between the sternal notch and xiphisternum
- The patient is rotated 45° towards the right, into the left anterior oblique position, and the arm on the side furthest from the image receptor is raised onto the pillow if semi-prone, or on the top of the image receptor if erect. A 45° radiolucent pad will assist in accurate positioning, and immobilisation, for the semi-prone position. For the semi-prone patient the knee on the raised side is flexed and used as additional immobilisation
- The sternum should lie coincident with the long axis of the image receptor
- A PA anatomical marker is usually used for this projection

> Expose on gentle respiration, using low mA and long-time selection
> This will blur the rib shadows on the image.

Beam direction and FFD
Perpendicular to the image receptor
100 cm FFD

Centring
To the centre of the image receptor, over the raised side of the thorax

Collimation
The sternum, sternoclavicular joints

Criteria for assessing image quality
- Sternum and sternoclavicular joints are demonstrated
- Sternum and sternoclavicular joints are clear of the vertebral column, and superimposed over the right lung
- Sharp image of the sternum in contrast with the soft tissues of the lung. Blurred rib shadows

Common error	Possible reason
Sternum partially overlying vertebral column and mediastinum	Inadequate obliquity. This most frequently occurs in the semi-prone position, when the 45° pads used to assess rotation (and aid immobilisation) are not pushed far enough under the thorax. Use of these pads to achieve a 45° rotation can be more effective if the patient lies in a lateral position initially, with the thin edge of the sponge wedge placed closely against the lowered side. The patient then lowers their right side down onto the pad, rather than raising this side from the prone position
	The weight of the patient can also compress the pad enough to affect angle of obliquity. Use of two pads or one long pad placed under the thorax may prove more effective

STERNOCLAVICULAR JOINTS

The sternoclavicular joints are examined for evidence of subluxation[4] of the joints.

If used, an 18 × 24 cm cassette is selected and placed longitudinally in the erect cassette holder for all projections of the sternoclavicular joints.

▇ PA sternoclavicular joints (Fig. 15.5A,B)

Positioning
- A lead rubber apron is applied to the back of the patient's waist
- The patient stands facing the image receptor
- The middle of the cassette, if used, is level with the sternal notch
- The feet are separated for stability
- The MSP is perpendicular to the image receptor, assessed by ensuring that the medial ends of the clavicles are equidistant from the image receptor
- A PA anatomical marker is usually used for this projection

> Expose on arrested respiration

Beam direction and FFD
Horizontal, 90° to the image receptor
100 cm FFD

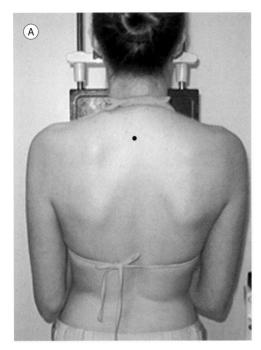

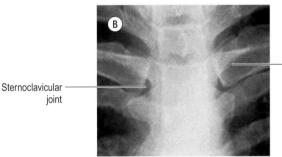

Sternoclavicular —
joint

— Clavicle

Figure 15.5   PA sternoclavicular joints

Centring
Over the middle of the body of T2 and to emerge through the sternal notch

Collimation
Both sternoclavicular (SC) joints

Criteria for assessing image quality
- Both sternoclavicular joints are demonstrated
- Medial ends of the clavicle are equidistant from the spinous processes of the thoracic vertebrae

Common error	Possible reason
Medial ends of clavicle not equidistant about the vertebral column; one joint only demonstrated	MSP not perpendicular to image receptor; the medial end of clavicle furthest from the vertebrae corresponds to the side rotated away from the cassette

- Sharp image demonstrating joints either side of the vertebral column in contrast to the vertebrae, medial ends of the posterior ribs, soft tissue of the lungs and sternum

■ Oblique sternoclavicular (SC) joints (Fig. 15.6A,B)

Both joints are examined for comparison.

If used, an 18 × 24 cm cassette is placed in the erect cassette holder.

Positioning
- A lead rubber apron is applied to the back of the patient's waist
- The patient stands facing the image receptor
- The middle of the cassette, if used, is level with the sternal notch
- *To demonstrate the left SC joint* the patient is rotated 45° towards the right, into the left anterior oblique position
- *To demonstrate the right SC joint* the patient is rotated 45° towards the left, into the right anterior oblique position
- The feet are separated for stability

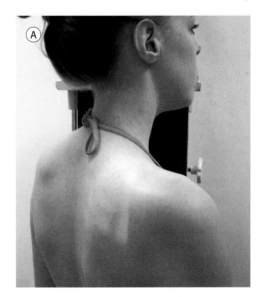

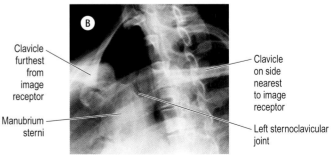

Clavicle furthest from image receptor

Manubrium sterni

Clavicle on side nearest to image receptor

Left sternoclavicular joint

Figure 15.6   **(A)** Anterior oblique SC joints; **(B)** oblique SC joints

- A PA anatomical marker is usually used for this projection. To avoid confusion, the PA anatomical marker should indicate the side of the joint under examination *and* be placed over to the relevant side on the image receptor

> Expose on arrested respiration

Beam direction and FFD
Vertical, 90° to the image receptor
100 cm FFD

Centring
Level with T2, over the side of the thorax furthest from the image receptor, to emerge through the sternal notch

Collimation
Both SC joints

Criteria for assessing image quality
- Both SC joints are demonstrated
- Sharp image demonstrating joint under examination contrast with clavicle and sternum

For the left joint
- Both joints are cleared from the vertebral column and shown overlying the lung apex on the right
- The right joint is shown with the medial end of the clavicle overlying the joint
- The left joint space is demonstrated as open

For the right joint
- Both joints are cleared from the vertebral column and shown overlying the lung apex on the left

- The left joint is shown with the medial end of the clavicle overlying the joint
- The right joint space is demonstrated as open

Common error	Possible reason
One or both joints are not seen clear of the vertebral column	Inadequate obliquity. A 45° pad assists in assessing angle of rotation more accurately

Anterior obliques have also been described with significantly less rotation – as little as 10°, the reason for this being that there will be clearance of the spine with minimum distortion of the joint.[7] However, it is noted from resulting images that this obliquity does not adequately clear the joint from the relatively high density of the upper mediastinum.

References
1. Helms CA. Fundamentals of skeletal radiology. 2nd edn. Philadelphia: WB Saunders; 1995.
2. Royal College of Radiologists working party. Making the best use of a department of clinical radiology: guidelines for doctors. 5th edn. London: Royal College Of Radiologists; 2003.
3. Nicholson DA, Driscoll PA. ABC of emergency radiology. Cambridge; BMJ Publishing: 1995.
4. Bontrager K, Lampignano JP. Textbook of radiographic positioning and related anatomy. 6th edn. St Louis: Mosby; 2005.
5. Whitley AS, et al. Clark's positioning in radiography. 12th edn. London: Hodder Arnold; 2005.
6. Sutherland R. Pocketbook of radiographic positioning. 2nd edn. Edinburgh: Churchill Livingstone; 2003.
7. Long BW, Rafaert JA. Orthopaedic radiography. Philadelphia: WB Saunders; 1995.

PRINCIPLES OF RADIOGRAPHY OF THE HEAD: CONVENTIONAL TECHNIQUE

Elizabeth Carver

INTRODUCTION

Radiography of the head is commonly termed 'skull radiography' but, since the word 'skull' refers to the cranial vault and its bones, the term 'skull radiography' would technically exclude facial bones, some paranasal sinuses, mandible and temporomandibular joints.

From the mid 1980s onwards there has been a reduction in the number of requests for plain radiography of the head, as computed tomography (CT) and magnetic resonance imaging (MRI) in particular have provided more detailed and useful information. These imaging methods now provide information which is either unlikely to be provided by plain radiographic images, or is only likely to be demonstrated by it in later stages of disease processes. There has also been a reduction in numbers of projections advocated per examination, in order to reduce radiation dose to patients.

Despite the drop in numbers of requests and projections undertaken, this section will include a full range of descriptions of projections for the head in order to provide information for regions where CT and MRI are less accessible or inaccessible. There does exist some argument to support plain radiographic examination of the cranial vault, despite RCR guidelines.[1] Where relevant, discussion on suitability of plain radiography versus specialised techniques will be presented throughout the section as each area is covered.

Techniques employed

There are two recognised types of approach to radiography of the head, the more *conventional* method which uses traditional X-ray equipment (with an erect or table-top prone/supine position for the patient, or examination on a trolley with the patient remaining supine) and the *isocentric* method using a dedicated isocentric unit which involves positioning the head at its 3D isocentre (see the introductory section on isocentrics in Chapter 17). Both methods will be described for each area of the skull in this text, with introductory sections for each given before individual chapters on specific examinations and projections.

CONVENTIONAL TECHNIQUE

Historically, radiographic texts have presented radiographers and students with information that has included up to approximately 50 projections.[2,3] This has proved daunting for radiographers in training, to say the least, and it is possible that the decline in frequency of use of plain radiography of the head is likely to exacerbate this.

However, if radiography of the head is approached logically it is realised that all projections are based upon a very few basic head positions, or projections, which require modification and variation by use of angulation and differing centring points. Collimation will also vary, according to area of interest for each projection. With reference to centring points, it will appear that there are as many of these as there are projections. However, on examination of radiographs, it becomes clear that centring points used are logically selected as being in the middle of the area of interest; so it is recommended that, if in doubt, ensure the area of interest lies centrally in the collimated field. Realistically the radiographer need only quote specific centring points when disseminating information to others.

Familiarity with the bony features of the skull and face, and their radiographic appearances, is vital when assessing radiographs for quality. The most important structures for recognition are:

- Orbits and the bones forming the orbits
- Bones of the vault and sutures
- Maxilla
- Sphenoid, including lesser and greater wings, sphenoid sinus, sella turcica and pterygoid processes/plates
- Petrous portion of temporal bone and its ridge
- Zygomae and arches
- Features of the mandible, temporomandibular joints
- Paranasal sinuses
- Nasal septum
- External and internal auditory meati
- Foramen magnum and atlantooccipital joints.

Description of basic projections relies heavily on the use of planes, baselines and surface markings, and the radiographer must be similarly familiar with these (Figs 16.1, 16.2).

Surface markings, planes and baselines
(Figs 16.1, 16.2)

Glabella
The glabella is situated in the midline of the forehead just above the level of the superior orbital margins; it lies over the frontal sinuses.

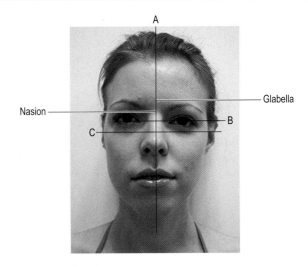

A. MSP
B. Interpupillary line
C. Infraorbital line

Figure 16.2 Surface markings, planes and baselines – 2

External occipital protuberance (EOP)
The EOP is situated in the midline and inferiorly over the occiput.

External auditory meatus (EAM)
The EAM is the hole surrounded by the pinna of the ear.

Nasion
The nasion is situated below the glabella, and is found as a depression between the orbits and above the nasal bone.

Coronal plane
The coronal place is coincident with the coronal suture and separates the body into anterior and posterior halves.

Infraorbital line
The infraorbital line connects the inferior orbital margins and lies parallel to the interpupillary line.

Interpupillary line
The interpupillary line is a horizontal line connecting the pupils of the eyes.

Median sagittal plane (MSP)
The MSP is a vertical plane in the midline of the head, separating the left and right sides.

Orbitomeatal baseline (OMBL)
The OMBL is an imaginary line extending from the outer canthus of the eye to the middle of the EAM. It is used in conventional radiography techniques of the head.

Anthropological baseline
The anthropological baseline is an imaginary line extending from the inferior orbital margin to the upper border of

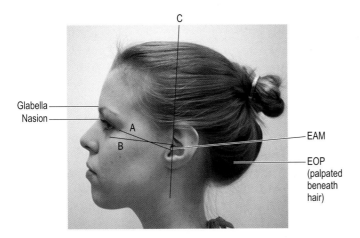

A. Orbitomeatal baseline (OMBL)
B. Anthropological baseline
C. Auricular line

Figure 16.1 Surface markings, planes and baselines – 1

the EAM. This baseline is mostly used in descriptions of isocentric techniques and has a difference of 10° from the OMBL.

Care must be taken when locating the orbital end of this line, as the level of the inferior orbital margin is frequently assessed inaccurately since it is common practice to assess its position visually. Palpation is the only accurate method for location of this structure; this will ensure the anthropological line is correctly assessed. At the meatal end of the baseline, error can occur when users misunderstand the location of the end of the line; it must be stressed that it should pass across the top of the EAM and not through its centre.

Auricular line
The auricular line crosses the anthropological baseline at 90°, passing through the EAM.

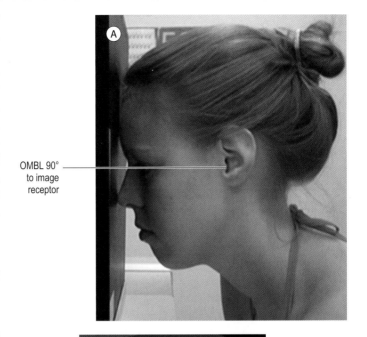

BASIC POSITIONS OF THE HEAD

In this text, names of projections are always given as representation of the direction of beam, so that this gives the radiographer information on the initial patient position. This is in preference to a system which uses names for some projections which reflect the original describer of the projection (for example, 'Towne's', 'Waters') but gives little or no information on the position. When such a name is very commonly used in everyday practice, the alternative name will be given in brackets.

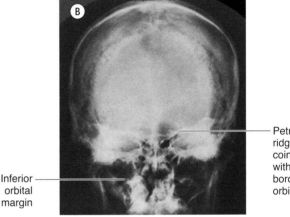

Figure 16.3   **(A)** Basic OF position; **(B)** OF

■ Occipitofrontal (OF) (Fig. 16.3A,B)

This is a posteroanterior (PA) position, with the forehead in contact with the image receptor and the OMBL at 90° to it. It is easiest to achieve with the patient seated erect. Traditionally it is referred to as a 'PA skull' position but, since the occipitomental (OM) position is also PA, this does not describe the true position of the head for the OF.

Tube angulation will affect the position of the ridge of petrous portion of temporal, caudal angulation lowering it in relationship to the orbits and cranial angulation raising it. Effects of caudal angulation can be compared using Figures 16.4A,B and C.

Common errors – OF projections	Possible reasons
Petrous ridge appears higher within the orbits than required, or appears above superior orbital margins	OMBL not 90° to the image receptor, chin down too far Caudal tube angle selected, if used, is less than required for projection Direction of angle incorrect
Petrous ridge appears lower within the orbits than required, or appears below inferior orbital margins	OMBL not 90° to image receptor, chin raised slightly Caudal tube angle selected, if used, is more than required for projection
Symmetry of the structures on either side of the head is a requirement of AP or PA radiographs of the head. Rotation of the head, away from the position with the MSP perpendicular to the image receptor, will affect this symmetry. The most obvious identifiable appearance suggestive of rotation is increased distance of the lateral orbital border from the lateral outer table of the vault on one side, when compared to the other	

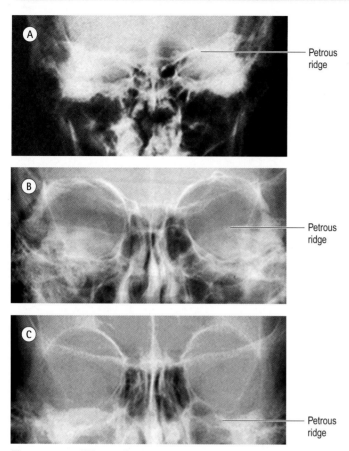

Figure 16.4 Effects of caudal angulation on petrous ridge in the OF position: **(A)** no angle; **(B)** 10° angle; **(C)** 20° angle

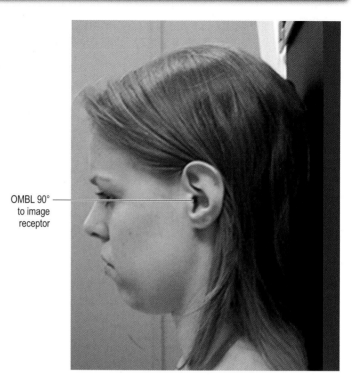

Figure 16.5 Basic FO position

These positions are reliant upon the accurate positioning of the OMBL at 90° to the image receptor and accurate angle selection. The effects of errors on the appearance of the petrous ridge in the OF position are outlined below.

It has been noted that it is common practice for radiographers to initially ask the patient to place their nose and forehead in contact with the image receptor and that nose size will affect OMBL relationship if this method is used.[4] For this reason it is advocated that the patient is asked to only place their forehead against the image receptor, with the radiographer adjusting OMBL position as necessary.

Frontooccipital (FO) (Fig. 16.5)

This is an anteroposterior (AP) position, with the occiput in contact with the image receptor and OMBL at 90° to it. It can be undertaken erect or supine. It is often used in cases of trauma when patient condition is not suitable for an OF projection; if this is the case any caudal angulation normally given in conjunction with the OF position is directed *cranially rather than caudally*. It is also used in imaging departments who do not have a skull unit facility

or erect bucky arrangement, and who avoid PA projections of the head due to potential difficulty in achieving and maintaining the correct position. Caudal angulation is also applied in the FO position routinely, as for the FO 30° half axial (Towne's) projection. (See Ch. 18 on the cranial vault.)

The appearance of the FO projection, with no tube angulation, should be identical to those for the OF, with the exception of relative orbital size. In the FO position the lateral orbital borders will appear very close to, or even superimposed over, the lateral outer table of the vault. The OF projection will show the lateral orbital borders well within the outer margins of the vault. (Fig. 16.6A,B) Clearly this is due to the difference in magnification of the orbits, since they lie close to the image receptor in the OF position and further away in the FO position; the distance of the lateral aspects of the vault to the image receptor will be similar for both.

Errors in positioning have the same effects as those for the OF projection, OMBL position affecting position of the petrous ridge and rotation affecting symmetry. A raised chin in the FO position will have the same effect as the same action in the OF position, which is that of lowering the petrous ridge, whilst a dropped chin will raise it. The FO with caudal angulation will show the petrous ridges rising above the orbital outlines, and becoming increasingly 'v' shaped as the angle increases. More specific guidelines on FO projectional errors are given in Chapters 18–21.

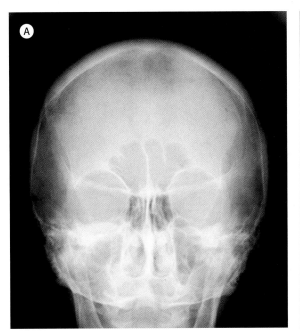
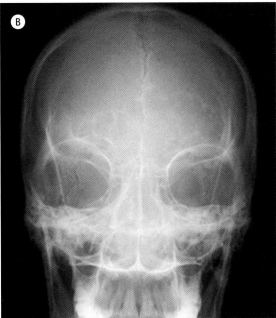

Figure 16.6 Appearances of OF and FO radiographs: **(A)** OF angled 20° caudally, showing lateral orbital margins further from the lateral skull than in **(B)** FO angled 20° cranially

Positioning of the OMBL at 90° to the image receptor can be difficult in this position, especially in the case of the patient who is of stocky build or is kyphotic. If sitting erect, the patient will find it easier to press the occipital area against the image receptor, and achieve the correct relationship of OMBL to it, if the chair they use is placed slightly forward of the receptor unit. Leaning back towards the unit initially until their shoulders come into contact with it, they are then asked to push the back of their neck against the unit, flexing their neck until the occipital area is also in contact. It has been noted that this method is more effective than asking the patient to simply put the back of their head against the image receptor, whilst dropping the chin, since the back of the head generally lies at the top of the occiput rather than in its centre.[4]

Positioning of the OMBL is more difficult for the supine patient; use of a non-opaque pad under the head may help facilitate the position but it is not considered ideal since the increase in object film distance (OFD) causes magnification unsharpness which increases in severity towards the vertex of the skull. For the non-neck-injured patient it is preferable to use a support under a cassette with stationary grid, positioned directly under the patient's head and at 90° to the OMBL (Fig. 16.7). Other solutions and suggestions will also be considered in Chapter 18 on the cranial vault.

▨ OM (Fig. 16.8A,B)

This is a PA position, with the chin raised and in contact with the image receptor. Relationship of the OMBL to the

image receptor varies, and is usually between 30° and 45° from the perpendicular, according to the requirements of the examination. With the OMBL at 30° the nose is close to, or even in contact with, the image receptor but this does vary according to shape of the nose; the chin is well elevated in order to achieve a 45° relationship to the image receptor and the nose is very unlikely to be in contact with it in this position.

As for the OF and FO projections, location of the petrous ridge on the image is also used to assess accuracy of positioning. The required level for most OM projections requires the petrous ridge to be seen at the midpoint or the lower border of the maxillary sinuses. Caudal angulation will further lower the position of the petrous ridge on this projection.

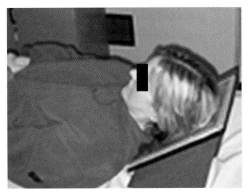

Figure 16.7 Cassette supported for supine patient

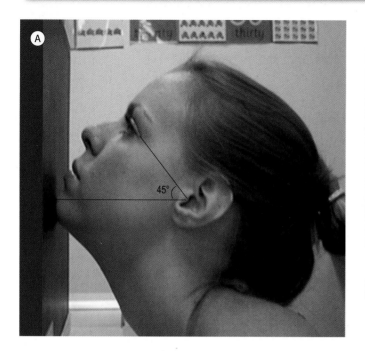

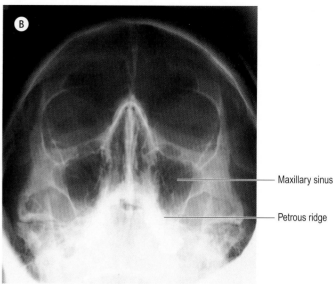

Figure 16.8   (A) Basic OM position: chin raised 45°; **(B)** OM 45°

With further reference to the assessment of projectional accuracy using the petrous ridge, as for the OF and FO positions, a higher level of the ridge than that required indicates that the chin is inadequately elevated. If the ridge is lower than required the chin is over-elevated. Again, evidence of rotation is assessed by symmetry of the facial structures, especially the distance of the lateral orbital margins and rami of mandible from the lateral aspect of the vault.

Lateral (Fig. 16.9A,B)

This is a familiar position, with the MSP parallel to the image receptor. Angulation can be used for some lateral oblique projections, such as those for mandible or temporomandibular joints. Both tilt and rotation will affect the appearance of the lateral projection. If this projection is undertaken with the patient seated or prone, it can be

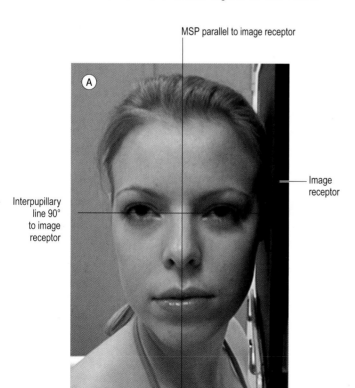

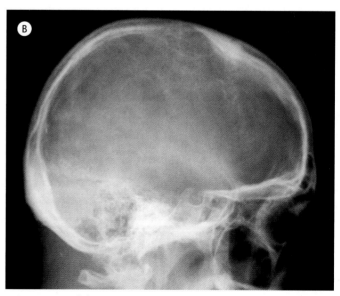

Figure 16.9   (A) Basic lateral position; **(B)** lateral

difficult for the patient to achieve the required position. If undertaken erect, the required rotation into position, whilst maintaining a vertical MSP which is parallel to the image receptor, may be more easily achieved with the chair placed very close to the image receptor and the patient's vertebral column vertically positioned. When a patient leans forward towards the unit there is more likelihood of tilt. Another solution lies in the use of a cassette with grid in the erect holder, or supported vertically against the side of the supine patient's head (which is elevated on a radiolucent pad), and enables the patient to be positioned with their whole MSP parallel to the image receptor. This reduces the difficulty associated with turning the head and obtaining an accurate position.

Submentovertical (Figs 16.10A,B)

The vertex of the skull is placed in contact with the image receptor for this projection, facilitated by the patient initially sitting facing the X-ray tube and extending the neck and head backwards. The OMBL is parallel to the image receptor. The projection is not in common use since the information it provides is minimal and even inadequate when compared to that given by CT and MRI. The projection can be quite difficult for some patients to achieve and maintain, especially as pressure on the vertex of the skull can be quite painful.

Table-top or erect technique?

Although radiographic examination of the skull can be undertaken erect or supine, erect positioning is easier for the patient for most positions, especially in the case of PA positions. As already mentioned, lateral projections can be difficult to achieve when the patient is erect with their head turned, but a supine horizontal projection, with the whole of the body's MSP parallel to the image receptor, is easier for the patient. Since this method usually uses a stationary grid, this could similarly be employed using an erect cassette support with the patient seated. The patient's shoulder fits comfortably under the support, without the patient needing to turn their head. A lateral with the patient prone can be very difficult and, in any case, any prone position is out of the question for the injured patient. Achieving the perpendicular relationship of the OMBL for the FO projection is also quite difficult for the supine patient. Because of this, the method selected for descriptions of radiography of the head (conventional method) is that of the erect technique.

SUMMARY

There is a small range of basic projections (OF, FO, lateral, OM, submentovertical) upon which radiography of the head is based and this range can be seen to be simplified when it is remembered that:

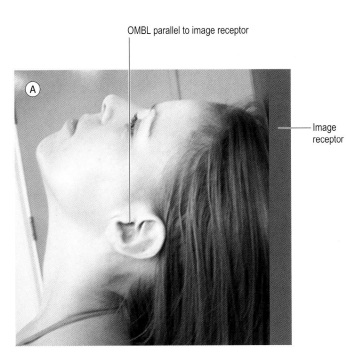

OMBL parallel to image receptor

Image receptor

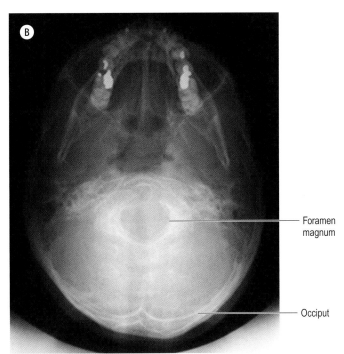

Foramen magnum

Occiput

Figure 16.10   (A) Basic SMV position; (B) SMV

- the OF and FO projections are simply the reverse of each other
- the lateral projection is a familiar concept and therefore not a difficult one
- the SMV projection is little used
- erect positioning is often easier to achieve.

Later chapters (18–21) give the relevant projections for specific areas of the head and these are described in more detail, showing use of these basic projections with modifications in angles used, centring points and collimation requirements. Isocentric techniques are also included, after the descriptions of conventional techniques. An introduction to isocentrics follows in Chapter 17.

References

1. Royal College of Radiologists working party. Making the best use of a department of clinical radiology: guidelines for doctors. 5th edn. London: Royal College of Radiologists; 2003.
2. Bontrager K, Lampignano JP. Textbook of radiographic positioning and related anatomy. 6th edn. St Louis: Mosby; 2005.
3. Whitley AS, et al. Clark's positioning in radiography. 12th edn. London: Hodder Arnold; 2005.
4. Unett EM, Royle AJ. Radiographic techniques and image evaluation. London: Chapman and Hall; 1997.

CHAPTER 17

PRINCIPLES OF RADIOGRAPHY OF THE HEAD: ISOCENTRIC TECHNIQUE

Amanda Royle

Isocentric radiography requires the use of specialist equipment which moves around the patient, rather than requiring movement of the patient, to adjust relationship of the head or other body part to the image receptor and central ray. The principle of putting the centre of the area under examination into the 3D isocentre of the unit requires tube and receptor movement in three dimensions, using rotation and tilt of the unit's components. Figure 17.1 shows a typical isocentric unit, identifying key components.

Isocentric radiography of the head offers the radiographer the opportunity to produce high quality, reproducible images of the head, irrespective of patient condition. Isocentric radiography really comes into its own in the A&E situation but only when the patient's condition allows for their transfer onto the X-ray table. Clearly patients with unstable injury anywhere in the body would not be suitable for such transfer.

In conventional radiography of the head, the patient is required to achieve many uncomfortable positions by raising or lowering the chin or rotating their head through as much as 90°. Most 'fit' patients find these positions difficult to attain and hold, and for the injured, immobile or unsteady patient it is virtually impossible. As a result, the radiographer may have to accept radiographs that would normally be considered below standard, leading to difficulty in interpretation for the casualty doctor and those making the radiological report.

In contrast, isocentric radiography allows the patient to remain supine with the head in a more natural, comfortable position. This leads to improved patient cooperation and a speedier, more accurate examination. Once the patient is on the table with the head in the base position, rotation and tilting of the head is simulated by angulation of the X-ray beam in the horizontal and vertical planes. Angulation in the third plane allows for craniocaudal angulations employed in conventional techniques.

As it is possible to obtain occipitofrontal (OF) projections of the injured patient using isocentric equipment, radiation dose to the radiosensitive lenses of the eyes is significantly reduced. This is favourably comparable to the patient who must be examined supine, on a trolley, and who cannot be examined in the OF (PA) position. This has implications for radiation dose to the lenses of the eyes and thyroid.

With the isocentric unit, the relationship of the image receptor with respect to the X-ray beam is always 90°, so no matter what beam angulation is applied in the craniocaudal direction there will be minimal distortion on the resultant image. This is particularly pertinent in the case of the conventional frontooccipital (FO) 30° skull projection, when additional or even excessive beam angulation is often required to compensate for patient position when the orbitomeatal baseline (OMBL) cannot be placed at 90° to the image receptor. This leads to further exaggeration of the elongated image of the vertex. The isocentric equivalent of the FO 30° produces, by comparison, a relatively more rounded appearance of the vault with no distortion.

As the isocentric unit is usually situated at the end of a conventional X-ray table with bucky and over-couch tube, examination of other areas is possible without further movement of the patient.

As previously stated, regarding conventional skull radiography techniques, (see Ch. 16) all isocentric projections are also based upon a few basic projections which require modification and variation by use of different angles and centring points. In the isocentric technique, the patient remains supine whilst the equipment is moved about them. Essentially, the patient's head is initially placed in one of the 'basic' or 'start' positions and the unit is moved around the patient until the centre of the part of the head under examination lies in the 3D 'isocentre' of the unit. Angulation is then applied.

HEAD POSITIONS

For some of the isocentric techniques, the head is positioned using the anthropological baseline as reference (see Fig. 16.1). This allows the head to be placed in a more natural, comfortable position, increasing patient comfort and reducing the risk of repeats due to movement.

With the anthropological baseline vertical, the OMBL will be raised by 10° from the basic OF/FO position used in conventional techniques. This requires different angles to be applied in order to produce projections equivalent to conventional skull techniques, namely OF 0°/10°/20° or FO 30°. Think of it as dealing with a patient who cannot lower their chin sufficiently when using the conventional technique; in this case the radiographer would have to compensate by adapting the beam angulation in order to produce the correct projection. Throughout the following isocentric descriptions, projections will be named according to the appearances of the images produced and not with reference to the angulation applied.

COLLIMATION, CENTRING, FOCUS FILM DISTANCE (FFD)

Collimation must be applied while the skull unit is in the anteroposterior (AP) position and the area of interest is visible within the light beam. Once the unit is turned into the posteroanterior (PA) position it is impossible to accurately collimate the beam to the area of interest.

Accurate centring is achieved by displacement of the X-ray table and the patient. FFD is not set by the radiographer but is governed by the position of the equipment once the isocentre is determined. The final act of the radiographer prior to pressing the exposure button is to slide the image receptor along the C-arm to achieve the smallest object film distance (OFD) possible and, therefore, reduce image magnification and unsharpness.

DESCRIPTION OF ISOCENTRIC TECHNIQUES IN THIS TEXT

In Chapters 18 to 21, examinations of the cranium, facial bones and paranasal sinuses are described in detail. As familiarity with the techniques develops, it will be seen that they are all an adaptation of the conventional techniques taught to everyone as part of their radiographic training.

When projections are named for isocentric technique descriptions in these chapters, they are named as for conventional technique. For example, the OF projection of the cranial vault which demonstrates the petrous ridge at the bottom of the orbits is the OF with 20° caudal angulation; the isocentric method which produces the required appearance of the petrous ridge utilises only a

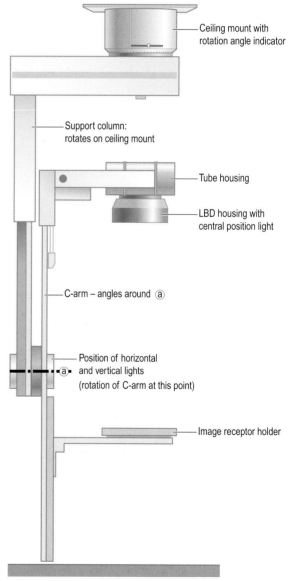

Figure 17.1   Isocentric unit

10° angle. However, the projection will be described as an *OF 20° equivalent*.

As the same rules apply to both conventional and isocentric techniques, the effects of caudal/cranial angulation on the level of the petrous ridge, as well as common errors and possible reasons, can be found in the introduction to conventional techniques and in the 'common faults' tables after descriptions of both conventional and isocentric techniques.

LINES AND BASELINES USED IN ISOCENTRIC RADIOGRAPHY

These are outlined in full in the introductory section on conventional techniques in Chapter 16, and as shown in Figures 16.1 and 16.2. For isocentric techniques the following planes or baselines are most commonly used.

Anthropological baseline
The anthropological baseline is an imaginary line extending from the inferior orbital margin to the upper border of the external auditory meatus (EAM). This baseline is mostly used in descriptions of isocentric techniques and has a difference of 10° from the OMBL.

Interpupillary line
The interpupillary line is a horizontal line connecting the pupils of the eyes.

Coronal plane
The coronal plane is coincident with the coronal suture, separating the body into anterior and posterior halves.

Median sagittal plane (MSP)
The MSP is a vertical plane in the midline of the head, separating the left and right sides.

TERMINOLOGY SPECIFIC TO ISOCENTRIC RADIOGRAPHY OF THE HEAD

◼ Tube and support column position

Lateral: the support column is at the side of the table, at 90° to its long axis (Fig. 17.2).
Medial: the support column is at the end of the table, in line with its long axis (Fig.17.3).
AP: the C-arm is vertical (0°) with the X-ray tube above the table and the image receptor below.
PA: the C-arm is vertical (0°) with the X-ray tube below the table and the image receptor above.

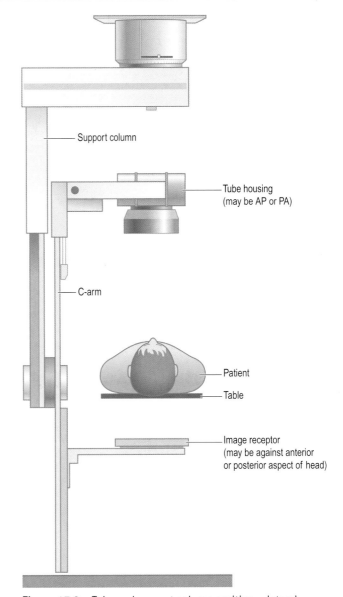

Figure 17.2   Tube and support column position – lateral

Horizontal: the C-arm is horizontal (Fig. 17.4), with the support column in the medial position

◼ Positional lights (Figs 17.5, 17.6, 17.7)

Central: the light shines on the front of the patient's head and face, coincident with the MSP. Lateral table movement alters the position of the light.
Horizontal: the light shines on the side of the patient's head, parallel with the coronal plane. It moves with table height movement.
Vertical: the light shines vertically on the front and side of the patient's head and face at 90° to the sagittal and coronal planes. It moves with table movement as the patient's head is fed in or out of the unit.

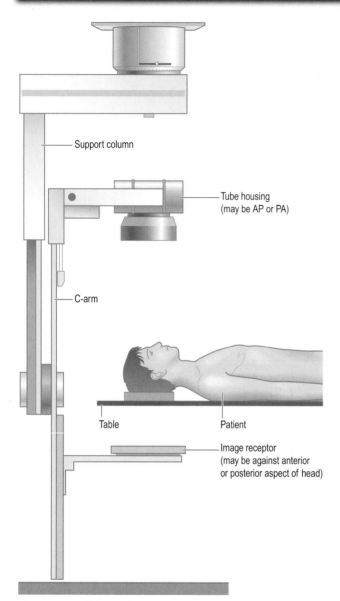

Support column

Tube housing
(may be AP or PA)

C-arm

Table

Patient

Image receptor
(may be against anterior
or posterior aspect of head)

Figure 17.3   Tube and support column position – medial

▮ Angulations

Support column in the **lateral** *position:* C-arm movement facilitates and simulates craniocaudal beam angulation.
Support column in the **medial** *position:* C-arm movement simulates rotation of the head.

BASIC PATIENT POSITIONS FOR ISOCENTRIC RADIOGRAPHY OF THE HEAD

The patient is set up in one of *three* base positions for all isocentric projections. In the following chapters base positions are described first, before the isocentric technique for the projections, followed by further instructions

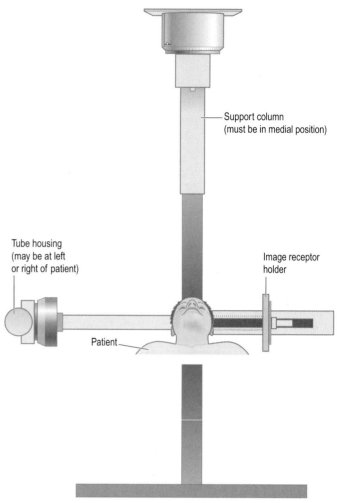

Support column
(must be in medial position)

Tube housing
(may be at left
or right of patient)

Image receptor
holder

Patient

Figure 17.4   Tube position – horizontal

for individual projections of the head, face and paranasal sinuses.

Preparation for positioning: all projections

- At the start of all examinations the isocentric unit is 'parked' in the lateral position, the angulation scales are set to 0° and the image receptor is at the far end of the C-arm to prevent damage to the patient/equipment during movement of the equipment
- For examinations of the skull and facial bones a 24 × 30 cm image receptor is used, while an 18 × 24 cm image receptor is used for paranasal sinuses and more specialised examinations of smaller areas. The correct receptor is attached to the unit prior to positioning of the patient
- For the purposes of radiation protection of the patient a sheet of lead rubber is placed on the table to correspond with where the patient's shoulders and upper thorax will rest
- The patient lies supine on the X-ray table, with the head resting in a radiolucent head pad on the centre of the head extension board. The MSP of the head and body is coincident with, and perpendicular to, the midline of the table

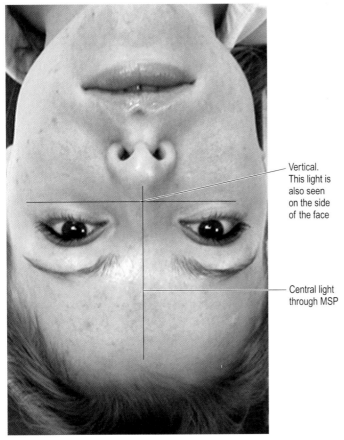

Vertical. This light is also seen on the side of the face

Central light through MSP

Figure 17.5 Skull base position. Position of positional light seen on the face. Lights that are seen on the face are shown here and in Figure 17.7 with the face upside down, as this is often the way the radiographer will view the patient whilst manipulating the equipment and the patient's head position

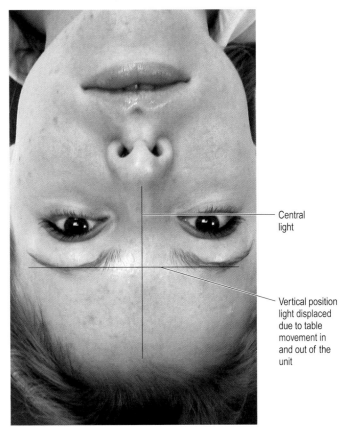

Central light

Vertical position light displaced due to table movement in and out of the unit

Figure 17.7 Movement of the table moves the vertical position lights position over the face. Once the start position has been achieved, movement of the table brings the isocentre of the unit coincident with the area under examination. This example shows how the position of the light alters from the skull 'base' position to bring the cranium's isocentre coincident with the unit's isocentre, as described for the cranium in Chapter 18

- The table is then raised to the correct working height for the isocentric unit

Post-positioning: all projections
- AP/PA anatomical markers are applied when the isocentric unit is finally positioned. This prevents confusion encountered when trying to correctly place a PA marker with the unit still in the AP position
- The final act before pressing the exposure button is to slide the image receptor along the C-arm to achieve the shortest possible OFD. Leaving this till last prevents accidents to the patient and/or equipment during movement/angulation of the unit

■ Base position 1: skull (Fig. 17.8)

Positioning
- The patient is positioned on the table as described above
- The central positional light is coincident with the MSP of the head

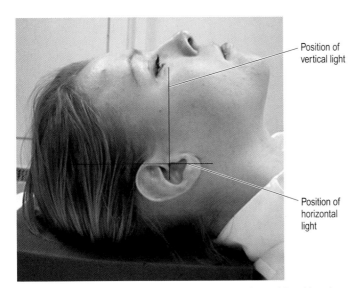

Position of vertical light

Position of horizontal light

Figure 17.6 Position of positional lights seen from side of head – (skull base position)

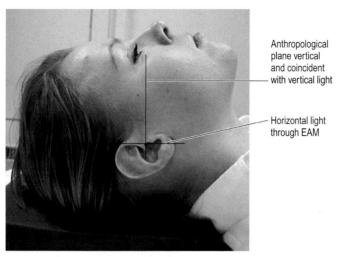

Figure 17.8 Base position for skull

- The chin is positioned to bring the anthropological baseline vertical, coincident with the vertical positional light
- The height of the C-arm is altered so that the horizontal positional light runs through the centre of the EAM

Base position 2: face (Fig. 17.9)

Positioning

- The patient is positioned on the table as described above
- The radiolucent head pad is removed
- The central positional light is coincident with the MSP of the head
- The chin is raised so that the OMBL is 45° to the horizontal. This can be accurately measured by ensuring that the horizontal positional light is passing directly through the EAM and then applying a 45° caudal angle. The chin is then raised so that the OMBL is coincident with the

light beam on the side of the face. The C-arm is then returned to the vertical position
- The height of the C-arm is altered so that the horizontal positional light is level with the outer canthus of the eye

Base position 3: submentovertical (SMV) (Fig. 17.10)

Positioning

- The patient is positioned on the table as described above
- For easier positioning, attach the stepped head extension board to the isocentric unit if one is available
- The radiolucent head pad is removed
- The central positional light is coincident with the MSP of the head
- The neck is flexed and the chin is raised to bring the OMBL as close to the horizontal as possible
- The height of the C-arm is altered so that the horizontal positional light runs through the centre of the EAM

With the patient in one of these three base positions any projection of the head, face or paranasal sinuses can be achieved by movement of the table, and therefore the patient, and by application of the required tube angulation. Angulation may be applied in two planes by angling the C-arm or the support column. In some of the supplementary projections, angulation may be applied in both planes to simulate patient rotation as well as beam angulation.

For descriptions of isocentric techniques there will be no specific centring point given at the end of the positioning section, as displacement of the patient after implementing the base position places the anatomical structure under examination into the isocentre of the unit.

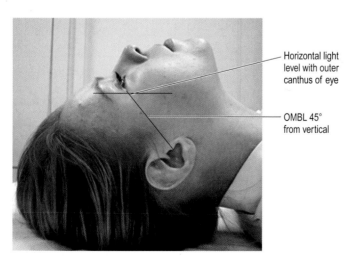

Figure 17.9 Base position for face

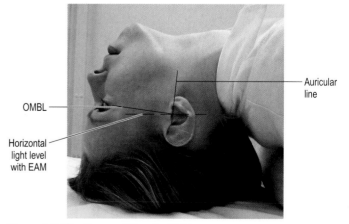

Figure 17.10 Base position for SMV

CHAPTER 18

CRANIAL VAULT

Barry Carver, Amanda Royle

Skull radiography is in decline. It is still in limited use for the investigation of some metabolic and bone disorders, and as part of the skeletal survey protocol for cases of suspected non-accidental injury (NAI). In cases of trauma, even where still utilised, fewer projections are recommended – two rather than the 'traditional' three being advised.[1]

Why is this? The easy answer appears to be radiation protection – minimisation of dose.

In 1978 Eyes & Evans, in a study of 504 patients in two Liverpool teaching hospitals, found a very low yield of positive findings on plain skull radiographs, suggesting that they are of limited value in the management of patients with head injury.[2] Earlier and later studies in the USA agreed with these findings, the yield of fractures varying but with a low of 2.7% in agreement with the above UK study.[3,4,5]

Head injuries are the cause of up to 1 million A&E department visits per year in the UK,[6] creating 100 000 admissions to hospital in England alone.[7] Imaging of the head injury patient is directed at detecting the nature of the underlying pathology; once this is accomplished the brain can be protected against greater damage. Optimal imaging is dependent on the nature of the injury, with evaluation of the brain normally being of paramount importance. The advent of CT has had a massive impact on the diagnosis and treatment of traumatic head injury, allowing rapid non-invasive identification of both diffuse injury and surgically treatable lesions.

It should be noted that cervical spine injury is relatively common in comatose patients with head injury,[8] hence it is important to exclude such an injury prior to mobilisation; the minimum examination being a high quality lateral examination C1–C7.

The Royal College of Radiologists (RCR) guidelines were produced to eliminate unnecessary skull radiographs, and have been successful in reducing the number of skull films being performed. The latest RCR guidelines[9] adopt the Canadian computed tomography (CT) head rule[10] eliminating the need for radiography of the skull in trauma, except for where CT is unavailable, or in the case of NAI in children.

RCR guidance has been added to in the UK by guidance issued by the National Institute for Clinical Excellence (NICE).[7] This guidance has been the subject of some debate and has caused concern in some imaging departments regarding implementation of the guidance, as greater use of CT is advocated. This has potential consequences on departmental management and staffing, as well as clear implications for patient dose. The National Radiological Protection Board (NRPB) report the effective dose for a skull series as approximately 0.06 mSv, compared to cranial CT which has an approximate dose equivalent of 2.0 mSv.[11] From this we can see that, put simply, cranial CT is equivalent to a skull film series of over 33 images.

It is suggested that patients with minimal external signs of injury, who are fully alert and orientated (Glasgow coma scale (GCS) 15), with normal neurological examination and no symptoms other than headache do not need a CT scan, but require close reliable observation over 24 hours.[12] Another school of thought is that 'head injury cards kill patients'. This is because, unfortunately, a small percentage of these patients with minimal evidence of trauma may have acute haematoma; these patients would certainly be observed more closely if skull fracture was demonstrated. About 50% of patients with compound depressed fractures do not suffer a loss of consciousness, and 40% of patients with intracranial haematoma do not have an initial loss of consciousness.[13] It has also been suggested that some patients with extradural haematoma present with normal conscious levels, this small group of patients may fail to be recognised by clinical evaluation alone, with potentially fatal results. The size of this group is open to debate. For the most part, in USA emergency departments, most patients are examined by CT regardless of whether it is clinically indicated or not.[14]

It has previously been suggested that if the mechanism of injury is such that there is a possibility of skull fracture, then skull X-ray (SXR) is indicated.[15] The emphasis is laid upon diagnosis of skull fracture due to the association between skull fracture and intracranial injury. However the 5th edition of the RCR guidelines suggests that this group also should proceed to CT (within 8 hours).[9]

Given its ability to demonstrate bony detail as well as much greater detail of the underlying soft tissues within the cranial vault, CT is the investigation of choice in an increasing number of circumstances.

Thus the use of skull radiography, particularly in trauma, is diminishing but its use is not yet obsolete and it is still necessary for the radiographer to be competent in X-ray examination of the cranial vault. Conventional techniques for the cranial vault may be undertaken erect with an erect bucky of the Lysholm or Schonander type units, and with the patient supine or prone with a table bucky. The technique described here uses erect positioning and the table-top or trolley technique must be modified by remembering that erect anteroposterior (AP) becomes supine and erect posteroanterior (PA) becomes prone, etc. For the *injured patient*, no projections are undertaken prone, and occipitofrontal (OF) projections must be adjusted to become frontooccipital (FO), with any cranial or caudal angulations directed in the opposite direction to those given for OF projection. For example, if an OF 20° with caudal angle is required, the FO employs a 20° cranial angle. Use of the isocentric unit is described separately.

■ OF cranium: conventional technique (Fig. 18.1A,B)

If used, a 24 × 30 cm cassette is placed vertically in the bucky, to coincide with the patient's median sagittal plane (MSP).

Positioning
- The patient is seated facing the bucky, their forehead in contact with it
- The orbitomeatal baseline (OMBL) and MSP are perpendicular to the image receptor. The MSP position can be checked by ensuring that the distances between both external auditory meatuses (EAMs) and the image receptor are equidistant
- The glabella is coincident with the middle of the cassette, if used

Beam direction and focus film distance (FFD)
There are a range of beam directions used, which affect position of the petrous ridge on the image produced (see Ch. 16); *20° caudal angulation* clears the ridge to the lowest border of the orbits and this angulation is probably that used most frequently, since it maximises the amount of vault shown above the maxilla

Centring
In the midline of the occiput, to emerge through the glabella

For erect bucky or table-top technique the cassette is displaced to coincide with the central ray.

Collimation
Vertex of vault, inferior border of occiput, lateral margins of vault

When a patient presents on a trolley, after a head injury, or when patients cannot turn face down for table-top technique, the FO projection (described later) is used and adapted by using a 20° cranial angle. Centring is over the glabella.

■ OF projections: isocentric technique

Positioning
- Base position: skull (see Fig. 17.8)
- The table is then moved caudally to bring the vertical central ray, the point at which the central and vertical positional lights intersect, over the glabella
- Collimate, using the iris diaphragm, to include the vertex of the skull, maxillae and parietal bones
- With the support column in the lateral position, the C-arm is put into the PA position
- The long axis of the 24 × 30 cm image receptor is coincident with the MSP

Beam angulation
Prior to making the exposure the image receptor is brought into contact with the head to minimise the object film distance (OFD)

Projection	Beam angulation
Image equivalent to OF 0°	10° cranial on C-arm
Image equivalent to OF 10°	0° on C-arm
Image equivalent to OF 20°	10° caudal on C-arm

Criteria for assessing image quality
- Vertex of vault, inferior border of occiput, and the lateral margins of vault are demonstrated
- Superior border of petrous ridge shown superimposed on inferior orbital margins if no angle is used. For tech-

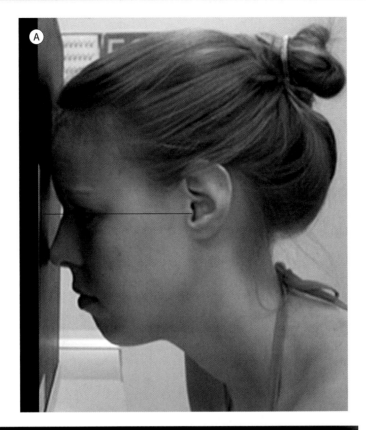

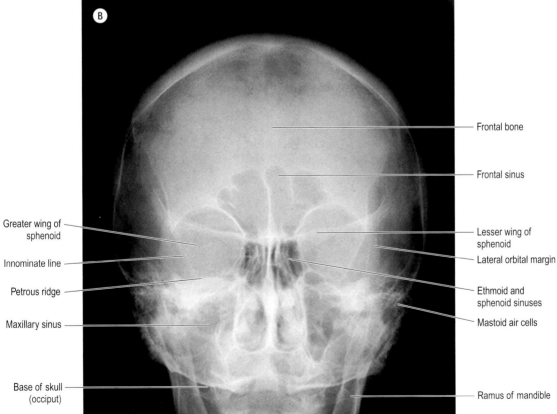

Frontal bone

Frontal sinus

Greater wing of sphenoid

Lesser wing of sphenoid

Innominate line

Lateral orbital margin

Petrous ridge

Ethmoid and sphenoid sinuses

Maxillary sinus

Mastoid air cells

Base of skull (occiput)

Ramus of mandible

Figure 18.1 **(A)** OF cranium **(B)** OF 20° cranium. The OF 20° projection shows the petrous ridge level with the bottom of the orbits, thus clearing as much of the cranial vault above the maxilla and petrous portion of temporal bone

niques using beam angulation, the petrous ridge should appear half way down the orbits for 10° caudal angle and at the bottom of the orbits for 20° angle

- Lateral borders of orbits equidistant from lateral borders of skull
- Sharp image showing the dense petrous ridge in contrast with the orbits and occiput, frontal bone in contrast with the adjacent air filled sinuses

Common errors	Possible reasons
Petrous ridge is seen above required level in relationship to orbits	Inadequate angle selected or baseline used is incorrectly positioned (chin down too far)
Petrous ridge is seen below required level in relationship to orbits	Angle selected is too great or baseline used is incorrectly positioned (chin not down enough)
Distance between lateral orbital margins is not equal	Rotation of the head; the orbit demonstrating the shortest distance between its lateral border and the lateral aspect of the vault coincides with the side towards which the head is rotated

■ FO 30° cranium: conventional technique
(Fig. 18.2A,B)

This projection is also referred to as the *Towne's* or *half axial* projection and may also be produced as an FO with a 30° cranial angle. The OF approach is seldom used in conventional skull technique as the projection is mostly used to show the occiput, which is positioned closest to the image receptor in the FO position. However, the OF position is easier to achieve if the patient is seated erect, and the risks associated with radiation dose to eye lens and thyroid dose are less severe.

If used, a 24 × 30 cm cassette is placed vertically in the bucky, to coincide with the patient's MSP.

Positioning
- The patient sits erect facing the X-ray tube
- The OMBL and MSP are perpendicular to the image receptor. The MSP position can be checked by checking that the distances between the EAMs and the image receptor are equidistant. Avoid using facial structures such as eyebrows to assess symmetry of the position, as such soft tissue structures generally are not symmetrical in their position

For notes on how to overcome difficulties when positioning the OMBL for the FO in conventional technique, see Chapter 16.

Beam direction and FFD
Initially horizontal, then angled 30° caudally

Centring
Traditional centring is often described as being approximately 5 cm above the glabella, but this has been found to cause unnecessary irradiation of the neck and thyroid.[16] Radiographers will be familiar with the instruction to 'centre at the hairline' but, unfortunately, not only do hairlines vary in their position but they are also non-existent in many males. Alternatively the central ray can be directed to a point above the glabella, ensuring that its path travels through the foramen magnum (found approximately midway between the EAM and mastoid process from the lateral perspective). Changing the centring point and central ray angle can have the effect of reducing thyroid dose. This was first described by Denton:[17]

1. The vertical beam is collimated to the size of the vault and angled 25° caudally
2. The beam is re-centred over the vault to include it in the collimated field; further longitudinal collimation may be possible at this point. It will be noted that the centring point is higher than when using the 30° angle

Collimation for conventional FO 30° projection
Occiput, parietal bones, foramen magnum, petrous temporal bone, lateral aspects of vault

■ OF with 30° cranial angulation 'reverse Towne's'

Positioning
- The patient is seated facing the bucky, their forehead in contact with it
- The OMBL is perpendicular to the image receptor as for other OF projections
- The MSP is perpendicular to the image receptor

Beam direction and FFD
30° cranial angulation
100 cm FFD

Centring
Below the EOP to emerge above the glabella. The beam should pass through the foramen magnum (found approximately midway between the EAM and mastoid process from the lateral perspective)

The image receptor will require cranial displacement to ensure its centre coincides with the central ray.

Figure 18.2 FO 30°

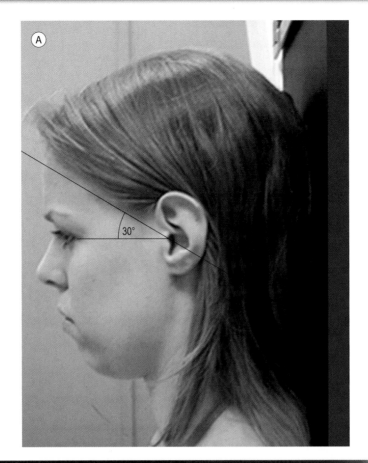

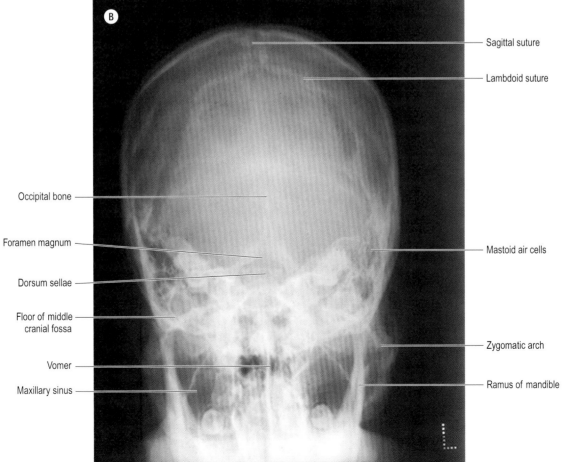

Sagittal suture

Lambdoid suture

Occipital bone

Foramen magnum

Dorsum sellae

Floor of middle
cranial fossa

Vomer

Maxillary sinus

Mastoid air cells

Zygomatic arch

Ramus of mandible

Collimation

Occiput, parietal bones, foramen magnum, petrous temporal bone, lateral aspects of vault

■ Towne's projection of the cranium: isocentric technique

Positioning

- Base position: skull (see Fig. 17.8)
- The table is then moved caudally to bring the vertical central ray, the point at which the central and vertical positional lights intersect, over the glabella
- Collimate, using the iris diaphragm, to include the vertex of the skull, maxillae and parietal bones
- With the support column in the lateral position, the C-arm is put into the PA position
- The long axis of the 24 × 30 cm image receptor is coincident with the MSP

Beam angulation

40° cranial on C-arm

Prior to making the exposure the image receptor is brought into contact with the head to minimise the OFD

Criteria for assessing image quality

- Occiput, parietal bones, foramen magnum, petrous temporal bone and lateral aspect of vault are shown
- Foramen magnum is demonstrated with dorsum sella seen centrally within its borders
- Petrous ridge is seen as a shallow 'v' either side of the foramen magnum
- Sharp image showing dorsum sella in contrast with the less dense foramen magnum; bones of the vault in contrast with the petrous portion of temporal bone

Common errors	Possible reasons
Foramen magnum appears short or is not evident. Dorsum sella may be visible above the portion of the foramen magnum that is seen	Angle selected is inadequate or baseline used is positioned incorrectly (chin not down enough)
Large foramen magnum seen but curve of the posterior arch of C1 is seen in its lower third, rather than the anvil shaped dorsum sella	Angle selected is too great or baseline used is not positioned correctly (chin down too far)
Dorsum sella not seen centrally in foramen magnum and petrous portions of temporal are asymmetrical	Rotated head; direction of rotation coincides with the direction of shift of the sella within the foramen

■ Lateral cranium: conventional technique
(Fig. 18.3A,B)

If used, a 24 × 30 cm cassette is placed transversely and vertically in the bucky, to coincide with the patient's MSP. A gridded cassette can be used in the erect cassette holder (see Ch. 16).

Positioning

- The patient is seated, facing the erect bucky
- The head is turned through 90°, away from the side of interest, and the side of the head is placed in contact with the image receptor or bucky
- The MSP is parallel to the image receptor

Beam direction and FFD

Horizontal, at 90° to the image receptor (must also be 90° to the MSP)
100 cm FFD

Centring

Midway between the glabella and external occipital protuberance

Collimation

Vertex of skull, occiput, frontal bone

■ Lateral cranium – isocentric technique

Positioning

- Base position: skull (see Fig. 17.8)
- The table is then moved caudally to bring the vertical central ray, the point at which the central and vertical positional lights intersect, over the glabella
- Collimate, using the iris diaphragm, to include the vertex of the skull, maxillae and parietal bones
- With the support column in the medial position, the C-arm is put into the horizontal position with the image receptor at the affected side
- The long axis of the 24 × 30 cm image receptor is vertical
- Check that the collimation includes the vertex of the skull, base of the occiput, glabella and external occipital protruberance

Beam angulation

90° on C-arm

Prior to making the exposure the image receptor is brought into contact with the head to minimise the OFD.

Criteria for assessing image quality

- Vertex of skull, occiput and frontal bone are demonstrated

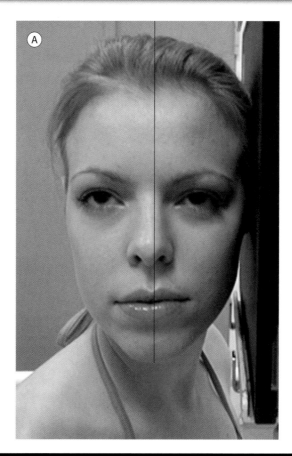

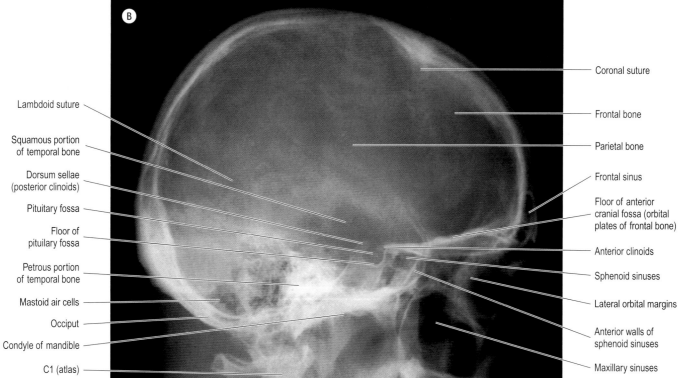

Coronal suture

Frontal bone

Parietal bone

Frontal sinus

Floor of anterior
cranial fossa (orbital
plates of frontal bone)

Anterior clinoids

Sphenoid sinuses

Lateral orbital margins

Anterior walls of
sphenoid sinuses

Maxillary sinuses

Lambdoid suture

Squamous portion
of temporal bone

Dorsum sellae
(posterior clinoids)

Pituitary fossa

Floor of
pituilary fossa

Petrous portion
of temporal bone

Mastoid air cells

Occiput

Condyle of mandible

C1 (atlas)

Figure 18.3   Lateral cranium

- There is superimposition of the floor of the anterior cranial fossa, superimposition of the outlines of the sphenoid and pituitary fossa; superimposition of the inner table of occiput; superimposition of the inner table of frontal bone, superimposition of the petrous portions of temporal
- Sharp image demonstrating bony detail of the vault in contrast with the less dense sutures, mastoid air cells and air-filled sphenoid sinus. The petrous portions of temporal should appear slightly underpenetrated as compared to the temporal bones and the EAMs should be identified within the dense area of the petrous portions of temporal

There are many structures which are identified for superimposition in the lateral skull projection and all are not included in the list of image criteria above. Those not listed here include temporomandibular joints, angles of mandible and orbital outlines. In the real world of clinical practice, experience has shown that these paired structures are almost never all superimposed on one lateral image. The main reason for this is the varying distance of these structures from the central ray, accompanied by the distance between the structures themselves; this serves to project the outline of the structure nearer the central ray away from the outline of the other structure in the pair. For example, consider the lateral orbital outlines which lie, on the average male adult, around 6 cm away from the centring point: at an FFD of 100 cm this would create obliquity of the ray passing through the lateral orbit. This obliquity can be assessed mathematically to be around 3.5°, which is enough to displace the image of the orbital outline furthest from the image receptor. Other structures, such as angle of mandible furthest from the image receptor, are even more remote from the central ray.

Common errors	Possible reasons
Vertical aspects of structures not superimposed and appear *side by side*. These include: Anterior clinoids, posterior clinoids, floor of pituitary fossa, anterior aspect of sphenoid sinus, lateral orbital margins, temporomandibular joints, petrous ridges	MSP not perpendicular to the image receptor; rotation of the head
Horizontal aspects of structures not superimposed and appear *one above the other*. These include: Floor of the anterior cranial fossa, anterior clinoids, posterior clinoids, floor of sphenoid sinus, orbital outlines, temporomandibular joints, petrous ridges	MSP not perpendicular to the image receptor; tilt of the head Note that the image produced may demonstrate both tilt *and* rotation

Frequently the pituitary fossa is used as the main focus for assessment of this position but it must be noted that a seriously tilted lateral may show a single pituitary fossa outline, suggesting good positioning. Severe tilt will displace one side of the fossa and lower its outline sufficiently so as to mask its outline with inferiorly positioned structure; this leaves one side of the fossa appearing to be a beautifully superimposed image of the full pituitary fossa. It is therefore recommended that the pituitary fossa is only used for position assessment in conjunction with at least one other pair of structures, for the lateral skull image.

Submentovertical (SMV) cranium: conventional technique (Fig. 18.4A,B)

If used, a 24 × 30 cm cassette is placed vertically in the erect bucky, to coincide with the patient's MSP.

This projection is not possible as part of table-top technique unless equipment is available that can support the patient's trunk and legs above the table-top and allow extension of the neck to bring the vertex of the head in contact with the table-top.

Positioning

- A chair or stool is placed in front of the erect bucky and pulled approximately 30 cm from it. If using a chair, its back should be perpendicular to the bucky, rather than parallel with it. Brakes must be applied if the stool or chair has wheels

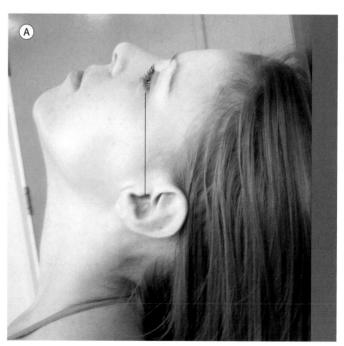

Figure 18.4   SMV

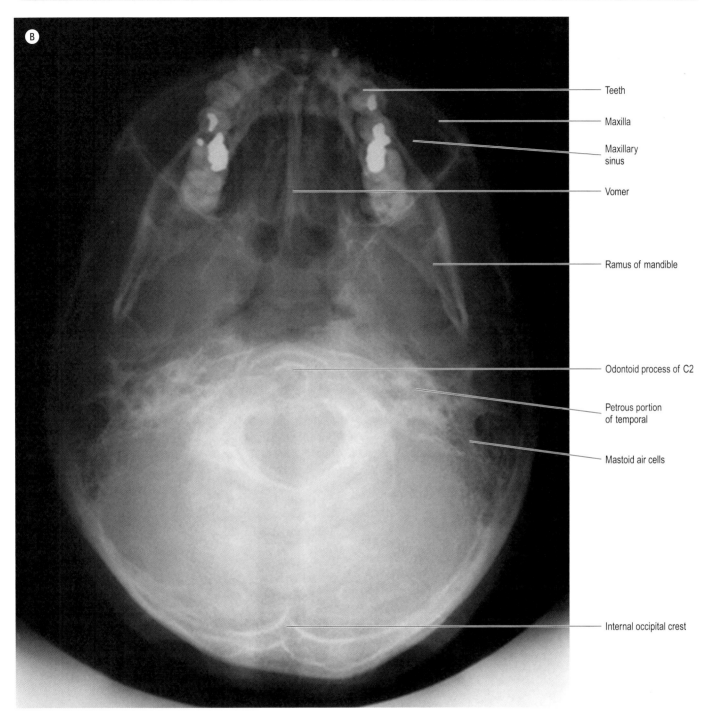

Teeth

Maxilla

Maxillary sinus

Vomer

Ramus of mandible

Odontoid process of C2

Petrous portion of temporal

Mastoid air cells

Internal occipital crest

Figure 18.4 cont'd

- The patient is seated with their back to the erect bucky
- The patient is asked to lean back and extend their neck; the radiographer should support their shoulders gently but should avoid taking the patient's full weight
- The patient is asked to place the vertex of their head in contact with the bucky
- MSP of the head is perpendicular to the image receptor and the OMBL parallel to it

Beam direction and FFD
Horizontal, then angled 5° cranially
100 cm FFD

Centring
Midway between the angles of the mandible

Collimation
Frontal bone, occiput, parietal bones

Maintenance of the required SMV position is very difficult for patients and their body weight is borne by the vertex of the skull; this is actually quite painful and can leave the patient feeling quite nauseous. The radiographer must position the patient confidently and efficiently, in order to ensure that their patient experiences minimum discomfort.

■ SMV cranium: isocentric technique

Positioning
- Base position: SMV (see Fig. 17.10)
- The table is moved to bring the vertical central ray, the point at which the central and vertical positional lights intersect, through the EAM
- With the support column in the lateral position, the C-arm is in the AP position
- The long axis of the 24×30 cm image receptor is coincident with the MSP
- Collimate to include the entire circumference of the skull

Beam angulation
90° to OMBL then a further 5° cranial on C-arm

Prior to making the exposure the image receptor is brought into contact with the head to minimise the OFD.

Criteria for assessing image quality
- Frontal bone, occiput and parietal bones are demonstrated
- Circular image of the odontoid process seen under the anterior rim of the foramen magnum
- Body of the mandible passes through the centre of the maxillary sinuses; symphysis menti is seen just inside the frontal bone
- Angles of the mandible are superimposed over corresponding temporomandibular joints

Common errors	Possible reasons
Body of the mandible below maxillary sinuses; odontoid process seen more elongated, similar to its appearance on the AP C1–C2 projection; symphysis menti seen through the sphenoid or ethmoid sinuses; angles of the mandible below temporomandibular joints	OMBL not parallel to the image receptor; inadequate chin elevation
Asymmetry of anatomical structures	MSP not perpendicular to the image receptor (tilt of the head)

- Sagittal suture is seen centrally and bisects the foramen magnum; the cervical vertebrae are superimposed centrally down the MSP
- Symmetry of bilateral structures of the skull

References
1. McGlinchey I, et al. Comparison of two or three radiographic views in the diagnosis of skull fractures. Clinical Radiology 1998; 53:215–217.
2. Eyes B, Evans A. Post-traumatic skull radiographs. Time for a reappraisal. Lancet 1978; 2(8080):85–86.
3. Balasubramaniam S, et al. Efficacy of skull radiography. American Journal of Surgery 1981; 142:366.
4. Strong I, et al. Head injuries in accident and emergency departments at Scottish hospitals. Injury 1978; 10:154.
5. St John EG. The role of the emergency skull roentgenogram in head trauma. American Journal of Roentgenology 1968; 76:315.
6. Wasserberg J. Treating head injuries. British Medical Journal 2002; 325:454-455.
7. NICE. Head injury – triage, assessment, investigation and early management of head injury in infants, children and adults guideline. National Institute for Clinical Excellence. June 2003. (www.nice.org.uk)
8. Zimmerman R. Head injury. In: Taveras J, Ferrucci J. Radiology on CD-ROM. June 2001; 3, Ch 37.
9. RCR. Making the best use of a department of clinical radiology. 5th edn. RCR;2003.
10. Steill I, et al. The Canadian CT head rule for patients with minor head injury. Lancet 2001; 357:1391–1396.
11. NRPB. Radiation exposure of the UK population from medical and dental x-ray examinations. NRPB; 2001.
12. Ingebrigtsen T, et al. Scandinavian guidelines for initial management of minimal, mild, and moderate head injuries. Journal of Trauma 2000; 48(4):760–766.
13. Jennett B, et al. Severe head injuries in three countries. Journal of Neurology, Neurosurgery and Psychiatry 1977; 40:291.
14. Hadley J. Over-utilization of imaging in the acute trauma setting (abstract). In: Radiological Society of North America scientific assembly and annual meeting program. Oak Brook Ill: Radiological Society of North America 2004; 372.
15. Nee P, et al. Biomechanical factors in patient selection for radiography after head injury. Injury 1993; 24(7):471–475.
16. Laudicina P. Head trauma. Seminars in Radiologic Technology 2000; 8(1):7–11.
17. Denton B. Improving plain radiography of the skull: The half axial projection redescribed. Synergy 1998; Aug:9–11.

CHAPTER 19

FACIAL BONES

Elizabeth Carver, Amanda Royle

The most frequent reason for radiological examination of the facial bones is trauma to the region; use of plain radiographic imaging of the area remains a popular and appropriate method of initial assessment in the acute setting, providing information relatively quickly and with a relatively low radiation dose in comparison to computed tomography (CT), the other imaging method best suited for providing information on bony injury to the area. Low dose CT is considered a suitable method for demonstration and assessment of orbital fractures, since plain radiographic images can sometimes be inconclusive and may not give the 3D information needed before treatment of fractures. Plain radiography has been suggested as useful only in cases which show clinical signs that clearly suggest surgical intervention[1] yet it has also been seen to correspond well with CT findings.[2] Magnetic resonance imaging (MRI) may also be considered but, since scans are undertaken supine, the teardrop effect of the herniating orbital tissue may not be as well demonstrated as in the prone CT scan with coronal sections. CT will provide better bony definition on the images.

CT may also be required as a method for provision of information in trauma cases when plain images in the general facial bones survey are inconclusive or are difficult to produce to a standard high enough to provide the required information; this is often due to difficulties associated with patient condition in severe trauma when excessive oedema may reduce image contrast.

The facial bones can be demonstrated by a general plain radiographic survey that includes the maxilla, mandible, orbits, nasal bones and zygomae. A combination of occipitomental (OM) and lateral projections are employed for this purpose. However, provision of specific information on some of these areas requires alternative or additional projections in order that diagnosis can be made. The mandible and zygomae both require individual examination, in case of injury, and plain radiography is the initial examination method of choice for these areas. Regarding non-trauma-related indications, the mandible may require CT examination for assessment of progress of dental implants.

Temporomandibular joints (TMJs) can also be imaged by plain radiographic examination, which will provide information on condylar dislocation and loss of joint space. MRI will give more useful information regarding the joint itself and, since internal disruption is the most commonly encountered problem in the joint, MRI is most suitable. Arthrography will provide dynamic information regarding the joint.

Injury to the nasal bones is not considered a reason for routine radiographic examination but clinical specialists (e.g. for ear, nose and throat, and maxillofacial follow up) may consider special nasal bones projections to be useful.[3] This would be the case when assessing fragment displacement and septal deviation.

Whilst a significant number of patients presenting with facial trauma will attend on a trolley, patients also frequently arrive as a 'walk in' case and can be examined erect at a skull unit or erect bucky. Erect examination with a horizontal beam is essential for some projections where it is necessary to demonstrate air-fluid levels and erect examination must be attempted whenever possible. This is particularly relevant in the case of blow-out fractures of the orbital floor, where fluid level in the maxillary sinus is used as an indicator of this type of injury.

As for the cranium, the severely injured patient will present on a trolley and any OM projections must be modified to a mentooccipital position, with angle direction in opposition to that for OM. Laterals can be undertaken with the image receptor supported vertically at the side of the face. Description of a modified projection for zygomatic arches on the trolley-bound patient is given after the routine examination, near the end of this chapter. Facial examinations in the A&E situation are also covered in Section 4 of this text.

GENERAL SURVEY OF FACIAL BONES

Requests that define the desired examination as 'facial bones' require a general OM and (sometimes) lateral survey of the area. OM projections are based on a position with the orbitomeatal baseline (OMBL) at 45°, using a range of caudal beam angles. More than one OM projection may be included in the survey and two examples are shown of the 45° OM: without angulation in Figure 19.1B and with 30° caudal angulation in Figure 19.1C.

If used, a 24 × 30 cm cassette is placed lengthwise in the erect bucky or skull unit, for all projections in the general survey.

■ OM facial bones: conventional technique
(Fig. 19.1A,B,C)

Positioning
- The patient is seated, facing the image receptor
- The chin is placed in contact with the midline of the image receptor and the chin position is adjusted until the OMBL has been raised 45° from the horizontal
- The median sagittal plane (MSP) is perpendicular to the image receptor, which is assessed by checking that the external auditory meati (EAMs) or lateral orbital margins are equidistant from it

Beam direction and focus film distance (FFD)
100 cm FFD

1. Horizontal, at 90° to the image receptor and making an angle of 45° with the OMBL *or*
2. Initially horizontal, with caudal angulation applied according to requirements of the examination

Centring
Above the external occipital protuberance (EOP), to emerge half way between the level of the superior orbital margins and angle of the mandible

When using caudal angulation, the description for centring is unchanged, as the beam must always emerge through the middle of the area of interest; the point of entry for the central ray will become higher as angulation increases.

If a cassette is used, it should be displaced until its centre coincides with the central ray; this will result in the

level of the centre of the cassette, if used, appearing to fall in a relatively low position in relationship to the emergent beam. This difference will increase as caudal angulation is applied to the central ray. If a digital receptor plate is used, the beam should at least fall within the boundaries of its perimeter.

Collimation
Orbits, zygomatic arches, mandible

■ OM facial bones: isocentric technique

- Base position: face (see Fig. 17.9)
- The table is then moved to bring the vertical central ray, the point at which the central and vertical positional lights intersect, level with the alae of the nose in the midline
- Collimate, using the iris diaphragm, to include the superior orbital margins, mandible, zygomae and lateral soft tissue outlines
- With the support column in the lateral position, the C-arm is in the posteroanterior (PA) position
- The short axis of the 24 × 30 cm cassette, if used, should be coincident with the MSP. (Using the cassette transversely will minimise the unavoidable object film distance (OFD) in the OM projections)

Beam angulation

Projection	Beam Angulation
OM	0° on C-arm
OM 15°	15° caudal on C-arm
OM 30°	30° caudal on C-arm

Prior to making the exposure the image receptor is brought into contact with the face to minimise the OFD.

Criteria for assessing image quality
- Orbits, zygomatic arches and mandible are demonstrated
- Symmetry of the facial bones on each side; equal distance of the lateral orbital margins from the outer table of temporal bones
- Odontoid process is visible between the angles of the mandible

Horizontal beam/0° beam angulation
- Upper border of the petrous portion of the temporal bone is level with the apex of maxillary antra
- Zygomatic arches seen as a tight 'C' and reversed tight 'C' laterally

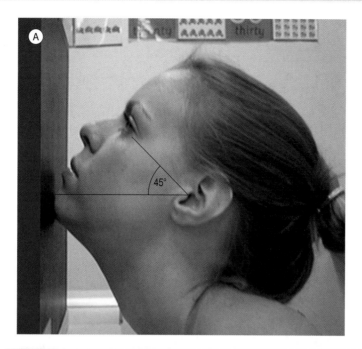

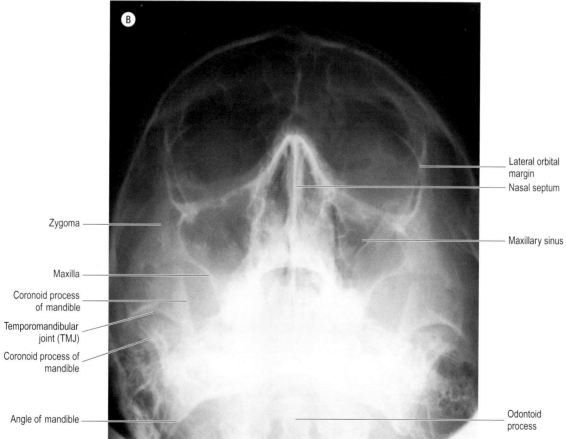

Lateral orbital margin

Nasal septum

Zygoma

Maxillary sinus

Maxilla

Coronoid process of mandible

Temporomandibular joint (TMJ)

Coronoid process of mandible

Angle of mandible

Odontoid process

Figure 19.1 **(A,B)** OM facial bones

Continued

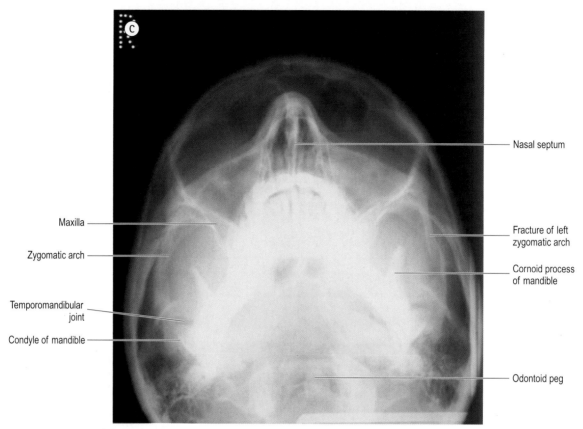

Nasal septum

Maxilla

Fracture of left zygomatic arch

Zygomatic arch

Cornoid process of mandible

Temporomandibular joint

Condyle of mandible

Odontoid peg

Figure 19.1 cont'd (C) OM facial bones with 30° caudal angulation

- Sharp image demonstrating the zygomae, nasal bones, orbits and mandible in contrast to the cranial vault, and the air-filled regions of the paranasal sinuses

15–20° caudal angle
- Zygomatic arches are more gently curved and elongated than with the perpendicular central ray
- Petrous ridge falls below maxillary antra and is likely to be indistinguishable
- TMJs are clearly demonstrated either side of the coronoid processes of the mandible
- Exposure factors are assessed as for the horizontal beam projection

30° caudal angle
- Zygomatic arches are slightly curved and elongated, when viewed from this inferior, half-axial, perspective
- Orbits appear almost closed
- Sharp image demonstrating contrast between the inferior orbital margins, maxillary sinuses and the zygomatic arches overlying the cranial vault. The frontal bone and upper orbital area may appear over-blackened but the nasal bones clearly seen

Common errors	Possible reasons
Asymmetry of facial structures	Rotation about MSP
Position of petrous ridge too high	Chin not raised enough. It has been noticed that, when using *conventional techniques*, radiographers frequently ask patients to put their nose and chin onto the erect image receptor for this projection; this will only serve to raise the chin approximately 30°. It has been noted that some imaging departments use this method with a 15° caudal angle, which only serves to clear the petrous ridge to the inferior margins of the antra; an identical image to the true OM 45° with horizontal beam will result

Lateral facial bones: conventional technique
(Fig. 19.2A,B,C)

Positioning
- The patient is initially seated, facing the image receptor
- The trunk is brought as close as possible to the receptor unit and the patient is asked to sit with their spine as erect as possible. This helps the patient turn their head more easily into the required lateral position
- The head is turned through 90° to bring the affected side in contact with the image receptor
- The MSP is parallel to the image receptor; there should be no tilt or rotation of the head. This can be assessed by checking the midline of the cranium over the top and symmetry of the frontal bone and orbits
- Asking the patient to gently close their eyes will assist in maintenance of the position; as the radiographer leaves the receptor unit, a patient will often follow this movement with their eyes and potentially affect the position of the head

Beam direction and FFD
Horizontal, at 90° to the image receptor
100 cm FFD

Centring
To the inferior border of the zygoma

Collimation
Superior orbital margins, symphysis menti, TMJs, nasal bones

Lateral facial bones: isocentric technique

- Base position: face (see Fig. 17.9)
- The table is then moved to bring the vertical central ray, the point at which the central and vertical positional lights intersect, level with the alae of the nose in the midline
- Collimate, using the iris diaphragm, to include the superior orbital margins, mandible, zygomae and lateral soft tissue outlines
- With the support column in the medial position, the C-arm is in the horizontal position with the image receptor at the affected side
- The long axis of the image receptor is vertical
- Check that the collimation includes the superior orbital margins, mandible, nose and soft tissue outlines

Beam angulation
90° on the C-arm

Prior to making the exposure the image receptor is brought into contact with the face to minimise the OFD.

Criteria for assessing image quality
- Superior orbital margins, symphysis menti, TMJs and nasal bones are demonstrated
- Superimposition of the malar processes of maxilla, orbital outlines and TMJs
- Sharp image demonstrating the malar processes of maxilla in contrast to the air-filled maxillary sinuses, and the orbits in contrast to other bones of the face. The mandible is seen in contrast to the soft tissues of the face. Nasal bones are over-penetrated

Common errors	Possible reasons
Non-superimposition of the floor of the anterior cranial fossa; malar processes seen as one above the other; orbital outlines seen as one above the other	MSP tilted, usually with the upper part of the head tilted towards the image receptor; this most commonly occurs with the conventional technique. If a patient cannot comply with the required position, a compensating caudal angle can be used to reduce the effects of the tilt
Lateral orbital margins seen side by side and not superimposed. Malar processes seen displaced in a horizontal direction	Head is rotated; this is often encouraged when the patient 'slumps' in their chair (conventional technique) rather than sitting with their spine erect, as described in 'positioning' for this projection

ORBITS

The orbits are examined for trauma or the presence and position of intraocular foreign body (IOFB). IOFB assessment may be made after penetrating injury or prior to MRI scanning as a safety measure to exclude presence of ferrous material in the eye.

A horizontal beam should be used wherever possible since demonstration of air fluid levels in the maxillary sinuses can be an indicator of orbital floor fracture. Air in the top portion of the maxillary antrum will also serve to provide contrast with any soft tissue teardrop appearance of a herniating inferior rectus muscle down through the fractured orbital floor. Clearly the OM orbital projection cannot be undertaken erect with a horizontal beam on the

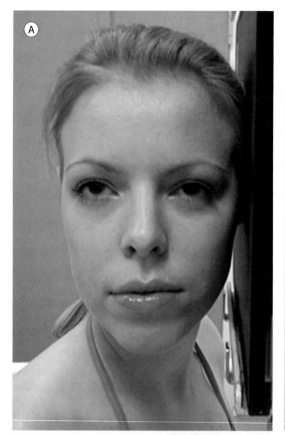

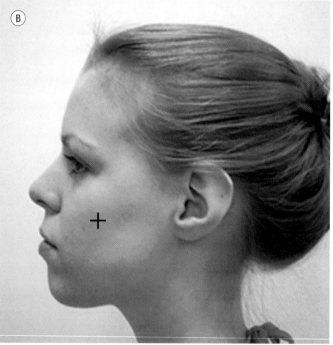

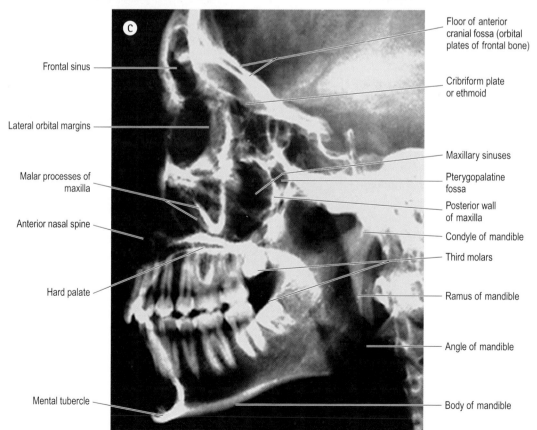

Floor of anterior cranial fossa (orbital plates of frontal bone)

Frontal sinus

Cribriform plate or ethmoid

Lateral orbital margins

Maxillary sinuses

Malar processes of maxilla

Pterygopalatine fossa

Posterior wall of maxilla

Anterior nasal spine

Condyle of mandible

Third molars

Hard palate

Ramus of mandible

Angle of mandible

Mental tubercle

Body of mandible

Figure 19.2 **(A)** Lateral facial bones; **(B)** centring for lateral facial bones; **(C)** lateral facial bones. (C) Reproduced with permission from Bryan GJ. Skeletal anatomy. 3rd edn. Edinburgh: Churchill Livingstone; 1996 and Gunn (2002)

seriously injured patient; at the very least a lateral with horizontal beam can be attempted whilst this type of patient is supine.

If used, an 18 × 24 cm cassette is placed in the erect bucky or skull unit, for both projections.

OM orbits: conventional technique (Fig. 19.3A,B)

Positioning
- The patient is seated, facing the image receptor
- The chin is placed in contact with the midline of the image receptor and the chin position is adjusted until the OMBL has been raised 30° from the horizontal
- The MSP is perpendicular to the image receptor, which is assessed by checking that the EAMs or lateral orbital margins are equidistant from the image receptor

Beam direction and FFD
Horizontal, at 90° to the image receptor
100 cm FFD

Centring
Above the EOP, to emerge level with the middle of the orbits

Collimation
Orbits, maxillary sinuses

OM orbits: isocentric technique

The importance of using air-fluid levels in the maxillary sinuses, as an indicator of blow-out fracture of the orbital floor, has already been mentioned. As the lateral produced on the isocentric unit employs a horizontal beam, presence of fluid levels should be demonstrated in this projection but cannot be utilised in the OM projection. Unfortunately, air-fluid levels are less distinctly shown than on the OM projection. However, this is also the case for the severely injured patient who presents in the imaging department on a trolley. It is recommended that erect OM projections be attempted if the patient condition allows; since the projection requires a 90° relationship between the central ray and image receptor, this can still be achieved on the isocentric unit (which should be positioned with a horizontal central ray and vertical image receptor). As already described, conventional X-ray units can also be used.

The supine procedure is as follows:

- Base position: face (see Fig. 17.9)
- The face position is modified as follows:
- The chin is raised so that the OMBL is 30° to the horizontal. This can be accurately measured by ensuring that the horizontal positional light is passing directly through the EAM and then applying a 30° caudal angle. The chin is then raised so that the OMBL is coincident with the light beam on the side of the face. The C-arm is then returned to the vertical position
- The table is then moved to bring the vertical central ray, the point at which the central and vertical positional lights intersect, over the interpupillary line in the midline
- The height of the isocentric unit is altered to bring the horizontal positional light level with the outer canthus of the eye
- Collimate, using the rectangular diaphragm, to include the outer margins of the orbits and the maxillary sinuses
- With the support column in the lateral position, the C-arm is in the PA position
- The short axis of the image receptor is coincident with the MSP

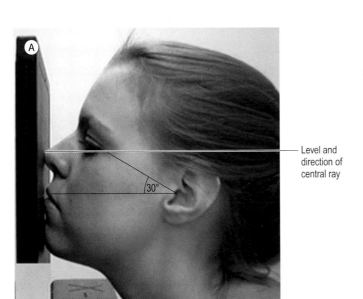

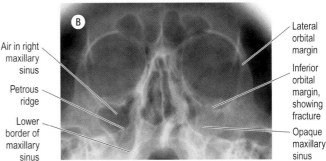

Figure 19.3   OM orbits

Beam angulation

0° on the C-arm

Prior to making the exposure the image receptor is brought into contact with the head to minimise the OFD.

Criteria for assessing image quality

- Orbits and maxillary sinuses are demonstrated
- Orbital margins are equidistant from the outer table of the temporal bones
- Petrous ridge seen half way down the maxillary sinuses
- Sharp image demonstrating contrast between the orbital outlines in contrast with the cranial vault and air-filled frontal and maxillary sinus. Fine detail of the orbital floor is seen at the top of the maxillary sinuses

Common errors	Possible reasons
Asymmetry of facial structures	Rotation about MSP
Petrous ridge level with inferior orbital margins or within orbital outline	Chin not raised enough
Petrous ridge in the lower half of the antrum, or even at its lower margin	Chin elevated too high. This will have a detrimental effect upon the ability of reporting personnel to diagnose blow-out fractures of the orbital floor, which is not well demonstrated on projections with the chin elevated more than 30°

■ Lateral orbits: conventional technique
(Fig. 19.4A,B)

Positioning

- The patient is initially seated, facing the image receptor and positioned with their head turned as for a lateral facial bones projection

Beam direction and FFD

Horizontal, at 90° to the image receptor

100 cm FFD

Centring

Over the outer canthus of the eye

Collimation

Orbits, frontal and maxillary sinuses

■ Lateral orbits: isocentric technique

- Base position: see isocentric OM orbits
- The table is then moved to bring the vertical central ray, the point at which the central and vertical positional lights intersect, level with the interpupillary line in the midline
- Unit height is adjusted to bring horizontal light level with the outer canthus of the eye
- With the support column in the medial position, the C-arm is in the horizontal position with the image receptor at the affected side

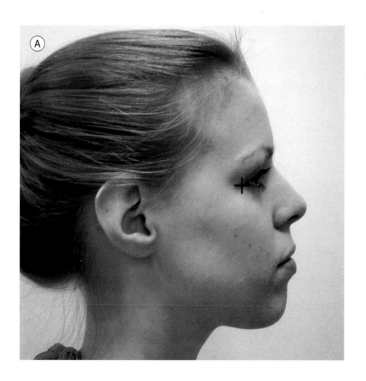

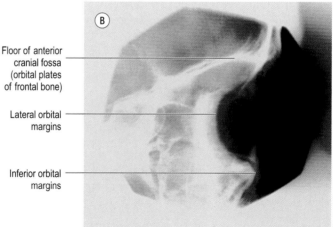

Floor of anterior cranial fossa (orbital plates of frontal bone)

Lateral orbital margins

Inferior orbital margins

Figure 19.4 (A) Centring for lateral orbits; (B) lateral orbits

- The long axis of the image receptor is vertical
- Check that the collimation includes the orbits

Beam angulation

90° on the C-arm

Prior to making the exposure the image receptor is brought into contact with the face to minimise the OFD.

Criteria for assessing image quality

- Orbits and maxillary sinuses are demonstrated
- Orbital outlines are superimposed
- Sharp image demonstrating orbital outlines in contrast to the air-filled maxillary sinuses and ethmoid sinuses

Common errors	Possible reasons
Overlap of orbital outlines in a vertical direction	MSP tilted. See notes on tilt in the errors section for facial bones
Overlap of orbital outlines in a horizontal direction	Head is rotated. See notes on rotation in the errors section for facial bones

NASAL BONES

◼ OM nasal bones; conventional technique
(Fig. 19.5A,B)

If used, an 18 × 24 cm cassette is placed in the erect cassette holder, for both OM and lateral projections. The lateral nasal bones projection can be undertaken using an occlusal dental film.

Positioning

- The patient is seated, facing the image receptor and positioned as for the OM facial bones

Beam direction and FFD

Horizontal, at 90° to the image receptor
100 cm FFD

Centring

Above the EOP, to emerge through the centre of the nasal bone

Collimation

Nasal bone, anterior nasal spine

◼ OM nasal bones: isocentric technique

- Base position: face (see Fig. 17.9)
- The table is then moved to bring the vertical central ray, the point at which the central and vertical positional lights intersect, over the nasal bones in the midline
- The height of the isocentric unit is altered to bring the horizontal positional light level with the alae of the nose
- Collimate, using the rectangular diaphragm, to include the nasal bones and anterior nasal spine
- With the support column in the lateral position, the C-arm is in the PA position
- The short axis of the image receptor is coincident with the MSP

Beam angulation

0° on the C-arm

Prior to making the exposure the image receptor is brought into contact with the face to minimise the OFD.

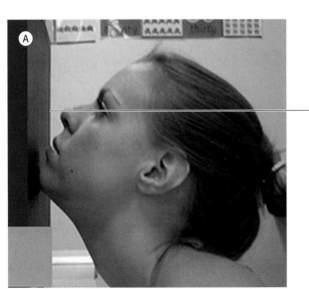

Level and direction of central ray

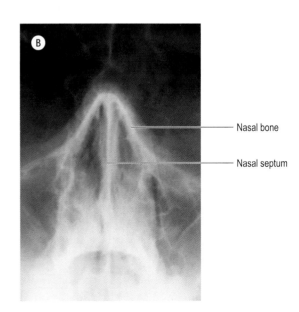

Nasal bone

Nasal septum

Figure 19.5 OM nasal bones

Criteria for assessing image quality

- Nasal bone and septum are demonstrated; there is evidence of frontal and maxillary sinuses superiorly and laterally
- Petrous ridge is evident as level with inferior maxillary antra
- Sharp image demonstrating the nasal septum centrally and the nasal bones laterally, in contrast with the air-filled ethmoid sinuses

■ Lateral nasal bones: conventional technique
(Fig. 19.6A,B)

Positioning
The patient is initially seated, facing the image receptor and positioned as for a lateral facial bones projection

Beam direction and FFD
Horizontal, at 90° to the image receptor
100 cm FFD

Centring
Over the nasal bone

Collimation
Nasal bone, anterior nasal spine, soft tissue of the nose

■ Lateral nasal bones: isocentric technique

- Base position: face (see Fig. 17.9)
- The table is then moved to bring the vertical central ray, the point at which the central and vertical positional lights intersect, over the nasal bones in the midline
- The height of the isocentric unit is altered to bring the horizontal positional light level with the alae of the nose

- Collimate, using the rectangular diaphragm, to include the nasal bones and anterior nasal spine
- With the support column in the medial position, the C-arm is in the horizontal position with the image receptor at the affected side
- Ensure that the collimation includes the nasal bones and anterior nasal spine

Beam angulation
90° on the C-arm

Prior to making the exposure the image receptor is brought into contact with the face to minimise the OFD. A grid must not be used for this examination.

Criteria for assessing image quality
- Nasal bone, anterior nasal spine and soft tissue of the nose are demonstrated
- Sharp image demonstrating bony detail of the nasal bone and anterior nasal spine, in contrast to the soft tissues of the nose and air-filled sinuses

MANDIBLE

The structure of the mandible makes it difficult to image accurately using the usual approach of obtaining two images at 90° to each other. As a result several projections are available for demonstration of this bone, none of which demonstrate it adequately in its entirety:

1. The PA mandible projection, which shows the rami relatively well but causes foreshortening over the body
2. The lateral which superimposes both sides of the mandible

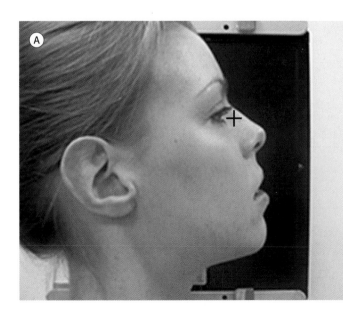
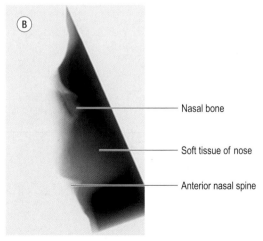

Nasal bone

Soft tissue of nose

Anterior nasal spine

Figure 19.6   Lateral nasal bones

3. The lateral oblique which clears the body on the side under examination from the opposite side but foreshortens the ramus. Both lateral obliques are undertaken in any one case, as the mandible is a recognised site for contrecoup fractures

A combination of all, or some, of these projections are used to provide information on the mandible as a whole.

Alternatively, orthopantomography (OPT) can be used to demonstrate the mandible. It is a method that clearly requires specialised equipment, which is not always available. Some units are unsuitable for patients in wheelchairs and the image does have some unsharpness. The main benefit of this method is its ability to demonstrate the whole mandible and TMJs on one image but it still may not be easy to see fractures; other projections may be required as supplement.[4]

■ PA mandible: conventional technique (Fig. 19.7A,B)

If used, an 18 × 24 cm cassette is placed longitudinally in the erect bucky.

Positioning

Note that, although described as a PA projection, the patient's head is positioned as for an occipitofrontal (OF) projection; since the beam will not travel through the occiput or frontal bone the projection cannot actually be named as OF.

- The patient is seated, facing the image receptor
- The forehead is placed in contact with the midline of the image receptor and the chin position is adjusted until the OMBL is perpendicular to it
- The middle of the cassette, if used, is level with the angles of the mandible
- The MSP is perpendicular to the image receptor, which is assessed by checking that the EAMs or lateral orbital margins are equidistant from it

Beam direction and FFD

Horizontal, at 90° to the image receptor
100 cm FFD

Centring

In the midline of the neck, midway between the angles of the mandible

Collimation

TMJs, angles of mandible, symphysis menti

■ PA mandible: isocentric technique

- Base position: skull (see Fig. 17.8)
- The table is then moved to bring the vertical central ray, the point at which the central and vertical positional lights intersect, level with the angles of mandible
- The height of the isocentric unit is altered so that the horizontal positional light passes through the angle of the mandible

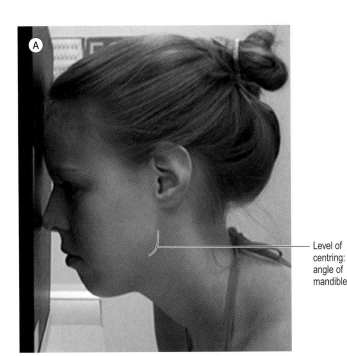

Level of centring: angle of mandible

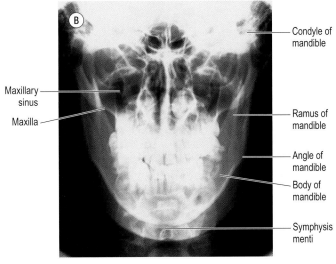

Condyle of mandible

Maxillary sinus

Maxilla

Ramus of mandible

Angle of mandible

Body of mandible

Symphysis menti

Figure 19.7   PA mandible

- Collimate, using the iris diaphragm, to include the symphysis menti and TMJs
- The support column is in the lateral position and the C-arm is in the PA position
- The long axis of the image receptor is coincident with the MSP

Beam angulation

10° cranial on the C-arm

Prior to making the exposure the image receptor is brought into contact with the face to minimise the OFD.

Criteria for assessing image quality

- TMJs, angles of the mandible and symphysis menti are demonstrated
- Petrous ridge is level with the top of the orbits
- Condyles are superimposed over the inferior aspect of the petrous bones laterally
- Symmetry of the mandible either side of the face and neck
- Mandible is seen as a 'U'
- Sharp image demonstrating the entire mandible in contrast to the soft tissues of the face and neck, and the bones of the cervical vertebrae

Common error	Possible reason
Pale area where the mandible overlies cervical vertebrae but contrast over rami is good	kVp too low to penetrate the area over the cervical vertebrae; mAs may need to be decreased if kVp increased

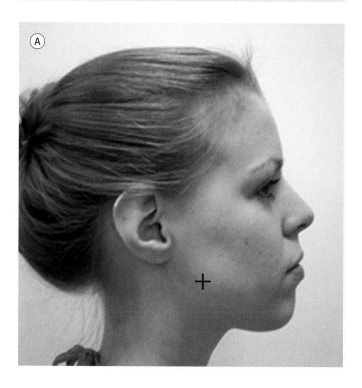

■ Lateral mandible: conventional technique
(Fig. 19.8A,B)

If used, an 18 × 24 cm cassette is placed longitudinally in the erect cassette holder.

Positioning

- The patient is seated, facing the image receptor
- The head is turned through 90° to place the affected side in contact with the image receptor
- The middle of the cassette, if used, is level with the angles of the mandible
- The chin is raised very slightly to decrease the density of the soft tissues of the throat which lie over the body of the mandible
- The MSP* is parallel to the image receptor, which is assessed by checking that the angles of the mandible are in alignment or superimposed

*Using the MSP of the head may not be appropriate for the lateral projection as the mandible may not lie in continuous alignment with the skull. It is suggested that, for this projection, the mandible should be considered to have an MSP that runs vertically down its midline and midway between the angles.

Beam direction and FFD

Horizontal, at 90° to the image receptor
100 cm FFD

Centring

Over the angle of the mandible

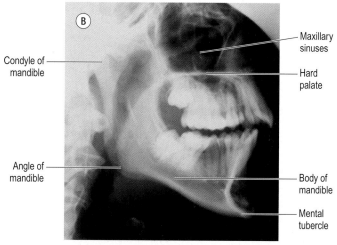

Figure 19.8 (A) Lateral mandible – centring; (B) lateral mandible

Collimation

TMJs, angles of mandible, symphysis menti

◼ Lateral mandible: isocentric technique

- Base position: skull (see Fig. 17.8)
- The table is then moved to bring the vertical central ray, the point at which the central and vertical positional lights intersect, level with the angles of the mandible
- The height of the isocentric unit is altered so that the horizontal positional light passes through the angle of the mandible
- Collimate, using the iris diaphragm, to include the symphysis menti and TMJs
- The support column is in the medial position and the C-arm is in the horizontal position with the image receptor at the affected side
- The long axis of the image receptor is vertical

Beam angulation

90° on the C-arm

Prior to making the exposure the image receptor is brought into contact with the face to minimise the OFD.

Criteria for assessing image quality

- TMJs, angles of mandible and symphysis menti demonstrated
- Condyles superimposed over each other; angles of mandible superimposed
- Mandible clear of the cervical vertebrae
- Sharp image demonstrating the entire mandible in contrast to the soft tissues of the neck and mouth

Common error	Possible reason
Non-superimposition of required structures	It is tempting to use the facial structures to assess the lateral position when employing conventional technique; see * at the end of the positioning section There may be some magnification of the side furthest from the image receptor on patients with wider mandibles, which will effectively take its outline outside that of the opposite side; this cannot be considered as radiographer error. Consider increasing FFD to compensate

◼ Lateral oblique mandible: conventional technique
(Fig. 19.9A,B)

If used, an 18 × 24 cm cassette is placed transversely in the erect cassette holder. Both obliques are undertaken in order to demonstrate the whole mandible.

Positioning

- The patient is seated alongside the image receptor with the side under examination nearest to it
- The middle of the image receptor is approximately level with the angles of the mandible but may require adjustment later in the examination (as described after the section on collimation below)
- The chin is raised very slightly, to decrease the density of the soft tissues of the throat which lie over the body of the mandible
- The MSP is initially parallel to the image receptor and the head then tilted towards it until the MSP is approximately 15° to it. Care must be taken not to rotate the head during the manoeuvre
- The chin is elevated as far as possible to clear the condyle from the neck

Beam direction and FFD

Initially horizontal, then directed 10° cranially
100 cm FFD

Centring

Midway between the angles of the mandible

Collimation

TMJ and angle of mandible on the side under examination, symphysis menti

Once collimation is complete, the image receptor position may require adjustment, until the radiation field lies within the boundaries and the central ray is coincident with its middle. The outline of the soft tissues overlying the mandible should be shown as a shadow within the light beam (and within the borders of the image receptor).

Unfortunately the combination of angle and obliquity for this oblique method does distort and foreshorten the ramus in particular. The body of the mandible is not in contact with the image receptor and this has implications for magnification and unsharpness of the body and lower portion of the ramus.

Since the lateral oblique position of the mandible itself will foreshorten the ramus of the mandible, an alternative method is to use a true lateral position of the head, with an increased cranial angle. For this the patient has been described as prone, with the head turned into the lateral position and a cranial beam angle of 25°.[5] Supine with the

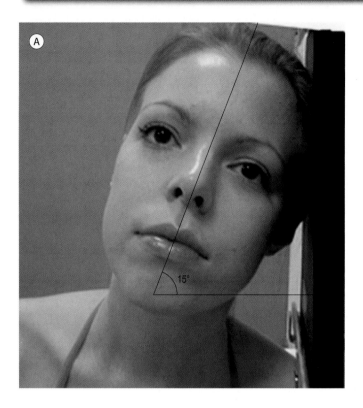

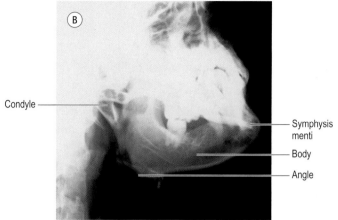

Figure 19.9   Lateral oblique mandible

head turned laterally has also been described, with a bucky and 35° central ray.[6] However, a prone lateral position often proves difficult for the patient, especially if injured. The supine lateral can be equally difficult but the patient's trunk can be obliqued to improve the situation; for both these supine and prone positions there is the potential for increased OFD which affects magnification of the image, although this could be improved upon by use of a stationary grid in conjunction with an image receptor which is supported on a pad on the table-top.[6] An increase in FFD will also reduce magnification.

Use of a 25° cranial angle in conjunction with a true lateral (seated patient position) requires the tube head to be in a relatively low position and the beam is frequently attenuated by the shoulder in larger patients; attempt to clear the shoulder can be made by effecting posterior rotation of the shoulder nearest the tube but this often causes rotation of the head. The shoulder can often lie within the primary beam, and be superimposed over the mandible, even with the prone lateral position.

The oblique position with cranial angulation can be deemed a general survey of the mandible and modifications have also been described which will provide more specific information of different aspects of the mandible.[7]

30° rotation towards the side under examination will demonstrate the body more adequately.

45° rotation demonstrates the symphysis menti.

It is also claimed that a rotation of 15° will give a general survey of the mandible but surely this rotation will cause the condyle to overlie the neck on the image?

Lateral oblique mandible: isocentric technique

- Base position: skull (see Fig. 17.8)
- The table is then moved to bring the vertical central ray, the point at which the central and vertical positional lights intersect, level with the angles of the mandible
- The height of the isocentric unit is altered so that the horizontal positional light passes through the angle of the mandible
- Collimate, using the iris diaphragm, to include the symphysis menti and TMJs
- The support column is in the medial position, and the C-arm is in the anteroposterior (AP) position
- The table is displaced to each side in turn so that the central positional light passes through the angle of the mandible of the side under examination
- The C-arm is then placed in the horizontal position with the image receptor at the side under examination
- The long axis of the image receptor is vertical

Beam angulation

1. X-ray beam is directed 10° upwards on the C-arm to prevent the tube head hitting the table when the second angle is applied
2. 25° cranially on support column

Criteria for assessing image quality

- TMJs, angles of the mandible and symphysis menti are demonstrated
- TMJ, condyle, ramus and body on the side under examination are cleared from the cervical vertebrae
- Sharp image demonstrating the entire mandible in contrast to the soft tissues of the neck and mouth

Common error	Possible reason
Condyle on the side under examination not cleared from the cervical vertebrae	Chin too low or Head is rotated towards the image receptor

■ OPT for mandible

Please refer to Chapter 23 for this examination.

TMJs

■ Lateral oblique: conventional technique
(Fig. 19.10A,B)

In the lateral position the TMJs are superimposed and an oblique central ray is used to clear the image of one TMJ to reveal the other. Both sides are examined for comparison.

If used, an 18 × 24 cm cassette is placed longitudinally in the bucky. Use of an erect bucky is more comfortable for the patient than using a table bucky.

Positioning

- The patient is initially seated, facing the image receptor and is then positioned as for the lateral facial bones; the TMJ under examination is in contact with the image receptor
- If a cassette is used, its middle is coincident with the TMJ; this is palpable anterior to the tragus of the ear. If the patient is asked to open their mouth the radiographer's finger will feel a depression over the mandibular fossa as the mouth opens, effecting the movement of the mandibular condyle forwards from the mandibular fossa
- The MSP is parallel to the image receptor; there should be no tilt or rotation of the head. This can be assessed by checking that the interpupillary line is perpendicular to the image receptor
- A legend is applied to the image receptor to indicate that the mouth is open or closed

Beam direction and FFD

Initially horizontal, then angled 25° caudally
100 cm FFD

Centring

Above the TMJ remote from the image receptor, with the beam emerging through the TMJ under examination

Collimation

TMJ, condyle of mandible

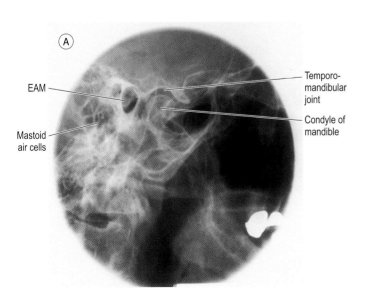
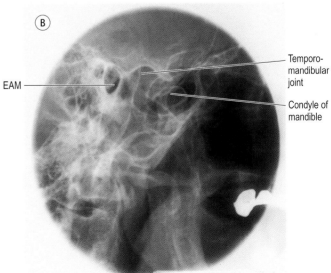

Figure 19.10   Lateral oblique TMJs with **(A)** mouth closed and **(B)** mouth open

Lateral oblique mandible: isocentric technique

- Base position: skull (see Fig. 17.8)
- The table is then moved to bring the vertical central ray, the point at which the central and vertical positional lights intersect, over the midline at the level of the TMJs
- The height of the isocentric unit is altered to bring the horizontal positional light through the TMJ
- The support column is in the medial position, and the C-arm is in the AP position
- The table is displaced to each side in turn so that the central positional light passes through the TMJ of the side under examination
- The C-arm is then placed in the horizontal position with the image receptor at the side under examination
- The long axis of the image receptor is vertical
- Collimate, using the iris diaphragm, to include the TMJ under examination (a diameter of approximately 5 cm on the side of the face remote from the image receptor)

Beam angulation

25° caudal on the support column

Prior to making the exposure the image receptor is brought into contact with the face to minimise the OFD.

Criteria for assessing image quality

- TMJ and condyle of mandible are demonstrated
- Other TMJ is clear from the area of interest
- TMJ under examination anterior to EAM

- Indication of whether the mouth is open or closed is clearly seen on the image
- Sharp image demonstrating the mandibular fossa in contrast to the temporal bone and condyle of mandible

Common errors	Possible reasons
Mastoid air cells of unaffected side overlying TMJ	MSP rotated, face turning towards image receptor
TMJ or ramus of mandible closest to tube not cleared from TMJ under examination	1. Inadequate angle used *or* 2. Head is tilted with its vertex towards the image receptor, which effectively reduces the effects of angulation

OF 30–35° TMJs: conventional technique
(Fig. 19.11A,B)

If used, an 18 × 24 cm cassette is placed transversely in the erect bucky.

Positioning

- The patient is seated, facing the image receptor
- The forehead is placed in contact with the midline of the image receptor and the chin position adjusted until the OMBL is perpendicular to it, as for the basic OF position
- The middle of the cassette, if used, is initially level with the glabella but will require displacement after accurate tube centring

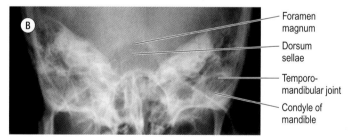

Figure 19.11   Temporomandibular joints – OF 30–35°

30°–35° Cranial central ray to pass through level of TMJs

- The MSP is perpendicular to the image receptor, which is assessed by checking that the EAMs or lateral orbital margins are equidistant from it

Beam direction and FFD
Initially horizontal, with 30–35° cranial angulation

The specific angle has not been suggested here as it does appear that there is some variation in practice.[8,9] *Selection of optimum exposure factors will ensure that the joints will be well demonstrated regardless of a 5° difference in angle.*
100 cm FFD

Centring
In the midline of the neck, to travel through the TMJs

The cassette, if used, is adjusted until its centre is coincident with the emerging central ray. Digital receptor plates should include the field of radiation and area of interest.

Collimation
TMJs

> Exposure is made with the mouth open and a legend should be applied to indicate this

Most texts describe the frontooccipital (FO) projection rather than the OF[5,6,8,9] but, as outlined in Chapter 16, the OF position is easier for the patient, especially if they can sit in an erect position. The OF position will also help reduce dose absorbed by the lenses of the eyes and the thyroid, although the close collimation required for TMJs does ensure that dose is minimised, even in the FO position. It is unlikely that the joints will lie significantly closer to the image receptor on either the OF or FO projections, therefore image sharpness should be similar on both.

■ FO 30–35° TMJs: conventional technique

If used, an 18 × 24 cm cassette is placed transversely in the erect bucky. Table-top technique may be used but the FO position is difficult to achieve with the patient supine.

This projection is essentially the same position as the 30° FO projection (Towne's) used for the cranial vault, with collimation to the area of interest and alteration of height of centring.

Positioning
- The patient is seated, with their back to the image receptor
- The back of the occiput is placed in contact with the midline of the image receptor and the chin position is adjusted until the OMBL is at 90° to it

- The MSP is perpendicular to the image receptor, which is assessed by checking that the EAMs or lateral orbital margins are equidistant from it
- It will be necessary to adjust the height of the image receptor after centring

Beam direction and FFD
A horizontal central ray is angled 30–35° caudally
100 cm FFD

Centring
In the midline above the glabella, with the beam travelling through the TMJs and then the lower occiput. The cassette, if used, is adjusted until its centre is coincident with the emerging central ray. The digital receptor plate should include the field of radiation

Collimation
Mastoid bones, TMJs, condyles of mandible, upper rami of mandible

■ OF 30–35° TMJs: isocentric technique

- Base position: skull (see Fig. 17.8)
- The table is then moved to bring the vertical central ray, the point at which the central and vertical positional lights intersect, over the midline at the level of the TMJs
- The height of the isocentric unit is altered to bring the horizontal positional light through the TMJ
- Collimate, using the rectangular diaphragm, to include the lateral margins of the skull and proximal thirds of the mandibular rami
- With the support column in the lateral position, the C-arm is in the PA position
- The short axis of the image receptor is coincident with the MSP

Beam angulation
40–45° cranial on the C-arm

Prior to making the exposure the image receptor is brought into contact with the face to minimise the OFD.

Criteria for assessing image quality
- Mastoid bones, TMJs, condyles of mandible and upper rami of mandible are demonstrated
- Symmetry of the petrous portion of the temporal bones on either side of the foramen magnum; the condyles of mandible are an equal distance from the lateral portions of the skull
- Dorsum sellae seen within the foramen magnum; arch of C1 may be demonstrated if a 35° angle has been used
- Sharp image demonstrating contrast between the TMJs and the denser petrous temporal and mastoids

Common errors	Possible reasons
Asymmetry of petrous temporal bones around the foramen magnum	Rotation about MSP
Pale image over the TMJ	Inadequate penetration

◼ Orthopantomography (OPT)

As in the case of the mandible, the TMJs are seen on the OPT examination of the mandible (see Ch. 23) but the joints are shown closed in the conventional mouth position. Open mouth exposure should also be made in order to adequately demonstrate the joint. This is a difficult manoeuvre for patients with dislocation and implementation of the TMJ may not be possible using the OPT technique.

ZYGOMATIC ARCHES

The zygomatic arches are demonstrated reasonably well in contrast to the cranium on the OM facial bones projections but they can be shown in profile over the soft tissues of the cheeks in the FO 30° projection.

◼ FO 30° zygomatic arches: conventional technique
(Fig. 19.12A,B)

As mentioned for the TMJ examination in this position, a technique with the patient supine may be used but is not recommended unless absolutely necessary (for example when the patient is injured seriously enough to present as supine on a trolley).

An alternative OF projection is not described as the zygomatic arches must show some magnification in order to demonstrate them laterally at either side of the cranial vault. To undertake an OF projection would minimise magnification of the arches since they lie closer to the image receptor in this position; the posterior half of the vault will be magnified and potentially overlie part, or all, of the zygomatic arches.

If used, an 18 × 24 cm or 24 × 30 cm cassette is placed transversely in the erect cassette holder.

Positioning
- The patient is seated with their back to the image receptor and positioned initially as for the FO 30° TMJ projection
- It will be necessary to adjust the height of the image receptor after centring

Beam direction and FFD
A horizontal central ray is angled 30° caudally
100 cm FFD

Centring
In the midline above the glabella, with the beam travelling through the zygomatic arches. The cassette, if used, is adjusted until its centre is coincident with the emerging central ray. The digital plate receptor should include the field of radiation

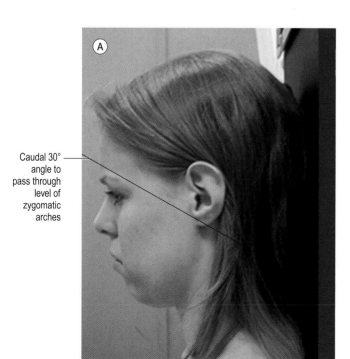

Caudal 30° angle to pass through level of zygomatic arches

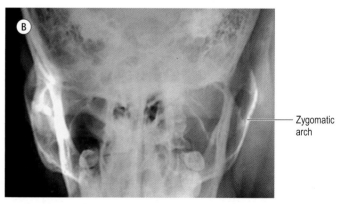

Zygomatic arch

Figure 19.12   **(A)** FO 30° zygomatic arches **(B)** OF 30° zygomatic arches. (B) Reproduced with permission from Ballinger PW, Frank ED. Merrill's atlas of radiographic positioning and radiologic procedures. 10th edn. St Louis: Mosby; 2003

Collimation

Mastoid bones, zygomatic arches, zygomae, upper rami of mandible

Exposure factors

Exposure factors must be set at significantly lower values than for other FO 30° projections of the cranial vault, mastoids and TMJs. This is due to the low density of the arches and the fact that no grid is necessary for the examination

■ Modified submentovertical (SMV) zygomatic arches for the injured patient: conventional technique (Fig. 19.13)

A 24 × 30 cm cassette is selected for this examination.

Positioning

- The patient lies supine on the table or trolley; it may be necessary to place a pillow under the patient's shoulders in order to elevate the area of interest
- The neck is flexed back as far as possible and the cassette placed in contact with the top of the head, its long axis resting on the table-top
- The cassette position is adjusted until parallel to the long axes of the zygomatic arches and supported in this position by pads and sandbags
- The MSP is perpendicular to the cassette and coincident with its midline

Beam direction and FFD

The beam should be perpendicular to the cassette and zygomatic arches

FFD 120 cm, or slightly more for patients with a large abdomen

Centring

In the midline, to travel through the midpoint of the zygomatic arches

Collimation

As for the FO 30° projection

■ FO 30° zygomatic arches: isocentric technique

- Base position: skull (see Fig. 17.8)
- The table is then moved and the height of the isocentric unit is altered so that the vertical and horizontal positional lights pass midway along the zygomatic arches
- Collimate, using the rectangular diaphragm, to include the zygomatic arches
- The support column is in the lateral position, with the C-arm in the PA position
- The short axis of the image receptor is coincident with the MSP

Beam angulation

40° cranial on the C-arm

Prior to making the exposure the image receptor is brought into contact with the face to minimise the OFD.

Criteria for assessing image quality – FO 30°

- Mastoid bones, zygomatic arches, zygomae and upper rami of mandible are demonstrated
- Symmetry of the petrous portion of the temporal bones on either side of the foramen magnum
- Dorsum sellae seen within the foramen magnum
- Sharp image demonstrating contrast between the low density zygomatic arch and the soft tissues of the face

Common errors – FO 30°	Possible reasons
Asymmetry of petrous temporal bones around the foramen magnum	Rotation about MSP
Dark image with poor contrast	Quite obviously, selection of mAs and kVp is too high. Density of the arch is frequently overestimated and it should be remembered that this density is less than that of a phalanx. There is an air gap between the zygomatic arch and the image receptor which will need consideration when selecting exposure factors

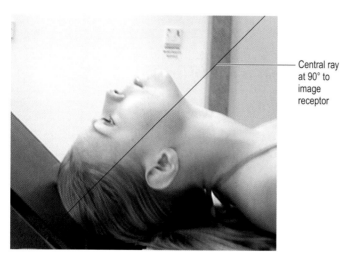

Central ray at 90° to image receptor

Figure 19.13   Modified SMV zygomatic arches

Essentially the FO 30° projection uses a tangential approach to demonstrate the zygomatic arches; other methods that employ the tangential approach have also been described as:

1. An SMV projection with the beam centred under the chin at the level of the midpoint of the zygomatic arches. Collimation includes both sides
2. An SMV with a 15° tilt of the head (the vertex turned away from the side under examination) and centring over the apex of the arch. Each side is exposed in turn[7]

Use of the SMV may prove difficult for the patient, especially those who present supine on a trolley. Maintenance of the position is also difficult for the patient. A more comfortable position is used in the modified SMV.

SMV zygomatic arches: isocentric technique

- Base position: SMV (see Fig. 17.10)
- The table is then moved and the height of the isocentric unit is altered so that the vertical and horizontal positional lights pass midway along the zygomatic arches
- Collimate, using the rectangular diaphragm, to include the zygomatic arches
- With the support column in the lateral position, the C-arm is in the PA position
- The short axis of the image receptor is coincident with the MSP

Beam angulation
90° to OMBL

Prior to making the exposure the image receptor is brought into contact with the face to minimise the OFD.

Criteria for assessing image quality (SMV)
As for the FO 30° projection

References
1. Bhattaychara J, et al. The role of plain radiography in the management of suspected orbital blow-out fractures. British Journal of Radiology 1997; 70:29–33.
2. Kim SH, et al. The usefulness of orbital lines in detecting blow-out fracture on plain radiography. British Journal of Radiology 2000; 73:1265–1269.
3. Royal College of Radiologists working party. Making the best use of a department of clinical radiology: guidelines for doctors. 5th edn. London: Royal College of Radiologists; 2003.
4. Scally P. Medical Imaging. Oxford: Oxford University Press; 1999.
5. Ballinger PW, Frank ED. Merrill's atlas of radiographic positioning and radiologic procedures, 10th edn. St Louis: Mosby; 2003.
6. Eisenberg R, et al. Radiographic positioning. 2nd edn. Boston: Little Brown and Company; 1995.
7. Bontrager K, Lampignano JP. Textbook of radiographic positioning and related anatomy. 6th edn. St Louis: Mosby; 2005.
8. Unett EM, Royle AJ. Radiographic techniques and image evaluation. London: Chapman and Hall; 1997.
9. Swallow RA, et al. Clark's positioning in radiography. 11th edn. London: Heinemann; 1986.

PARANASAL SINUSES

Elizabeth Carver

X-ray examination of the sinuses is rarely undertaken in the 21st century as acute symptoms should be diagnosed and treated clinically. X-ray examination should only be undertaken in circumstances when treatment has failed to improve the symptoms.[1] Computed tomography (CT) is a useful tool in the investigation of chronic sinus symptoms.

The projections must be undertaken erect, with horizontal beam, to demonstrate any fluid levels that might be present in the sinuses. Isocentric technique is therefore not undertaken in the supine position and the isocentric unit is used in the same way as an erect X-ray unit; isocentric technique is therefore not described in this chapter.

▌ Occipitomental (OM) sinuses (Fig. 20.1A,B)

If used, an 18 × 24 cm cassette is placed longitudinally in the erect bucky.

Positioning
- The patient is seated, facing the image receptor
- The chin is placed in contact with the midline of the image receptor and the chin position is adjusted until the orbitomeatal baseline (OMBL) has been raised 45° from the horizontal
- The median sagittal plane (MSP) is perpendicular to the image receptor, which is assessed by checking that the external auditory meatuses (EAMs) or lateral orbital margins are equidistant from it

Beam direction and focus film distance (FFD)
Horizontal, at 90° to the image receptor and making an angle of 45° with the OMBL
100 cm FFD

Centring
Above the external occipital protuberance (EOP), to emerge at the level of the inferior orbital margins

Collimation
Frontal sinuses (the upper border of these sinuses vary with each individual and a specific border description cannot be given), maxillary sinuses

Criteria for assessing image quality
- All paranasal sinuses are demonstrated
- Symmetry of facial bones on each side; equal distance of lateral orbital margins from outer table of temporal bones
- Upper border of the petrous portion of the temporal bone is level with the apex of the maxillary antra
- Images of premolars and molars are medial to, and clear of, the medial aspects of the maxillary sinuses
- Zygomatic arches are seen as a tight 'C' and reversed tight 'C' laterally
- Sharp image demonstrating the air-filled regions of the paranasal sinuses in contrast with the bones of the skull

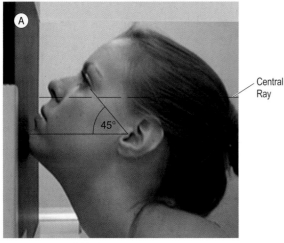

Figure 20.1   OM sinuses

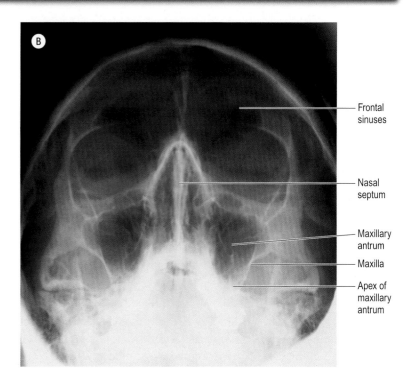

Common errors	Possible reasons
Asymmetry of the facial structures	Rotation about MSP
Position of the petrous ridge is too high; it is seen through the maxillary sinuses	Chin is not raised enough. (see further notes in Ch. 19, OM facial bones)
Petrous ridge is below the maxillary sinuses; image of crowns of premolars overlying the medial aspects of the maxillary sinuses. The frontal sinuses are foreshortened and may appear over-dark	Chin is raised too high
Position appears acceptable; frontal sinuses are over-darkened	Collimation might not be tight enough around the area of interest, thus scatter may blacken the upper anterior aspect of the frontal bone

Lateral sinuses (Fig. 20.2A,B)

Positioning
- The patient is initially seated, facing the image receptor
- The trunk is brought as close as possible to the receptor unit and the patient is asked to sit with their spine as erect as possible. This helps the patient turn their head more easily into the required lateral position
- The head is turned through 90° to bring the affected side in contact with the image receptor
- The MSP is parallel to the image receptor; there should be no tilt or rotation of the head. This can be assessed by checking the midline of the cranium over the top and symmetry of the frontal bone and orbits
- Asking the patient to gently close their eyes will assist in maintenance of the position; as the radiographer leaves the receptor unit, a patient will often follow this movement with their eyes and this will potentially affect the position of the head

Beam direction and FFD
Horizontal, at 90° to the image receptor
100 cm FFD

Centring
Over the midpoint of the OMBL

Collimation
Paranasal sinuses, including the sphenoid posteriorly

Criteria for assessing image quality
- All paranasal sinuses are demonstrated
- Orbital plates of frontal bone (floor of the anterior cranial fossa) are superimposed; superimposition of the malar processes of maxilla; superimposition of pterygopalatine fossae, which is seen as a 'v' behind the maxillary sinuses
- Sharp image demonstrating the air-filled sinuses in contrast with the bones of the face and cranium

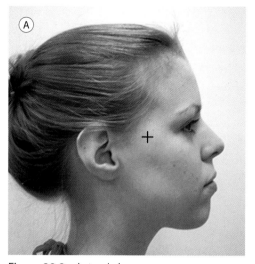

Figure 20.2   Lateral sinuses

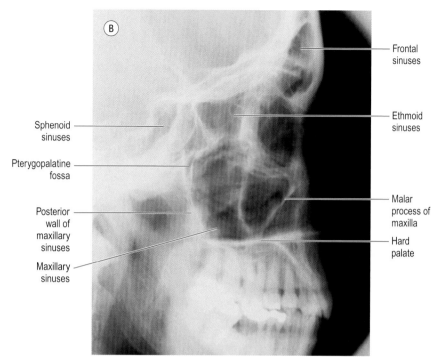

Frontal sinuses

Ethmoid sinuses

Sphenoid sinuses

Pterygopalatine fossa

Posterior wall of maxillary sinuses

Maxillary sinuses

Malar process of maxilla

Hard palate

Common errors	Possible reasons
Non-superimposition of the floor of the anterior cranial fossa; malar processes seen as one above the other; orbital outlines seen as one above the other	MSP is tilted, usually with the upper part of the head tilted towards the image receptor. If a patient cannot comply with the required position, a compensating caudal angle can be used to reduce the effects of the tilt
Lateral orbital margins are seen side by side, not superimposed. Pterygopalatine fossae has double edges	Head is rotated; this is often encouraged when the patient 'slumps' in their chair rather than sitting with their spine erect, as described in 'positioning' for this projection

▪ Lateral postnasal space (Fig. 20.3A,B)

If used, an 18 × 24 cm cassette is placed in the erect cassette holder. A grid is not required as this technique examines an area consisting of soft tissues which are demonstrated in contrast with air-filled structures.

Positioning
- The patient stands or sits with the side of their head next to the image receptor and their MSP parallel to it

- The ramus of the mandible is brought over the middle of the cassette, if used
- The MSP is parallel to the image receptor; there should be no tilt or rotation of the head. This can be assessed by checking the midline of the cranium over the top and symmetry of the frontal bone and orbits
- The chin is raised slightly, to reduce the density of the soft tissues of the throat and clear as much of the mandible as possible from the air-filled regions

Beam direction and FFD
Horizontal, at 90° to the image receptor
100 cm FFD

Centring
Below the midpoint of the OMBL, half way between the level of the temporomandibular joint (TMJ) and angle of the mandible

Collimation
Angle of the mandible and 3 cm anterior to this, TMJ, pharynx and down to the level of the thyroid cartilage

Criteria for assessing image quality
- Postnasal space, the posterior wall of the maxillary sinuses, the TMJ and thyroid cartilage are demonstrated

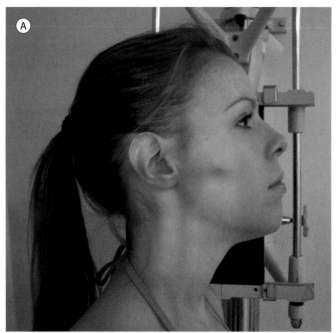

- Clear joint spaces are shown between the cervical vertebrae
- Sharp image demonstrating the darker air-filled pharynx in contrast with the soft tissues of the surrounding area and the mandible. Cervical vertebrae appear pale and low in contrast

■ Occipitofrontal (OF) maxillary and anterior ethmoid sinuses (Fig. 20.4A,B)

If used, an 18 × 24 cm cassette is placed longitudinally in the erect bucky.

Positioning
- The patient is seated, facing the image receptor
- The forehead is placed in contact with the image receptor and the chin position is adjusted until the OMBL is at 90° to it
- The inferior orbital margins are level with the middle of the cassette, if used
- The MSP is perpendicular to the image receptor, which is assessed by checking that the EAMs or lateral orbital margins are equidistant from it

Beam direction and FFD
Horizontal, at 90° to the image receptor
100 cm FFD

Centring
In the midline of the occiput, to emerge at the level of the inferior orbital margins

Collimation
Frontal sinuses (the upper border of these sinuses vary with each individual and a specific border description cannot be given), maxillary sinuses

Criteria for assessing image quality
- All paranasal sinuses are demonstrated
- Equal distance of the lateral orbital margins from the outer table of the temporal bones on each side
- Upper border of the petrous portion of the temporal bone is level with the superior orbital margins
- Sharp image demonstrating the air-filled regions of the paranasal sinuses in contrast with the bones of the skull. The petrous portion of the temporal appears underpenetrated

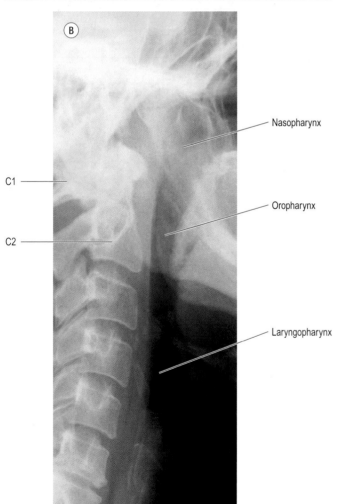

Nasopharynx

C1

Oropharynx

C2

Laryngopharynx

Figure 20.3 Lateral postnasal space

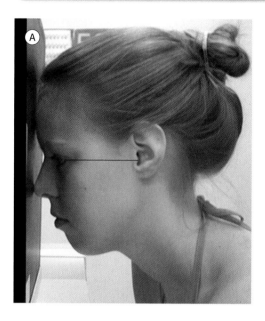

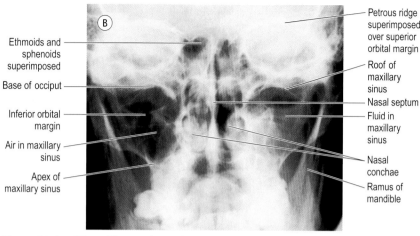

Petrous ridge superimposed over superior orbital margin

Ethmoids and sphenoids superimposed

Base of occiput

Inferior orbital margin

Air in maxillary sinus

Apex of maxillary sinus

Roof of maxillary sinus

Nasal septum

Fluid in maxillary sinus

Nasal conchae

Ramus of mandible

Figure 20.4   OF maxillary and anterior ethmoid sinuses

Common errors	Possible reasons
Distance of the lateral orbital margins from the lateral borders of skull differs on each side	Rotation about MSP
Position of the petrous ridge is too high; it is seen above the superior orbital margins	OMBL is not perpendicular to the image receptor; chin is too far down
Petrous ridge is too low; it is seen within the outline of the orbits	OMBL is not perpendicular to the image receptor; the chin is raised slightly
Maxillary sinuses are over-blackened with poor contrast between the air-filled sinuses and maxilla. Petrous temporal shows good contrast and detail	Over-penetration. The maxilla itself is not a particularly dense bone and this is often overlooked

Positioning

- The patient is positioned initially as for the OF maxillary sinuses projection, with the middle of the cassette level with the nasion
- The chin is raised 10° and a radiolucent pad placed between the forehead and image receptor for immobilisation. If a Lysholm or Schonander type skull unit is used, the bucky can be tilted by moving its upper border 10° towards the patient and positioning the head with the OMBL at 90° to the bucky

Beam direction and FFD

Chin raised 10° from perpendicular
Horizontal, at 90° to the image receptor

■ OF (10°) frontal sinuses (Fig. 20.5)

In the OF projection for maxillary and anterior ethmoid sinuses the frontal sinuses are foreshortened, whilst in the OM projection they are magnified and distorted. For a more accurate representation of these sinuses, the OMBL is raised to bring the vertical axis of the frontal sinus into a position where it is more parallel to the image receptor. 10° caudal angulation will achieve the required effect but a horizontal beam is advised in order to demonstrate fluid levels more accurately.

If used, an 18 × 24 cm cassette is placed longitudinally in the erect bucky.

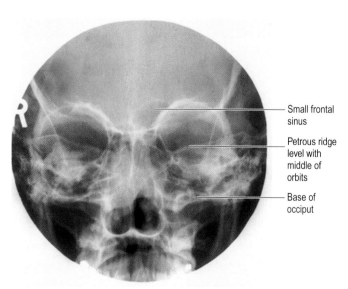

Small frontal sinus

Petrous ridge level with middle of orbits

Base of occiput

Figure 20.5   OF frontal sinuses

If the chin is to be elevated 10° then a guide must be used to assess this accurately; it is arguable that the human eye can accurately estimate a small angle such as 10°. Use of a 10° radiolucent pad for immobilisation would be appropriate. Alternatively a large protractor, or a large piece of clear plastic marked with angles, can be placed against the OMBL. 100 cm FFD

Lysholm or Schonander unit, bucky tilted 10°
Horizontal
100 cm FFD

Centring
In the midline of the occiput, to emerge through the nasion

Collimation
Frontal, ethmoid, sphenoid sinuses

Criteria for assessing image quality
- Frontal, ethmoid and sphenoid sinuses are demonstrated
- Symmetry of structures around the midline
- Upper border of the petrous portion of the temporal bone half way down the orbits
- Sharp image demonstrating the air-filled frontal and ethmoid sinuses in contrast with the frontal and ethmoid bones

■ OF ethmoid and sphenoid sinuses (Fig. 20.6)

Positioning
- As for the frontal sinuses, these sinuses can be seen on an *OF projection*, this time with *the chin lowered* until

the *OMBL moves through 10°*. If using a Lysholm or Schonander type skull unit, the lower border of the bucky is tilted towards the patient whilst the OMBL is positioned at 90° to the bucky

Beam direction, centring and collimation
As for the OF for frontal and anterior ethmoid sinuses

Criteria for assessing image quality
- Ethmoid and sphenoid sinuses are demonstrated
- Symmetry of structures around the midline
- Upper border of the petrous portion of the temporal bone is shown above the superior orbital margins; the petrous ridges start to elevate obliquely towards the outer table of the vault, rather than appearing horizontal
- Sphenoid and ethmoid sinuses seen in the midline, slightly above the orbits and between the petrous portions of the temporal bones
- Sharp image demonstrating the air-filled ethmoid and sphenoid sinuses in contrast with the bones of the vault and petrous portions of the temporal bones

Reference
1. RCR Working Party. Making the best use of a Department of radiology: guidelines for doctors. 5th edn. London: The Royal College of Radiologists; 2003.

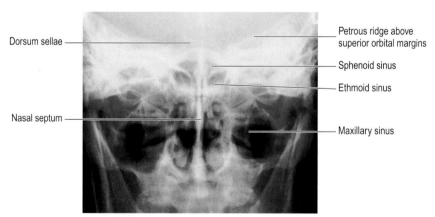

Dorsum sellae

Nasal septum

Petrous ridge above superior orbital margins

Sphenoid sinus

Ethmoid sinus

Maxillary sinus

Figure 20.6 OF sphenoid and ethmoids

SPECIALISED PROJECTIONS OF THE SKULL

Elizabeth Carver, Amanda Royle

In the 21st century, the majority of hospitals in the Western world have access to specialised imaging modalities. Of these, computed tomography (CT) and magnetic resonance imaging (MRI) have largely replaced plain radiography in diagnosis of diseases which were originally only assessed with plain radiography. Unfortunately, plain radiography frequently only provides information when disease is very advanced; CT provides more detailed and high quality information and MRI has the advantage of providing information on neurological and other soft tissues (with no patient dose from ionising radiation) before any bony effects are seen.

Information on plain radiography is still provided in this text, as support for radiographers working in areas with limited or no access to MRI and CT.

SELLA TURCICA (PITUITARY FOSSA)

To clarify the use of terms in this text, the name 'pituitary fossa' refers to the depression within the sella turcica, in which lies the pituitary gland. The sella turcica itself forms the top of the central portion of the sphenoid bone, lying over the sphenoid sinus in the midline.

An enlarged and eroded sella can be a sign of a pituitary tumour or raised intracranial pressure but this appearance is an effect of long-term disease.

Lateral sella turcica: conventional technique
(Fig. 21.1A,B)

If used, an 18 × 24 cm cassette is placed longitudinally in the erect or table bucky.

Positioning
- The patient is initially seated facing the image receptor
- The trunk is brought as close as possible to the receptor unit and the patient is asked to sit with their spine as erect as possible. This helps the patient turn their head more easily into the required lateral position
- The head is turned through 90° to bring the side of the head in contact with the image receptor
- The median sagittal plane (MSP) is parallel to the image receptor; there should be no tilt or rotation of the head. This can be assessed by checking the midline of the cranium over the top and symmetry of the frontal bone and orbits
- The temporal bone lies over the middle of the cassette, if used

Beam direction and focus film distance (FFD)
Horizontal, at 90° to the image receptor
100 cm FFD

Centring
Midway between the posterior tubercle of the first cervical vertebra and the glabella *or* 2.5 cm anterior to the external auditory meatus (EAM), along the orbito-meatal baseline (OMBL), and 2.5 cm above this point

The second centring point will have variable efficacy due to variation in the skull size of the individual patient.

Collimation
Sphenoid bone from lesser wing (anterior clinoid processes) anteriorly and posterior clinoids posteriorly

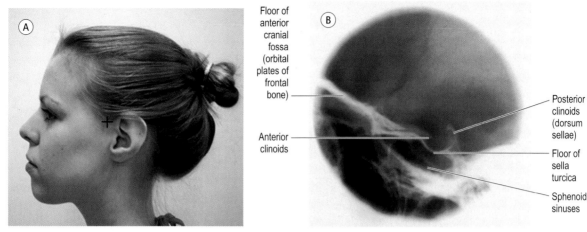

Figure 21.1   Lateral sella turcica

Lateral sella turcica: isocentric technique

- Base position: skull (see Fig. 17.8)
- The table is then moved to bring the vertical central ray, the point at which the central and vertical positional lights intersect, over the midline and 2.5 cm superior to the level of the EAMs
- The height of the isocentric unit is altered to bring the horizontal positional light 2.5 cm anterior to the EAM
- Collimate, using the iris diaphragm, to include the sella turcica
- With the support column in the medial position, the C-arm is in the horizontal position
- The short axis of the image receptor is vertical

Beam angulation
90° on the C-arm

Prior to making the exposure the image receptor is brought into contact with the face to minimise the object film distance (OFD).

Criteria for assessing image quality
- Anterior and posterior clinoid processes, sella turcica, sphenoid sinus and dorsum sellae are demonstrated
- Superimposition of both sides of the floor of pituitary fossa and floor of the anterior cranial fossa
- Anterior clinoid processes are superimposed
- Posterior clinoid processes are superimposed
- Sharp image demonstrating outline of the clinoids and pituitary fossa in contrast with the temporal bones and sphenoid sinus

Common errors	Possible reasons
Both pairs of clinoid processes overlapped, seen one above the other	Tilted skull
Both pairs of clinoid processes overlapped, seen side by side	Rotated skull
'Double' floor of sella turcica; two lines over floor area	Tilted skull or floor is eroded on one side by tumour

Occipitofrontal (OF) sella turcica: conventional technique (Fig. 21.2A,B,C)

The OF 20° projection will demonstrate the floor of the sella turcica, indicating asymmetry if the floor is eroded on one side. The OF 30° projection has limited value, demonstrating the dorsum sella through the foramen magnum; the dorsum will appear as low density if it is eroded.

If used, an 18 × 24 cm cassette is placed longitudinally in the erect or table bucky.

Positioning
- The patient is seated facing the bucky, their forehead in contact with it
- The OMBL and MSP are perpendicular to the image receptor
- The nasion is coincident with the middle of the cassette, if used, for demonstration of the floor of the pituitary fossa
- The glabella is coincident with the middle of the cassette, if used, for demonstration of the dorsum sella

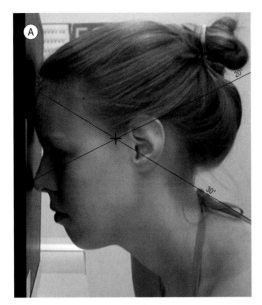

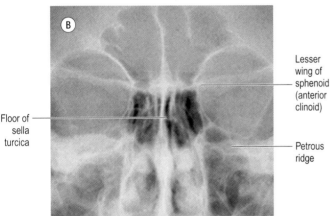

Lesser wing of sphenoid (anterior clinoid)

Floor of sella turcica

Petrous ridge

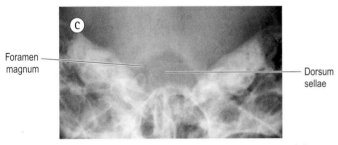

Foramen magnum

Dorsum sellae

Figure 21.2 (A) OF sella turcica; (B) OF 20° sella turcica; (C) OF 30° sella turcica

Beam direction and FFD

(a) Initially horizontal, a *20° caudal* angle will demonstrate the floor of the pituitary fossa through the ethmoid and sphenoid sinuses

(b) A *30° cranial* angle will demonstrate the dorsum sella over the frontal bone and through the foramen magnum

100 cm FFD

Centring

(a) Above the external occipital protuberance (EOP) to emerge through the nasion

(b) Below the EOP, on the neck, to emerge through the glabella

Collimation

OF 20°: Lesser wing of sphenoid, sphenoid and ethmoid sinuses

OF 30°: Ethmoid sinus, foramen magnum

Collimate to include (a) floor of pituitary fossa through sphenoid and ethmoid sinuses and lesser wings of sphenoid or (b) dorsum sellae and posterior clinoid processes within foramen magnum.

▌ OF sella turcica: isocentric technique

- Base position: skull (see Fig. 17.8)
- The table is then moved to bring the vertical central ray, the point at which the central and vertical positional lights intersect, over the midline and 2.5 cm superior to the level of the EAMs
- The height of the isocentric unit is altered to bring the horizontal positional light 2.5 cm anterior to the EAM
- Collimate, using the iris diaphragm, to include the sella turcica
- With the support column in the lateral position, the C-arm is in the posteroanterior (PA) position
- The long axis of the image receptor is coincident with the MSP

Beam angulation

OF 20° equivalent	10° caudal on the C-arm
OF 30° equivalent	40° cranial on the C-arm

Prior to making the exposure the image receptor is brought into contact with the face to minimise the OFD.

Criteria for assessing image quality

OF 20°:

- Lesser wing of the sphenoid, sphenoid and ethmoid sinuses are demonstrated
- Medial aspects of the superior border of petrous ridge are shown superimposed on the inferior orbital margin
- Lesser wing of sphenoid seen medially and symmetrically across the upper portion of the orbits
- Medial borders of the orbits are equidistant from nasal septum
- Floor of pituitary fossa is seen as a horizontal line across the ethmoid sinuses. In cases of erosion of the floor of the fossa, this line may deviate from horizontal orientation

- Sharp image showing the fine line indicating the floor of the pituitary fossa in contrast with the air-filled ethmoid sinus

OF 30°:

- Foramen magnum is demonstrated
- Dorsum sella is seen in the centre of the foramen magnum
- Sharp image showing dorsum sella in contrast with the less dense foramen magnum

Common errors OF 20°	Possible reasons
Petrous ridge seen above the level of the inferior orbital margins	Inadequate angle selected *or* baseline used is incorrectly positioned (chin down too far)
Petrous ridge seen below the level of the inferior orbital margins	Angle selected is too great *or* baseline used is incorrectly positioned (chin not far enough down)

Common errors OF 30°	Possible reasons
Foramen magnum appears short or is not evident. Dorsum sella may be visible above the portion of the foramen magnum that is seen	Angle selected is inadequate *or* baseline used is positioned incorrectly (chin not far enough down)
Large foramen magnum seen but curve of the posterior arch of C1 is seen in its lower third, rather than the anvil shape of dorsum sellae	Angle selected is too great *or* baseline used is not positioned correctly (chin too far down)

MASTOIDS

Lateral oblique mastoids: conventional technique
(Fig. 21.3A,B)

Positioning for this projection is identical to that for lateral oblique temporomandibular joints (TMJs), although the centring point differs. The pinna of the ear must also be cleared from the mastoid area. Both sides are examined for comparison.

If used, an 18 × 24 cm cassette is selected and placed longitudinally in the erect bucky.

Positioning

- The patient is initially seated, facing the image receptor
- The trunk is brought as close as possible to the receptor unit and the patient is asked to sit with their spine as erect as possible. This helps the patient turn their head more easily into the required lateral position
- The head is turned through 90° to bring the mastoid on the side under examination over the middle of the cassette, if used. Location of this bone can be detected by palpating the mastoid process which lies inferiorly and posteriorly to the EAM
- The pinna of the ear on the side nearest the image receptor is then gently pulled forward and the head rests against the image receptor to keep the pinna forward. This clears the image of the pinna from the area of interest
- The MSP is parallel to the image receptor; there should be no tilt or rotation of the head. This can be assessed by checking the midline of the cranium over the top, symmetry of the frontal bone and orbits and that the interpupillary line is perpendicular to the image receptor

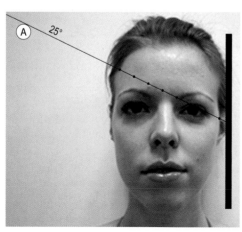

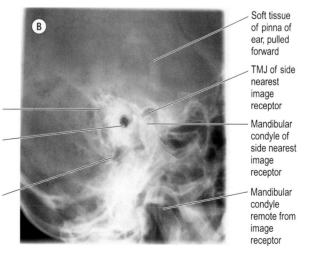

Figure 21.3   Lateral oblique mastoids

- Asking the patient to gently close their eyes will assist in maintenance of the position; as the radiographer leaves the receptor unit, a patient will often follow this movement with their eyes and potentially affect the position of the head

Beam direction and FFD

Initially horizontal, angled 25° caudally
100 cm FFD

Centring

Above the mastoid process on the side remote from the image receptor, to emerge over the mastoid process on the side nearest the image receptor

Collimation

EAM, mastoid process, air cells behind the pinna of the ear

▮ Lateral oblique mastoids: isocentric technique

- Base position: skull (see Fig. 17.8)
- The table is then moved to bring the vertical central ray, the point at which the central and vertical positional lights intersect, over the midline at the level of the EAMs
- The height of the isocentric unit is altered to bring the horizontal positional light through the EAM
- The support column is in the medial position, with the C-arm in the anteroposterior (AP) position
- The table is displaced to each side in turn so that the central positional light passes through the mastoid air cells of the side under examination
- The C-arm is then placed in the horizontal position with the image receptor at the side under examination
- The long axis of the image receptor is vertical
- Collimate, using the iris diaphragm, to include the mastoid air cells under examination (a diameter of approximately 10 cm on the side of the face remote from the image receptor)

Beam angulation

25° caudal on support column

Prior to making the exposure the image receptor is brought into contact with the face to minimise the OFD.

Criteria for assessing image quality

- EAM and air-filled mastoid are demonstrated posterior to the EAM
- Condyle of mandible and mastoid air cells of the opposite side are projected clear from those under examination

- Pinna of ear is folded forward and cleared from the mastoid
- Air cells of the mastoids are seen in contrast to bone; bony detail of the mastoid bone is demonstrated

Common errors	Possible reasons
Mastoid closest to tube not cleared from mastoid under examination	1. Inadequate angle used *or* 2. Head is tilted with its vertex towards the image receptor, which effectively reduces the effects of angulation
TMJ of opposite side not cleared from mastoid	Inadequate angle, or tilt as above *or* the head is rotated with the face away from the image receptor

▮ Profile of mastoid process: conventional technique
(Fig. 21.4A,B)

Both sides are examined for comparison.

If used, an 18 × 24 cm cassette is placed longitudinally in the erect holder.

Positioning

- The patient is initially positioned as for an OF projection, with the centre of the cassette, if used, below the outer canthus of the eye and level with the mastoid process, on the side under examination
- The head is rotated approximately 30° away from the side under examination, until the process is in profile and cleared from ramus of the mandible

Beam direction and FFD

Initially horizontal, angled 25° caudally
100 cm FFD

Centring

Over the mastoid process under examination (nearest the image receptor)

Collimation

Mastoid air cells, mastoid process

▮ Profile of mastoid process: isocentric technique

- Base position: skull (see Fig. 17.8)
- The table is then moved to bring the vertical central ray, the point at which the central and vertical positional lights intersect, over the midline at the level of the EAMs

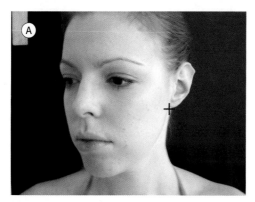

Figure 21.4   Profile of mastoid process

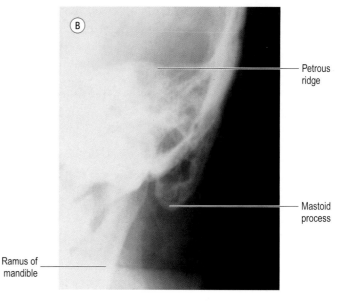

Petrous ridge

Mastoid process

Ramus of mandible

- The height of the isocentric unit is altered to bring the horizontal positional light through the EAM
- The support column is in the lateral position, with the C-arm in the AP position
- The FFD is set at 100 cm with the image receptor immediately below the head board
- The long axis of the image receptor is coincident with the MSP
- The patient's head is rotated through 30°, away from the side under examination
- The table is then moved to bring the vertical central ray, the point at which the central and vertical positional lights intersect, over the mastoid air cells nearest the image receptor
- Collimate, using the iris diaphragm, to include the mastoid air cells and mastoid process

Beam angulation
25° caudal on the C-arm

Prior to making the exposure the image receptor is brought into contact with the head to minimise the OFD.

Criteria for assessing image quality
- Mastoid and mastoid process are demonstrated
- Mastoid process is cleared from the mandible and zygoma
- Mastoid bone is seen in contrast to air-filled cells and soft tissues of the neck

Common errors	Possible reasons
Mandible and/or zygoma overlying mastoid process	Inadequate obliquity
Occiput overlies mastoid process	Excessive obliquity

OF 30° mastoids: conventional technique
(Fig. 21.5A,B)

If used, an 18 × 24 cm cassette is selected and placed transversely in the erect bucky.

Positioning
- The patient is seated facing the bucky, their forehead in contact with it
- The OMBL and MSP are perpendicular to the image receptor
- The glabella is coincident with the middle of the cassette, if used

Beam direction and FFD
Initially horizontal, angled 30° cranially
100 cm FFD

Centring
In the midline of the neck, to travel through the mastoid processes

It may be necessary to further displace the cassette, if used, to ensure the beam emerges at its centre. For the digital plate receptor, the field of radiation should be included.

Collimation
Temporal bones, mastoid processes

OF 30° (equivalent): isocentric technique

- Base position: skull (see Fig. 17.8)
- The table is then moved to bring the vertical central ray, the point at which the central and vertical positional lights intersect, over the midline at the level of the EAMs

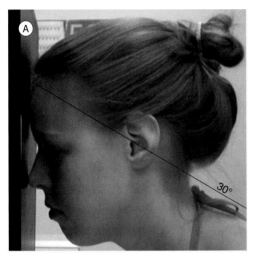

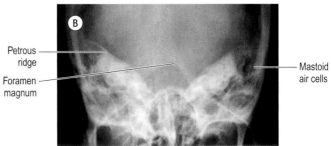

Petrous ridge

Foramen magnum

Mastoid air cells

Figure 21.5 **(A)** OF 30° mastoids – conventional technique; **(B)** OF 30° mastoids

- The height of the isocentric unit is altered to bring the horizontal positional light through the EAM
- Collimate, using the rectangular diaphragm, to include the lateral margins of the skull and proximal halves of the mandibular rami

Beam angulation

40° cranial on the C-arm

Prior to making the exposure the image receptor is brought into contact with the face to minimise the OFD.

Criteria for assessing image quality

- Air-filled mastoid bones are demonstrated on the lateral portions of the temporal bones
- Dorsum sellae and posterior clinoid processes are projected through the centre of the foramen magnum
- Petrous temporals seen as a slight 'v' shape about the foramen magnum
- Symmetry of the petrous portions of the temporal around the midline
- Sharp image demonstrating the air-filled mastoids in contrast to the denser bones of the vault

Common errors	Possible reasons
Foramen magnum appears short or is not evident. Dorsum sellae may be visible above the portion of the foramen magnum that is seen	Angle selected is inadequate *or* baseline used is incorrectly positioned (chin not far enough down)
Large foramen magnum seen but curve of the posterior arch of C1 is seen in its lower third, rather than the anvil shape of dorsum sellae	Angle selected is too great *or* baseline used is incorrectly positioned (chin too far down)

TEMPORAL BONE (PETROUS PORTION FOR INTERNAL AUDITORY MEATUS (IAM))

OF 5° IAMs: conventional technique
(Fig. 21.6A,B)

If used, an 18 × 24 cm cassette is selected and placed longitudinally in the erect bucky.

Positioning

- The patient is seated facing the bucky, their forehead in contact with it
- The OMBL and MSP are perpendicular to the image receptor
- The nasion is coincident with the middle of the image receptor

Beam direction and FFD

Initially horizontal, angled 5° caudally
100 cm FFD

A central ray perpendicular to the image receptor has previously been described[1] for this projection but, since the petrous ridge lies coincident with the upper border of the orbits, location of the IAM can be difficult. Use of the 5° caudal angle brings the ridge just below the upper border of the orbits; this acts as a distinguishable landmark, below which lies the low density channel for the IAM (Fig. 21.6B).

Centring

Above the EOP to emerge through the nasion

Collimation

The whole of the orbits

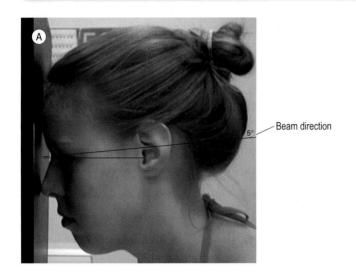

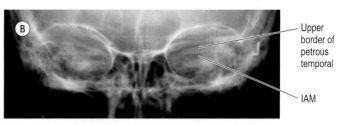

Figure 21.6   OF 5° IAMs

OF 5° (equivalent) IAMs: isocentric technique

- Base position: skull (see Fig. 17.8)
- The table is then moved to bring the vertical central ray, the point at which the central and vertical positional lights intersect, over the midline at the level of the EAMs
- The height of the isocentric unit is altered to bring the horizontal positional light through the EAM
- Collimate, using the rectangular diaphragm, to include the outlines of the bony orbits
- With the support column in the lateral position, the C-arm is in the PA position
- The short axis of the image receptor is coincident with the MSP

Beam angulation

5° cranial on the C-arm

Prior to making the exposure the image receptor is brought into contact with the face to minimise the OFD.

Criteria for assessing image quality

- Both orbits are demonstrated
- Petrous ridge is seen within the orbits, approximately a quarter of the way down their length
- Symmetry of structures is seen through the orbits; semi-circular canals seen at the outer limits of the IAMs can be assessed as to their equidistance from the lateral orbital outlines
- Sharp image demonstrating contrast of the petrous portions of temporal bones with the outline of the orbits and the less dense IAMs lying within the petrous portion

Common errors	Possible reasons
Petrous ridge seen above required level in orbits	Inadequate angle selected *or* baseline used is incorrectly positioned (chin too far down)
Petrous ridge seen below required level in orbits	Angle selected is too great *or* baseline used is incorrectly positioned (chin not far enough down)

Anterior oblique (OF oblique) IAMs: conventional technique (Fig. 21.7A,B)

This projection is also known as *Stenver's projection*.[1] The projection aims to place the petrous portion of temporal parallel to the image receptor, whilst utilising the cranial angle to clear the image of the petrous bone above the zygomatic arch and over the flatter, less detailed, image of the temporal and parietal bones. The obliquity of the petrous portion of the temporal bones for the Stenver's position is given as approximately 45° but variations according to build have been highlighted as ranging from 40° in the dolicocephalic head (long narrow vault as seen from above), through 47° in the mesocephalic ('average') and as much as 54° in the brachycephalic (short and broad vault when seen from above).[2]

If used, an 18 × 24 cm cassette is placed longitudinally in the erect bucky.

Positioning

- The patient is initially positioned in an OF position; the middle of the cassette, if used, is coincident with the midpoint of the inferior orbital margin on the side under examination

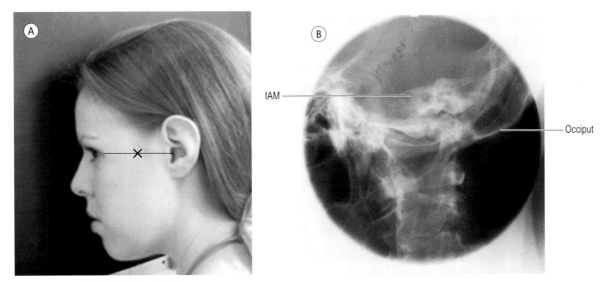

Figure 21.7 AO (OF oblique) IAMs

- The head is rotated 45° away from the side under examination

Beam direction and FFD
Initially horizontal, angled 12° cranially
100 cm FFD

Centring
Midway between the EOP and the EAM remote from the image receptor, to emerge midway between the EAM nearest the image receptor and outer canthus of the eye

The cassette, if used, is adjusted until its centre is coincident with the central ray.

Collimation
Temporal bone under examination

Anterior oblique (OF oblique) IAMs: isocentric technique

Application of a double angle using the isocentric technique can lead to confusion. The trick is for the radiographer to stand back and take a look prior to exposure. Imagine how the patient's head would look in relation to the image receptor and X-ray beam in the conventional technique; rather than rotating the patient's head the image receptor has moved, and the craniocaudal angulation should still be in the same direction. Familiarity with the anatomy for demonstration is a distinct advantage here; the intention of the projection is for the central ray to strike the petrous portion of temporal at 90° and to project it through the anterior portion of the lateral vault (but cleared above the zygomatic arch) between the orbit and the EAM. Thus, the beam must travel, (1) in one plane, approximately 45° obliquely across the MSP to strike the petrous portion of temporal at 90° and (2) in the second plane, cranially to project the petrous portion above the zygomatic arch.

The procedure is as follows:

- Base position: skull (see Fig. 17.8)
- The table is then moved to bring the vertical central ray, the point at which the central and vertical positional lights intersect, over the midline at the level of the EAMs
- The height of the isocentric unit is altered to bring the horizontal positional light through the EAM
- The support column is in the medial position, with the C-arm in the AP position
- The table is displaced to each side in turn so that the central positional light passes through the centre of the orbit of the side under examination
- Collimate, using the iris diaphragm, to include the petrous portion of temporal of the side under examination (a diameter of approximately 10 cm)
- The long axis of the image receptor is coincident with the MSP
- With the support column remaining in the medial position, the C-arm is then turned into the PA position

Beam angulation
1. 45° towards the side under examination on the C-arm
2. 25° cranial on the support column

Criteria for assessing image quality
- Orbits, base of occiput and petrous portion of the temporal bone are demonstrated

- Mastoid air cells of the side under examination projected shown laterally in relationship to semicircular canals
- Image of the curve of the occipital outline (of the side not under examination) travels through the mastoid air cells
- Lines representing the right and left sides of the base of the skull are horizontal and at the same level
- IAM, semicircular canals and vestibule of the ear are seen below the arcuate eminence, above the head of mandible
- Sharp image demonstrating the dense petrous portion of temporal in contrast to the IAM, semicircular canals and the vestibule

Common error	Possible reason
Short meatus	Incorrect rotation in conventional technique; inadequate rotation will show the internal occipital crest crossing the meatus or semicircular canals

OF 30° petrous temporal: conventional technique
(Fig. 21.8A,B)

If used, an 18 × 24 cm cassette is selected and placed transversely in the erect bucky.

Positioning
- The patient is seated facing the bucky, their forehead in contact with it
- The OMBL and MSP are perpendicular to the image receptor
- The middle of the image receptor is initially approximately 5 cm above the glabella

Beam direction and FFD
Initially horizontal, angled 30° cranially
100 cm FFD

Centring
In the midline of the neck, to travel through the level of the EAMs. It may be necessary to further displace the cassette, if used, to ensure the beam emerges at its centre. The digital plate receptor should include the radiation field

Collimation
Temporal bones to include petrous portion

OF 30° (equivalent): Isocentric technique

- Base position: skull (see Fig. 17.8)
- The table is then moved to bring the vertical central ray, the point at which the central and vertical positional lights intersect, over the midline at the level of the EAMs
- The height of the isocentric unit is altered to bring the horizontal positional light through the EAM
- Collimate, using the rectangular diaphragm, to include the outlines of the bony orbits
- With the support column in the lateral position, the C-arm is in the PA position
- The short axis of the image receptor is coincident with the MSP

Beam angulation
40° cranial on the C-arm

Prior to making the exposure the image receptor is brought into contact with the face to minimise the OFD.

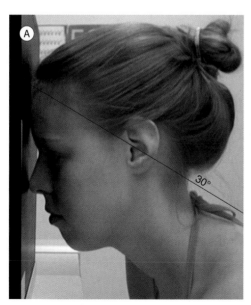

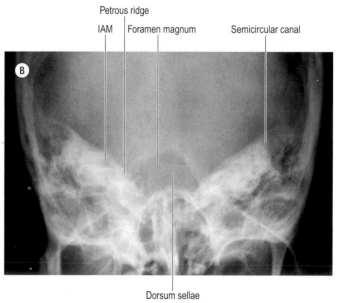

Petrous ridge
IAM Foramen magnum Semicircular canal

Dorsum sellae

Figure 21.8 OF 30° petrous temporal

Criteria for assessing image quality

- Temporal bones, including petrous portions, are demonstrated
- Dorsum sellae and posterior clinoid processes are projected through the centre of the foramen magnum
- Petrous temporals are seen as a slight 'v' shape about the foramen magnum
- Symmetry of petrous portions of temporal around the foramen magnum
- Sharp image with dense petrous portions of temporals seen in contrast to the less dense acoustic meati and the occiput

Common errors	Possible reasons
Foramen magnum appears short or is not evident. Dorsum sellae may be visible above the portion of the foramen magnum that is seen	Angle selected is inadequate *or* baseline used is incorrectly positioned (chin not far enough down)
Large foramen magnum seen but curve of the posterior arch of C1 is seen in its lower third, rather than the anvil shape of dorsum sellae	Angle selected is too great *or* baseline used is incorrectly positioned (chin too far down)

OPTIC FORAMEN

Occipitomental (OM) oblique/anterior oblique (AO) optic foramen: conventional technique
(Fig. 21.9A,B)

Both optic foramina are examined for comparison.

If used, an 18 × 24 cm is selected and placed longitudinally in the erect bucky.

Positioning
- The patient is seated, facing the image receptor
- The chin is placed in contact with the midline of the image receptor; the middle of the cassette, if used, is coincident with the midpoint of the inferior orbital margin of the eye under examination
- The chin position is adjusted until the OMBL has been raised 30°; the head is then rotated through 30°, away from the eye under examination
- The orbit should overlie the centre of the cassette, if used

Beam direction and FFD
Horizontal, at 90° to the image receptor
100 cm FFD

Centring
Behind and above the mastoid process nearest the X-ray tube, to emerge through the middle of the orbit under examination

Collimation
Bony outline of the orbit under examination

Optic foramen anterior oblique: isocentric technique

> As for the isocentric technique for petrous portion of temporal, understanding of anatomical structure (direction of travel of the foramen in relationship to the rest of the skull and orbit) assists with understanding of the double angulations used. The foramen follows an oblique path, medially and superiorly to take the optic nerve towards the optic chiasma. Angulations used therefore ensure the central ray follows this path.

The procedure is as follows:

- Base position: skull (see Fig. 17.8)
- The table is then moved to bring the vertical central ray, the point at which the central and vertical positional lights intersect, in the midline at the level of the centres of the orbits
- The height of the isocentric unit is altered to bring the horizontal positional light to the outer canthus of the eye
- With the support column in the medial position, the C-arm is in the AP position
- The table is displaced to the side under examination so that the central positional light passes through the centre of the orbit under examination
- Collimate, using the iris diaphragm, to the outline of the bony orbit under examination
- With the support column remaining in the medial position, the C-arm is then turned into the PA position
- The long axis of the image receptor is coincident with the MSP

Beam angulation
1. 40° towards the side under examination on the C-arm
2. 25° caudal on the support column
   Prior to making the exposure the image receptor is brought into contact with the head to minimise the OFD.

Criteria for assessing image quality
- Outline of orbit is demonstrated in full

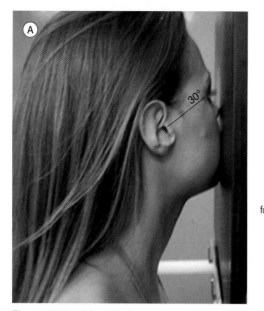

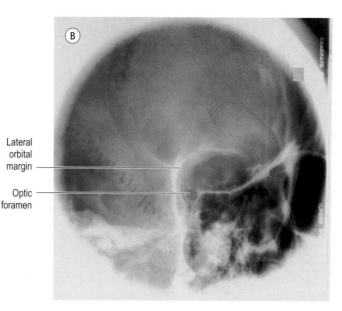

Figure 21.9   AO optic foramen

- Optic foramen seen as a low density circle within the orbit, level with its midpoint and nearer the lateral margin of the orbit
- Sharp image demonstrating the low density foramen in contrast to the bones forming the orbit and the overlying bones of the vault

> **Note on errors relating to isocentric technique**
> It is assumed that accurate angulations are selected.

JUGULAR FORAMINA

Submentovertical (SMV) 20° jugular foramina: conventional technique (Fig. 21.10A,B)

If used, an 18 × 24 cm cassette is selected and placed transversely in the erect bucky.

Positioning

- A seat is placed midway between the X-ray tube and erect bucky; the patient sits on the stool, facing the X-ray tube

Common errors	Possible reasons (related to conventional technique)
Lateral orbital margin obscuring part, or all, of the foramen	Head is rotated too far
Inferior orbital margin obscuring part, or all, of the foramen	Chin is raised too far
Foramen appears elliptical and is located nearer to the medial aspect of the orbit than is required	Inadequate rotation
Foramen appears to be cylindrical and is located in the upper half of the orbit	Inadequate raising of the chin

Common errors	Possible reasons (related to isocentric technique)
Lateral orbital margin obscuring part, or all, of the foramen	MSP is not vertical – the head is rotated away from the side of interest
Inferior orbital margin obscuring part, or all, of the foramen	Chin is raised too far
Foramen appears elliptical and is located nearer to the medial aspect of the orbit than is required	MSP is not vertical – the head is rotated towards the side of interest
Foramen appears to be cylindrical and is located in the upper half of the orbit	Inadequate raising of the chin

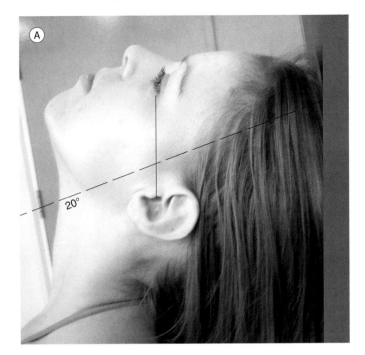

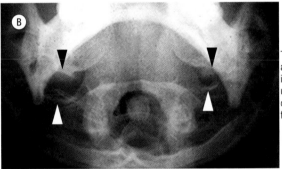

The 2 black arrows indicate the upper aspect of the jugular foramina

Figure 21.10 **(A)** SMV – jugular foramina; **(B)** SMV 20° jugular foramina. (B) Reproduced with permission from Ballinger PW, Frank ED. Merrill's atlas of radiographic positioning and radiologic procedures. 10th edn. St Louis: Mosby; 2003

- The patient leans back gently onto the radiographer's arm and flexes their neck and back until the vertex of their head can be placed in contact with the bucky
- The middle of the cassette, if used, is level with the angles of the mandible

Beam direction and FFD
20° cranially
100 cm FFD

Centring
Midway between the angles of the mandible

Collimation
Angles of mandible, symphysis menti, foramen magnum

▨ SMV jugular foramina: isocentric technique
- Base position: SMV (see Fig. 17.10)
- With the support column in the lateral position, the C-arm is in the AP position
- Collimate, using the rectangular diaphragm, to the angles of the mandible and symphysis menti
- The short axis of the image receptor is coincident with the MSP

Beam angulation
1. 90° to the OMBL
2. 20° cranial on the C-arm

Prior to making the exposure the image receptor is brought into contact with the underside of the head to minimise the OFD.

Criteria for assessing image quality
- Angles of the mandible, symphysis menti and foramen magnum are demonstrated
- Odontoid process of C2 is demonstrated, through the upper half of the foramen magnum
- Mandible is raised clear of the jugular foramina and superimposed as an arch over the petrous temporal bones
- Both jugular foramina are demonstrated symmetrically on either side of the midline, midway between the edge of the foramen magnum and angle of mandible
- Sharp image demonstrating dense bone of the skull base, in contrast with the jugular foramina

Common errors	Possible reasons
Mandible overlying foramina	Chin is not elevated enough
Mandible is clear but foramina not clear	Chin is elevated too much

References
1. Swallow RA, et al. Clark's positioning in radiography. 11th edn. London: Heinemann; 1986.
2. Eisenberg R, et al. Radiographic positioning. 2nd edn. Boston: Little, Brown; 1995.

DENTAL RADIOGRAPHY

Elizabeth Carver

Dental radiography is still a widespread imaging technique required by dentists and oral surgeons in dental surgeries and hospitals. Intraoral techniques, in particular, are low dose in relation to examinations undertaken elsewhere in the body but this does not mean that dose should be considered an irrelevance in examinations of the teeth and mouth.

DOSE REDUCTION AND RADIATION PROTECTION

As long ago as 1994 in the UK, the National Radiological Protection Board (NRPB) issued guidelines stating that there was no justification for the routine use of lead rubber aprons.[1] In practice, the artefacts caused by incorrect placement of lead rubber aprons during orthopantomography (OPT) were considered to be a common cause of repeat radiographs, doubling the radiation dose received by the patient. At this stage the NRPB also concluded that dental radiography posed no risk to female patients at any stage during pregnancy; however, since the use of lead rubber does not actually increase the dose to patients, it could be suggested that its use for any intraoral or cephalometry technique may be of 'psychological' benefit to the patient. This may be especially appropriate in the case of the patient who is aware of the risks associated with ionising radiation but who is not reassured by the radiographer's explanation that there is no likelihood of danger when undergoing dental radiographic examinations. Since the 1994 NRPB document there have been key documents issued regarding guidelines and regulations on use of radiation for medical exposure, each referring less specifically to the use of lead rubber for dental examinations but emphasising the responsibility of the radiographer to reduce the radiation dose wherever possible.[2,3,4] In view of this, and the previous comments on the 'psychological' benefits to the patient, it may be more appropriate to offer all patients lead rubber aprons for intraoral and cephalometric examinations.

DIFFICULTIES IN PROVIDING ACCURACY OF DENTAL ASSESSMENT

The teeth themselves provide the radiographer with problems of accurate imaging, due to the nature of their various shapes. This, added to their positions within the alveolar ridges of the maxilla and the mandible, their arched arrangement in the mouth and the varying positions of the teeth with each individual, shows that implications for accurate representation of dentition are complex.

TERMINOLOGY ASSOCIATED WITH DENTAL RADIOGRAPHY

Dental techniques require understanding of some terms that are not encountered in radiography of the rest of the body and that are outlined in the following table. [Table 22.1]

Table 22.1 Dental Terminology	
Buccal/labial (Fig. 22.1)	The (outer)aspect of the teeth that lies between the teeth and the cheeks or lips
Lingual/palatal (Fig. 22.1)	The (inner) aspect of the teeth that lies between the teeth and the tongue

Continued

Table 22.1 cont'd

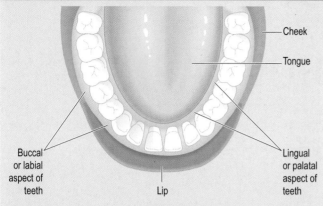

Figure 22.1 Buccal/labial, lingual/palatal aspects of the teeth

Distal (Fig. 22.2)	The direction of the dental arch towards the molars, posteriorly and outwards away from the MSP. Used to describe beam shift, tube shift or angulation
Mesial (Fig. 22.2)	The direction of the dental arch towards the incisors, anteriorly and inwards towards the MSP. Used to describe beam shift, tube shift or angulation and is in the opposite direction to distal movement

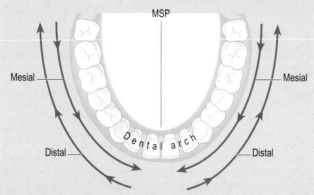

Figure 22.2 Distal and mesial

Alatragal line (Fig. 22.3)	An imaginary line from the tragus of the ear to the middle of the ala of the nose (the flare of soft tissue around the nostril)
Occlusal plane (upper) (Fig. 22.3)	The line of the biting surfaces of the upper teeth. When the mouth is closed this is deemed to be the occlusal plane rather than the upper occlusal plane. The line lies parallel to the anthropological baseline and the alatragal line. It lies approximately 4 cm below the alatragal line

Cont'd

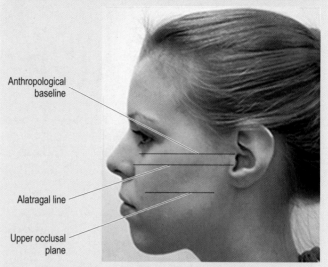

Figure 22.3 Reference lines used in dental radiography

Occlusal plane (lower)	*With the mouth open*, this line lies parallel to, and approximately 2 cm below the line which lies between the tragus of the ear and the outer canthus of the mouth. Because all radiography of the teeth should be undertaken with the mouth closed around an image receptor holder or occlusal film, this plane is not actually used in this text and is therefore not illustrated
MSP (Fig. 22.4)	Plane running vertically down the middle of the face, separating the left and right sides

Figure 22.4 MSP

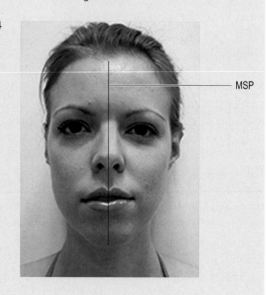

TECHNIQUES USED IN DENTAL RADIOGRAPHY

Intraoral techniques

Bitewings: Demonstrate the crowns and interproximal surfaces of the teeth
Periapicals: Demonstrate the whole tooth
Occlusals: Demonstrate a range of structures and aspects of the mouth including the hard palate, incisors and canines, unerupted canines, confirmation of position of unerupted canines, premolars, submandibular salivary glands and ducts and the symphysis menti

Extraoral techniques

Orthopantomography (OPT or OPG)/dental panoramic tomography (DPT): Demonstrates the whole mouth including dentition, mandible, maxillary sinuses and temporo-mandibular joints. This technique is covered in Chapter 23.
Lateral cephalometry: Mainly used to assess the extent of malocclusions and facial deformities prior to and post surgery. This technique is covered in Chapter 24.

RECORDING AND DISPLAYING THE IMAGES

At the time of publication, use of digital units for dental radiography is not the most frequently encountered imaging system and use of film is still very widespread. This is likely to change in the foreseeable future, possibly more quickly than digitisation for all other radiographic examinations. This is because replacement of dental equipment is less expensive than for conventional radiographic equipment and also because its replacement does not involve digitising a whole imaging department. It is therefore necessary to still give direction on use of film and display of film images.

Digital dental units utilise small image receptors which are connected to the digital unit (Fig. 22.5) and are similar in size to films used in dental radiography.

Film sizes (Fig. 22.6)

There is a range of film sizes available, *size 0* is the smallest and is used in periapical examinations for children and adults with small mouths. *Size 1* is also used in periapical examinations, usually for adults, and also for parallax technique. *Occlusal* films are larger than size 0 and 1, since they are designed to cover a larger area of dentition. Intraoral techniques do not use a film screen system as the

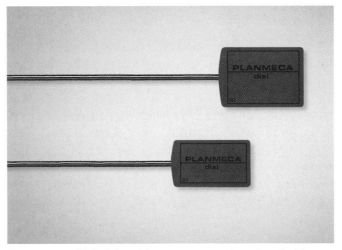

Figure 22.5 Digital dental image receptors. Reproduced with permission from Xograph Imaging Systems

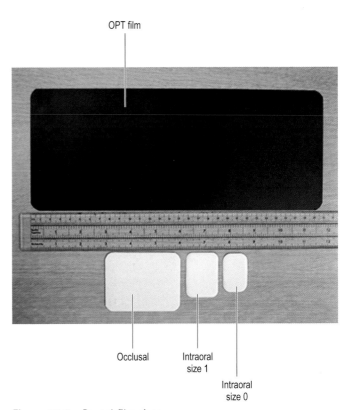

OPT film

Occlusal

Intraoral size 1

Intraoral size 0

Figure 22.6 Dental film sizes

area under examination is of low density, and exposure factors used are relatively low, so that intensifying screens are not necessary.

Film used in OPT is usually of a specific size designed solely for this examination and is approximately 14–15 × 30 cm in size. These are used in conjunction with cassettes and intensifying screens since the area under examination is significantly denser than individual teeth. Lateral cephalometry film is 18 × 24 cm or similar.

Film orientation

There must be a consistent method used to orientate the film in the mouth, since it is impossible to tell whether teeth are from the left or right side, from the mandible or maxilla. The most popular method is to use the orientation 'pimple', which is a tiny but palpable raised lump on the tube side of the film (Fig. 22.7). The pimple is always positioned towards the crowns of the teeth in periapical and occlusal examinations. For bitewings the pimple is usually orientated towards the roots of the upper teeth. Digital image receptors are always used with the lead leaving the edge of the receptor, which is outside the mouth.

Displaying film images

Films are usually mounted with patient and tooth/ projection identification in clear holders or stapled to clear film or translucent mounting medium. The 'pimple' must face outwards, towards the viewing radiographer. Left and right teeth are also clearly indicated. Before the widespread use of OPT for whole mouth examinations, whole mouth periapical images were displayed in the format of the mouth itself.[5]

Intraoral techniques: bitewings

These demonstrate the crowns, interproximal surfaces and gingival margins of the premolars and molars. If using film, bitewing film is available which is a small dental film with a centralised flap of paper on the tube side of the film. Film size is equivalent to size 1. The patient's teeth bite on

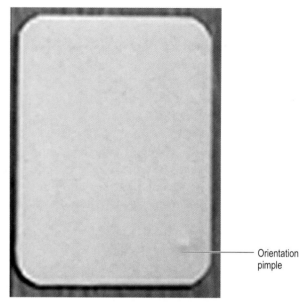

Figure 22.7   Orientation pimple

the flap in order to immobilise and maintain position (Fig. 22.8A). Bitewing holders are also available, these are a disposable device into which the film is inserted; a plastic flap at 90° to the film is placed between the patient's teeth.

Positioning
- The patient is seated with their neck leaning on a support
- A bitewing film or bitewing holder is placed with its tube side in contact with the lingual surface of the teeth under examination and the flap between the occlusal surfaces of the teeth

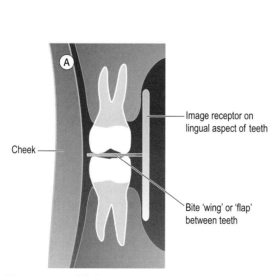

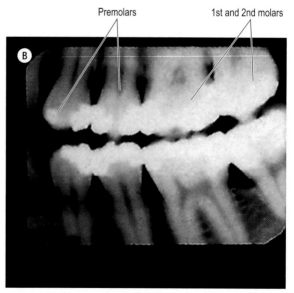

Figure 22.8   **(A)** Position of image receptor for bitewings and relationship to teeth; **(B)** bitewing image.
(B) Reproduced with permission from Whaites E. Essentials of dental radiography and radiology. 3rd edn. Edinburgh: Churchill Livingstone; 2002

- The patient closes their teeth over the flap
- The median sagittal plane (MSP) is vertical and the upper occlusal plane horizontal

Beam direction

Initially horizontal, then angled 5° caudally

Centring

To the middle of the image receptor, over the occlusal plane

Include

Crowns of the teeth under examination and alveolar crests

Criteria for assessing image quality

- Crowns of the teeth and alveolar crests are demonstrated
- No evidence of elongation or foreshortening of teeth
- No overlap of adjacent teeth
- Slight separation of occlusal surfaces of teeth
- Sharp image demonstrating enamel in contrast with pulp cavity and the alveolar crests

Common errors	Possible reasons
Foreshortening of the teeth	Poor beam selection or the image receptor has slipped away from the lingual surface of the teeth
Overlap of the crowns at their interproximal surfaces	Beam not at 90° in the mesiodistal direction

Intraoral techniques: periapicals

Periapical examinations are generally used to demonstrate individual or small groups of teeth. Before the introduction of OPT/OPG or DPT the whole of the mouth was examined in this way, with images mounted to represent the layout of the dentition.[5] OPT examination has almost exclusively superseded this approach.

As already mentioned in the introduction to this section, the structure and position of teeth cause problems for the radiographer when attempting to provide high quality images of the area. Ideally the radiographer places any body part so that its long axis is parallel to an image receptor and the X-ray beam is 90° to the body part and the image receptor.

More specifically, the most significant problems can be identified as:

1. The teeth are surrounded at their neck and root by the bones of the maxilla or mandible, which are additionally surrounded by the gum. This reduces the proportion of the tooth that can be placed in close contact with the

image receptor. When added to the arched construction of the hard palate, positioning of the image receptor parallel to the tooth becomes problematic. The teeth themselves are arranged in a variation of angles within the mouth, with the incisors being at a much greater angle than the molars.
2. The size of the patient's mouth will affect the possibility of positioning the image receptor, since a narrow dental arch may not accommodate the image receptor.
3. Overlapped teeth when the dentition is overcrowded will mean that it is impossible to provide images of some teeth without some superimposition.

Two techniques are available for periapicals, *bisecting angle technique* and *paralleling technique*. Each aims to reduce the effects of the obliquity of the teeth and problems outlined in the introduction to this section. There are advantages and disadvantages associated with each method, which will be discussed after descriptions of these techniques.

Periapicals: bisecting angle technique

It is already acknowledged that there will be an angle made between the long axis of the image receptor and the long axis of a tooth if the image receptor is placed on the labial aspect of the tooth and gum surrounding the root. Rather than directing the beam at 90° to either the tooth or the image receptor, for this technique the beam is aimed 90° to the bisector of the angle made by the tooth and image receptor; in other words, reaching a compromise (Fig. 22.9).

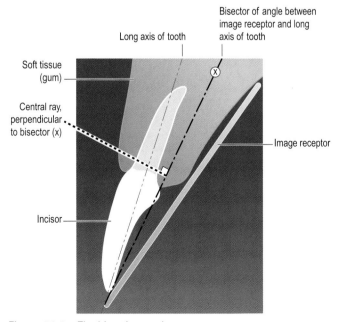

Figure 22.9   The bisecting angle

For this method, the angle of the individual patient's teeth must be estimated before commencing the examination. Although texts and dental radiography units list suggested beam angulation for this technique,[5,6] human dentition varies widely and each patient must be assessed as a result. Visual examination of the dentition in a mesiodistal direction will give the radiographer an idea of beam direction in order to ensure the beam will pass through the teeth at 90° and avoid overlap of the crowns at their interproximal surfaces. When assessing the angle of the long axis of the tooth in premolars, the centre of the crown must be assessed, rather than the longest (labially positioned) cusp, which is usually curved, and does not give an accurate indication of the tooth as a whole.

If film is used, a size 0 or 1 dental film is selected for this examination. The film should always be used with the 'pimple' facing outwards towards the X-ray tube and orientated towards the crowns of the teeth under examination. When film is used, a bisecting angle holder (Figs 22.10, 22.11, 22.12A) must always be used since use of the patient's finger for support is not acceptable.

Positioning
- The patient is seated with their neck supported
- The image receptor has its tube side in contact with the lingual aspect of the crowns of the teeth. The image receptor is vertically aligned for incisors and canines and transversely for premolars and molars
- The tooth under examination is centred to the image receptor, or the midpoint of the range of teeth intended for inclusion is centralised
- The patient closes their teeth over the holder for incisors and canines, and closes their lips over the holder for the other teeth, to immobilise the image receptor and maintain its position
- The head is adjusted until the MSP is vertical and the occlusal plane is horizontal

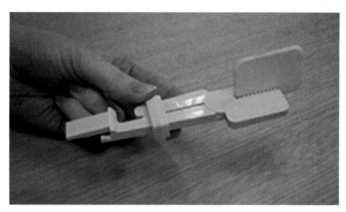

Figure 22.11   Bisecting angle holder – film in holder for molars and premolars

Beam direction
Initially horizontal, which is then adjusted until at 90° to the bisector of the angle formed between the long axis of the tooth and the long axis of the image receptor *and* 90° to the image receptor mesiodistally

Centring
Over the buccal surfaces of the teeth, to the centre of the film. A guide for *approximate* angles for 'normally positioned' teeth is given in Table 22.2

Collimation
Crowns and roots of the teeth under examination, surrounding bone

Criteria for assessing image quality
- Crowns, roots of the teeth and surrounding bone are demonstrated
- Minimal evidence of elongation or foreshortening* of tooth/teeth, or overlap of adjacent teeth *if there is no overcrowding of teeth in that region*
- Sharp image showing contrast of the alveolar bone and its trabeculae, pulp cavity and enamel of the tooth/teeth

*Ideally there would be no evidence of foreshortening or elongation but, since there will always be opportunity for this due to the arrangement of the teeth and gums, their exclusion cannot be expected.

Common errors	Possible reasons
Foreshortening of teeth; cusps of premolars and molars seen en face and crown appears 'squat'	Beam not at 90° to the bisecting angle in the craniocaudal direction
Overlap of crowns at their interproximal surfaces	Beam not at 90° in the mesiodistal direction *unless* there is actual overlap of teeth in the mouth

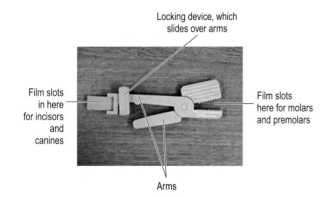

Figure 22.10   Holder for bisecting angle technique

Locking device, which slides over arms

Film slots in here for incisors and canines

Film slots here for molars and premolars

Arms

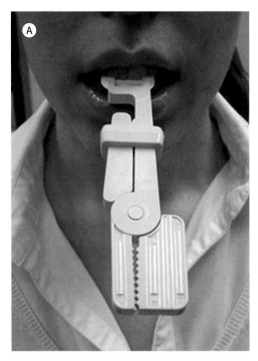

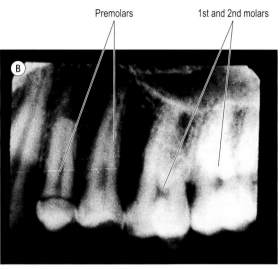

Premolars   1st and 2nd molars

Figure 22.12 **(A)** Bisecting angle holder – film in position for incisors; **(B)** bisecting angle periapical. (B) Reproduced with permission from Whaites E. Essentials of dental radiography and radiology. 3rd edn. Edinburgh: Churchill Livingstone; 2002

Table 22.2 Suggested approximate angulations for bisecting angle periapical technique (the alatragal line must be horizontal for use with these angles)

Upper teeth		Lower teeth	
Incisors	55–60° caudal angle	Incisors	25–30° cranial angle
Canines	45–50° caudal angle	Canines	15–20° cranial angle
Premolars	35–40° caudal angle	Premolars	10° cranial angle
Molars	25–30° caudal angle	Molars	Horizontal beam

Periapicals: paralleling technique (Figs 22.13, 22.14, 22.15, 22.16, 22.17A)

This technique also attempts to tackle the problems associated with producing accurate images of the teeth in this difficult body area. It also makes use of holders that maintain the position of the image receptor parallel to the long axis of the tooth and enables accurate selection of the central ray at 90° to the image receptor.

Positioning
- The patient is seated with their neck supported
- The image receptor is placed in a paralleling holder, longitudinally for incisors and canines, transversely for premolars and molars (Figs 22.13, 22.14)
- The holder, is placed in the mouth with the tube side of the image receptor facing the lingual surface of the teeth
- The image receptor is parallel to the long axes of the teeth under examination but is distant from the surface

of the teeth; this may appear to be a significant distance to the radiographer, being toward the soft palate for incisors and into the opposite half of the mouth for premolars and molars
- The tooth under examination is centred to the image receptor, or the midpoint of the range of teeth intended for inclusion is centralised
- The patient closes their mouth over the holder to immobilise the image receptor and maintain its position (Figs 22.15, 22.16)

Beam direction and centring
The beam is aligned to the centre of the indicator on the paralleling holder, in the direction indicated by the holder

Collimation
Crowns and roots of the teeth under examination, surrounding bone

Figure 22.13   Paralleling technique holder – film (incisors and canines)

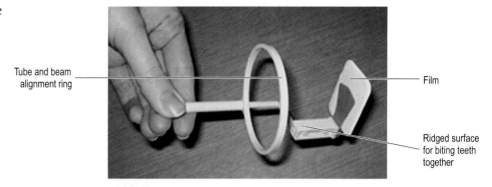

Tube and beam alignment ring

Film

Ridged surface for biting teeth together

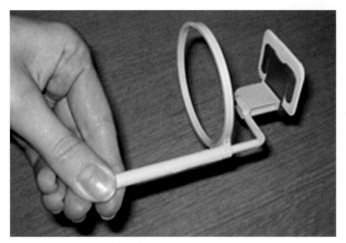

Figure 22.14   Paralleling technique holder – film (molars and premolars)

Criteria for assessing image quality

This is as for the bisecting angle technique; the teeth will appear slightly larger than with the bisecting angle technique but will be less distorted

■ Which to use, bisecting angle or paralleling technique?

The two periapical techniques described each have advantages and disadvantages. These are briefly outlined in the list below, which is intended to provide a résumé of the points that should be considered by the radiographer before selecting a suitable method. However, since these points for consideration may be likely to lead to an equivocal opinion, the final decision may be based solely in the availability of equipment, familiarity with one technique or user preference for a particular type of film holder. Some digital units may not provide equipment that offers a choice.

■ Occlusals

As identified at the start of this chapter, occlusals have many uses, which are more specifically identified in Table 22.3.

There is one basic patient position used for most occlusals and this is described first, followed by the

Advantages and disadvantages of periapical techniques; a comparison of Figs 22.9 and 22.17C and D will help illustrate these points	
Bisecting angle	*Paralleling*
Object film distance (OFD) varies along the length of the teeth, as the image receptor becomes more remote from crown to root; however, at no point is it as distant from the tooth as in paralleling technique. Magnification (and therefore unsharpness) increases towards the root	Relatively long OFD along the entire length of the tooth = implications for magnification and unsharpness. Also, large teeth may not fit within image receptor's periphery
Some image distortion as beam is not perpendicular to any structure	Minimum image distortion as the film is always parallel to the long axis of the tooth and the beam perpendicular to the image receptor
Selection of angle is less likely to be as accurate as for paralleling technique, since it requires estimation of the bisecting angle. Centring may also be less accurate	Use of the alignment and centring indicator on the paralleling holder ensures accuracy of beam centring and angulation
Holders are relatively small compared to the paralleling holders	Holders are more bulky for patients; however, their use is more widespread than bisecting angle holders and radiographers may prefer their use due to familiarity with the technique and equipment

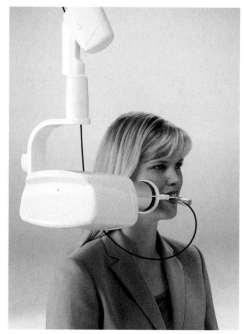

Figure 22.15 Paralleling technique – digital receptor. Reproduced with permission from Xograph Imaging Systems

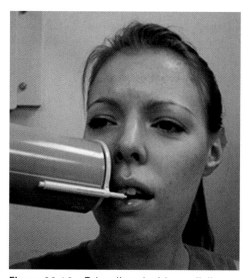

Figure 22.16 Tube aligned with paralleling holder

modification in position for the only exception, the submental occlusal. Relevant tube displacements and angulations are listed after the description of the basic position, alongside the area demonstrated for each (Table 22.4).

If used, occlusal film is selected for all these examinations.

Table 22.3 Occlusal projections

Projection	Demonstrates
70° maxillary occlusal (also known as standard anterior oblique maxilla)	Upper incisors, canines, hard palate
Oblique maxillary occlusal (also known as posterior oblique lateral maxilla)	Unerupted upper canines; upper premolars
Oblique mandibular occlusal (also known as posterior true mandible)	Unerupted lower canines; lower premolars
45° submandibular occlusal (also known as anterior oblique mandible)	Lower incisors, symphysis menti of mandible
Submental occlusal (also known as anterior true mandible)	Lower incisors, submandibular and sublingual ducts

Positioning (basic head position)

- The patient is seated with their neck leaning on a support
- The image receptor is in the mouth, tube side upwards for maxillary teeth and down for mandibular teeth
- The image receptor is pushed back as far as possible, at least to the first molars and to include the incisors
- The midline of the image receptor is coincident with the MSP
- The teeth are closed over the image receptor and the MSP is vertical
- The *occlusal plane is horizontal* for most examinations
- *Submental occlusal* (for submandibular ducts) requires extension of the neck as far as possible to bring the occlusal plane towards the vertical. The head and neck are supported in this position
- The basic position is shown in Figures 22.18A, 22.19A, 22.20A, 22.21A

General comment on errors

Errors most commonly occur when the occlusal plane is not maintained in the correct relationship to the beam, or when the image receptor slips from the position prepared by the radiographer. For this reason it must be emphasised that initial patient preparation must include explanation of the procedure to follow, reinforced by stressing the importance of immobilisation. The radiographer should also express understanding that the procedure may be uncomfortable for a short time.

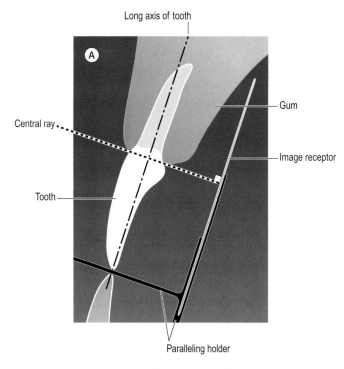

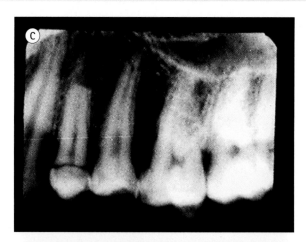

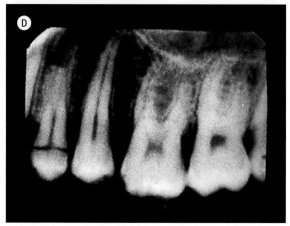

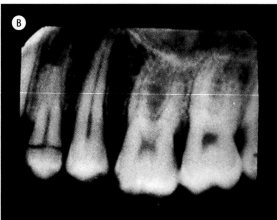

Figure 22.17   **(A)** Position of image receptor for paralleling technique; **(B)** paralleling periapical. Comparison of bisecting angle and paralleling technique on periapical images – **(C)** bisecting angle technique and **(D)** paralleling technique. (B), (C) and (D) Reproduced with permission from Whaites E. Essentials of dental radiography and radiology. 3rd edn. Edinburgh: Churchill Livingstone; 2002

Table 22.4 Beam direction and centring for occlusals

Area under examination	Projection identification	Beam direction and centring
Upper incisors, canines, hard palate	70° maxillary occlusal (Fig. 22.18A,B)	*Beam direction* 1. Initially vertical central ray; the tube head is in front of the patient's face, coincident with the MSP 2. The tube is then angled 20° towards the face, making a 20° angle with the image receptor *Centring* Over the nasal bone in the midline, to emerge over the middle of the image receptor
Unerupted upper canines; upper premolars	Oblique maxillary occlusal (Fig. 22.19A,B)	*Beam direction* 1. Initially a horizontal central ray; the tube head is at the side of the head under examination, next to the eye and perpendicular to the MSP 2. The tube is angled 65° caudally, and then angled distally 45° until at 45° to the MSP

Table 22.4 cont'd

		Centring Over the edge of the ala of the nose on the side under examination, to emerge over the middle of the image receptor
Unerupted lower canines; lower premolars	Oblique mandibular occlusal (Fig. 22.20A,B)	*Beam direction* 1. Initially a horizontal central ray; the tube head is at the side of the head under examination, next to the corner of the mouth and perpendicular to the MSP 2. The tube is angled 45° cranially, and then angled distally 45° until at 45° to the MSP *Centring* Under the inferior aspect of the mandible below the corner of the mouth, to emerge over the middle of the image receptor
Lower incisors, symphysis menti of mandible	45° submandibular occlusal (Fig. 22.21A,B)	*Beam direction* 1. Initially a horizontal central ray; the tube head is in front of the patient's face, coincident with the MSP 2. The tube is then angled 45° cranially *Centring* Under the symphysis menti, to emerge over the middle of the image receptor
Lower incisors, submandibular ducts	Submental occlusal (Fig. 22.22A,B)	*Beam direction* Initially horizontal, central ray is angled cranially until 90° to the occlusal plane *Centring* Under the symphysis menti to emerge over the middle of the image receptor

Criteria for assessing image quality – occlusals	
70° maxillary occlusal	Anterior arch of the maxillary teeth back to the first molars are demonstrated Incisors and canines are foreshortened; premolars and molars are demonstrated axially Symmetry of the maxillary arch
Oblique maxillary occlusal	Full length of incisors, canines and premolars including alveolar bone surrounding roots is demonstrated (on the side under examination) Incisors, canines and premolars are elongated (on the side under examination) Dental arch on the side under examination appears flattened Superimposition of teeth on the side that is not under examination
Oblique mandibular occlusal	Canines and premolars of the side under examination are demonstrated Mandibular arch on the side under examination appears flattened Superimposition of teeth on the side that is not under examination
45° submandibular occlusal	Symphysis menti and mandibular arch back to first molars are demonstrated Foreshortening of lower incisors Superimposition of the teeth over the mandible
All projections except submental occlusal	Sharp image demonstrating detail of the teeth under examination and their roots, in contrast to alveolar bone, pulp cavity and enamel
Submental occlusal	Mandibular arch from incisors to first molars is demonstrated Mandibular arch is demonstrated axially (i.e. from below); incisors and canines are foreshortened Medial aspect of distal premolars overlying lingual aspect of the mandible Sharp image demonstrating the soft tissues of the floor of the mouth in contrast with the mandible

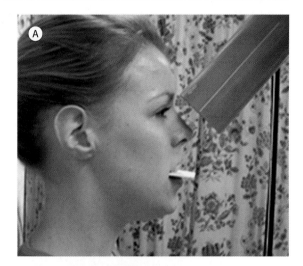

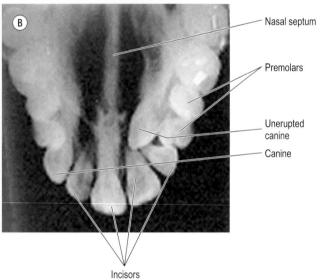

Nasal septum

Premolars

Unerupted canine

Canine

Incisors

Figure 22.18   70° maxillary occlusal

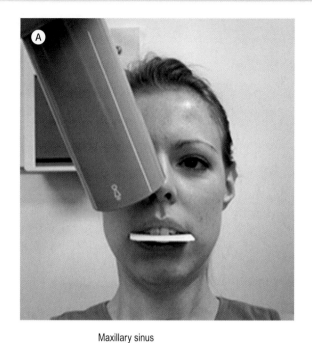

Maxillary sinus

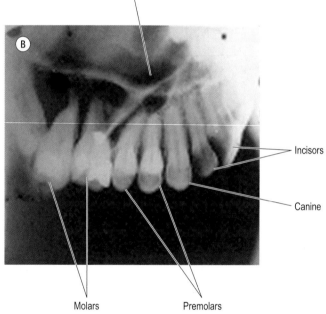

Incisors

Canine

Molars   Premolars

Figure 22.19   Oblique maxillary occlusal

LOCATION OF POSITION OF UNERUPTED CANINES ('PARALLAX' PROJECTION)

It is sometimes necessary to produce images that provide information in addition to that provided by occlusal projections. Specifically, these may be required to help identify the position of an unerupted canine, in relationship to other anteriorly placed teeth in an anterior or posterior direction. The method is only recommended for the area from the incisors to the first premolars.

An initial orthopantomograph may initially be required to show the orientation of the unerupted tooth, since they can sometimes be found lying horizontally and high within the maxilla. The principle of so-called parallax projections is to take two intraoral images, using tube shift (angulation) between the two images, to provide slightly varying images which allow assessment of the position of the unerupted tooth. An occlusal or periapical approach can be used and, although periapical images are likely to be easier to interpret, occlusals will prove beneficial in demonstrating the high, horizontally positioned canine.

Once tooth orientation has been ascertained, the next stage of the examination is based on two, separate, bisecting angle or occlusal examinations.

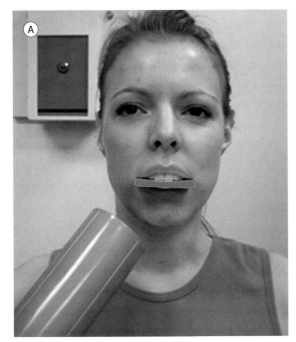

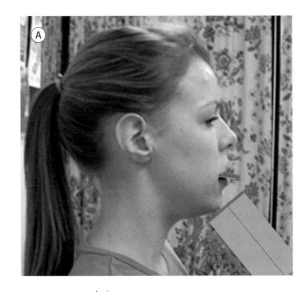

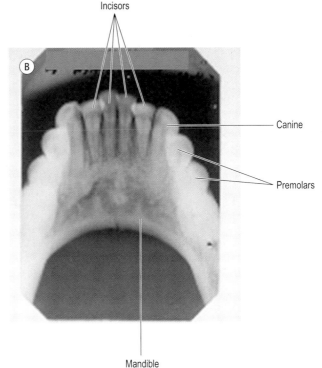

Figure 22.21   45° submandibular occlusal

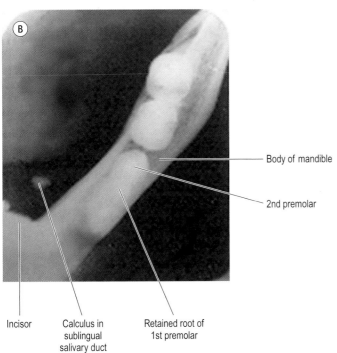

Incisor   Calculus in   Retained root of
sublingual   1st premolar
salivary duct

Figure 22.20   Oblique mandibular occlusal

Bisecting angle approach for parallax

The first examination uses a basic bisecting angle technique and the second employs bisecting angle technique plus tube shift to project the more anteriorly placed teeth (or tooth) laterally when compared to the initial image (Fig 22.23). In other words, a labially positioned unerupted canine will move further in the direction of angle (towards the MSP) than the erupted teeth on the second image; a palatally positioned unerupted canine will appear to shift away from the direction of angle (away from the MSP).

Positioning
- The patient is seated with their neck supported
- The image receptor has its tube side in contact with the lingual aspect of the crowns of the teeth. The image receptor is vertically aligned for incisors and canines and transversely for premolars and molars

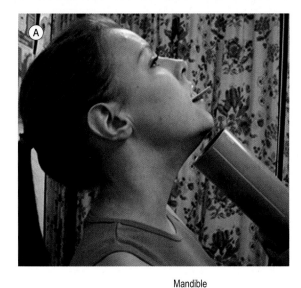

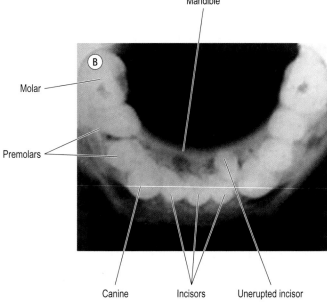

Figure 22.22 Submental occlusal

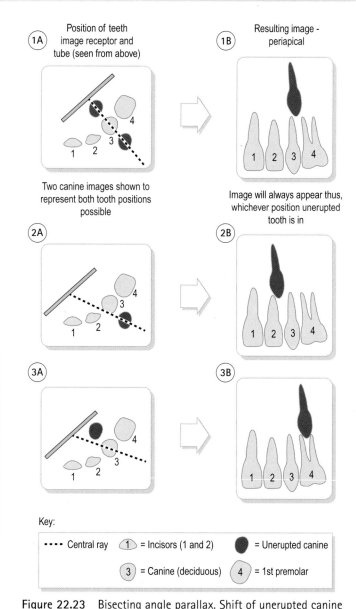

Figure 22.23 Bisecting angle parallax. Shift of unerupted canine related to its position: the left hand column (A) shows position of teeth, image receptor and tube (seen from above); the right hand column (B) shows the resulting periapical image. *(1A)* shows the (left) teeth from above, with unerupted canines anteriorly or posteriorly positioned (either way will give the periapical appearance seen in *(1B)*. An erupted canine tooth is included in this illustration and this would be a deciduous tooth; however, a deciduous canine tooth may not be present in all cases. *(2A)* shows the teeth from above, with an anteriorly positioned unerupted canine. The beam angulation created by tube shift will move this unerupted tooth further mesially (as in image *2B*) than the erupted canine, making it appear nearer to the 2nd incisor than on the original periapical seen in *(1A)*. *(3A)* shows the teeth from above, with a posteriorly positioned unerupted canine. The beam angulation created by tube shift will move the erupted teeth further mesially (as in *3B*) than the unerupted canine, making the unerupted canine appear nearer to the 1st premolar than on the original periapical seen in *(1A)*

- The tooth under examination is centred to the image receptor, or the midpoint of the range of teeth intended for inclusion is centralised
- The patient closes their mouth over the holder to immobilise the image receptor and maintain its position
- The head is adjusted until the MSP is vertical and the occlusal plane is horizontal

Beam direction and FFD

First image: initially horizontal, which is then adjusted until at 90° to the bisector of the angle formed between the long axis of the tooth and the long axis of the image receptor

Second image: from the angle and direction selected for the first image, the tube is shifted 25–30° in a distal direction (to form a mesially directed angle of 25–30° to the beam used for the first image)

Centring

Over the buccal surfaces of the teeth to the centre of the film; for the second image, the image receptor is displaced slightly in a mesial direction to ensure its centre is coincident with the central ray

The main purpose of the two exposure tube shift/angulation technique is to use geometric principles in order to ascertain the position of the unerupted tooth. This applies to both periapical and occlusal approaches.

Occlusal technique for parallax

If the occlusal method is used, tube shift is undertaken on the second exposure, as in the periapical method. The occlusal approach may be advisable if the unerupted tooth has a horizontal orientation and lies high in relationship to the erupted teeth and some authors recommend only this method for position location.[7] The tube movement can be either horizontal (distal tube head movement to form a mesial angle) or vertical (creating a more caudal angle) in relationship to the first exposure.[7]

If horizontal tube shift is used, a labially positioned unerupted canine will move further in the direction of angle (towards the midline) than the erupted teeth on the second image; a palatally positioned unerupted canine will appear to shift away from the direction of angle (away from the midline). If a vertical tube shift is used for the second exposure, a labially positioned unerupted canine will appear to shift down over or towards the erupted teeth and a palatally positioned unerupted canine will show the erupted

tooth to fall even lower in comparison to their position on the first image (opening up any space between them and the unerupted tooth above).

Identification of images and location of position of the unerupted tooth

Although it is essential that procedures for correct identification and image orientation are followed for all dental and other imaging procedures, parallax images need special attention to detail. It is vital that each image produced for the parallax examination is identified as to whether it is the initial, or second image with tube shift. Only with accurate identification can assessment be made regarding position of the unerupted tooth. Images should be displayed side by side in order to assess relative positions of the teeth.

References

1. Royal College of Radiologists NRPB. Guidelines on radiology standards for primary dental care. Documents of the NRPB 5;3 Didcot: NRPB; 1994.
2. European Commission. European Guidelines on Quality Criteria for Diagnostic Radiographic Images. Office for Official Publications of the European Communities. Brussels: 1996.
3. Statutory Instrument 1999 No. 3232. The Ionising Radiations Regulations 1999. London: HMSO; 1999.
4. The Ionising Radiation (Medical Exposure) Regulations 2000. London: HMSO; 2000.
5. Swallow RA, et al. Clark's positioning in radiography. 11th edn. Oxford: Heinemann; 1986.
6. Unett EM, Royle AJ. Radiographic techniques and image evaluation. London: Chapman and Hall; 1997.
7. Whaites E. Essentials of dental radiography and radiology. 3rd edn. Edinburgh: Churchill Livingstone; 2002.

ORTHOPANTOMOGRAPHY

Elizabeth Carver

ORTHOPANTOMOGRAPHY (OPT OR OPG) OR DENTAL PANORAMIC TOMOGRAPHY (DPT)

This technique requires the use of a specialised OPT unit (Fig. 23.1A,B), the tomographic principle being that which is used to produce the image of the full mouth and its dentition. The moving tube effectively blurs out the shadow of overlying structures by placing the dental arch in the axis of the tomographic movement. Structures not lying within this axis are effectively blurred and thus their detail does not overlie the image of the teeth and mandible. However, the area of interest does show some element of unsharpness when compared to radiographic images of other body parts when a non-moving tube is used.

The technique opens out the image of the dental arch to appear in a linear arrangement on the final image. It has long been employed in the dental setting and has largely replaced full mouth periapical examinations. As mentioned in Chapter 19, the OPT examination can be used to demonstrate the temporomandibular joints and mandible.

The tomographic movement of the unit attempts to follow the dental arch, which it keeps within the tomographic axis of the beam as it travels around the patient's face. Because of this, accurate positioning aims to place the dental arch within this axis and horizontally to follow the plane of tube movement. Positioning also aims to keep unwanted structures such as the cervical vertebrae clear from the tomographic axis.

Some tomographic units use a system of slit light beams that are aligned with the incisors, median sagittal plane (MSP), anthropological baseline or alatragal line. Lights are also used to assess the patient's position in an antero-posterior (AP) direction; these vertical slit beams are seen as superimposed when the patient is in the optimum position but are separated if the patient is too far forward or not forward enough. Since all these light arrangements are used in varying ways for each manufacturer, it is difficult to describe the use of each different system. Suffice to say, use of these light systems will ensure that the patient is actually in the position as described in the positioning section below. It can often be difficult to align the baselines with the lights on the OPT unit once they are switched on. Visually assessing the baselines *before* switching the lights on often helps, the radiographer using the lights to check height and positioning accuracy afterwards.

The X-ray beam leaves the tube housing via a slit collimator and the thin beam moves around the dental arch and across the image receptor; this arrangement reduces the inevitable penumbra which would be caused by a wider beam. However, some penumbral effect is unavoidable.

The tomographic movement travels around the head with a horizontal beam, in opposition to traditional tomographic units that move over the supine patient and use a beam which is initially vertical and moves longitudinally or in a circular, elliptical or helical movement.

Due to the nature of this horizontal movement around the patient, use of the OPT unit may be distracting for the patient during exposure. Advance preparation must include demonstration of tube movement for the patient, using the 'test' setting. The unit is then returned to the start position.

If used, an OPT cassette is inserted into the cassette holder on the unit.

Positioning (Fig. 23.2)

- A disposable bite rod is inserted into the chin rest, or a disposable plastic cover is applied to the permanent bite rod
- The patient is seated or standing with their chin resting on the chin support and in the correct position to facilitate the dental arch being placed in the correct tomogra-

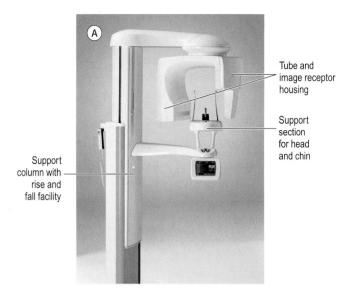

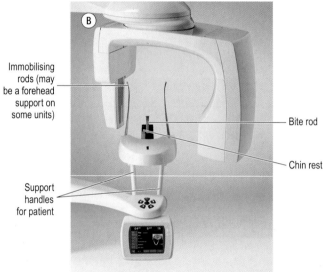

Figure 23.1   OPT unit. Reproduced with permission from Xograph Imaging Systems

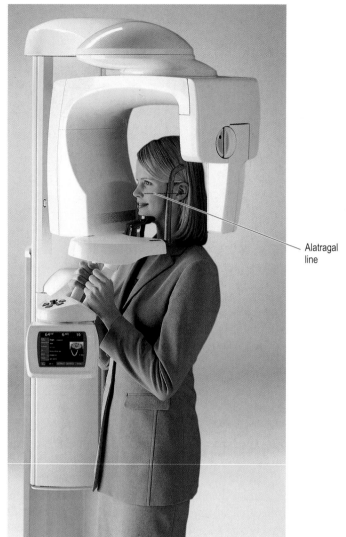

Figure 23.2   Patient positioned in OPT unit. The patient's MSP is vertical and there must be no rotation. The alatragal line is horizontal as indicated by the black line on the model. Note how the patient has stepped forward to bring the cervical vertebrae into the correct position. Reproduced with permission from Xograph Imaging Systems

phic plane (with the anthropological baseline and ala-tragal line horizontal and the head far enough forward, often indicated by slit light indicators as designed by the manufacturer)

- The patient bites with their incisors in the groove on the bite rod, to effect separation of teeth on the image
- The MSP is vertical and perpendicular to the bite rod. The height of the unit is adjusted until the occlusal plane is horizontal (assessed by checking that the alatragal line or anthropological baseline are horizontal)
- The patient holds onto the support handles and is asked to step forward slightly to bring the cervical spine vertical. If seated, their chair is pulled forward by the radiographer. Throughout this manoeuvre the head must not tilt or rotate and the chin must not lift or drop
- The head clamp is applied for immobilisation

- The patient is asked to close their lips and press their tongue forwards against the teeth and the roof of the mouth for the duration of the exposure
- Exposure is made after a reminder to the patient to keep still during tube movement

Criteria for assessing image quality

- All of the mandible, including symphysis menti inferiorly and condyles superiorly, is demonstrated. The hard palate and lower part of the maxillary sinuses are demonstrated
- Dentition is demonstrated in a horizontal line
- Bite rod is shown between upper and lower central incisors with separation of occlusal surfaces of all teeth
- All teeth are seen relatively sharply

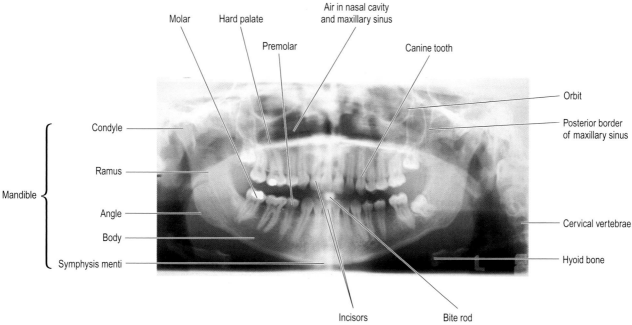

Figure 23.3   OPT image

• Slightly blurred shadow of the anterior aspect of the neck structures is superimposed over images of the incisors; sharper image of bodies of the cervical vertebrae seen at both lateral edges of the image, cleared from the area of interest

• Mandible outline is continuous and not 'stepped'

Reference

1. Iannucci Haring J, Jansen Lind L. Radiographic interpretation for the dental hygienist. Philadelphia: Saunders; 1993.

Common errors	Possible reasons
Step appears in the image, particularly noticeable over the mandibular outline	Patient may have moved chin during exposure
Part of the image is blurred whilst the rest appears sharp	Patient movement at some point during exposure, but not throughout exposure
Dentition layout not seen as horizontal, mouth appears to smile; mandibular incisors may be blurred and slightly magnified	Occlusal plane not horizontal; chin is lowered slightly
Dentition layout not seen as horizontal, mouth appears upturned (sulking); maxillary incisors may be slightly blurred and magnified	Occlusal plane not horizontal; chin is raised slightly
Dentition layout not seen as horizontal, appears tilted. Unsharp posterior teeth	MSP not vertical
Middle section of the mandible not seen sharply, outer sections appear more sharp. Unsharp posterior teeth	MSP rotated
Very narrow incisors; cervical vertebrae may be seen centrally	Patient's chin too far forward into the unit
Broad, unsharp incisors; these are sometimes likened to 'piano keys'	Patient's chin not far enough into the unit
Sharper image of cervical vertebrae superimposed over the incisors (some OPT units may produce some cervical shadowing as normal)	Patient's head too far forward in the unit and the cervical vertebrae are further towards the panoramic axis. Patient may not have stepped forward to reduce the cervical curve; the middle vertebrae may protrude into the axis[1]
Dark band seen across the roots and upper aspect of crowns of upper teeth	Tongue not depressed against roof of mouth during exposure; lips may not be closed

CEPHALOMETRY

Elizabeth Carver

Prior to maxillofacial surgery and orthodontic treatment it is usually necessary to examine the relationship of the soft tissues of the face to facial bones and teeth. After treatment further assessment is made and it is therefore essential that all images in the series are comparable. To ensure that this is the case, specialised equipment is used to produce consistent images.

The unit (Fig. 24.1) can be an independent unit or form part of a unit which has dual function for orthopantomography (OPT) and lateral cephalometric applications. The example given here actually forms part of the OPT unit shown in Chapter 23. In any case the cephalometry unit usually includes:

1. Fixed focus film distance (FFD) (minimum 150 cm to minimise magnification and geometric unsharpness). If the object film distance (OFD) can be altered in a unit, the distance of the median sagittal plane (MSP) from the image receptor must be registered to allow accurate assessment; measurement facility may be found on the nasion support (see point 3, below).
2. Head clamps with ear plugs. These are inserted into the external auditory meati (EAMs) to ensure accurate and consistent positioning.
3. Nasion support which slides in an anteroposterior (AP) direction in relationship to the patient. This ensures that different sized heads can be immobilised in the unit. They also slide along a measured scale and measurements from this scale are used in units with automatic filter positioning, to ensure that the filter lies in a position that is accurate for each patient.
4. A filter which is used to compensate for the range in density from facial soft tissue to facial bones. This filter can be permanently situated in the tube head (both free-

standing and OPT units) or, in older equipment, an aluminium wedge is attached to the light beam diaphragm. The latest equipment uses a digital image receptor.

If used, a lateral cephalogram cassette or 24 × 30 cm cassette is placed longitudinally in the erect cassette holder on the unit.

Positioning (Fig. 24.2)
- The patient is erect with their MSP parallel to the cassette
- The height of the unit is adjusted until the earplugs can be placed in the EAMs
- The occlusal plane is horizontal
- The nasion support is positioned in contact with the nasion
- If not permanently situated within the tube housing, the wedge filter is inserted over the light beam diaphragm with its thicker end aligned over the soft tissues of the face
- The patient is asked to close their back teeth and relax the lips; this is maintained during exposure

Beam direction
Horizontal, at 90° to the image receptor; this is fixed for most units

Centring
Over the earplugs and the middle of the image receptor; this is fixed for most units

Collimation
Fixed collimation is usually found in most units and includes soft tissue outlines of the forehead, face/nose and mandible

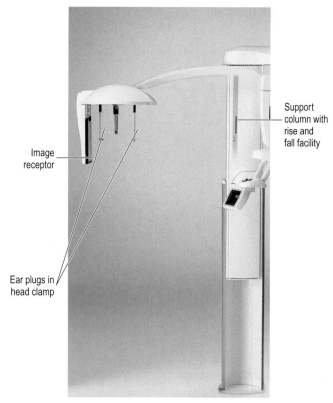

Figure 24.1 Cephalometry unit. Reproduced with permission from Xograph Imaging Systems

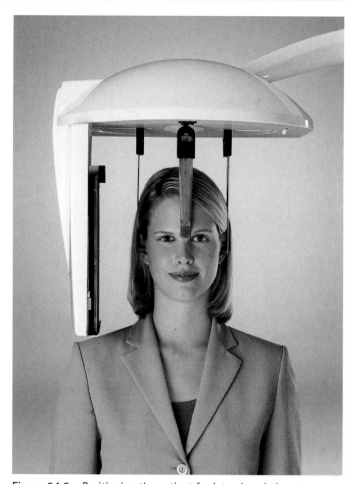

Figure 24.2 Positioning the patient for lateral cephalometry

Criteria for assessing image quality

- Soft tissue outline of face including forehead, nose, lips and chin are demonstrated
- Whole of mandible and ear plugs are demonstrated
- Superimposition of both the ear plugs and of the right and left facial structures
- Anthropological baseline is horizontal
- Sharp image demonstrating detail of the facial bones *and* soft tissues of the face

Common errors	Possible reasons
Soft tissues of the face too dark	Filter not applied, or not selected on the unit
Denser soft tissues below the chin in comparison with the other soft tissues of the face	Anthropological baseline not horizontal; the chin is down and increases the density of the soft tissues under the mandible
Projection is usually acceptable on lateral cephalogram images, since the use of the ear plugs ensures accuracy. If the ear plugs are not inserted fully this is likely to impinge upon positioning of the MSP	

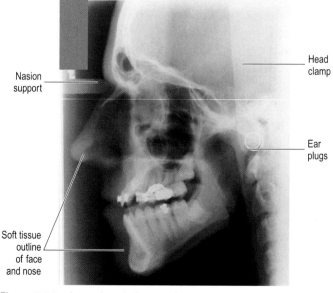

Figure 24.3 Lateral cephalometry image

CHEST AND ABDOMEN

CHEST AND THORACIC CONTENTS

Elizabeth Carver

Plain radiographic examination of the chest, in particular the posteroanterior (PA) projection, is considered to be the most commonly performed examination in the imaging department and is still a valid and useful diagnostic tool.[1] This remains the case at the start of the 21st century, despite a reduction in the number of requests for the examination, resulting from efforts to cut the numbers of unnecessary referrals for examinations using ionising radiations.[2,3]

Common findings on the chest image

Common findings on the chest image include: abscess; atelectasis; bullae; calcifications; cardiomegaly; consolidation; emphysema; empyema; fibrosis; haemothorax; hiatus hernia; hilar enlargement or displacement; mastectomy; mediastinal enlargement (including lymph node enlargement); metastasis; neoplasm; pleural effusion; pleural plaques; pneumonectomy; pneumonia; pneumoperitoneum; pneumothorax; pulmonary oedema; raised diaphragm/s; rib fractures; thyroid goitre; tracheal shift; vertebral collapse.

Note that this is not a list of indications for referral for chest radiography; it is a résumé of commonly encountered appearances.

THE PA CHEST PROJECTION AND COMMENTS ON ITS IMPLEMENTATION

The PA chest projection is the primary method for demonstration of the thoracic contents. It is universally acknowledged that the gold standard for demonstrating the chest is to execute it with the patient in the erect, PA position. Reasons for this are straightforward and logical:

Erect

1. Undertaking the projection in the erect position allows for demonstration of unnaturally located fluid, which finds its natural level within the thoracic cavity and is well demonstrated as more dense in appearance in contrast to the air-filled lung tissue. In the supine position this pleural fluid will lie posteriorly in a layer which will show as an increased density over the hemithorax in which it lies; this density may overlie other pathology.[4] Wherever possible radiographers should undertake chest radiography erect; in the case of the infirm patient an erect sitting projection is a suitable alternative and this can be achieved using a stool or, preferably, a commercially built chair which is designed for stability and versatility. These chairs have wheels for manoeuvrability, wheel locks for stability and removable back and arms for versatility of use. A PA erect chest can therefore be undertaken with the chair back removed but chair arms in place (Fig. 25.1A,B,C,D). For patients who must remain in a wheelchair, on a trolley or bed, an erect anteroposterior (AP) projection can be undertaken.

2. Inspiratory effort is more effective when the thorax is in the erect position.

PA

1. The PA projection allows forward tilt of the thorax to elevate the lung apices above the clavicles. Tuberculosis (TB) frequently manifests itself in the lung apex, thus indicating the importance of clearing this area from the image of the clavicles (although a lordotic projection will clear the clavicles entirely above the apices, allowing visualisation of the lung apex without superimposition of the clavicles over the lower apical

portion). Numbers of reported cases of TB in the 21st century are relatively insignificant in the UK, when compared to the 17th, 18th and 19th centuries and the first half of the 20th century, but it is by no means non-existent. Indeed, internationally there are still areas where TB causes concern and numbers have been rising at an average of 0.4% globally in recent years.[5] In the UK, numbers of recorded TB cases fell to their lowest level in 1987, reaching the low plateau of 5–6000 cases per year for some years afterwards; the first signs of a

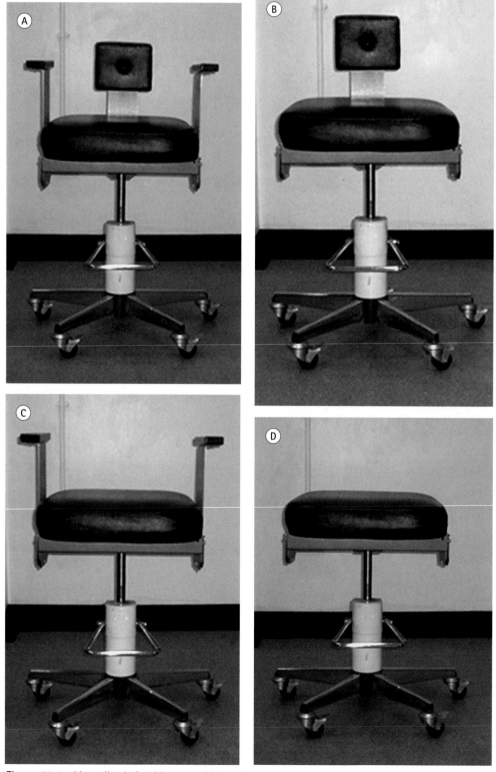

Figure 25.1 Versatile chair with removable back and arms

very slight increase were noted around the year of 1997.[6] Forward tilt also avoids a lordotic appearance of the image; lordosis affects accuracy of cardiothoracic ratio (CT) assessment for cardiomegaly.

2. The chin can be supported clear of the apices by its position resting upon the upper border of the cassette.

3. Since the heart lies anteriorly within the thorax (Fig. 25.2) the degree of magnification of this organ is minimised in the PA position; again, in assessment of the CT ratio, minimal magnification is preferred.

4. In the case of the adult female, compression of breast tissue against the cassette will reduce body thickness and ensure the lowest exposure factor settings can be used.

5. It is acknowledged that the use of PA projections reduces the dose to anteriorly positioned radiosensitive organs, due to the higher average beam energy, after travelling through the posterior portions of the chest (and therefore producing less absorption in these anterior organs). The sternum and female breasts lie within the field of primary radiation, and will also benefit from reduction of dose in the PA position.

6. Obliquity of the X-ray beam at the periphery of the thorax will assist projection of the scapulae away from the area of the lung fields. Angle of this obliquity is likely to vary, as the distance of the scapulae from the central ray will differ according to chest width but it is likely that this angle will be quite small, even in the patient who has a wide chest. Examples of such angles of obliquity of the beam at 2 m focus film distance (FFD), at different points around the beam centre (when using a central ray at 90° to the cassette) and using geometric calculations, are given as approximate figures in the following table (figures are given to the nearest decimal point).

Distance from centring point	Angle of oblique rays at this point (2 m FFD)
12 cm	3.4
17 cm	4.8
21.5 cm	6.2

Comments on exposure technique selection

In order to adequately image the lung tissue in contrast to air within the thorax, exposure factors with a fairly low kVp were traditionally selected for chest radiography. These were usually in the range of 60–75 kVp and accompanied by values of 6–12 mAs. However, structures overlying dense areas such as the heart failed to be

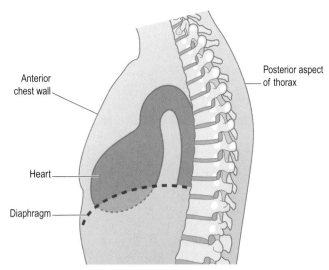

Figure 25.2   Heart in relationship to anterior chest wall

demonstrated due to the low penetration of the beam. EC guidelines in 1996 not only stressed the importance of using a high energy beam in order to penetrate such areas but emphasised the reduction of absorbed dose by using high kVp techniques, namely 125 kVp.[7] These high kVp techniques may well require use of an anti-scatter grid or bucky and use of automatic exposure chambers (AECs) is recommended in the 1996 EC guidelines, using the right AEC.[7]

Positioning choices for the PA projection

Text in this chapter has already referred to the relatively high frequency of requests for the PA chest examination and it is seen as a routine examination. This possibly explains why little published comment has been made in the past regarding actual positioning techniques (although there has been reasonably frequent comment on exposure factor techniques, radiation protection and dedicated chest radiology systems).

Historically, and internationally, descriptions for PA chest techniques have included a confusing range of centring points (T4–T7), suggestions for caudal angulation or use of the horizontal beam. This range of techniques should be questioned, especially as consistency of approach is desirable when aiming to provide a quality-led service.

Caudal angulation

On the issue of angulation it appears that, internationally, this is not in widespread employment and the UK appears to be the most likely area where its use is found.[8] Caudal angulation has been suggested as inappropriate since the (minimal) obliquity of the beam used is actually likely to reduce the amount of posterior, inferior lung tissue demonstrated above the diaphragm on the image (this is despite the common belief that its use 'opens out the lung fields' or maximises the amount of lung tissue seen above the diaphragm.[9] The effectiveness of small angles has also been challenged.[10] In addition, caudal angulation takes the beam direction towards the abdomen, thus potentially increasing radiation dose to this region. On consideration of these points, instruction for use of a horizontal beam will be given in this text.

Centring method

As indicated, suggestions for centring have varied from T4 to T7,[11,12,13,14] with mention of the middle of the image receptor, chest or thorax also given in some texts.[13,14,15] In some cases more than one suggestion is given. So which is most appropriate? An additional question is: do texts specifying a vertebral level mean the body *or* spinous process of that which is indicated? This is an important point when it is remembered that the body of a thoracic vertebra lies level with the spinous process of the one above it. It is also important that a suggested centring point be located as a palpable surface marking, so spinous process will be referred to in this text.

One suggestion for accurate assessment of T7 as a centring point involves use of a ruler to practise measuring the radiographer's hand span in order to accurately locate this centring point (given in centimetres and inches from T1) for use on the 'average' male and 'average' female;[16] but how can this be standardised or accurate when the assessment of 'average' is likely to vary from radiographer to radiographer, and any set measurement in centimetres or inches varies in its distance down each individual spine from a given point?

So which spinous process *can* be considered most suitable for suggestion? Centring points are most effective when simply in the centre of the area of interest, whether or not tube angle is used, and this should similarly apply to the chest region. This suggests a move from traditional centring points as high as T6 (which lies only one-third of the distance from apices to costophrenic angles). Study of PA chest images has shown that the vertebral body which most frequently lies level with the midpoint of the lungs is the body of T8 (spinous process of T7).[17] This has influenced the decision to select this point for the central ray in this text.

Yet the reality of actually visualising this centring level accurately, and at a distance of 2 m, can also be questioned, despite accurate palpation at the skin surface. Of course, a mark can be made at the appropriate level on the patient's gown after palpation but, realistically, only female patients undergo chest radiography in an examination gown. Would marking of the skin on a male patient be ethical? It probably would not be. Alternatively, a removable sticker could be applied to the back of male patients but this may also not be acceptable to every individual.

In support of the question regarding ability to accurately select a centring point at 2 m, it has been found that radiographers frequently believe that they use a specific centring point for PA projection of the chest but, in reality, ensure that the area of interest lies centrally over the cassette. They then centre to the middle of the cassette and area of interest.[18] This provides a well-centred image and suggests that radiographers are accurate at centring appropriately at 2 m but not at selecting the point they believe they use. For this reason the description of technique and centring point reflects a combination of this second method and selection of a specific centring point.

■ PA chest projection (Fig. 25.3A,B,C)

When using cassettes, size selected for this projection is determined by patient size, which is most frequently 35^2 for females and 35×43 cm for males. An erect cassette holder is used; for higher kVp techniques a grid may be used with the cassette. Alternatively the cassette may be placed in an erect bucky. Orientation of the 35×43 cm cassette will depend on the build of the patient. For patients known to suffer from conditions that cause hyperinflation of the lungs, such as emphysema, the longest dimension of the cassette should be used in order to maximise available space for this hyperinflation.

Positioning

Cassette technique: direct exposure (including cassette with grid)

- A horizontal X-ray beam is centred over the midpoint of the cassette; the beam is collimated to the dimensions of the cassette; further collimation to account for patient size will be required once positioning is completed
- A lead rubber apron is applied to the patient's waist
- The anterior aspect of the chest is placed in contact with the cassette; the feet are slightly separated for stability
- The height of the cassette is adjusted until the whole of the thorax is included in its perimeter. Checking that the middle of C7 is level with the upper border of the cassette will ensure lung apices are included at the top of the image and ensure maximum cassette length is available for inclusion of costophrenic angles on the image. If an appropriate cassette size is used, this will also ensure that the midpoint of the chest lies relatively close to the middle of the cassette

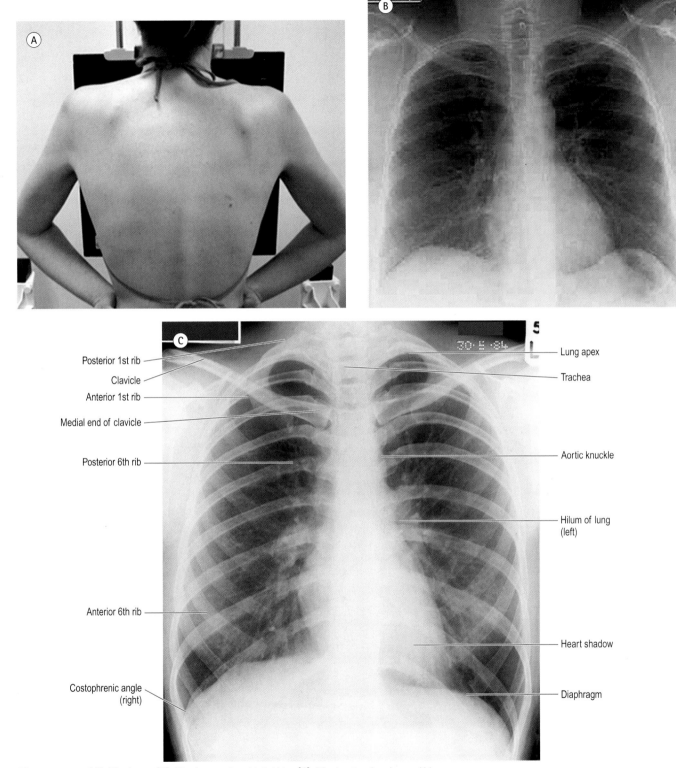

Posterior 1st rib
Clavicle
Anterior 1st rib
Medial end of clavicle
Posterior 6th rib
Anterior 6th rib
Costophrenic angle (right)

Lung apex
Trachea
Aortic knuckle
Hilum of lung (left)
Heart shadow
Diaphragm

Figure 25.3 **(A)** PA chest; **(B)** PA chest using high kVp; **(C)** PA chest using lower kVp

Bucky or digital technique system
- A lead rubber apron is applied to the patient's waist
- With the patient facing the image receptor and their chest in contact with it, the beam is collimated to the

patient's thorax; the centre of the image receptor is then centred to the central ray to ensure the thorax is included within the perimeter of the digital receptor. Adjustments may be necessary after positioning has been completed.

In dedicated digital chest units the central ray is often fixed as centred to the centre of the image receptor
- The patient's feet are separated slightly, for stability

All methods
- The patient leans forward and the chin is raised slightly; the chin is supported on the top of the cassette, if used
- The median sagittal plane (MSP) is coincident with the longitudinal midline of the cassette
- The MSP is perpendicular to the image receptor; this is checked by ensuring the sternoclavicular joints are equidistant from the image receptor
- The elbows are flexed and the backs of the hands are placed on the sides of the waist, resting on the lateral aspects of the iliac crests. The elbows are then gently pressed forwards towards the cassette, to clear the scapulae from the lung fields on the image. Ensure that the hands are actually on the lateral aspect of the waist as this maximises forward movement of the shoulders; positioning of the hands on the posterior aspect significantly reduces the range of forward movement
- A PA marker is most frequently used, on the upper aspect of the image receptor and usually on the opposite side to the area used for marking identification

Beam direction and FFD
Horizontal
2 m FFD

Centring
To the middle of the thorax and cassette, over the spinous process of T7 (body of T8)

Collimation
1st thoracic vertebra, 1st rib, lateral margins of ribs 2–10, costophrenic angles

---

Expose on arrested inspiration; maximum effort required

Before exposure the radiographer should check that the shoulders are not raised during the inspiratory effort, or that the arms and shoulders have not relaxed backwards. The time lapse between initially pressing the arms forward during positioning and exposure may seem relatively short, yet patients frequently, and usually imperceptibly, relax their arms enough to superimpose at least some scapular outline over the upper lung fields during this short time.

Criteria for assessing image quality
- 1st thoracic vertebra and 1st rib, lateral rib margins and costophrenic angles are demonstrated. The costophrenic angles must be demonstrated above the collimated field
- 3–5 cm of apical tissue is demonstrated above the clavicles
- Posterior aspect of the ribs are slightly inclined from the thoracic spine down towards their lateral borders
- Anterior aspects of the ribs are inclined more steeply than the posterior aspects, from their lateral borders down towards the midline
- Medial ends of the clavicles are equidistant from the midline of the thoracic vertebrae
- Scapulae are cleared from the lung fields
- 6 anterior or 9 posterior ribs are demonstrated above the diaphragms
- Sharp image demonstrating the vascular pattern of the lungs to the periphery in contrast to the air-filled lung tissue and dense structures of the hilae and mediastinum (heart, aorta). Trachea and proximal bronchi should be visible as should the retrocardiac lung and mediastinum. The thoracic vertebrae (intervertebral disc spaces) should be evident through the cardiac image. Diaphragms and costophrenic angles should be clearly seen. These exposure factor criteria relate to high kVp technique as outlined by EC 96 regulations.[7] For images produced with kVp lower than 85–90, penetration is assessed by checking that the spinous process of T4 is adequately seen in the midline as in Figure 25.3C. (Note that the patient position in Fig. 25.3C is superior to that in Fig. 25.3B.)

Adherence to quality standards outlined above are particularly important in the PA chest radiograph:

- *Poor inspiratory effort, lordosis and rotation* will all affect the accuracy of CT ratio assessment. *Rotation* will also cause hilar markings to appear to be more prominent on one side of the thorax and potentially mimic suggestion of pathology. Lung density in each lung will appear to be different in the rotated patient. A rotated position will also cause the mediastinum to appear widened and the trachea to appear shifted laterally.[4,19]
- It is vital to include *all* the outline of the whole of the costophrenic angle on each side, as a significant volume of 100 mL of pleural effusion may be present before blunting of the costophrenic angle will be demonstrated.[4] This is related to the fact that the diaphragm level sits lower on the posterior aspect of the thorax, in relationship to its anterior portion. Pleural fluid can collect in this lower posterior portion, before it is actually demonstrated in the anterior portion and on

the PA erect chest radiograph, when it is seen to cause blunting of the costophrenic angle as its earliest appearance.[19] Although the lateral radiograph is more sensitive than the PA when demonstrating pleural effusions, most often a good quality PA is the first indication that the lateral will be necessary.[19] It is therefore essential that the PA image includes the whole costophrenic angle to ensure the earliest radiographic signs of pleural effusion can be noted as soon as possible.

Common errors	Possible reasons
Medially positioned soft tissue shadow, between and/or overlying the apices	Chin not raised adequately
Apices inadequately cleared above the clavicles; posterior and anterior aspects of the ribs flattened	Patient is lordotic; i.e. not leaning forward towards the image receptor
Medial ends of the clavicles not seen at an equal distance from the thoracic vertebrae	Patient is rotated. The medial end of the clavicle furthest from the vertebrae corresponds to the side rotated away from the image receptor Any evidence of scoliosis? If the patient has scoliosis, it may not be possible to ensure the clavicle lie equidistant from the midline[20]
Scapulae overlying upper, lateral aspects of lung fields	Elbows and shoulders not pushed forward adequately, or patient has relaxed their arm position Patients with limited shoulder movement may not find it possible to fully comply with the required action; try extending the patient's arms in forward abduction, with internal rotation at the shoulder
Less than 6 anterior or 9 posterior ribs are demonstrated above the diaphragms	*Miscounted ribs*; check again. The first and second ribs cross over superiorly on the image and can sometimes be erroneously counted as one, rather than two ribs. Counting the thoracic vertebrae to identify posterior ribs confirms rib number *Poor inspiratory effort.* Obese patients or patients with dyspnoea may find improvement difficult Any evidence or history suggestive of infective or cardiac disease, lobar collapse, lobectomy, subphrenic abscess, phrenic nerve paralysis or upper abdominal mass? These are likely to affect diaphragm height and improvement may not be possible

■ AP erect chest (Figs 25.4, 25.5)

As in the PA projection, if used, cassette size for this projection is determined by patient size.

Positioning
- For a patient who can sit on a chair, the patient sits with their back to the image receptor (Fig. 25.4)
- For a patient who presents on a trolley the image receptor is placed in (a) the erect cassette holder or (b) supported by a large 45° pad which rests on the raised back of a trolley or bed (Fig. 25.5). This method may be used with a dedicated digital system if the patient can sit erect at the digital unit
- The posterior aspect of the chest is placed in contact with the image receptor

Cassette/independent digital plate technique: direct exposure (including cassette with grid for larger patients)
- The height of the image receptor is adjusted until the whole of the thorax is included in its perimeter. Ensuring that the 1st thoracic vertebra is below the upper border of the receptor will ensure lung apices are included at the top of the image

Bucky or digital technique system
- The patient sits, supported with their back against the image receptor
- The beam is collimated to the patient's thorax and its upper border positioned level with the upper border of T1; the centre of the image receptor is then centred to the central ray

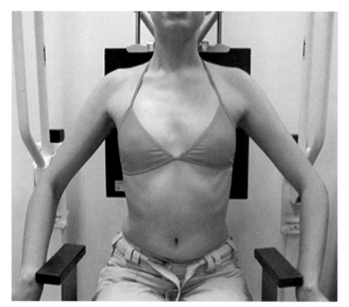

Figure 25.4   AP chest for patient in chair

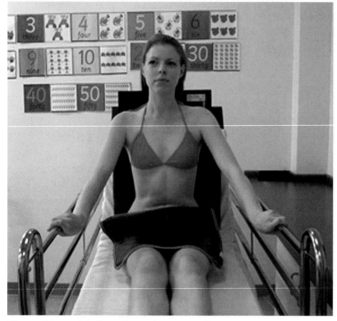

Figure 25.5   AP chest for patient on trolley

All methods

- A lead rubber apron is applied to the patient's waist
- A small radiolucent pad is placed behind the shoulders, to reproduce the slight elevation of the lung apices above the clavicles achieved in the PA position. The chin is raised slightly and the MSP is coincident with the longitudinal midline of the cassette
- MSP is perpendicular to the image receptor; this is checked by ensuring the sternoclavicular joints are equidistant from the receptor
- For the patient who is sitting on a chair, the elbows are flexed and the backs of the hands are placed on the

sides of the waist, resting on the lateral aspects of the iliac crests. The elbows are then gently pressed forwards towards the cassette, to clear the scapulae from the lung fields on the image. Some patients in bed or on a trolley may be able to achieve this position

- For patients unable to clear the scapulae by the above method, the arms are abducted and, if possible, rotated internally at the shoulders. Resting the forearms on the trolley or bed sides, whilst maintaining some internal rotation, is an effective method for achieving and maintaining this position
- An AP marker is used, on the upper aspect of the cassette and usually on the opposite side to the area outlined for identification
- If the patient has electrocardiogram (ECG) leads attached to their chest, or is using an oxygen mask, care must be taken to clear these artefacts from the field. ECG leads should leave the chest area by the 'shortest route' if they cannot be temporarily detached (Fig. 25.6)
- An 'erect AP' legend is applied next to the anatomical marker

Beam direction and FFD

Horizontal

2 m FFD

A caudal angle may be used to reduce the effect of lordosis if the patient unavoidably leans back. The angle

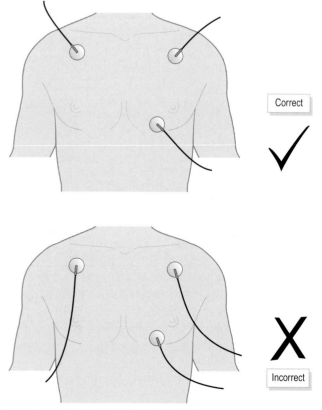

Figure 25.6   Position of ECG leads for chest radiography

should be selected by assessment of the degree of recumbence, although an example of approximately 5° has been suggested.[16] Use of such an angle should be considered carefully since significant deviation from the use of a horizontal beam may affect demonstration of fluid in the chest cavity.

Centring

To the middle of the thorax and image receptor (approximately midway between the sternal angle and xiphisternum)

Collimation

1st thoracic vertebra, 1st rib, lateral margins of ribs, costophrenic angles

> Expose on arrested inspiration; maximum effort required

Criteria for assessing image quality

Criteria are identical to those for the PA projection but it should be remembered that elevation of the apices above the clavicles may be less successful than on a PA image, despite use of the radiolucent pad suggested in the positioning description. There is the likelihood that there will still be some lordosis as it is tempting for the infirm patient to lean back, using the cassette for support. Elevation of the chin is often difficult for the infirm patient and is made more difficult if the thorax is tilted slightly forward by the radiolucent pad. Forward tilt will also cause some magnification of the upper thorax.

Lordosis is more likely to occur in the case of the bed- or trolley-bound patient, where the cassette is supported by a sponge and the legs of the patient extend forward, increasing the tendency of the thorax to lean back. The possibility of lordosis increases further when no pad is used or pillows are substituted for the pad. The potential risk of lordosis in the AP position does not validate approval of its presence on the image and maximum effort should be made to avoid its incidence.

Common errors (see also errors outlined under PA projection)	Possible reasons
Lordosis	Patient using cassette as support. If lordosis cannot be improved, a compensating caudal angle may be effective in reducing the effect
Soft tissue shadow over lower lung fields	Abdominal tissue may be superimposed; usually seen in lordotic patients on a trolley or bed

Supine AP chest

As in the PA or AP projection, cassette size for this projection is determined by patient size. Two people are required to facilitate safe manual handling whilst positioning the image receptor.

Positioning

- The patient's trunk is elevated from the bed or trolley and the cassette is placed underneath the chest. The top of the cassette should be level with the middle of C7
- The midline of the cassette should be coincident with the MSP, which is perpendicular to the cassette
- A lead rubber apron is applied over the abdomen, below the diaphragm
- A vertical X-ray beam is centred over the midpoint of the cassette
- The chin is raised slightly
- The arms are abducted and, if possible, rotated internally at the shoulders
- An AP marker is used, on the upper aspect of the cassette and usually on the opposite side to the area outlined for identification
- A 'supine AP' legend is applied next to the anatomical marker
- Artefacts should be moved as described for the AP erect projection

Beam direction and FFD

Vertical; however, a caudal angle of 5° will reduce the appearance of lordosis on the image
FFD as high as possible – up to a maximum of 2 m

Centring

To the middle of the thorax and cassette, as for erect AP chest

Collimation

1st thoracic vertebra, 1st rib, lateral margins of ribs 2–10, costophrenic angles

> Expose on arrested inspiration; maximum effort required

For patients on a ventilator it may be necessary to ask for suitably designated staff to facilitate suspension of respiration by controlling the ventilator.

Considerations for radiation protection

Although some patients will be examined in the supine position on a trolley in the imaging department, the majority of supine chest examinations are undertaken as mobile examinations on the ward, i.e. in a radiation supervised area rather than a controlled area. Therefore the radiographer's responsibility regarding radiation exposure is of paramount importance, particularly regarding protection of personnel and other patients in the vicinity.

Criteria for assessing image quality

Criteria are identical to those for the PA and AP projections, with the risk of lordosis similar to that for the AP projection. Suspension of adequate inspiration is likely to be more difficult in the case of the unconscious patient who is breathing independently, therefore a maximum attempt to achieve an adequately inspired, sharp image must be made.

Unfortunately it is often not possible to achieve the optimum FFD of 2 m for the supine projection, due to equipment or environment restrictions. This will cause magnification that is greater than for examinations undertaken at 2 m FFD. With the additional consideration of the fact that the heart is already magnified in the AP position, assessment of CT ratio is further compromised. The mediastinum will also appear enlarged.

▉ Lateral decubitus PA chest (Fig. 25.7)

This projection should be employed when it is vital that a horizontal beam is utilised in order to demonstrate pleural effusions; ultrasound can also be employed for confirmation or exclusion of this condition.[4] Occasionally small pneumothoraces require demonstration using this method.[14]

Cassette size is selected as for PA or AP projections.

Positioning

- The patient lies on a radiolucent pad *on their affected side*, to allow for the settlement of pleural fluid in the lateral portion of the lung. The patient lies *on their unaffected side* to allow the demonstration of air in the pleural cavity. The knees are flexed for comfort and stability and the arms raised to clear them from the area of interest and primary beam
- The image receptor is placed vertically in a portable erect holder, its long axis parallel to the long axis of the table-top, trolley or bed
- The anterior aspect of the chest is placed in contact with the image receptor and the position is adjusted until the whole of the thorax is included in its perimeter, with the 1st thoracic vertebra included. The MSP is coincident with the longitudinal midline of the receptor
- A lead rubber apron is applied to the patient's waist
- The chin is raised slightly to clear it from the lung apices. The MSP is perpendicular to the cassette; this is checked

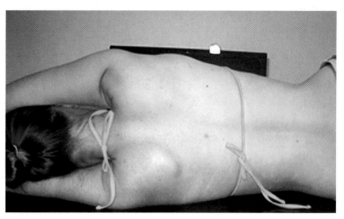

Figure 25.7 Lateral decubitus PA chest

by ensuring the sternoclavicular joints are equidistant from the cassette
- A PA marker is applied

Beam direction and FFD

Horizontal
2 m FFD

Centring

To the middle of the thorax and image receptor, over the spinous process of T7 (body of T8)

Collimation

1st thoracic vertebra, 1st rib, lateral margins of ribs 2–10, costophrenic angles

Criteria for assessing image quality

Criteria follow those for the PA erect chest. However, if the suspected pathologies outlined as reasons for use of this projection are found, it may not be necessary to repeat the examination in the case of rotation, poor inspiration, poor scapular clearance or lordosis. The most important criterion for this projection is that of inclusion of the whole area of interest, especially inclusion of the lateral border of the hemithorax related to the pathology in question.

▉ Lateral chest (Fig. 25.8A,B)

Unless there is known pathology related to a particular side of the chest, the PA projection should be examined to determine pathology site, prior to taking the decision to undertake this projection. Decision on the appropriate lateral is made on the basis that the side with the most significant pathological feature is selected as the aspect for positioning closest to the cassette.

Under no circumstances should a lateral projection be undertaken as 'routine' or without relevant clinical reason.

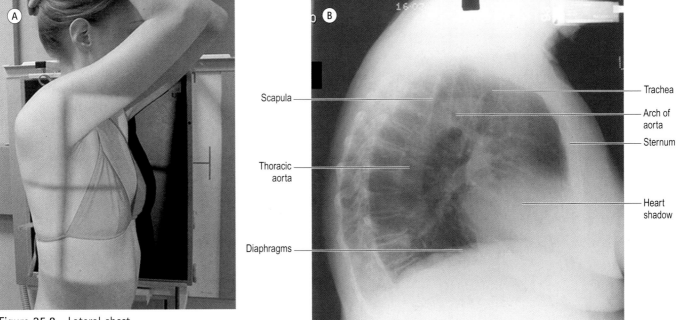

Scapula

Thoracic aorta

Diaphragms

Trachea

Arch of aorta

Sternum

Heart shadow

Figure 25.8   Lateral chest

EC guidelines, as for the PA chest, also recommend use of anti-scatter grid in conjunction with 125 kVp exposure technique and AEC device,[7] although this is not, as yet, widespread in practice. Commonly, a grid is only utilised for larger patients and kVp is often lower than 125.

Again, cassette size (if a cassette is used) should be assessed by the radiographer, and the range of suggested sizes is from 30 × 40 cm, 35^2 to 35 × 43 cm.

Positioning

Cassette technique: direct exposure (including cassette with grid)

- The cassette is placed in the erect cassette holder, its longer axis vertical
- A horizontal X-ray beam is centred over the midpoint of the cassette; the beam is collimated to the dimensions of the cassette. Further collimation to account for patient size will be required once positioning is completed
- A lead rubber apron is applied to the patient's waist
- The arms are raised and the lateral aspect of the chest is placed in contact with the image receptor
- The height of the cassette is adjusted until the top of the cassette is level with the top of the patient's shoulder

Bucky or digital technique system

- A lead rubber apron is applied to the patient's waist
- The arms are raised and the lateral aspect of the chest is placed in contact with the image receptor
- The beam is collimated to the patient's thorax, the top of the collimated field level with the top of the patient's shoulder

All methods

- The midline between the anterior and posterior chest walls is coincident with the vertical midline of the image receptor; the feet are slightly separated for stability
- The elbows are flexed and the hands clasped at the back of the head; the humeri are adducted medially until parallel. Upper arm tissue and humeri must be cleared from as much of the apices and upper lungs as possible
- A slight forwards tilt of the trunk will bring the thorax into a vertical position on the image
- The MSP is parallel to the cassette

Patients who cannot comply with the positioning described above can be examined with modifications listed in the following table.

Difficulty	Modification or adaptation
Patient cannot maintain position of raised arms, cannot raise arms or cannot flex elbows comfortably	Patient holds vertical structure with raised hands. Commonly a drip stand is used for this
Patient cannot stand	Projection can be undertaken using a stool or chair (Fig. 25.9)
Patient needs support at their back	A radiolucent pad can be placed behind the patient's back as in Figure 25.10

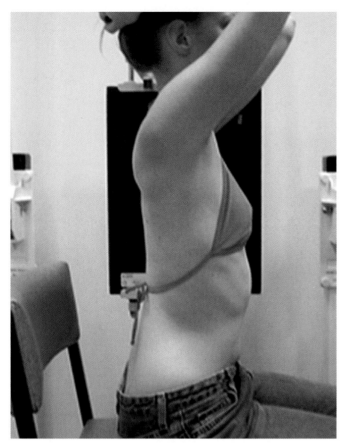

Figure 25.9   Lateral chest in chair

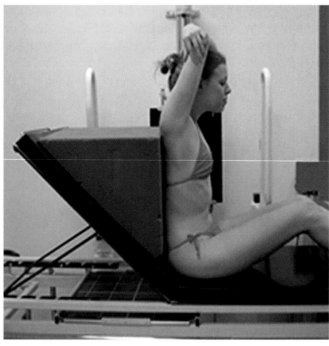

Figure 25.10   Lateral chest on trolley

Beam direction and FFD
Horizontal
2 m FFD

Centring
To the middle of the cassette

Collimation
Shoulder, sternum, spinous processes of thoracic vertebrae, posterior and anterior costophrenic angles

Criteria for assessing image quality
- Shoulder, sternum, spinous processes of thoracic vertebrae, posterior and anterior costophrenic angles are demonstrated
- Shoulder and soft tissue of upper arms overlying lung apices only
- Condyles on posterior aspect of thoracic vertebrae are superimposed; posterior aspect of ribs are superimposed
- Intervertebral joint spaces are clear
- Image of left diaphragm seen slightly above right
- T11 is demonstrated above the posterior diaphragm
- Sharp image demonstrating lung markings in contrast with the heart, aorta, air-filled trachea and ribs. The sternum, posterior heart border, diaphragms, anterior and posterior costophrenic angles and thoracic vertebrae should also be demonstrated

Common errors	Possible reasons
Non-superimposition of condyles of vertebral bodies; non-superimposition of posterior aspects of ribs	Rotation; MSP not parallel to cassette
Intervertebral joint spaces not cleared	Patient tilt; MSP not parallel to cassette or patient has scoliosis. PA chest image will confirm this
Pale shadow over upper lungs	Unavoidable at extreme upper lung area (apices); soft tissue shadow lower than this is almost certainly due to the upper arms dropping from their required position. Take care not to confuse the appearance with pathology

LUNG APICES

Suspected lesions in the lung apex may well be seen above the clavicle on a PA chest image but there is some risk that the clavicle itself will overlie some appearances. The lung apex can be cleared from the clavicle by one of the following methods:

1. With the patient initially AP or PA, the thorax is tilted in extreme lordosis, to elevate the clavicles above the lung apices. A horizontal beam is used (Figs 25.11A,B, 25.12)
2. With the patient initially PA, a horizontal beam is angled 30° caudally to project the lung apices below the clavicles (Fig. 25.13)
3. With the patient initially AP, a horizontal beam is angled 30° cranially to project the clavicles above lung apices. Selection of an appropriate method to clear the clavicles from the apices should be made after consideration of imaging principles and dose implications

Method 1 (lordotic AP or PA with horizontal beam)

The horizontal beam image has less distortion than methods using angulation but the AP position has implications for increased dose to the thyroid, eye lens, breast and sternum when compared to the PA position. In the AP position the patient can lean back onto the cassette for support but, unless there are suitable structures for the patient to hold onto, the PA method can be unstable. In the AP position the apical region is closer to the cassette, whereas there is increased lung apex to film distance in the PA position which has implications for magnification unsharpness of the area. An air gap will also exist, requiring some increase in exposure. However, the air gap will have the effect of some reduction in scatter and therefore improved image quality.

Method 2 (PA position with 30° caudal angulation)

Benefits of using the PA position are as those for method 1 but the 30° angulation will cause some image distortion.

Method 3 (AP position with 30° cranial angulation)

Disadvantages of using the AP position are as those outlined in method 1 but in addition to this the angulation will cause some image distortion as in method 2. Since the angle is directed cranially, this has implications for the dose to the lenses of the eyes and thyroid which is greater than those for AP method 1.

This method will be more acceptable to patients who cannot comply with requirements for sitting or standing in a PA position, as for the routine chest PA projection. It can be used in the supine position, with a vertical central ray directed 30° cranially.

A lordotic projection can also be used to demonstrate right middle lobe collapse, using the PA position described in method 1, and a full-sized cassette as for the routine PA chest projection, centring at the level of T8.

Apparent lesions adequately seen above the clavicle on the PA projection can be demonstrated in a different plane by utilising a lordotic apical projection, since information on lung apices cannot be gleaned from a lateral chest image. Use of beam angulation will provide a more distorted image and is therefore of limited value. Current recommendation for investigation of suspicious lesions in this region is for CT investigation, whenever readily available.

Exposure factors

Since the apices are not overshadowed by dense structures, such as the mediastinum, in apical projections, it is not necessary to utilise a high kVp technique or anti-scatter grid. Selection of lower kVp will help reduce scatter and increase contrast quality. The projections should be well collimated which will reduce dose and therefore also ensure optimum contrast by assisting with scatter reduction.

▪ Lung apices: AP lordotic (Fig. 25.11A,B)

If used, a 24 × 30 cm cassette is placed transversely in the erect cassette holder.

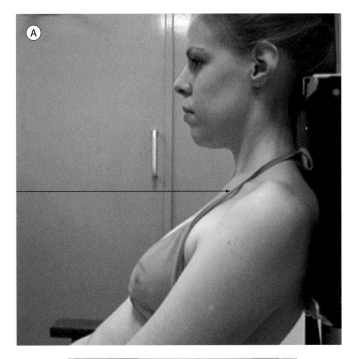

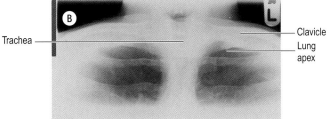

Figure 25.11   AP lung apices with lordosis

Positioning

- A horizontal X-ray beam is centred over the midpoint of the image receptor; the beam is collimated to the dimensions of the cassette, or lung apices with the patient sitting with their back to the image receptor
- A lead rubber apron is applied to the anterior aspect of the patient's waist
- The patient initially sits erect in the AP position, with their seat approximately 25–35 cm from the image receptor. Distance varies according to patient height; taller patients will need to sit further away than shorter patients
- The patient leans back to rest the backs of their shoulders upon the image receptor; the clavicle should lie horizontally level with the C7/T1 region
- The cassette, if used, is adjusted until its midpoint lies level with the sternal angle
- The MSP is coincident with the midline of the image receptor
- The sternoclavicular joints are equidistant from the image receptor
- Scapular clearance is required as for the PA chest projection
- An AP marker is used

Beam direction and FFD

Horizontal

2 m FFD

However, magnification reduction is not as great an issue as in the full PA chest projection, since the CT ratio is not relevant to the projection.

Centring

To the middle of the cassette, if used *or* over the sternal angle for the digital plate receptor

A visual check that the shadow of the upper border of the soft tissue above the shoulder and clavicle lies within the light beam field will ensure that the top of the lung apices are included.

Collimation

Upper border of T1, clavicles, lung apices, lateral borders of ribs 1–5, 5th thoracic vertebra

▉ Lung apices: PA lordotic (Fig. 25.12)

If used, a 24 × 30 cm cassette is placed transversely in the erect cassette holder.

Positioning

- *Cassette:* A horizontal X-ray beam is centred over the midpoint of the cassette and the beam is collimated to its dimensions

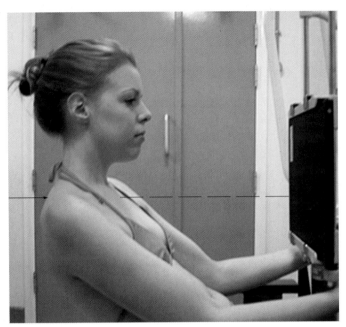

Figure 25.12   PA lung apices with lordosis

- *Digital plate:* Collimate to the lung apices, with the patient sitting with their back to the X-ray tube and facing the image receptor
- A lead rubber apron is applied to the posterior aspect of the patient's waist
- The patient initially sits erect in the PA position, with their seat directly in front of the image receptor
- The patient leans back, away from the image receptor, until their clavicles lie horizontally level with the C7/T1 region
- The patient holds onto the unit, bucky housing or handles for stability
- The cassette height is adjusted until its midpoint is level with the sternal angle
- If a digital system is used the beam should be centred at this point in the examination (see below), then is further collimated from the initial settings, to include the upper border of T1, lateral borders of ribs 1–5 and the 5th thoracic vertebra
- The MSP is coincident with the midline of the cassette
- The sternoclavicular joints are equidistant from the cassette
- Scapular clearance is required
- A PA marker is used

Beam direction and FFD

Horizontal

2 m FFD

In contrast to the AP method, this distance is essential in order to reduce magnification and unsharpness.

Centring

Cassette: to the midline of the patient, to emerge through the sternal angle and coincident with the midline of the cassette
Digital plate: to the midline of the patient, to emerge through the sternal angle

Collimation

Upper border of T1, clavicles, lung apices, lateral borders of ribs 1–5, 5th thoracic vertebra

For both the PA and AP lordotic projections of the apices, a visual check that the shadow of the upper border of the soft tissue above the shoulder and clavicle lies within the light beam field will ensure that the top of the lung apices are included.

◼ Lung apices: PA with 30° caudal angulation
(Fig. 25.13)

Most dedicated digital chest units have a fixed central ray which is perpendicular to the image receptor; this method, and the AP with cranial angulation, is therefore unsuitable for use with this type of unit.

If used, a 24 × 30 cm cassette is placed transversely in the erect cassette holder.

Positioning

- A lead rubber apron is applied to the posterior aspect of the patient's waist
- The patient sits erect in the PA position and the image receptor is adjusted until its midpoint lies level with the sternal notch; the MSP is coincident with the midline of the image receptor
- The sternoclavicular joints are equidistant from the image receptor
- Scapular clearance is required
- A PA marker is used

Beam direction and FFD

Initially horizontal, which is then directed 30° caudally
2 m FFD

Centring

Over the vertebral column, to emerge at the sternal notch

Collimation

Upper border of T1, clavicles, lung apices, lateral borders of ribs 1–5, 5th thoracic vertebra

A visual check that the shadow of the upper border of the soft tissue above the shoulder and clavicle lies within the light beam field will ensure that the top of the lung apices are included.

◼ Lung apices: AP with 30° cranial angulation (Fig. 25.14)

If used, a 24 × 30 cm cassette is placed transversely in the erect cassette holder.

Positioning

- A lead rubber apron is applied to the anterior aspect of the patient's waist

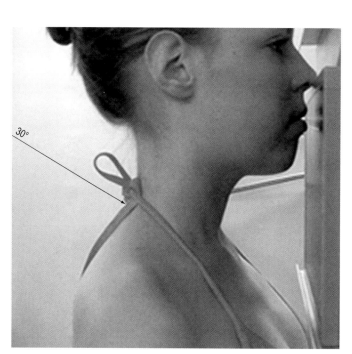

Figure 25.13 PA lung apices with 30° caudal angulation

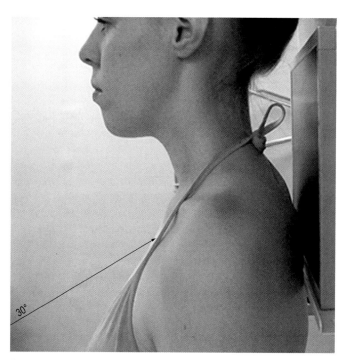

Figure 25.14 AP lung apices with 30° cranial angulation

- The patient sits erect in the AP position and the cassette, if used, is adjusted until its midpoint lies level with the sternal angle; the MSP is coincident with the midline of the image receptor
- The sternoclavicular joints are equidistant from the image receptor
- Scapular clearance is required
- An AP marker is used

Beam direction and FFD
Initially horizontal, which is then directed 30° cranially
1 m FFD

Centring
To the sternal angle

Collimation
Upper border of T1, clavicles, lung apices, lateral borders of ribs 1-5, 5th thoracic vertebra

A visual check that the shadow of the upper border of the soft tissue above the shoulder and clavicle lies within the light beam field will ensure that the top of the lung apices are included.

All methods

> Expose on arrested inspiration

Criteria for assessing image quality
- Upper border of T1, clavicles, lung apices, lateral borders of ribs 1–5 and 5th thoracic vertebra are demonstrated on the image
- Clavicles cleared above the top of the lung apices

Common errors	Possible reasons
Overall image density low	Insufficient exposure given; the projection requires an increase from that used for the PA projection as the beam travels through an increased thickness due to lordosis or beam angulation. If PA lordotic method used, has the increased air gap been considered?
One lung apex more dense than the other	Rotation
Clavicles overlying lung apices	Lordosis or beam angle is insufficient

- Flattened appearance of the ribs
- Medial ends of clavicles equidistant from the midline of the thoracic vertebrae
- Scapulae cleared from the lung fields

OBLIQUE PROJECTIONS OF THE CHEST

Prior to the widespread use of CT, oblique projections of the chest were valuable for demonstration of the estimated 40% of lung tissue obscured by dense structures in the chest.[21] In addition, oblique projections can be used to demonstrate the mediastinum, heart and great vessels, trachea, hilae and pleural plaques evident in cases of mesothelioma.

■ 45° anterior oblique chest (RAO, LAO)
(Fig. 25.15A,B,C,D)

If used, cassette size for this examination is selected after consideration of patient build and size. It is recommended that cassettes are used in the vertical cassette holder or bucky, with vertical orientation unless a 35^2 cassette is used.

Positioning
- A horizontal X-ray beam is centred over the midpoint of the image receptor

Cassette technique
- The beam is collimated to the dimensions of the cassette; further collimation to account for patient size will be required once positioning is completed

Digital technique
- The beam is collimated to the size of the patient's thorax, with the patient standing either with the back or the front of their chest in contact with the receptor

All techniques
- A lead rubber apron is applied to the patient's waist
- The image receptor height is adjusted until the midpoint is level with the patient's 8th thoracic vertebra
- From a PA position, with their MSP perpendicular to the image receptor, the patient rotates 45° to the left for the RAO or 45° to the right for the LAO projection
- The feet are slightly separated for stability
- The arms are raised at the sides of the head and then flexed at the elbows; the forearms are then rested across the top of the head. This clears the arms from the field

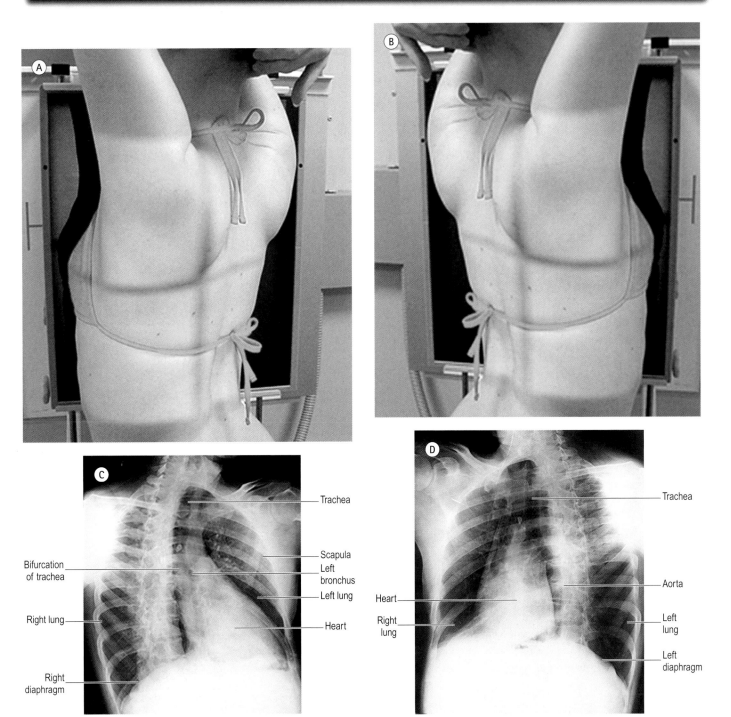

Figure 25.15   (A) RAO chest; (B) LAO chest; (C) RAO chest; (D) LAO chest. (C) and (D) Reproduced with permission from Ballinger PW, Frank ED. Merrill's atlas of radiographic positioning and radiologic procedures. 10th edn. St Louis: Mosby; 2003

- Without leaning forward, the patient is immobilised by resting the shoulder nearest the image receptor on the upper part of the receptor
- A PA marker is most frequently used, on the upper aspect of the image receptor. An RAO should bear a right marker and an LAO a left marker, which should always lie above the side nearest the cassette

Beam direction and FFD

Horizontal

2 m FFD

Centring

To the middle of the image receptor, at the level of the spinous process of T7 (body of T8), midway between the vertebral column and the lateral borders of ribs on the side furthest from the cassette

Collimation

1st thoracic vertebra, 1st rib, lateral margins of ribs 2–10, costophrenic angles

Criteria for assessing image quality

- 1st thoracic vertebra and 1st rib, all rib outlines and diaphragms are demonstrated
- Arms are cleared from the lung fields
- Vertebral column shown closer to the lateral border of the thorax on the side positioned nearest the cassette
- Heart shown in its entirety over the vertebral column and side positioned furthest from the cassette
- 7 anterior ribs are demonstrated above the diaphragms. These should be counted on the side positioned nearest to the cassette
- Sharp image demonstrating the dense mediastinal structures in contrast with air-filled lungs

Common errors	Possible reasons
Heart shadow slightly overlapping onto side nearest cassette	Less than 45° rotation on the thorax
Appearance of space between heart shadow and vertebral column on side furthest from cassette	More than 45° rotation on the thorax

◼ Other anterior oblique chest positions

The 45° obliques described are probably the most useful obliques in the 21st century, since they are most appropriate for a general oblique survey of the chest and adequate for demonstration of pleural plaques when ongoing assessment may not require CT at every stage. Other obliques are suggested for demonstration of more specific structures:

1. Trachea, great vessels and cardiac outline will best be seen with a greater angle of rotation (60°) on the RAO projection.[13,16] The structures are seen well clear of the vertebral column, as is the descending aorta
2. Bifurcation of the trachea and arch of aorta can be demonstrated by use of a 70° rotation on the LAO projection.[13] Structures are seen cleared from the vertebral column but the descending aorta is seen to overlie it

THORACIC INLET

The trachea can appear as deviated or compressed on plain radiographic images, due to tumour or thyroid goitre. It can also deviate from the midline towards the side of lobar collapse on AP or PA projections. Rotation when positioning the patient will cause apparent deviation of the trachea from the midline. In the 21st century, examination of the area covered by the thoracic inlet is largely undertaken by MRI, CT or RNI studies

◼ PA thoracic inlet (Fig. 25.16A,B)

If used, a 23 × 30 cm cassette is used lengthwise in the erect cassette holder for this projection.

Positioning

- A lead rubber apron is applied to the patient's waist
- The patient faces the image receptor; the feet are slightly separated for stability
- The MSP is coincident with, and perpendicular to, the long axis of the image receptor
- The height of the cassette, if used, is adjusted until its centre is level with the sternal notch
- The chin is raised until the occiput and mandible are superimposed, to maximise the amount of upper trachea demonstrated on the image
- A PA marker is most frequently used, on the upper aspect of the cassette or image receptor

Beam direction and FFD

Horizontal
100 cm FFD

Centring

To the centre of the cassette, if used, through T2 to emerge through the sternal notch

---

Expose on arrested inspiration or Valsalva manoeuvre
The Valsalva manoeuvre is forced exhalation against a closed upper airway; i.e. not actually exhaling but forcing air from the lungs into a closed mouth and nasal passage. It has been likened to the bearing down action of defaecation. The action serves to fill the trachea with air in order to provide a contrast with the soft tissues surrounding it.

Use of the Valsalva manoeuvre has traditionally been advocated for use with projections of the thoracic inlet but this action may be difficult whilst asking the patient to maintain a particular position. It must therefore be suggested that the Valsalva manoeuvre is exercised with caution on the patient who is standing erect. It must also be considered that, since the trachea is a structure that does not naturally rest with closed walls, as in the case of the oesophagus, it will in fact always contain air even if the patient's lungs are not in an inspirational phase. So, for lower thoracic inlet demonstration, is the Valsalva maneouvre actually necessary?

Collimation

C4–T6 longitudinally, lateral soft tissue outlines of the neck

Criteria for assessing image quality

- Trachea down to its bifurcation and lateral soft tissue outlines of the neck are demonstrated
- Spinous processes of vertebrae and the trachea are demonstrated down the centre of the vertebral bodies and medial ends of clavicles equidistant from the spinous process
- Mandible and occiput are superimposed

- Sharp image demonstrating air-filled trachea in contrast to the soft tissue of neck and vertebral column

Common errors	Possible reasons
Symmetrical dense white shadow of occiput obscuring upper trachea	Chin raised too high
Symmetrical shadow of mandible obscuring upper trachea	Chin not raised enough
Asymmetrical shadow of occiput and/or mandible superimposed over upper neck	Head is rotated. If appearances are accompanied by rotation of the trunk (see next comments on line below) the whole of the MSP is incorrectly positioned
Trachea not centralised over vertebral column	MSP not perpendicular to image receptor or some deviation may be due to external common compression (for example in cases of thyroid enlargement). This, of course, is not due to radiographer error

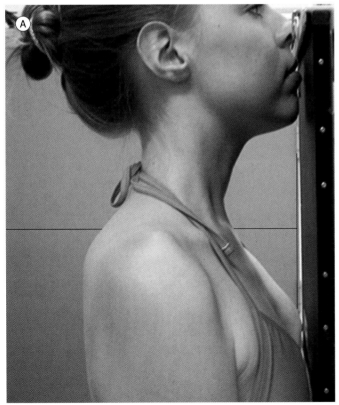
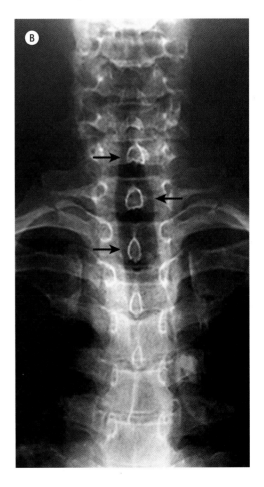

Figure 25.16 PA thoracic inlet. **(B)** the arrows outline the lateral margins of the air-filled trachea. (B) Reproduced with permission from Ballinger PW, Frank ED. Merrill's atlas of radiographic positioning and radiologic procedures. 10th edn. St Louis: Mosby; 2003

Lateral upper respiratory tract and thoracic inlet
(Fig. 25.17A,B)

If used, a 23 × 30 cm cassette is placed lengthwise in the erect cassette holder for this projection.

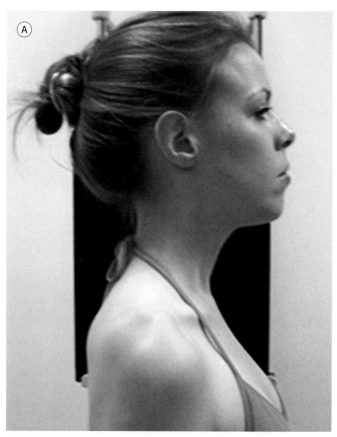

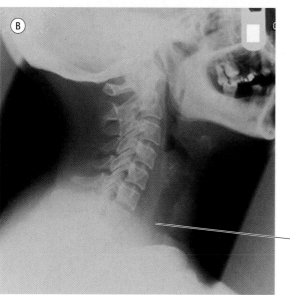

Air-filled trachea

Figure 25.17   Lateral upper respiratory tract

Positioning
- A lead rubber apron is applied to the patient's waist
- The patient stands erect with their MSP parallel to the image receptor; the feet are slightly separated for stability. This projection may be undertaken with the patient sitting
- The height of the cassette, if used, is adjusted until its centre is level with the thyroid eminence
- The chin is raised until the mandible is cleared as far as possible from the upper trachea
- The shoulders are relaxed downwards to clear them from the inlet into the thorax

Beam direction and FFD
Horizontal

200 cm FFD. This is an increase from the 100 cm used for the PA projection. It aims to reduce magnification of the trachea which lies further from the cassette due to the shoulder's position against the cassette or image receptor

Centring
To the middle of the neck, at the level of the thyroid eminence

Collimation
Nasopharynx and down to include medial end of clavicle, anterior soft tissue outline, vertebral bodies of cervical vertebrae, T1

Good collimation, avoiding irradiation of the orbits, can be improved by slightly rotating the light beam diaphragm so that its long axis follows the angle of the neck.

> Expose on arrested inspiration

Criteria for assessing image quality
- Nasopharynx, oropharynx, upper trachea, medial end of clavicle and anterior aspect of soft tissues of neck are demonstrated
- Mandible is elevated to clear it from as much of the trachea as possible (but there will still be some superimposition)
- Sharp image demonstrating air-filled trachea in contrast to the soft tissue of the neck. The vertebral column will be underpenetrated

Common error	Possible reason
Soft tissue shadow obscuring clavicle and trachea	Poor patient posture during exposure (shoulders not relaxed). This may be a problem with kyphosed patients

Lateral lower trachea and thoracic inlet (Fig. 25.18A,B,C)

If used, a 23 × 30 cm cassette is placed lengthwise in the erect bucky for this projection. A cassette with a station- ary grid may also be used in the erect cassette holder.

Positioning
• A lead rubber apron is applied to the patient's waist

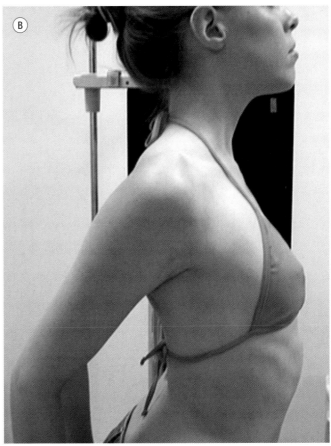

Figure 25.18 Lateral lower trachea and thoracic inlet with **(A)** arms raised and **(B)** arms pulled back; **(C)** lateral lower trachea and thoracic inlet

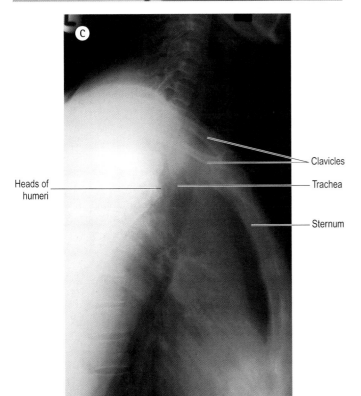

Clavicles

Trachea

Heads of humeri

Sternum

- The patient stands erect with their MSP parallel to the image receptor; the feet are slightly separated for stability. This projection may be undertaken with the patient sitting
- The position of the cassette, if used, is adjusted until its middle is level with the sternal angle and midline coincident with the long axis of the neck
- The arms are extended and raised either side of the head, until vertical. The chin is raised to further effect this manoeuvre, which aims to clear the humeral heads from the retrosternal area of the trachea

The method described for clearance of humeral heads from the area of interest may seem contrary to those previously described,[13] where the hands are clasped behind the back and the shoulders pulled back (Fig. 25.18B). This method is difficult for many patients, particularly those with degenerative disease of the joints and for some who are overweight. The method using raised arms has previously been suggested as an alternative for patients with stiff shoulders[12] and is a viable first choice due to its easy implementation. It must be remembered, however, that failure to raise the chin adequately and bring the arms vertical will limit effectiveness of the manoeuvre.

Beam direction and FFD
Horizontal
200 cm FFD. As for the lateral of the upper region, this FFD is selected to counteract magnification caused by increased object film distance (OFD)

Centring
Below the sternal notch, at the level of the sternal angle

Collimation
Thyroid eminence and carina of trachea, soft tissue anterior to trachea in neck and thorax, bodies of cervical vertebrae, lung tissue posteriorly

It is important that the whole of the trachea is demonstrated by the combination of the two lateral projections described for the trachea and thoracic inlet. As a result, the crossover area which is that of the inlet of the trachea into the thorax level with the sternal notch, must be seen adequately on both images. Since two exposures are made this has implications for dose to the patient; it is possible to undertake one projection of the whole area, using a high kVp technique and suggested centring at the level of C6–C7 whilst collimating to include the whole of the trachea.[16]

Expose on arrested inspiration

Criteria for assessing image quality
- Trachea from above the sternal notch down to its bifurcation, manubrium sterni, lung tissue anterior and posterior to the trachea are demonstrated
- Soft tissue of shoulders and heads of humerii are cleared from the trachea
- Sharp image demonstrating air-filled trachea in contrast to the lung tissue, clavicle and manubrium

Common error	Possible reason
Density overlying trachea on image	Arms and shoulders inadequately raised or not pulled back

References
1. Manning D, Cooper A. Chest X-ray image quality: relationships between physical measurements and observer grading. Radiography Today 1993; 59(678):12–15.
2. The Ionising Radiation (Medical Exposure) Regulations 2000. London: HMSO; 2000.
3. Radiation Protection 118. Referral Guidelines for Imaging. European Commission: Luxembourg; 2000.
4. Scally P. Medical imaging. Oxford: Oxford University Press; 1999.
5. World Health Organisation Report. Global tuberculosis control. Geneva: WHO; 2003.
6. Walford D, Noah N. Emerging infectious diseases– United Kingdom. Center for Disease Control–Prevention 1999; 5:298.
7. European Commission. European guidelines on quality criteria for diagnostic radiographic images. Brussels: Office for Official Publications of the European Communities; 1996.
8. Sjovall A. (*Correspondence*) PA chest films. British Journal of Radiology 1982; 55:168.
9. Smith RF. (*Correspondence*) Radiography. 1982; April:80.
10. Dimmick R. (*Correspondence*) Radiography. 1981 March:79.
11. Clark KC. Positioning in radiography. 4th to 10th edns. London: Heinemann;1945–1979.
12. Unett EM, Royle AJ. 1997. Radiographic techniques and image evaluation. London: Chapman and Hall; 1997.
13. Swallow RA, et al. Clark's positioning in radiography. 11th edn. London: Heinemann; 1986.
14. Ballinger PW, Frank ED. Merrill's atlas of radiographic positioning and radiologic procedures, 10th edn. St Louis: Mosby; 2003.
15. Watkins P. A practical guide to chest imaging. Edinburgh: Churchill Livingstone; 1984.
16. Bontrager K, Lampignano JP. Textbook of radiographic positioning and related anatomy. 6th edn. St Louis: Mosby; 2005.

17. Unett E, Carver B. The chest X-ray: centring points and central rays – can we stop confusing our students and ourselves? Synergy 2001; Nov:14–17.
18. Unett E, Carver B. The chest X-ray: centring points and central rays – can we stop confusing our students and ourselves? Synergy 2001; Dec:8–9.
19. Meholic A, et al. Fundamentals of chest radiology. Philadelphia: WB Saunders; 1996.
20. McQuillen Martensen K. Radiographic critique. Philadelphia: WB Saunders; 1995.
21. Chotas H, Ravin C. Chest radiography: estimated lung volume and projected area obscured by the heart, mediastinum and diaphragm. Radiology 1994; 193:403–404.

ABDOMEN

Elizabeth Carver

Plain radiography of the abdomen is often used for assessment of gross anatomical deviation, such as displacement of organs in the case of abdominal tumours or obstruction of the alimentary tract. Provision of information on the urinary system can be given by the plain abdomen image, preceding other imaging procedures, also providing information on gross anatomical deviation within the urinary system. Appearance of radiopaque calculi will be demonstrated on the image but urography, ultrasound, RNI or CT will be required to provide information on renal function, site of urinary obstruction or extent of obstruction.

▌ Supine abdomen (Figs 26.1, 26.2)

If used, a 35 × 43 cm cassette is placed in the table bucky *or,* in the case of trolley-bound patients, in the trolley cassette tray (with stationary grid).

Positioning
- The patient is supine with the arms slightly abducted from the trunk
- The median sagittal plane (MSP) is coincident with the long axis of the table and the centre of the bucky
- Lead rubber or lead gonad protection is applied, below the symphysis pubis, to male gonads
- ASIS are equidistant from the table-top
  (a) The iliac crests are level with the middle of the image receptor *or:*
  (b) Using the calibrated markings on the light beam diaphragm, collimate to the cassette size and orientation selected; in the case of most adult patients a 35 × 43 cm cassette is placed longitudinally in the bucky tray. With digital units collimate to a maximum field size of 43 × 43 cm. For both, ensure that the lower edge of collimation lies just below the lower border of the symphysis pubis
- Because of magnification, due to the significant distance from the symphysis pubis to the image receptor, the symphysis pubis should lie well above the lower boundary of the image receptor
- Central ray and the middle of the image receptor should be accurately aligned

Beam direction and focus film distance (FFD)
Vertical, at 90° to the cassette
FFD 100–120 cm, selected to ensure magnification is at its minimum and include the maximum amount of abdominal tissue on the image

Centring
For positioning (a) over a point in the midline of the abdomen, level with the iliac crests. Note that this point refers to the actual *highest point of the crests at the back*, rather than the lower level palpated on the lateral aspect of the abdomen
Positioning for (b) is to the centre of the cassette
  The midline of the abdomen, or MSP, can be identified by palpating the middle of the upper border of the symphysis pubis and the xiphisternum. The line joining these surface markings will represent the position of the MSP.

Collimation
Symphysis pubis, as much upper abdomen as possible, lateral soft tissue outlines

Comments on centring, collimation and area of interest
It has been stated that the 11th thoracic vertebra should be included in the collimated field since it lies above the renal outlines, and at the tip of the right lower lobe of

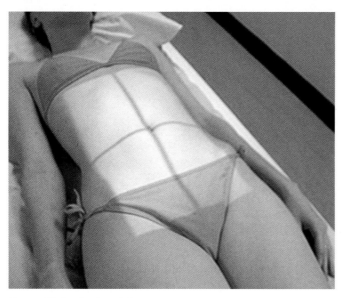

Figure 26.1 Supine abdomen

liver and spleen.[1] It is noted that this would not usually allow for the inclusion of all the upper abdominal contents in most adults; however, with the exception of examination of the upper gastrointestinal (GI) tract, ultrasound is the most appropriate imaging modality for the upper abdomen. This would negate the necessity for the inclusion of abdominal tissue immediately below the diaphragm. When the supine abdomen position is used to demonstrate the kidneys, ureter and bladder (KUB), and additional abdominal information is not required, lateral collimation can be made to the ASIS on each side to more effectively reduce radiation dose.

Traditionally a specific centring point has been given when describing the anteroposterior (AP) supine abdomen. This has usually been stated as level with the iliac crests in the midline, as in centring 'a' above.[2] Unfortunately, the continuing trend for an increase in average height, noted especially in Europe and the western world and estimated

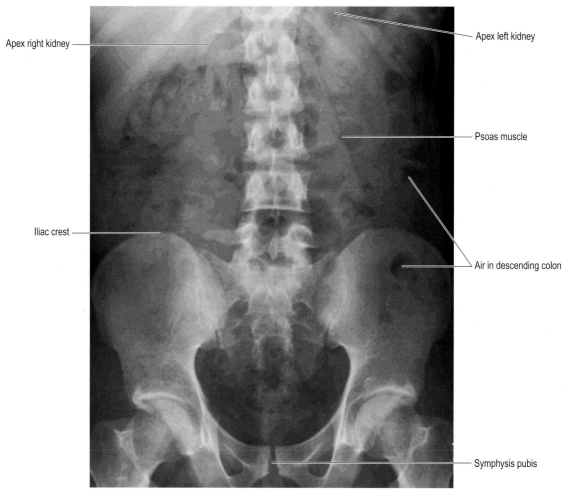

Figure 26.2 Supine abdomen

currently to be increasing by between 10 and 30 mm per decade,[3] is likely to have begun to affect the amount of body tissue which can realistically be included on the image. Although the iliac crests do appear midway between the diaphragms and symphysis pubis on the image, centring point 'a' will only be useful in smaller patients, i.e. those whose abdominal tissue will actually 'fit' within the maximum (43 cm) receptor length. Selection of the centring point/positioning method will therefore depend upon the radiographer's assessment of the patient's size.

An additional complication occurs with larger patients, whose adipose tissue will cause further elevation of the symphysis pubis above the table-top; this increases the effect of magnification, potentially adding to the risk of the image of the symphysis being projected below the lower border of the film. Using the second suggested method of centring will reduce the risk of projecting the symphysis pubis off the lower end of the image in these cases.

Compensation for magnification may be made by increasing the FFD[4] but this may still not be effective for very tall patients. Unfortunately in these cases it may be necessary to undertake an additional projection of the upper abdomen if this area is essential for inclusion in the examination. Indeed, it has been suggested that the hypersthenic patient requires two, separately centred, radiographic exposures using two 35 × 43 cm cassettes placed crosswise in the bucky.[5] This does seem somewhat excessive and would result in a higher radiation dose to the patient than undertaking an additional, well-collimated, upper abdomen projection.

When considering the issue of the increase in average height of a population, if larger image receptors, cassettes, films, buckys and cassette trays/holders were made available in the future, the issues raised in this discussion would be easily addressed and result in the reduction of unnecessary additional radiation exposure to the patient. At present, digital plates available have a maximum size of 43 × 43 cm; this provides an increase in size across the width from the conventional 35 × 43 cm cassette, but an increase in length is clearly necessary.

> Expose on arrested respiration during exposure

Clearly, exposure must be made on arrested respiration to reduce the risk of movement unsharpness on the image, caused by the shift of abdominal organs during diaphragmatic movement. There exists a range of recommendations on phase of respiration to suspend[1,6] and questions regarding the most appropriate choice arise from this. Suspension of respiration after exhalation cannot be excluded since it facilitates lower density of abdominal tissue, necessitating selection of lower exposure factors and therefore reducing dose when compared to exposure in the opposite phase of respiration. Unfortunately, when this issue is considered alongside that of the tall patient, as previously discussed in this chapter, it can be argued that exhalation will exacerbate the problems of inclusion of the whole required area on the image.

Therefore the concept of exposure on arrested inspiration to compress abdominal contents into an apparently shorter area may become more acceptable since it reduces the area covered by the abdominal contents (i.e. the area from the diaphragm to the symphysis pubis), increasing the chance of a single exposure examination. This is clearly an opportunity for the reflective practitioner to base their decision on practice using a benefit versus risk approach.

Criteria for assessing image quality

- Symphysis pubis, as much of the upper abdomen as possible, and lateral soft tissue outlines of the abdomen are included on image
- Spinous processes of vertebrae seen coincident with the midline of the image and centralised and aligned down the middle of the vertebral bodies
- Symmetry of the iliac crests
- Sharp image demonstrating soft tissue in contrast with bowel gas and bony structures

Note that scoliosis will affect symmetry of the vertebral column and position of the vertebrae coincident with the long axis of the film. It is distinguishable from rotation due to position error by the distinct lateral curve of the column and potential variation of rotation down its length.[1] If inclusion of the relevant body area on the image is acceptable, a repeat should not be considered. In the case of positional rotation it must be remembered that correction will be possible and will improve accuracy in the appearance of organ position within the abdominal cavity.

Common errors	Possible reasons
Symphysis pubis is not included on the image	Inaccurate centring/positioning *Or tall patient?*; centring point at the level of the iliac crests may have been used. (Try centring method 'b')
Upper abdomen is not included; symphysis pubis is well above the lower edge of the film	May have been centred using the lateral borders of iliac crest rather than the highest point at the back
Vertebral column is not coincident with the midline of the film	Xiphisternum to symphysis line is inaccurately positioned *or* scoliotic patient
Spinous processes are not demonstrated in the midline of the vertebral bodies	MSP is not perpendicular to the table-top; palpate ASIS to ensure it is equidistant from the table *or* the patient is scoliosed

Erect abdomen

Validity of use of this projection

The erect abdomen has traditionally been requested to diagnose/exclude obstruction of the bowel, alimentary perforation or the effects of stab injury. The erect position allows air to rise, above fluid levels in the obstructed bowel where the inferior level of the air shadow appears flat, or under the right diaphragm in cases of perforation. Towards the close of the 20th century, the validity of requests for the erect abdomen examination began to be questioned as it was recognised that other projections demonstrate appearances suggestive of obstruction or perforation. More specifically, in the case of the supine acute abdomen, these appearances are:[7]

- *Sentinel loop sign:* an isolated loop of distended bowel indicates the effects of inflammatory processes such as appendicitis or pancreatitis, causing ileus
- *Dilated small bowel loops:* indicate small bowel obstruction. Loops are centrally sited and there is absence of faecal matter; eventually the distal bowel becomes airless as it collapses but the stomach may still contain air. Air in the distended small bowel may appear as a ladder or stack of coins
- *Dilated colon:* points to obstruction. Dilation of the colon with air is noted, up to the site of obstruction. The bowel is much distended, with distended haustra and the appearances are notable around the edges of the abdomen, rather than the more centralised loops as in the case of the obstructed small bowel
- *Volvulus:* obstruction appears as a distended portion of looped bowel. The obstruction is caused by the closed ends of the loop, which may have a 'coffee bean' appearance

As the right diaphragm lies at a higher level than the left, in cases of perforation, gas or air in the peritoneal cavity will rise to lie under the right diaphragm. The appearance is that of a dark line under the diaphragm, often following its curve, created by the contrast of the gas itself against the dense abdominal tissue. In addition, it should be remembered that heart and chest disease may give rise to symptoms which mimic an acute abdomen; myocardial infarction, dissecting aortic aneurysm, pneumonia and pulmonary embolism in particular.[7] What necessity is there to irradiate the whole abdomen simply to demonstrate the subdiaphragmatic area? Indeed, this is supported by guidelines from the Royal College of Radiologists in their referral guidelines for imaging, where a supine abdomen accompanied by an erect chest examination is recommended for patients with symptoms suggestive of the acute abdomen. A lateral decubitus projection of the abdomen *is* suggested if the patient cannot be examined erect for the chest film;[8] this projection is described in Chapter 34. The erect chest radiograph itself should not be forgotten as a useful projection for this region; apparent upper abdominal pain can be due to lower lobe pneumonia and an erect chest radiograph will provide evidence of either, on one image and with one exposure, which is clearly lower than that for an abdomen radiograph. Prior to positioning and exposure, the patient must always have been in an erect position for at least 5 minutes to allow air to rise to the highest point in the abdominal cavity, which is under the right diaphragm.

In cases of infirm patients, an erect projection of the chest can be attempted in the AP position with the patient sitting supported, in bed or on a trolley (Ch. 25). For some patients even this will prove difficult; in these cases a left lateral decubitus (right side raised) projection of the upper abdomen can be undertaken. This is described in Chapter 34 on the examination of the gastrointestinal tract.

The Royal College of Radiologists do suggest that, in circumstances where a patient's clinical symptoms and signs strongly suggest obstruction, yet X-ray examination proves negative, an erect AP abdomen may be considered. The projection may be undertaken standing or sitting.

Positioning

If used, a 35 × 43 cm cassette is placed in the erect bucky or a grid may be used if the patient is sitting on a trolley.

- The patient is sitting, or standing erect with legs separated for stability
- MSP is perpendicular to the image receptor and coincident with its long axis
- The middle of the image receptor is level with the iliac crests *or* its upper border should include the upper abdomen if this area is required

Beam direction and FFD

Horizontal, at 90° to the image receptor

FFD 100–120 cm, selected to ensure magnification is at its minimum and include the maximum amount of abdominal tissue on the image

Centring

To the centre of the cassette

Collimation

As much upper abdomen as possible, lateral soft tissue outlines

The symphysis pubis need not be included as it should be included on the supine abdomen projection.

Exposure factors

Exposure factors will require an increase from the supine AP projection, to allow for increased density due to sagging of the abdominal tissue in this position.

Image quality

Image quality is assessed as for the supine abdomen but there may be a reduction in contrast, compared to the AP projection, due to increased exposure factors and abdomen sag. The symphysis pubis need not be included.

References

1. McQuillen Martensen K. Radiographic critique. Philadelphia: WB Saunders; 1995.
2. Eisenberg R, et al. Radiographic positioning. 2nd edn. Boston: Little Brown and Company; 1995.
3. Cole TJ. Secular trends in growth. Nutrition Sociology. 2000; 59(2):317–324.
4. Gunn C. Radiographic imaging: a practical approach. 3rd edn. Edinburgh: Churchill Livingstone; 2002.
5. Bontrager K, Lampignano JP. Textbook of radiographic positioning and related anatomy. 6th edn. St Louis: Mosby; 2005.
6. Swallow RA, et al. Clark's positioning in radiography. 11th edn. London: Heinemann; 1986.
7. Nicholson DA, Driscoll PA. ABC of emergency radiology. Cambridge: BMJ Publishing; 1995.
8. RCR Working Party. Making the best use of a Department of radiology: guidelines for doctors. 5th edn. London: The Royal College of Radiologists; 2003.

SECTION

4

ACCIDENT AND EMERGENCY IMAGING

ACCIDENT AND EMERGENCY

Jonathan McConnell, Elizabeth Carver

This chapter will evaluate the position of the imaging professional within the multidisciplinary team, consider the advancing role of the radiographer and review how an understanding of injury mechanisms and pattern recognition informs the choice of projection and technique adaptation in the traumatised patient. Special considerations for techniques, in addition to radiographic equipment choice, will also be considered for this wide field of service provision.

THE ROLE OF THE RADIOGRAPHER IN THE MULTIDISCIPLINARY TEAM

The advent of highlighting abnormalities through the use of a 'red dot' system,[1] development of the advanced trauma and life support (ATLS)[2] approach to dealing with the patient with multiple injuries and the inception of the four tier system[3] of working in Britain have advanced the position of the radiographer within the accident and emergency (A&E) multidisciplinary team. Gradual development of service provision through advanced training to create the reporting radiographer has further assured the value of this team member in the A&E department.

The enhanced role of the reporting radiographer has ensured an invaluable service can now be provided instantly in the A&E department. Acting as report writer, advanced A&E imaging practitioner, advisor to junior radiographic staff or students and other professionals within the multidisciplinary team, the reporting radiographer keys in neatly with (at a minimum) the advanced practitioner stage of the four tier system of work which is under development at the start of the 21st century.

Although the advanced practitioner may be seen as a key representative for imaging within the multidisciplinary team, it should be remembered that the radiographer has a developing responsibility to ensure they contribute fully to the trauma service. As a member of the ATLS team, the imaging practitioner must take command of their aspect of the service provided for the patient. A highly experienced team may not necessarily always provide this service and, in a stressful situation, the radiographer must control their contribution through being confident and assertive; this ensures a good outcome is achieved whilst maintaining safety for patients and the wider ATLS team. In this way the radiographer becomes an advocate for all those who come into contact with ionising radiation in the resuscitation room.

It is not only in the ATLS situation that the radiographer will display the versatility to cope with the demands of the varied A&E patient presentations, across widely ranging age groups and varying requirements for adaptation of techniques. The radiographer also displays their value to the multidisciplinary team for all A&E cases in which they are involved. However, admission of lack of knowledge or ability should not be seen as a suggestion of general inability; examples of this are most likely to lie in unusual circumstances, difficult patient presentations or difficulty with highlighting perceived abnormalities. Admission of lack of knowledge or ability, and acceptance that another more experienced or skilled member of the team may provide a better service, is the most responsible and appropriate action for this situation. This may be reflected in discussing A&E images, or requests for imaging, with the referrer (be they nurse practitioner or A&E doctor) or radiologist so that the best patient outcome may be achieved. Also, knowledge and its application in the form of advising alternative imaging, perhaps with a protocol driven application of the Ionising Radiation (Medical Exposure) Regulations [IR(ME)R 2000],[4] is further evidence of the extended service provision of the radiographer within the multidisciplinary team. Indeed, acting as a gatekeeper of ionising radiation exposure to the general public is one of the more demanding roles, expected even of the newly qualified radiographer.

It is necessary that the radiographic professional understands the following:

• trauma mechanisms
• most common injury presentations associated with trauma mechanisms
• how trauma mechanism and presentation may influence projection or technique selection
• how trauma mechanism and presentation may influence technique adaptation, in varied situations

Being able to draw on a wide experience base that has been developed through reflecting on practice (be this formalised or in an intuitive way) is another expectation of the A&E radiographer. With this in mind it is the professional and medicolegal responsibility of radiographers to ensure that they maintain and continually develop their skills. Ensuring participation in continuing professional development (CPD) is paramount for even the most experienced – change can occur and trap the unwary, especially where the future requirements of the Health Professions Council is anticipated. For instance, 'red dotting'[5] has become an accepted norm for the practising radiographer and now features in many undergraduate radiography courses in the UK. However, the full medicolegal position of 'red dotting' and the radiographer may not be appreciated until a patient attempts to prove negligence; CPD will help protect the practitioner from this ill wind. The referring practitioner also needs assurance that this abnormality highlighting service is reliable and that a reasonable standard of care is exercised. An example of an unreliable service is when the radiographer sends an image to the referrer without a red dot marker, believing that non-application of the dot means responsibility for diagnosis (potentially made wholly via clinical reasoning and without radiological input) and treatment decisions will transfer to the referrer. The referrer may believe that the absence of the red dot implies that there is no perceived abnormality in the eyes of the radiographer. This situation illustrates the importance of ensuring that a reliable and standardised service is provided. Similarly, radiographers who provide a reporting service, and have necessarily undergone significant postgraduate education should offer the same standard of report – because they are not radiologists is it acceptable that a lower standard of report is provided?[6]

Even if a radiographer is not held responsible in civil proceedings, there is no reason why disciplinary or professional conduct hearings will not find the radiographer guilty of negligent conduct, especially if it was felt that radiographers, with their general training and experience, would be expected to identify common abnormalities. Vicarious liability by the employing hospital trust expects reasonable standards of care to have been exercised when

supporting its employees in the execution of their duties. This includes operating within recognised protocols, working to professional standards but also, on the part of the employer, provision of appropriate educational support and safe working practices agreed by all participants.[7]

Experience also plays a significant role in the perceived mundane activities of service provision, especially on the ancillary equipment selection front. Frequently, selection of this type of equipment for support to the A&E imaging department is often made without inclusion of the radiographer in the purchasing exercise. As an example, choices of trolleys that are widely used across disciplines often results in difficulties not only for radiology staff but also for the patient and the wider team in the A&E department. In the end, a poor quality service is delivered because of a lack of foresight in operating as a cohesive team. Holistic care demands cooperation across boundaries seen as traditional divides; however, borders are created where they are inappropriate.[8] This is particularly a problem where professions not forming the majority in an area of operation are perceived as lacking in appreciation for what is best for that department area or the patient. Advocacy for the patient and service can take many different forms that are frequently not recognised.

MECHANISMS OF INJURY

A range of reasons exists as to why the patient will present in A&E. There are the common occurrences, being just that, although many injuries present themselves after apparently minor trauma or as a result of seemingly ridiculous circumstances. In addition, people frequently abuse themselves through use of socially acceptable drugs such as alcohol, or in today's more liberal society, with relatively mild narcotic agents. Obviously more serious class A type drugs frequently lead to more demanding clinical presentations that are beyond the scope of this chapter and indeed outside the remit of the radiographer.

Certain patterns of trauma present themselves time and again, i.e. the 'common occurrences'. Probably the most famous of all causes of injury is the 'fall onto out-stretched hand' or FOOSH. Also, twisting the ankle may generate injury patterns that are again linked as force is transmitted along the whole of the leg. Certain age groups, due to involvement in specific activities, or alternatively as a result of pathological processes influencing bone integrity, display unexpectedly severe presentations of injury following apparently innocuous trauma forces. The following table attempts to draw together injuries linked to the mechanism so that potential plain film skeletal imaging projections can be determined and expected injury patterns anticipated.

Mechanism of injury related to examination requirements

Mechanism	Part injured	Plain film imaging	Further or alternative projections	Alternative imaging
FOOSH	Carpometacarpal joint	DP, DPO, lateral hand	Ball catcher's hand	
	Scaphoid	PA wrist/scaphoid with ulnar deviation PA oblique Lateral wrist Stecher (banana view)	If scapho-lunate dissociation stress projections similar to standard scaphoid images may be needed later in treatment	RNI or MRI for occult scaphoid waist fracture MRI or US for suspected ligament damage
	Distal radius (Colles #)	PA and lateral wrist		
	Radial Head	AP elbow Lateral elbow	Specific radial head projections – see Chapter 6	
	Glenohumeral joint	AP shoulder Axial or Y view of scapula	Modified axial	CT, MRI or US to evaluate for Bankhart lesion of glenoid labrum or rotator cuff damage US or MRI for longstanding injury – used to also evaluate rotator cuff
	Acromioclavicular joint	AP A/C joint AP stress/weight bearing		
	Coracoid process	AP Axial	Inferosuperior	
Inversion at ankle	Ankle	Mortise/AP ankle Lateral	Internal or external oblique ankle Stress projections for ligament integrity evaluation	US to examine ligament integrity
	Base of 5th metatarsal	DP foot DP oblique foot		US may be used to evaluate peroneus brevis or related ligaments
	Fibula neck	AP tibia and fibula	Lateral tibia and fibula	
Falls from a height	Calcaneum	Axial and lateral calcaneum	Standing axial (if possible) Subtalar oblique projections	CT to evaluate fracture fragments
	Ankle	Mortise/AP ankle Lateral		CT to evaluate fracture fragments
	Pelvis	AP pelvis Lateral hip (if indicated)	Judet's view of acetabulum Sacrum/sacroiliac joint	CT to evaluate fracture component relationship/3D reconstruction
	All spinal regions	AP Lateral	Horizontal beam lateral Obliques	CT to evaluate fracture component relationship/3D reconstruction
Flexion/extension or compression of spine	Cervical spine	Odontoid process (open mouth) AP and lateral C Spine	Horizontal beam lateral Obliques (Rarely) flexion and extension laterals Lateral skull for C1 crush	CT and MRI to evaluate bone fracture relations and soft tissue damage respectively
Flexion/extension or compression of spine	Thoracic spine	AP and lateral T spine	Horizontal beam lateral	CT and MRI to evaluate bone fracture relations and soft tissue damage respectively

Continued

Mechanism of injury related to examination requirements—cont'd				
	Lumbar spine	AP and lateral L spine	Horizontal beam lateral	CT and MRI to evaluate bone fracture relations and soft tissue damage respectively
Rotation forces	Knee	AP and lateral knee	Intercondylar notch Internal/external obliques of knee	
	Elbow	AP and lateral elbow	90° flexed elbow Forearm parallel with cassette *or* Humerus parallel with cassette	CT to evaluate fracture component relationships US to evaluate ligament damage MRI for longer-term soft tissue damage evaluation
	All spinal regions	AP Lateral	Oblique projections of area as required to evaluate intervertebral articulations and neural foraminae	CT to evaluate bone relations and soft tissue damage MRI for soft tissue damage

An awareness of the developmental anatomy of the skeleton is equally important as injury patterns change with age. Young children may not yet possess the skeletal components that would generate adult injury characteristics, or indeed the maturity of bone may be responsible for causing variation in presentation. It is with this in mind that the radiographer can act as a resource of information for the referrer, such that an appropriate examination is embarked upon with least detriment to the child radiologically.

It is with all the above in mind, and the need to deal with the psychological aspects of the traumatised patient and accompanying relatives or friends, that the role of the radiographer is a wide-ranging one, acting as the advocate for holistic imaging management. Following recognition of the above it would now be pertinent to consider the more esoteric projections or adaptations to standard plain film imaging that may be considered as useful adjuncts to the trauma radiographer's range of skills.

FURTHER PROJECTIONS AND ADAPTED TECHNIQUES

Working around the patient in non-standard and trauma situations is one of the greater skills of the experienced radiographer in the A&E department and an understanding of how radiographic equipment or body parts may be moved (although it may not be safe to move the limb/body part in question) to achieve the required positions is of major importance. As well as appreciating these subtleties, the radiographer has a further responsibility for ensuring that appropriate radiation protection methods can be achieved for the patient, staff or relatives who may have to be present in these situations. Good collimation, selection of appropriate imaging equipment and radiation protection techniques, that would normally be considered run of the mill, will require adaptation to ensure successful application. Clean technique approaches will also be required where open wounds present, with appropriate protection for the radiographer and supplementary considerations for equipment and the cleaning of this thereafter. Cling film is often employed in the A&E department to wrap equipment, as protection from blood and other body fluids, and appropriate cleaning agents employed thereafter to attend to any pieces of equipment that may not have escaped exposure. Alternatively, special plastic sheaths may be made for foam immobilisation pads or cassettes, however, care must be taken to ensure that these covers are also kept clean and do not cause problems through artefact generation on any images.

The upper limb

Common mistakes made in obtaining projections of the hand and finger frequently occur as a result of the mistaken belief that the radiographer is being kinder to the patient by not causing excessive pain. Another example is when the radiographer attempts to obtain several finger projections in a single exposure. In both these instances it becomes immediately apparent that a less than acceptable image might be obtained, resulting in increased risk of misdiagnosis from the projection provided for radiological opinion. This lack of foresight and poor practice serves no purpose except to place the patient at risk and to lay the practitioner open to claims of negligent practice. Although hand injuries may not appear as severe, the actual effects of the injury may be quite significant. By understanding this, the radiographer should realise that the highest standard of imaging possible must be achieved. Realisation of this requires assertiveness (with respect to encouragement of achieving an ideal position when the patient may resist) in order to gain the best result, or implementation of adaptation of technique to allow an image to be obtained in less than ideal circumstances. Further up the upper limb, towards the elbow and shoulder, similar demands surface to ensure that unambiguous radiographic representation of the traumatised limb or joint is achieved. Of particular concern are the supracondylar and radial head regions of the elbow, whilst adequate evidence of the relatively rare, but easily missed, posteriorly dislocated shoulder is vital.

Adapted projections of the hand

Frequently the patient requiring hand radiography will present to the X-ray department on a trolley, as a result of shock after experiencing trauma, and being able to see the effects of the damage inflicted upon the limb. It is possible that routine projections of the hand may be undertaken with the arm extended across onto a table or platform but adaptation may be necessary if other injuries prevent this. At this point the radiographer must consider adaptation of technique to ensure a diagnostic image is produced, without the serious compromise of increased radiation dose to radiosensitive tissues. However, there are other methods for provision of images of the hand and this section identifies a range of these.

Lewis[9] identified a way to address the problems of the inadequacy of hand projections by suggesting that the dorsipalmar (DP) projection is obtained with the forearm medially rotated at the elbow so that the ulnar border of the hand is lifted from the cassette surface. A 15° radiolucent foam pad is placed under this aspect of the hand to immobilise the limb and the vertical central ray is centred over the head of the 3rd metacarpal and collimated to include all the hand (as for routine DP hand projection, described in Ch. 6) and the distal radioulnar joint (Fig. 27.1).

As patients are reluctant to flatten their hand and extend their fingers following trauma, or soft tissue swelling prevents this from happening, this small change to technique allows the interphalangeal, metacarpophalangeal and carpal joints to be displayed squarely so that a true representation of the bony relationships can be gathered.

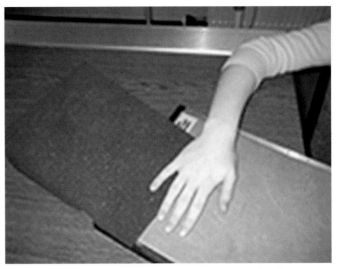

Figure 27.1   Clear joint presentation in the injured hand. Placing a 15° pad under the 5th metacarpal enhances the joint visualisation of the injured hand

The elevation of the medial aspect of the hand also places the little finger and 5th metacarpal into a DP position, rather than the oblique position in which they lie in the routine DP hand position.

Lewis continues to make further suggestions about hand radiography that would improve visualisation of certain digits.[10] Of the thumb he makes the point that, in the normal anteroposterior (AP) and lateral projections, the thenar eminence and other structures medial to the thumb are frequently superimposed over the first metacarpophalangeal joint, preventing clear visualisation due to imperfect achievement of radiographic density. He suggests, for the AP projection, that the radiographer simply angles the central X-ray beam 10–15° along the long axis of the thumb, towards the wrist, so that the soft tissue structures are projected away from the area of interest. Using this technique helps to reveal the proximal joint region without juggling with exposure factors that may blacken the distal part of the thumb whilst attempting to reveal the proximal aspect (Fig. 27.2). Alternatively, the supine AP thumb technique described in Chapter 5 is most suitable, especially for the patient who presents on a trolley.

In a third suggestion about hand technique modifications Lewis describes another projection of the 5th metacarpal, a bone which is difficult to demonstrate, due to the anatomical relationship of the bones or soft tissues of the hand in the dorsipalmar oblique (DPO) or lateral projections.[11] He recommends further external rotation of the hand from the lateral position by an extra 5–10° so the overlying 2nd to 4th metacarpals no longer superimpose. The central ray is directed towards the middle of the 5th metacarpal and angled so that the ray is parallel with the thumb, which

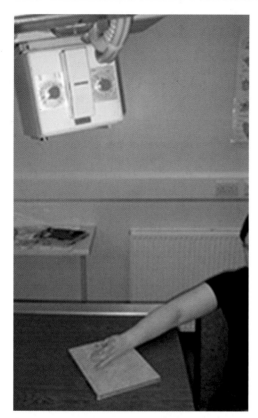

Figure 27.2 Angulation to clear the thenar eminences of the thumb. Angulation 10° cranially along the long axis of the first metacarpal ensures the thenar eminences do not superimpose and a good view of the articular surface of the metacarpal base is achieved

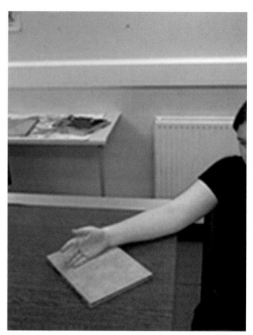

Figure 27.3 Fifth metacarpal neck projection. Slight over-rotation of the lateral hand allows visualisation of the neck of the 5th metacarpal. The thumb is further abducted before exposure

has been extended and abducted such that it does not overlie the 5th metacarpal (Fig. 27.3). Although an elongated projection is generated, almost the whole of the 5th metacarpal becomes visible.

Normally used for visualising the small joints of the fingers in the arthritic patient, the ball catcher's (Noorgaards)[12] projection may be employed to show the extent of damage in the fight bite situation (Fig. 27.4). Puncture of the assailant's skin by the tooth of the victim may allow for generation of osteomyelitis. Other than the clinical signs of the puncture wound or soft tissue swelling, little evidence of such an injury may be noted. However, the tangential representation of the metacarpal heads generated by this projection allows the viewer to see the indentation caused when the tooth has impacted with the metacarpal during a punching injury.

To achieve the image the patient sits with the palms of their hands cupped, as if preparing to catch a ball, with the dorsal aspects of the hands forming an approximate angle of 40–45° relative to the image receptor face. Note that the angle of the hands must be at this angle, rather than the 30° described for the palmar dorsal oblique ball catcher's

projection described in Chapter 5. A vertical central ray is centred between the heads of the 5th metacarpals and the beam is collimated to include both hands. Exposure factors similar to those for the DP hand projection are used.

Adapted projections of the thumb

Injuries to the thumb are highly debilitating as the ability to grip is affected. Assessment of the integrity of the ulnar

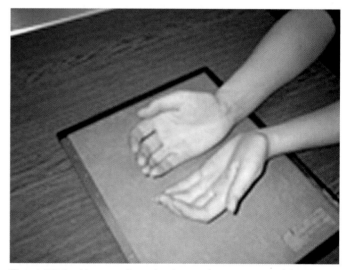

Figure 27.4 Noorgaards projection to show metacarpal heads tangentially. The contour of the spreading X-ray beam aligns with the articular surfaces of the metacarpal heads to allow tangential viewing to reveal subtle puncture wounds

and radial collateral ligament at the metacarpophalangeal joint is achievable through the use of self-applied stressing forces in the posteroanterior (PA) projection. This is achieved by using the index finger of the affected hand to generate adduction and abduction forces. The patient is asked to adduct the thumb by placing their index finger over the distal surface of the tip of the thumb and pulling the thumb medially towards the finger; abduction is achieved by placing the tip of the index finger against the medial aspect of the tip of the thumb before pushing the tip of the thumb laterally, away from the index finger. Through stressing in a horizontal direction, the ulnar and radial collateral ligaments are strained to reveal their integrity. Rupture is revealed by widening of the respective side of the metacarpophalangeal joint that is associated with the damaged ligament. (Fig. 27.5A,B)

Should a true lateral projection of the base of the first metacarpal be required to reveal subtle fractures, the Gedda-Billings projection can be used.[13] Simply position as for the lateral thumb projection and angle the central ray 10° along the axis of the metacarpal, towards the forearm. This will free the articular surface of any superimposition from the trapezium (Fig. 27.6).

Adapted projections of the wrist and forearm

As noted with the hand, occasionally there is the need to adapt the positioning of the patient to achieve the correct projection. One of the neatest tricks that may be employed in obtaining PA and lateral projections of the wrist require encouragement of the patient to extend their arm as far as possible; this makes external rotation for the lateral projection easier. This is reasonably easy to achieve on a trolley-bound patient, with the arm abducted to lie over a table. Indeed, the ulna will only turn through 90° between

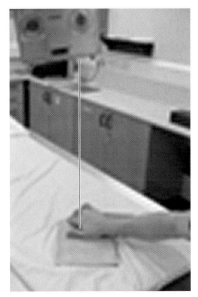

Figure 27.6 The Gedda-Billings lateral projection of the thumb. The Gedda-Billings projection that gives an uninterrupted lateral perspective of the base of the first metacarpal

PA and lateral projections if the lateral is undertaken with the arm extended in this way. Alternatively, where this cannot be achieved, position the patient relative to the examination table (whether seated or on a trolley) in such a way as to allow horizontal beam projections of either view to be obtained with minimal risk of exposing other body areas to primary radiation. Appropriate upper arm support may be required, or manipulation of patient vehicles (trolley/wheelchair), to allow the radiographer and patient

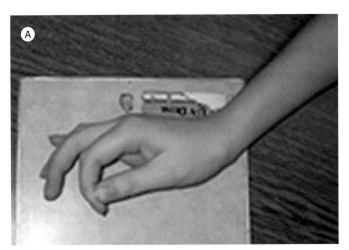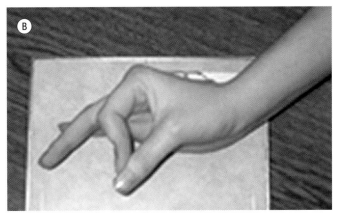

Figure 27.5 Stress projections of the thumb. **(A)** shows the stressed thumb being pulled towards the hand by the index finger while **(B)** shows the opposite stressing force. These are used to show radial and ulnar collateral damage respectively around the first metacarpophalangeal joint

to achieve satisfactory positions from a radiographic and comfort perspectives. This may require the use of copious amounts of sandbags or radiolucent foam pads; these, at times, may seem rather insecure in their construction of a supporting cradle for the injured limb.

When the patient presents with an injury to the forearm, it is often extremely difficult for the patient to assume the standard (anatomical position) attitude required for radiography. If this is the case the forearm is best treated as two separate objects for imaging, although the individual joint aspects will manifest themselves as correct radiographic presentations on the resultant images. Handling of the limb is recommended as follows (this requires shoulder movement and the radiographer should ascertain that this is safely possible):

- At commencement of positioning ensure the table is level with the shoulder
- Abduct the limb from the trunk at the shoulder, whilst encouraging the patient to extend their elbow so that the whole arm may be rested on the table-top
- Externally rotate the shoulder to bring the elbow joint into a true AP position as the arm is supinated
- Often the patient will naturally want to rest the arm, when in this position, with the wrist very close to the lateral position; this will allow an AP elbow and lateral wrist projection to be obtained on one image. Clearly there will be crossover of shaft of radius over ulna
- After obtaining the previous image, the arm is internally rotated at the shoulder and the elbow flexed. The medial aspects of the upper arm and elbow are placed in contact with the table-top. The positions of radius and ulna in relationship to the humerus do not alter. The forearm thus assumes a position that now generates lateral elbow and, through natural pronation of the hand, PA wrist projections. Again, there will be crossover over radial and ulnar shafts
- For both positions described, centre to the mid forearm and collimate to include the whole of the lower forearm

Although this is not an anatomically correct approach, at least two views of the injured forearm at 90° to each other are obtained so some approximation of the anatomical relationship can be gleaned (Fig. 27.7A,B).

Shoulder injury is likely to affect the ability to achieve some of the positions described above and horizontal beam technique may be required if this is the case. This technique is highly valued in such limiting situations but is very dependent upon the position that the patient's forearm and image receptor can be supported in. The approach must be taken from the perspective that minimal patient movement is required and similar results can be obtained as

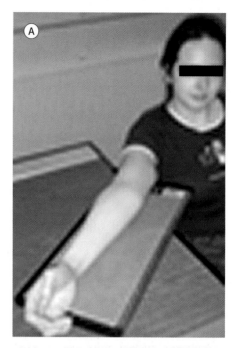

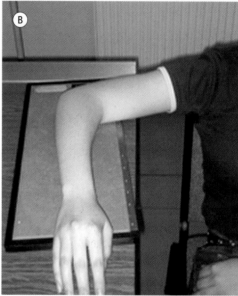

Figure 27.7 Trauma projections of the forearm. Non-standard positions of the forearm to aid the patient who is injured by obtaining projections that are **(A)** lateral wrist with AP elbow and **(B)** vice versa

indicated above with least induction of pain to the patient. Care, however, must be exercised with respect to achieving these projections without unnecessary exposure to primary radiation from the horizontal beam technique, since there are implications for its direction towards the trunk. Careful use of appropriate thickness of lead rubber over the trunk, collimation and turning the patient's head away from the

X-ray tube are all essential measures which must not be ignored.

Adapted projections of the elbow and humerus

The elbow is noted as one of the most difficult areas to examine adequately following trauma, due to concerns about exacerbating neurovascular damage that may have occurred. Frequently the patient will present with the elbow flexed and will resist attempts to extend the limb due to pain. To negotiate this problem individual images of each half of the elbow joint, i.e. proximal radius and ulna or distal humerus, should be obtained. In this way a relationship between major elbow components is noted but the articular surfaces are shown to advantage.[13] If cassettes are used, an 18 × 24 cm size may be employed (the relatively small size is the most practicable in trolley situations and, at time of going to press, such small direct digital receptors are not available) with the forearm and humeral aspects of the elbow imaged in turn, thus allowing the radial and ulnar joint surfaces to be seen tangentially or the trochlear/capitellar surfaces of the humerus to be displayed clearly for each projection (Fig. 27.8A,B). A vertical central ray, or beam perpendicular to the joint portion of interest if a horizontal beam technique has to be used, is centred in turn at a point in the middle of the two articulation areas, i.e. over the proximal radio ulnar joint for the forearm projection and through the coronoid/olecranon fossae region for distal humerus. Whichever approach is adopted, remember to place the area of interest in the midpoint of the cassette so that all regions can be captured on the image. As already stated, at the time this text is going to press, digital image receptors are not available in very small sizes and the body part is more easily included within the perimeter of the receptor; as long as collimation is correctly applied, the area of interest will almost certainly be included. However, it must be noted that the larger digital receptors may not be as versatile as the 18 × 24 cm cassette when a patient is lying on a trolley.

As noted earlier, patients with significant elbow injury often present with the *elbow held in flexion* as this guards the elbow against excessive pain. There is an association between this position and the likelihood of there being a fracture to the supracondylar region of the humerus, particularly in the younger patient. In these instances any attempt to extend the arm would be inappropriate as this could cause further damage to the soft tissue structures in the area. The worst case scenario would be permanent disability, as in Volkmann's ischaemic contracture. Instead of extending the elbow for the AP projection, take an image of the elbow with the arm still flexed but held in an AP distal humerus or elbow position, resting the posterior aspect of the upper arm on the cassette, which has been placed on the examination table. The upper arm should be positioned with the elbow level with the shoulder (Fig. 27.9A) and the vertical beam is centred midway between the humeral epicondyles. Collimate to the area of interest but use exposure factors modified (increased) to make allowance for the greater thickness of the tissue overlying the elbow; higher kVp selection should be used to even out the range of densities that are required for demonstration. The distal radius and ulna can be similarly demonstrated in the flexed elbow by positioning the posterior aspect of the forearm in contact with the image receptor. This time the elbow and wrist lie in the same plane (Fig. 27.9B). Centring remains as for the projection for distal humerus, as do considerations for exposure factor selection.[14] Use

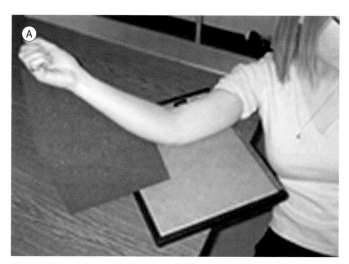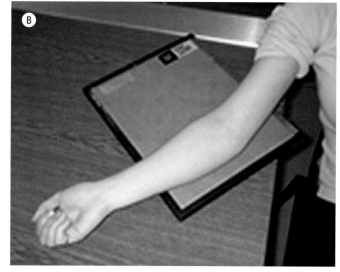

Figure 27.8   The semi-flexed projections of the elbow. Obtaining the semi-flexed elbow image from the frontal aspect as two separate projections allows the tangential viewing of the articular surfaces to be achieved thus providing a detailed examination of the injured joint

of both projections to demonstrate the elbow adequately may be necessary but justification of this must be ascertained, since there are implications for radiation dose increase due to use of two exposures. It must be noted that the image of the elbow joint will not be as accurate as in the routine AP projection. However, elbow flexion *is* required for the lateral projection of the joint, and this projection is likely to be produced well. Positioning of the arm into the correct position for the lateral is also relatively easy, therefore lessening the risk of further injury to the joint. Using an adapted technique to demonstrate the radial head, as described later in this chapter and in Chapter 6, is also possible with the elbow retained in a flexed position.

Still considering examination of the elbow in flexion, if the patient is unable to place the appropriate aspect of the arm in contact with the cassette (e.g. if information on radius and ulna is required, the patient is supine and cannot sit to put their forearm in contact with the image receptor, or if information on distal humerus is required and the posterior aspect of the upper arm carries significant abrasion) then modification of the flexed elbow position can be achieved. For proximal radius and ulna, when the posterior aspect of the forearm cannot be placed in contact with the image receptor, place the posterior aspect of the humerus in contact with the image receptor and employ a beam angle perpendicular to long axis of radius and ulna (Fig. 27.9F). For distal humerus, when it is not possible to place the posterior aspect of the upper arm in contact with the image receptor, place the posterior aspect of the forearm in contact with the image receptor and angle the central ray until it is perpendicular to the humerus (Fig. 27.9E). The centring point for each is midway between the humeral epicondyles. Note that the angle for either will vary greatly with each patient, due to variations in upper arm build, degree of elbow flexion the patient holds the injured arm in, and the amount of abduction achievable at the shoulder.

Clearly the patient who presents on a trolley is unlikely to be able to sit next to a table for flexed elbow projections but it is possible to reproduce them with the patient supine and the flexed joint positioned on the trolley, the arm abducted from the supine trunk. A horizontal beam technique may be necessary if the shoulder rotation to bring the elbow into the correct position is not possible; this would be appropriate for both AP and lateral projections.

With more specific reference to the lateral projection for the injured elbow, obtaining a satisfactory lateral image frequently demands ingenuity in adaptation if the patient is unable to sit at the end of the table. The general rule, however, is to ensure that the elbow is supported on the image receptor so that the shoulder and elbow are at the same level, as in the routine lateral elbow position. This may be quite easy in a supine patient if the shoulder is mobile.

However, it may not be possible to achieve, even in a patient who is able to sit at the table and often it is the extent of required external rotation at the shoulder which limits this; often the patient is limited to a position where their wrist and elbow joints lie lower than their shoulder. To reduce the effects of this, modification of the lateral elbow projection can be made by supporting the image receptor and arm with wedge-shaped pads and using a beam angle which will strike the image receptor at 90°. (Fig. 27.10). Similarly, adaptation for the AP projection can be made, which does not require the extent of external rotation at the shoulder. This is a horizontal beam approach where the elbow lies in a lateral position in relationship to the table-top, but has the image receptor supported vertically behind its posterior aspect (Fig. 27.11). Again this may require the support of several immobilisation foam pads and care should be taken to ensure that the arm lies parallel to the table-top.

When the patient cannot move their upper arm, but can stand or sit, a useful alternative technique for the lateral elbow projection is to position them erect PA and facing a vertical cassette holder as if positioning for a full lateral humerus projection. The flexed elbow, supported at the forearm by the hand of the uninjured side, should be abducted away from the body so that, viewed from the posterior aspect of the patient, the medial aspect of the elbow is visible (Fig. 27.12). The humerus can be maintained in position by a radiolucent foam pad between the humerus and thorax but this will not maintain elbow flexion if the patient cannot achieve this with the injured limb alone. Centre a horizontal ray to a point approximately 3–5 cm above the elbow joint, along the humeral shaft and on the medial aspect. Collimate to include the whole joint and distal humerus. This relatively high centring point will use oblique rays to traverse the joint and reveal a clearer joint space. This approach may also be adopted for the patient who might present on a trolley but is able to sit with their legs over the side. With the trolley placed close to the erect image receptor stand a similar result to that described may be obtained.

Elbow injury that also involves the bones of the forearm is relatively common and frequently creates damage that may not be identified. Rotating the elbow externally from the true AP position so the humeral epicondyles lie at 45° relative to the image receptor cassette allows visualisation of the *radial head, neck and tuberosity* without superimposition of other bones (Fig. 27.13). An image of this is shown in Figure 6.5B. The humeral capitellum will also be clearly displayed. Internal rotation of the elbow from the AP position will advantageously display the coronoid of the ulna, the trochlea and an elongated medial epicondyle of the humerus (see Fig. 6.8A,B).

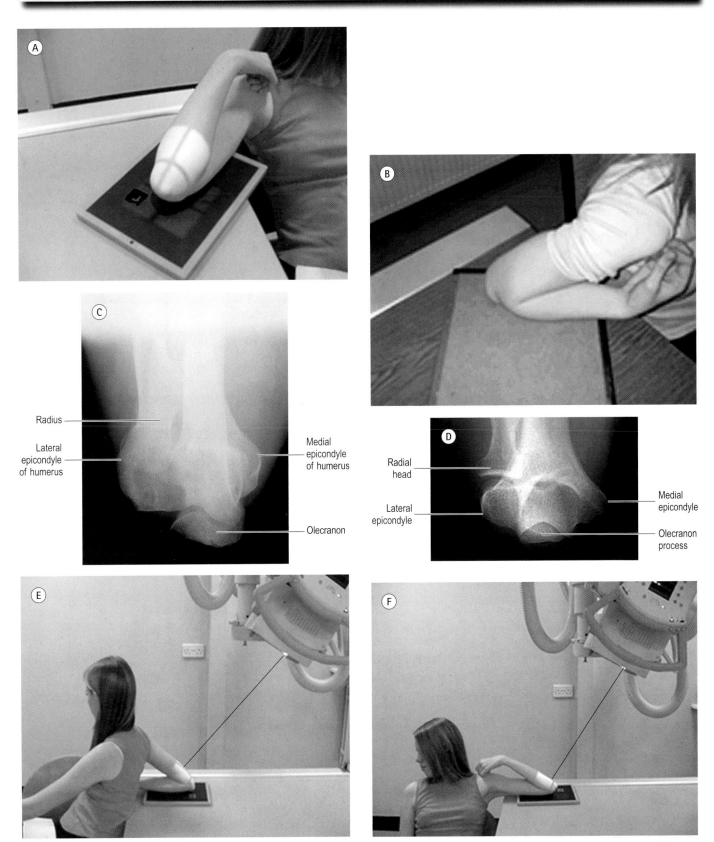

Figure 27.9 (A,B) Fully flexed projections of the traumatised elbow show (A) the position to demonstrate the distal humerus and (B) the proximal radius and ulna; (C) flexed elbow projection to demonstrate humerus; (D) flexed elbow projection to demonstrate radius and ulna; (E) elbow in flexion – forearm in contact with image receptor, with beam angulation – this projection will show distal humerus; (F) elbow in flexion – upper arm in contact with receptor, with beam angulation – this projection will show proximal radius and ulna

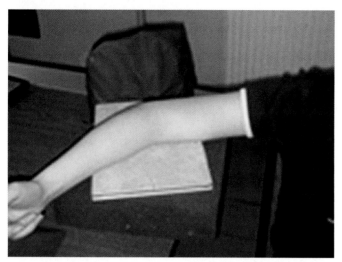

Figure 27.10   Reduced movement lateral projection of the elbow. Note the image receptor is supported obliquely to ensure a comfortable but accurately positioned limb. The hand and shoulder are in the same plane and the hand supported to maintain this. In this case a slight mediolateral angle will ensure that the beam is perpendicular to the image receptor. This projection can be used for trolley-bound patients

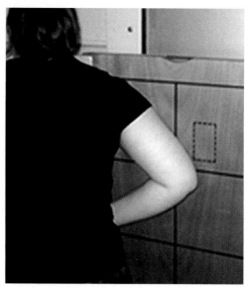

Figure 27.12   The PA erect lateral elbow projection. The erect lateral elbow, performed in much the same way as the lateral full length humerus

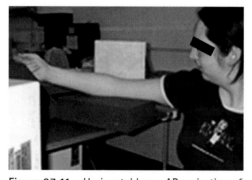

Figure 27.11   Horizontal beam AP projection of the elbow. This is used when the patient cannot externally rotate the shoulder for a routine AP, in conjunction with horizontal beam. This figure shows how the projection can be used for partially flexed elbows as well as extended elbows. The projection can be achieved for trolley-bound patients

The radial head can also be further visualised in the lateral position by rotating from the lateral start point. Four exposures can be made with the forearm displaying, in the lateral position, maximum supination, lateral with the ulna border of the forearm in a comfortable position, pronation of the hand and hyperpronation of the hand with the hand positioned as if attempting an AP projection of the thumb. This gradually rotates the radial head so that aspects of the proximal radial profile are displayed (see Ch. 6, Figs 6.6A,B and 6.7A,B). Finally the Coyle projection[15] of the radial head employs lateromedial angulation of 45° across the forearm, which is in a lateral position. This projection separates the

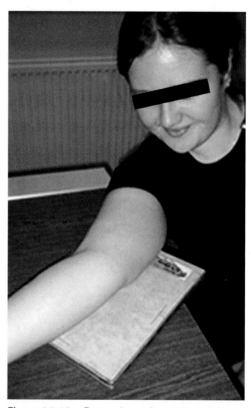

Figure 27.13   External rotation to reveal proximal forearm details. Further external rotation from the AP elbow position will allow visualisation of the radial head, neck and tuberosity

radial head and capitellum from superimposing structures to reveal indistinct injuries that may be too subtle to detect on the normal lateral image (Fig. 27.14A,B).

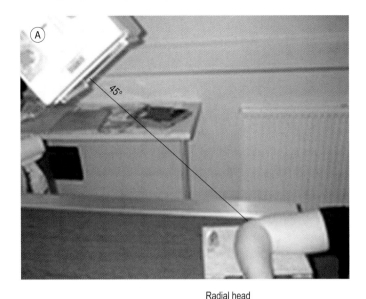

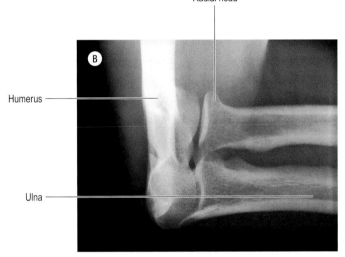

Radial head

Humerus

Ulna

Figure 27.14   (A) Coyle radial head projection – the Coyle projection – by angling 40–45° lateromedially, this view separates the radial head from the superimposing ulna for suspected radial head/neck fractures; **(B)** Coyle radial head X-ray – the Coyle projection – by angling 40–45° lateromedially, this view separates the radial head from the superimposing ulna for suspected radial head/neck fractures

Fractures of the *humerus* frequently appear ugly due to deformation of the limb and demand the utmost care from the imaging practitioner when obtaining radiographs. In cases like this the patient is best examined erect so that the most information can be obtained by using a single projection, in the same way as follow-up images would be achieved. However, if the patient presents on a trolley or has to be examined on the X-ray table, provision of immobilisation pad support will be necessary to obtain a true projection of the limb. Although images reveal their best information by being taken with the cassette in close proximity to the limb, using the bucky tray or under trolley cassette tray may be an option that is desired to minimise

movement of the arm and reduce patient discomfort. The associated projection at 90° to the first can be obtained using a combination of overlapping horizontal beam projections from the shoulder down and elbow up. Moving the arm away from the body and elevating it on supporting pads to allow clear visualisation of the limb may be necessary for these projections. Good communication techniques with appropriate analgesia are the most helpful additions that can be offered in this setting – as in most trauma imaging approaches (Fig. 27.15A,B,C).

Adapted projections of the shoulder joint

The shoulder joint (specifically the glenohumeral joint) has been the source of the generation of many tailored projections to prove various injury and degenerative processes. This section will consider the supplementary projections of value following trauma.

Confusion is occasionally apparent regarding the degree of external rotation that is required for the frontal projection of the shoulder. Ideally, appropriate clinical evaluation will result in the indication by the referrer; for example, if the *clavicle* is the injured component for which a radiological opinion is sought, this would necessitate a clavicular projection. Where this is not the case, and foreshortening of the clavicle is not a consideration, appropriate external rotation of the trunk to the affected side should be attempted so that the glenoid edge will be projected in profile. This will allow the viewer to scrutinise the *glenohumeral joint* effectively so that the image can be correctly evaluated for the presence of subtle dislocation or fracture characteristics. This rule also applies for patients who present in a supine position, depending of course on the potential for causing further injury through rotating the patient.

The modified axial projection is one such projection that can be used in the patient in any situation. Essentially the projection is obtained by positioning the patient as for an AP shoulder, with 30–45° caudal angulation from the original perpendicular beam direction (Fig. 27.16). This can also be undertaken with 45° rotation on the trunk; this is sometimes known as the Garth projection or Garth Apical Oblique[16] and is used to assess dislocation by examining the position of the humeral head relative to the glenoid of the scapula. The projection can be undertaken erect or supine. On the resulting image, if the humeral head lies inferiorly to the glenoid then the dislocation is anterior, with the positions of the anatomical structures reversed for posterior dislocations, i.e. the glenoid edge is lower in relationship to the humeral head. This is also discussed in Chapter 7.

Another alternative is based on the Wallace & Hellier projection,[17] which is suitable for patients who can sit, either on a chair or wheelchair. The patient is positioned with their back towards the examination table, upon which the

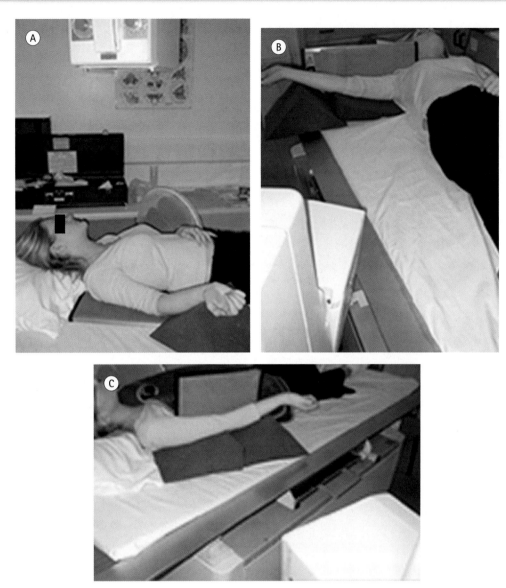

Figure 27.15 Supine projections of the injured humerus. Several options are available for obtaining images of the injured humerus with differing impacts on the patient from a movement **(A,B)** and potential radiation dose **(C)** perspective

image receptor is placed horizontally. They are seated facing the X-ray tube. The vertical X-ray beam is angled 30° towards the shoulder and centred over the superior surface of the glenohumeral joint (Fig. 27.17). The table is lowered until it allows for the central ray to emerge from the shoulder to coincide with the centre of the image receptor. To ensure an accurate projection is obtained, the patient may have to be rotated slightly towards the affected side so that the blade of the scapula is parallel with the long edge of the image receptor. Remember, magnification effects will be encountered due to the excessive object–receptor distance so an increase in the focus film distance (FFD) will be required to reduce these effects. This, in addition to the air gap created between the shoulder and image receptor, will have a concomitant effect on the required

exposure factors so that a fine balance needs to be struck between the selection of kVp and mAs in order that appropriate density and contrast are maintained within the image. Clearly, modification of exposure factors will require careful calculation using the inverse square law.

This technique can be adapted with trolley-bound patients whereby the length of the trolley can serve as an examination table behind the seated position of the patient, thus minimising movement; however, the patient will be required to sit erect without support behind their back.

Where the patient is unable to be seated and presents on the trolley, true inferosuperior or superoinferior projections may be achieved using gentle encouragement of the patient to abduct the arm so an imaging cassette may be placed in the axillary space. Alternatively the cassette is

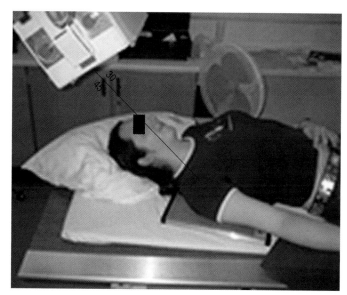

Figure 27.16   The Garth projection. The Garth projection to reveal dislocation of the glenohumeral joint. This projection produces a half axial view of the shoulder and is one option to consider where a true axial image might not be possible. It can also be undertaken sitting or standing

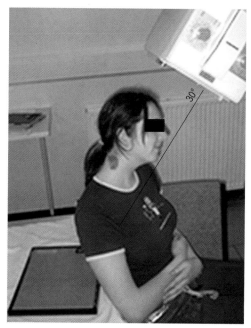

Figure 27.17   The Wallace & Hellier half axial shoulder projection. Another option for a half axial shoulder projection

placed above the shoulder and the central ray directed from below the joint. This may be feasible, while minimising pain, as relatively small amounts of movement are required following the performance of the AP projection that complements the above.

Due to the structure of the shoulder, the *coracoid process* has other structures superimposed over it on the image. This may be a particular problem in younger patients, where

Further discussion on the options for production of shoulder projections, including considerations for implementation in trauma situations, can be found in Chapter 7.

secondary ossification of the coracoid tip could mimic a fracture, thus necessitating clear visualisation of this aspect of the shoulder. Depending on if any kyphosis of the thoracic region is present, simply angle 20–30° cranially, with the patient in the normal AP shoulder position (Fig. 27.18). Greater kyphosis will require greater angulation. This image can also be helpful in the evaluation of the *acromioclavicular joint*.

Adapted projections of the foot, ankle and leg

Where injuries of the *foot* are concerned, radiographers frequently have to work around the patient, depending heavily at times on the versatility of the radiographic equipment. This means that, although projections are standardised or similar, the equipment must be manoeuvred into various positions, rather than moving the patient's limb. Horizontal ray techniques are often used to create a projection that is at least similar to the one obtained in the less injured patient.

When the patient presents in a *wheelchair* for foot examinations, consider placing the image receptor on the floor or a small step for the patient to place the injured foot upon (Fig. 27.19). In this way the frail patient does not have to be moved and a relatively standard projection is possible. Slight extension of the ankle, required to clear

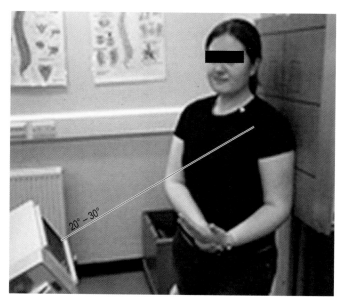

Figure 27.18   Inferosuperior projection to show the coracoid of the scapula. The coracoid projection – note the cranial angulation – also allows good visualisation of the acromioclavicular joint, projected clear of other shoulder structures

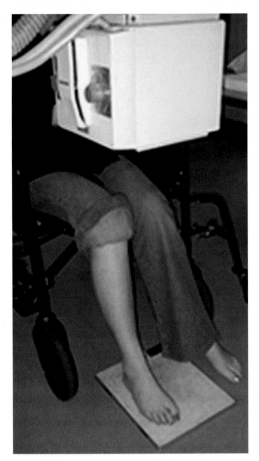

Figure 27.19 DP foot for the non-ambulant patient. A simple modification of technique which minimises movement of the patient, therefore reducing risk of distress and further injury to the patient. It also reduces the risks associated with manual handling. The DPO projection can also be achieved this way

the tibia and fibula from the majority of the tarsus, is also easier in this position. *The trolley-bound patient* can be examined with the leg fully extended or with the hip and knee slightly flexed. The image receptor is supported under the plantar aspect of the foot; it does not matter at what angle the image receptor and foot lie, as long as the central ray is correctly angled until it is perpendicular to the image receptor. In some cases it may be necessary to elevate the foot slightly, by resting the back of the heel on a radio-lucent pad, in order that trolley components or patient anatomy are not projected over the image. This would be most likely in the patient whose leg is fully extended. The practitioner's skills are of paramount importance here, with respect to angling the beam and accurately positioning the image receptor.

Working in this way indicates that the patient probably requires no more than the equivalent of the basic 'two views at right angles' series. That said, orthopaedic colleagues may request further projections such as views of the *subtalar* joints. The best projections that would reveal the most information of the whole region are the medial and lateral ankle obliques where the foot is rotated internally and exter-nally respectively from the AP ankle position, to form an angle of 45° to the image receptor (Fig. 27.20A,B). 20° cranial angulation is placed on the central ray, which is directed towards the talus. Collimate to include the ankle joint, talus calcaneum and both malleoli.

Examinations for injury related to areas more proximal than the ankle can usually be obtained by using a combi-nation of routine and horizontal ray techniques. The use

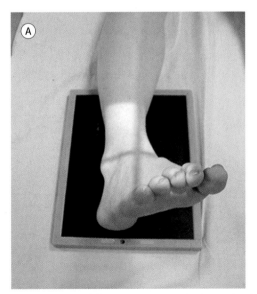 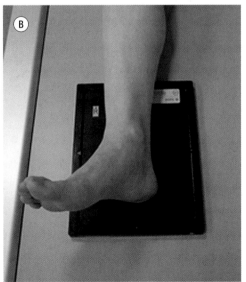

Figure 27.20 **(A)** The 'common' subtalar projection – the 'common' subtalar view, whereby a midpoint angle of 45° internal and external rotation of the ankle is accompanied by 20° cranial angulation of the central ray to reveal the majority of the subtalar articulation in a pair of images; **(B)** 45° external oblique ankle

of splinting devices will become more evident and, where possible, these should be removed to avoid artefact generation. Should the leg be so badly injured that gross rotation of one part relative to another is displayed (e.g. shaft of tibia and fibula rotated in relation to the ankle joint), then obtain projections that ensure that at least one part of the limb is projected with its joint in the correct orientation, so that the associated portion of the injured body part can be assessed relative to the part that is correctly projected. Using the lower leg as an example this would mean:
AP knee and lateral ankle obtained by vertical X-ray beam. Lateral knee and AP ankle obtained by horizontal ray technique.

Not all leg injuries will be as remarkable as the example above. When the patient is able to climb onto the examination table, further simple projections may be helpful in elucidating subtle injuries. Internal and external oblique projections of the ankle can be performed with the foot rotated through the axis of the ankle to form an angle of 45° to the table-top for the respective views. The vertical central ray is centred on the ankle joint and collimated as described for the AP ankle (Ch. 8). The internal oblique will show the *distal tibiofibular joint* and *lateral malleolus* clearly, with the external oblique displaying the *medial malleolus* and *talus* to advantage. Under- and over-rotation of the ankle joint in the lateral position are also useful images to obtain from the perspective of displaying (a) the posterior tibial lip in the under-rotated lateral and (b) the posterior margin of the fibula in the over-rotated lateral.

Stress projections to reveal ligament integrity in the ankle may also be required. The inversion stress view shows the integrity of the *lateral collateral complex* while the eversion stress view is helpful for showing the integrity of the *deltoid* or *medial collateral complex*. As the referring clinician is normally responsible for the action of stressing of the joint in each direction, the radiographer must control the situation by taking care to ensure any lead rubber protective devices used do not impinge on the region being radiographed. One such example would be to ensure that the clinician's hands and the lead rubber gloves, worn whilst applying stress to the joint, do not overlie the area of interest. It is also relatively easy for the clinician to inadvertently move the ankle from the mortise position, which is adopted as a baseline, so that the area under examination is projected incorrectly; this would make detection of subtle injury difficult. Alternatively, some radiology departments have developed stressing devices as a variation on the Thomas wrench, that the patient may control manually, though usually this device is operated by the medical practitioner.[18] This may produce the desired result, however care is required so that the patient does not over-stress the joint and cause more injury. More likely, however, is the chance that the patient will not exert enough force on the joint to achieve a diagnostic result.

To assess the *tibiotalar* and *talofibular ligaments* of the ankle using the lateral projection, the anterior draw stress view can be attempted without the presence of the medic and is a variation on that described by Horsfield & Murphy.[18] Rest the back of the heel of the patient's affected limb on a wooden block that has been placed on the table-top. A cassette is supported in a vertical position, on the medial aspect of the ankle and alongside the block, so that the ankle joint is raised away from the table-top. A horizontal X-ray beam is aligned with the lateral malleolus. Rest a medium sized sandbag on the mid shaft of the tibia so that the ankle joint is gently stressed for approximately 1 minute. Centre the horizontal central ray to the lateral malleolus and collimate to include the whole of the ankle joint, with at least 5 cm of the distal tibia included. Be sure the malleoli are equidistant from the block as for the mortise position (although malleoli are positioned relative to the *block* rather than the image receptor) (Fig. 27.21). A positive response to stressing the joint shows the talus to have subluxed anteriorly, indicating damage to the ligaments indicated. Remember to remove the weight as soon as possible as this examination is often uncomfortable for the patient.

Adapted projections of the knee, thigh and hip

Knee injuries are usually best evaluated via the routine AP and horizontal ray lateral so that subtle soft tissue signs such as lipohaemarthrosis may be detected. This also has added advantages: that (a) the patient need not be moved in more serious trauma situations and (b) any radiographic evidence that may indicate an effusive collection in the suprapatellar region will not be disturbed. That said,

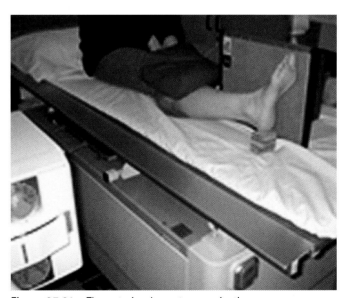

Figure 27.21 The anterior draw stress projection

the presence of an effusion should merely prompt the search for an underlying, more serious, bony cause.

Fractures of the *patella* are most commonly in the transverse direction, which should not be disturbed by bending the knee to achieve a lateral projection. However, the vertical fracture pattern that may not be obvious on the frontal projection may require a tangential/skyline projection to reveal its nature. In these situations a projection with a small (around 30°) angle of flexion at the knee, the degree of flexion probably being governed by the extent of compliance attainable by the patient, should be attempted. Unfortunately this minimal flexion will require the central ray to be directed quite closely towards the body and head of the patient; however, this problem may be navigable by asking the patient to lie on the affected side with the flexed knee resting in a lateral position close to the examination table edge (see patellar projections in Ch. 9). The head should be tilted back to clear the eyes as far as possible from the primary beam. In this way a grazing angle tangential to the patella is achieved which allows the patient to lean back from the track of the central ray, thus reducing the likelihood of exposing the torso and head of the subject being examined.

Femoral fractures are normally the result of significant force and are often accompanied by other injuries, so that adapted techniques are frequently required in order to obtain the images necessary for patient management. As with earlier examples, the use of horizontal beam techniques is vital in these situations, as is negotiating splinting devices that have been used to support the patient's limb to ease pain. The lateral is best undertaken with the horizontal beam and image receptor supported vertically at the side of the thigh. Lateromedial projections are favoured when it is difficult or inadvisable to raise the other leg to clear it from the femur under examination, although the lateromedial approach will involve the primary beam being directed towards the leg not under examination. Frontal projections can be obtained with the image receptor either in the bucky or trolley tray, in order that the limb is not unnecessarily moved. Image magnification is likely to be a problem if the image receptor is placed in a tray under the patient for the AP projection. An increase in FFD will help compensate for this. The approach to the lateral projection will mean that the image receptor may not sufficiently extend far enough along the thigh to include the injury site for evaluation in a single projection. The long femur may also not actually fit within the boundary of the image receptors available (see Chs 9 and 26 where the issue of patient length is discussed) and the only option in this instance is to obtain overlap images from the frontal perspective so that minimal movement of the patient is maintained. Also note that the femur is an area with a range of densities along its length, necessi-

tating the use of a higher kVp non-gridded technique. To summarise these suggestions, an acceptable compromise must be reached that may result in some loss of the contrast and detail in the image but allowing a single projection to be obtained with concomitant reduction in radiation dose to the patient.

Most hip fractures are found in the elderly; however, some younger patients may present with such conditions as slipped upper femoral epiphysis (SUFE) or after involvement in high energy accidents that may have caused dislocation at the hip. Patients who have undergone total hip replacement may present with dislocation of the femoral portion from such simple manoeuvres as standing from a seated position in a low chair. Occasionally, young athletes may present with stress injury to the neck of femur or, more rarely, a true fracture of the same region.

When the neck of femur has been fractured, two projections at right angles are necessary and usually require a whole AP pelvis, to allow full evaluation of the girdle for other injuries, and a horizontal beam lateral of the hip. A common error made with the horizontal ray lateral projection is to allow the thigh of the unaffected side to obstruct the X-ray beam, thus creating a soft tissue artefact. Proprietary devices, such as clamp-on stirrup type supports, are available to help the patient keep the uninjured limb suitably raised; the hip and knee are flexed until the thigh is as near vertical as possible, so the thigh is cleared from the beam path. See Chapter 10 for a description of this technique. A less expensive alternative to using a specialist support is to use a large radiolucent foam pad, which can be positioned appropriately under the leg. Another alternative advocated by some practitioners is to rest the patient's foot on the light beam diaphragm housing and then encourage them to externally rotate the limb to clear the soft tissue shadow from the X-ray beam. Care must be exercised if using this option; the weight of the patient's leg may push the X-ray tube out of alignment with the image receptor, thus exposing the patient to an unnecessary dose of radiation if the image produced is unacceptable and warrants a repeat examination. There is also a risk of patient injury if the tube is unstable and slips whilst the unaffected leg is resting on it.

These methods of producing a horizontal beam lateral are possible when the patient is able to elevate the unaffected limb. Often patients will resist such movement, usually because of pain and confusion. There may also be the valid reason of a recent hip replacement in the currently unaffected hip; there is a risk that the movements described above may cause dislocation of the unaffected side, which would be a disastrous result. When this is the case a type of axial oblique that will give lateral orientation information can be attempted. For this the patient remains supine with the image receptor initially positioned as for the horizontal beam lateral. From this position the cassette is tilted backwards 25° and supported with sandbags and foam pads. The horizontal central ray is angled 25° caudally and rotated on the ceiling mount until the central ray is perpendicular to the image receptor. Centre the beam over the medial aspect of the upper thigh at the level of the greater trochanter, to pass through the hip level with the femoral pulse (Fig. 27.22). Collimate the beam appropriately and select exposure factors slightly lower than those indicated for the horizontal beam lateral.

Adapted projections of the pelvis and hips

An AP examination of the pelvis is standard in the major trauma series associated with the ATLS protocols. However, in a trauma situation there are likely to be inherent problems that will require additional care in undertaking the examination. The fractured pelvis carries serious risks associated with unstable bony components and vascular damage, requiring movement of the patient to be minimised, especially until haemodynamic stability is achieved. As a result the patient must be examined on the trauma trolley, using a gridded cassette or cassette with grid or 'grid lid' in the tray beneath the trolley. Often, accurate centring of the cassette to coincide with the median sagittal plane (MSP), area of interest and central ray is difficult, since the positioning of the cassette under the patient is undertaken by 'guess' or estimation. Patients rarely present perfectly centralised on a trolley and often lie obliquely across its central long axis. Some practitioners peer down the gap

between the trolley top and cassette tray to assess the alignment of the cassette and MSP; unfortunately this does not prove to be the most accurate way of assessing the situation, since the narrowness of the slit between the trolley and tray means the cassette and patient cannot be seen at the same time. Where space permits, the following is a useful tip to ensure accurate alignment:

- Ensure the trolley is parallel to the wall of the X-ray room and the tube ceiling track
- At the head end of the trolley, find the midpoint of the trolley top or central handle (not the mattress, which is often not centralised on the trolley) and position the vertical central ray over this point
- Move the tube down the trolley, towards the patient's pelvis and without any crosswise shift of the tube
- When level with the pelvis, assess the distance between the patient's MSP and the central ray; this will give the practitioner a good indication of how far to displace the cassette laterally, if the MSP is displaced from the midline of the trolley; it may be necessary to turn the cassette slightly if the patient's pelvis is lying diagonally
- Reposition the tube to lie over the midline of the pelvis and the correct centring point
- Collimate as for routine pelvis or hips AP

Note that this tip can prove useful for any supine AP projection of the spine, abdomen or pelvis.

Less severely traumatised trolley-bound patients may also be examined whilst on the trolley; attention to detail will ensure the correct projection is obtained and that the body part is centralised to the cassette. Some imaging departments prefer to move the patient on the trolley mattress across to the examination table to ensure that a degree of imaging standardisation is achieved. However, this does expose practitioners and patients to risk of injury through accidents.

When the resuscitation room is not being used as the examination area, other projections beyond the AP pelvis may be requested if the patient has been stabilised haemodynamically. These include:

- Judets iliac oblique acetabulum (may be performed as a whole pelvis examination)
- Judets obturator oblique acetabulum (may be performed as a whole pelvis examination)
- Posterior oblique of ilium
- AP pubis
- Inlet view of pelvis
- Outlet view of pelvis

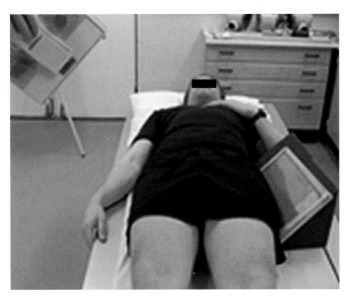

Figure 27.22 The half axial hip projection. The half lateral/semi-axial hip projection for patients unable to elevate the opposite side to produce a horizontal ray lateral. Use of a larger image receptor will facilitate inclusion of the upper third of femur to provide a lateral projection of the shaft

- Lateral pelvis (very rarely required following the widespread use of computed tomography (CT))

Judets projections involve 45° rotation of the patient, (a) towards the affected side to reveal the *iliac* portion of the hemipelvis and away from the affected side to show the *obturator* aspects. Respectively the projections show (a) the posterior or ilioischial column and anterior acetabular rim (when the affected side is lowered) and (b) the anterior or iliopubic column and posterior acetabular rim. When undertaken in order to show each half of the pelvis the whole hemipelvis should be included and the central ray directed to the acetabulum in both projections.[19] See Chapter 10 for a full description of the obliques.

Good visualisation of the anterior portion of the iliac bone and the crest are achieved by positioning as for the iliac oblique, but centring the vertical central ray over the iliac wing, remembering to collimate and adjust exposure as appropriate. A supplementary projection of the *pubis* may be helpful especially where the syndesmosis is 'bobbly' or it is unclear as to whether or not a fracture is present. Position the patient as for the AP projection of both hips. Centre the X-ray beam to the bucky or grid but with 20° cranial angulation applied for males and 30° cranial angulation for females (to allow for the differences in the pelvic shape). Centre to the lower border of the symphysis pubis and collimate to include the pubic and ischial rami. The view gives an apparently elongated (although, in fact, more accurate) projection of the pubic and ischial rami, when compared to the AP pelvis, as the effects of the natural tilt of the pelvis are countered by the cranial angle, so preventing foreshortening.

The pelvic inlet and outlet projections provide added information for the evaluation of the degree of pelvic component movement after a fracture to the area.[20] For the *inlet* projection, position the patient as for the AP pelvis with a film cassette in the bucky tray. Use a central ray angled 40° caudally, already centred to the bucky tray/grid to enter the patient at the level of the ASIS, along the midline. Collimate the beam to include the whole of the pelvis. This view is used to assess the degree of posterior displacement of the hemipelvis or inward/outward rotation of the anterior pelvis following trauma. The pelvic ring should be clearly demonstrated, though, when properly exposed for the anterior and posterior structures; the iliac wings are usually over exposed. For the *outlet* view, position as above but angle the central X-ray beam 40° cranially, centring the central ray to a point at the inferior border of the symphysis pubis. This view is again used in the assessment of trauma. As with the pubic bone AP view, the effect of pelvic tilt is countered, so the view shows these unforeshortened bones

clearly. Visualisation of the iliac wings is poor because of superimposition of the acetabulae over them.[21]

The lateral pelvis may rarely be required to support the postresuscitation regime although it could be helpful in identifying the position of foreign bodies. If it is a necessary projection, this is achieved by simply using a horizontal beam technique. The cassette and grid are supported vertically in a proprietary device, next to the patient's side on the table- or trolley-top and parallel to the patient's MSP. A radiolucent mattress is used as an elevating device to lift the area of interest clear of the examination table. Ensure both anterior superior iliac spines are equidistant from the table-top. The midpoint of the cassette is centred directly above the greater trochanter, in the midaxillary line; this then becomes the centring point for the horizontal beam central X-ray. Collimate the beam to include from iliac crests down to lesser trochanters and from ASIS to sacrum. If a cassette is used, rather than a digital receptor, a 35^2 size is usually adequate for an adult pelvis.

Finally, the *SUFE* presentation requires the use of the frog lateral in conjunction with the AP pelvis projection. Starting in the position for AP pelvis, flex the knees and externally rotate the hips through approximately 40–60° and bring the soles of the feet into contact with each other. Support the legs at the knees with foam immobilising pads and sand bags. Place an appropriately sized image receptor or cassette into the bucky tray and centre a vertical X-ray beam to the cassette and grid. Centre at a point 1–2.5 cm proximal to the symphysis pubis, (according to the size of the child) in the midline, and collimate the beam to include both hips/femoral necks. In this view the pelvis is shown as an AP projection. The proximal femora are projected laterally as for the 'turned' lateral (Lowenstein) projection, however, when visualised together this view may be termed the modified Cleaves projection.[22] This may be a first attendance for this presentation so apply gonad protection carefully so that essential aspects of anatomy, particularly the heads of the femora, are not obscured.

Adapted projections of the spine

Although this section will consider the adapted projections of the spine, it should be apparent that the majority of regions of the spine require just the AP and lateral projections to be obtained following trauma. Indeed, trauma is suggested by the Royal College of Radiologists guidelines as being the key need for radiography of the spine.[23] Often trauma is severe and complete evaluation of the spine may not have been possible without radiographic confirmation; indeed, further examination using CT is usually a necessary adjunct.

The cervical spine

Standard AP and lateral projections are usually obtained following whiplash type injuries, frequently with the patient able to sit or stand for the lateral view. Horizontal beam lateral is required for the patient who is at risk from movement and the lateral image must always be examined before a decision on further patient management is made. The common belief is that the lateral cervical projection takes preference as the first projection undertaken in the multiple injury series; this is entirely appropriate especially if there is serious concern that significant neck trauma has occurred. However, if the AP cervical spine projection is required and is undertaken first *without moving the patient's neck*, then moving to the lateral projection, would this really be considered dangerous practice?

The problems of shoulder shadow impingement upon the cervicothoracic region are typically similar to those encountered in the patient attending for examination of the cervical spine to evaluate degenerative changes and, as such, may be treated with similar techniques. Where more severe injuries necessitate patient presentation on a trolley, either in the imaging department or in the resuscitation room, then adaptation will be necessary to negotiate the shoulder superimposition problem described above. Frequently, where the patient is conscious, explanation of what the radiographer is attempting to achieve enables the patient to reach down towards their feet with their arms and clear the soft tissue of the shoulders from the lower cervical vertebrae. This is especially effective if coupled with an expiration breathing technique prior to exposure. If the patient is in pain and hence holds the shoulders in spasm, or should the patient be unconscious, then different techniques are required. Some resuscitation room practitioners may advo-

cate a pulling of the arms technique by a member of the medical staff who is wearing appropriate radiation protection garments. This at face value may seem sensible; unfortunately risk of further damage to either the neck or the upper limbs is possible. Also, personnel are frequently not strong enough to achieve sufficient movement of the shoulders, or the arms are held by the distal portions of the limb, so that laxity within the joints means the arms cannot be physically pulled sufficiently far to remove the shoulder from the projection. An alternative is to fold the patient's arms across their chest and pull from the distal humeral portion of the arms, the slight anterior abduction of the humerii more efficiently clears the soft tissue of the shoulder in an anterior direction (and away from the lower cervical vertebrae) (Fig. 27.23A,B).[24] Use of these shoulder clearance techniques assumes that the patient's arms are not injured and can be subjected to such forces.

When the arms are injured, possibly the best approach is to adopt a high kVp technique that will reduce contrast whilst ensuring that the whole lateral projection can be visualised on a single image. Many departments will immediately adopt the swimmers position, which can be undertaken supine as well as erect, as described in Chapter 11 (see Fig. 11.4A,B,C), but validity of its use can be questioned since it necessitates significant movement of the shoulders for the neck-injured and multiple-injured patient, carries somewhat confusing information due to overlying structures, and is often low in quality due to scatter produced by area density and increased exposure factors (also see Ch. 11). In any case, this projection is most suited to the conscious patient, since its use in the unconscious patient would require someone to hold the limbs in the required position, very close to the primary radiation beam, which is clearly unac-

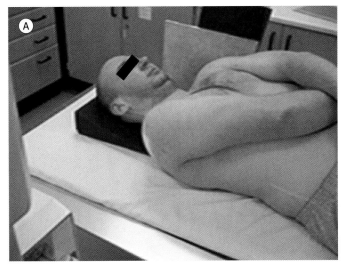 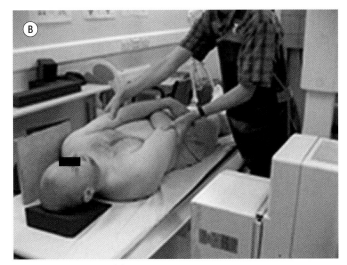

Figure 27.23 Arm folding may help reveal the cervicothoracic junction. The **(A)** folded and **(B)** pulled folded arm technique to reveal the lower cervical spine in the lateral projection

ceptable from a radiation protection standpoint. Typically, many practitioners find evaluation of patient size difficult in terms of selecting appropriate exposure factors – this may be compounded by the high-energy trauma situation, but even the recent 'cure all' suggestions made regarding digital imaging techniques appears to have missed the mark with respect to easing exposure selection decisions.

So a dichotomy exists in more difficult cases, with respect to how some kind of adequate projection might be obtained to reveal possible injuries to the cervical spine. Suggestions regarding the performance of trauma obliques have been made,[25] but unfortunately this is often met with resistance from some (usually the inexperienced, non-radiologic or non-radiographic) personnel, which indicates that reading the images is 'difficult'.[26] To produce the oblique cervical projection, the patient is supine on the examination table (but usually on a trolley). A maximum sized 24 × 30 cm

image receptor should be placed longitudinally in the trolley tray or directly on the table-top so that the edge of the cassette's furthest lateral edge aligns with the outer border of the shoulder. This may mean the cassette is pushed partially under the head when the table- or trolley-top method is used. This should only be done under supervision but will not be a problem for the cassette tray method. Angle the X-ray tube 45° in a lateromedial direction, the central ray entering the side of the neck at the level of C4 (Fig. 27.24A,B,C). Both obliques are undertaken. No grid is necessary but if one is required for a large patient ensure the grid lines are running parallel with the direction of the central ray. This avoids grid 'cut off'. To produce a more elongated image of the posterior spinal elements and the vertebral bodies, perform the same projection as above but with the lateromedial angulation at 60°. Although the bodies will not be projected in good relief, the posterior elements will

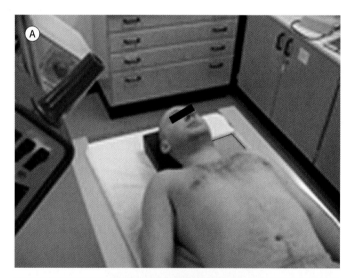

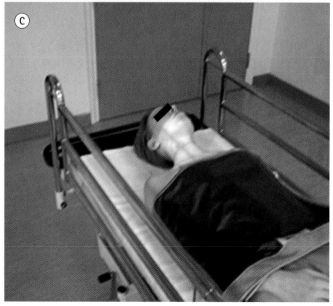

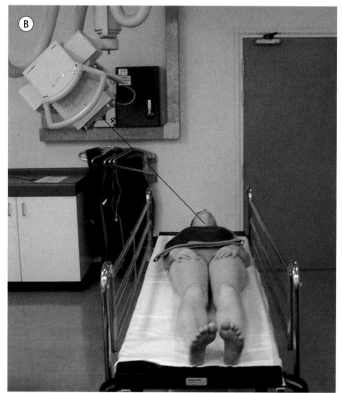

Figure 27.24   The trauma oblique cervical spine projection

be shown to advantage, so that injury to these regions will be revealed. In both techniques, images should be obtained from each side of the neck.

See Chapter 11 for further discussion on the cervical spine and the spine in trauma.

The thoracolumbar spine

Generally speaking, most images of these regions can be obtained by appropriate use of the AP vertical ray techniques with the patient on the trolley or examination table and grids placed on cassettes when the bucky tray is not used. Horizontal ray techniques allow the lateral projections to be obtained without the need to move the patient. Care is required, however, to ensure cassettes are held in appropriate positions without risk of injury to the patient and the projection of table- or trolley-top artefacts onto the image. The latter is most problematic as objects built into the trolley or table impinge upon the posterior spinal elements.

Adapted projections of the craniofacial skeleton

Chapters 16 to 19 have indicated techniques that were once the mainstay of craniofacial imaging in the radiology department. Table-top skull technique is mentioned in these chapters and it is this approach which is now the only method available in many A&E imaging departments, where the isocentric skull unit has been disposed of. Often the patient requiring skull radiography will present in a non-compliant state for various reasons, which questions the value of skull imaging from two perspectives, (a) can this imaging reveal anything of value to the patient's management and (b) will degradation of the image caused by non-compliance result in excessive radiation dose when compared to the benefit received?

All skull and facial examinations can be achieved using the trolley- or table-top method when embarked upon with a modicum of care and attention to detail. Whereas many projections have been described in this text as being obtained from a PA direction to enhance radiation protection considerations, simple reversal of angles through 180° allow images to be obtained from the AP perspective, as outlined in Chapter 16. Obviously, magnification will cause differences in the appearances of some projections; for example, the orbits are particularly affected by magnification. Care must also be taken where the image receptor has to be placed under the head, for all the reasons cited earlier in this chapter, with respect to moving the patient and performing the examination in relatively clean conditions.

The cranial vault

As with the descriptions in earlier chapters, the ability to achieve skull projections hangs on the fact that the orbito-

meatal baseline (OMBL) is perpendicular to the imaging cassette. If this is not always possible, and when the patient can be easily moved, a large radiolucent support can be an advantage when used under the neck or spine. This is particularly useful for kyphotic individuals. Placing this wedge beneath the shoulders will aid patient comfort whilst encouraging the head to fall naturally into a position that will place the OMBL perpendicular to the image receptor, which is placed directly under the skull (Fig. 27.25). The radiographer should avoid placing the image receptor under any support as this increases the object film distance. It is just a small matter then to ensure the central ray forms the required angle to the OMBL. If it is still not possible to position the OMBL at 90° to the image receptor, compensation can be made by initially aligning the central ray with the OMBL and then adding the appropriate angle for the relevant projection. As a more specific example, consider a patient whose chin is raised so that the OMBL is raised 10° from the perpendicular: for a projection that requires a 20° cranial angle the central ray will initially be selected as 10° caudally to coincide with the OMBL and then angled 20° cranially from this point to achieve the correct 20° to the OMBL. On examination the beam will be 10° cranially. The frontooccipital (FO) 30° (Towne's) projection of the occipital region is essentially an AP projection anyway and position of the OMBL is obtained as through the use of pads as for other FO projections. As mentioned in Chapter 16,

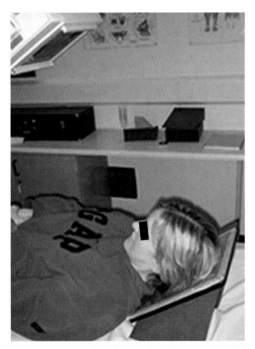

Figure 27.25 An adaptation for the FO skull. The AP table-top projection of the skull, where the patient is unable to lie flat. Note the pad lies under image receptor and patient, rather than under the head and on top of the image receptor

pads must never be placed under the head and must be placed under the image receptor (see Ch.16). A 30° wedge support system may be used for the FO 30° (Fig. 27.26), using a support which has an accurate 30° angle. As the image receptor is tilted 30° in this method, it is merely a simple matter of using a vertical central ray passing through the midline to exit the inferoposterior aspect of the skull to produce the required FO 30° projection. This is dependent upon the OMBL being accurately positioned in relationship to the image receptor.

Lateral projections are fairly straightforward, with the image receptor supported vertically at the side of the head, which is supported on a radiolucent pad (Fig. 27.27). However, if a neck-injured patient cannot be moved to raise the head on a pad, the image receptor must be supported in an erect cassette holder which may create an increased object film distance if this has to be positioned at the side of the trolley rather than directly next to the head. Compensation for this can be made by increasing FFD.

Facial bones

Similar rules may be employed for the facial skeleton as the ones identified above. However, it is clear that the use of the wedge support suggestion encourages lowering, rather than raising of the chin. Fortunately it is much easier for patients to raise the chin until the OMBL lies at the required angle to the image receptor. If it is too difficult for the patient

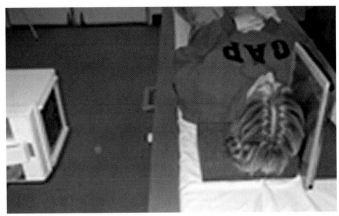

Figure 27.27 Continuing to work around the patient to generate a table-top lateral skull. The horizontal beam lateral projection of the skull with the head elevated on a radiolucent pad

to lift the chin adequately, one solution, where presentation permits, is to place supports under the shoulders so room is made for the head to be tilted backwards to allow the OMBL to form an appropriate angle relative to the image receptor (Fig. 27.28A,B). The centring point is in the midline, level with the midpoint of the facial structures required for inclusion on the image. When this modification is not possible, an alternative has been described.[27] The head is supported on a radiolucent rectangular pad and the image receptor is supported vertically at the vertex of the skull. The OMBL is parallel to the image receptor. The X-ray tube is initially horizontal and then the caudal angle is applied according to the requirements of the projection. For this the tube has to be positioned close to the chest of the supine patient for some angulations and this may be difficult with units with bulky tube housings. Increasing FFD, with the adjustment of exposure factors and use of a parallel grid, will act as a means to overcome this. Another alternative involves slight tilting of the image receptor, in conjunction with chin adjustment (if possible) to ensure the OMBL lies parallel to it. This allows the tube to be used in a higher position; of course, the initial tube position will change from horizontal to a relationship of 90° to the image receptor.

TRAUMA IMAGING EQUIPMENT SELECTION

A&E and its associated imaging department should, ideally, be sited as close neighbours if not in the same departmental area. The rooms themselves should display features that will enable them to handle the wide variation in patient presentation that spans ages from cradle to grave. X-ray rooms should be spacious, with a large 'footprint', so that enough room is available for practitioners to work around

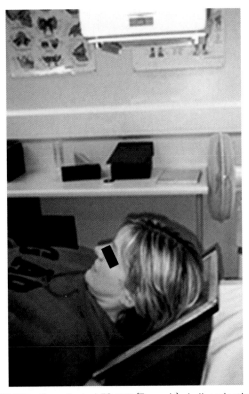

Figure 27.26 The adapted FO 30° (Towne's) skull projection

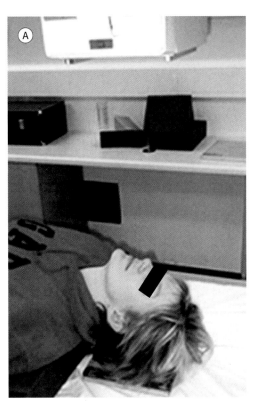

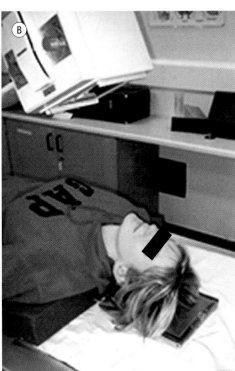

Figure 27.28   Adapted facial techniques where patient can extend the neck. Tilted head projections to show the facial bone structures as equivalent OM and OM 15° projections

the patient in relative ease, while using X-ray equipment capable of performing the maximum range of movement possible. This is often in the face of fairly tight budgetary constraints. However, despite likely restrictions on cost, employment of a rise and fall table is a must for the range of patients who may be examined in A&E (many of the projections identified in the earlier sections necessitate this versatility), and who must be worked around to obtain the required images. Figure 27.29 shows a fairly simple example of the type of equipment required.

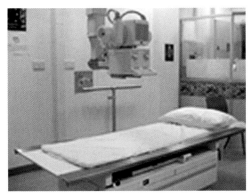

Figure 27.29   A general X-ray room for trauma. A general X-ray room capable of handling the traumatised patient. Note rise and fall table, large amount of room space and some decoration to help calm or distract the paediatric patient during the procedure

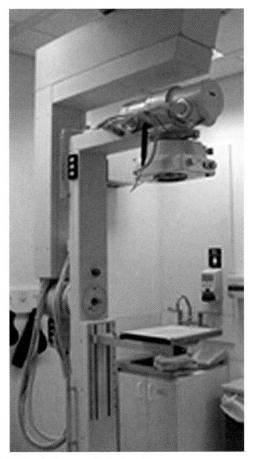

Figure 27.30   An isocentric skull unit

As stated earlier, ancillary equipment should be chosen to meet the demands of adaptability and ease of use;[28] however, support equipment must also be robust and available either as static units in the examination room or reliably mobile if the decision is made to share facilities. Ideally, piped gases and suction should be provided in any newly built department and all staff should be trained in the use of this and other general equipment. Short-handedness through lack of education in a moment of demand will not carry any weight in a court of law, should litigation be instigated as a result of neglect.

Many A&E imaging departments will show signs of age through the degree of obsolescence of X-ray equipment in use. Isocentric skull units are an example of this (Fig. 27.30); due to their versatility these were once popular but are now falling out of favour owing to the change in imaging preferences due to expanded and improved modalities such as CT. Initiatives such as the guidelines generated by the National Institute for Clinical Excellence (NICE)[29] for evaluation and treatment of head injuries have contributed to the death knell of plain film evaluation in these situations. Some practitioners will miss isocentric skull units, as they

have greater uses than easing the difficulty in obtaining plain films of the skull and facial bones in the emergency setting. This has resulted in the revival of table-top techniques described in the skull sections in this and Chapters 16 to 21 – some may argue that all this is for the better as it enhances the role and art of radiography, however, there is necessarily a loss in image quality in these instances.

That said, when equipment breaks down the versatility of the experienced practitioner comes to the fore with their ability to instantly translate static techniques to mobile equipment. Therefore patients can still expect to receive a service that, although adapted, will provide the answers needed in a traumatic situation. Advances in mobile X-ray unit technology have enabled the mobile ward service, breakdown situations in A&E or in some departments the imaging service in the resuscitation room, to move from good to excellent. Indeed, the use of mobile equipment support in the resuscitation room is seen by many to be advantageous over static units, particularly in the USA, as evidenced by television documentaries, etc. By offering versatility and manoeuvrability with an X-ray tube and generator that can provide almost identical qualities to that

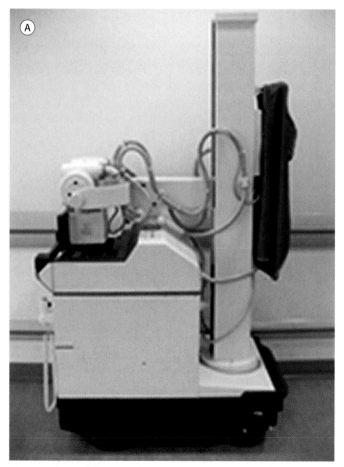

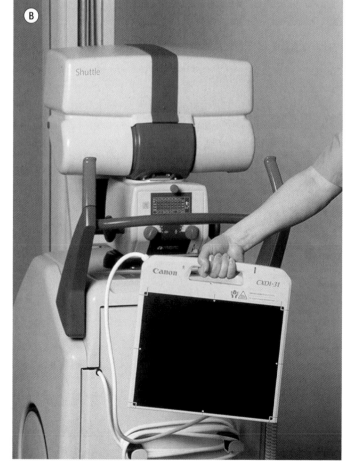

Figure 27.31 (A) The mobile unit – a motorised A&E department?; (B) mobile direct digital equipment. Reproduced with permission from Xograph Imaging Systems

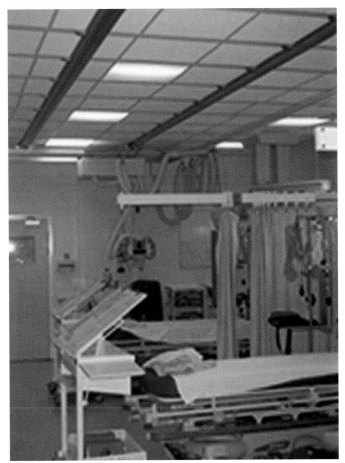

Figure 27.32 Modern thinking in the resuscitation room. The newly commissioned resuscitation room arrangement – note how lead rubber curtains provide radiation protection between bays that can be reached by the X-ray tube along the ceiling track that spans the whole room

offered by static equipment, the mobile unit is perceived as superior. Another bonus for mobile radiography is the availability of digital mobile units, with versatile image receptor sizes (Fig. 27.31A,B). Although state of the art equipment may be built into a new establishment, anecdotal experience of the author and others has shown implementation of this still does not always meet the demands of the service or its users. Much depends upon the activity of the hospital and how assertive staff may be in the resuscitation area. Resuscitation is for just that – for very ill patients – radiation protection issues and the impact of image quality on performing radiographic examinations in an area not fully designed for X-ray imaging makes us ask why radiography is performed in an area out of context. Even so, many radiographers do appreciate the identification that their needs are being recognised by commissioning of such equipment (Fig. 27.32). However, they are able to perform perfectly well when a breakdown occurs and mobile machinery has to be employed.

References

1. Berman L, et al. Reducing errors in the accident department: a simple method using radiographers. Radiography 1986; 52(603):143–144.
2. American College of Surgeons 2003. Advanced trauma life support student manual. 7th edn. Chicago, USA.
3. Department of Health. A health service of all the talents: developing the NHS workforce. London: HMSO; 2000.
4. Health and Safety Executive. The Ionising Radiation (Medical Exposure) Regulation 20. (Statutory Instruments, 2000; no.1059). London: HMSO; 2000.
5. Society and College of Radiographers. Reporting by radiographers: a vision paper. London: SCoR; 1997.
6. Dimond BC. Red dots and radiographer's liability. Health Care Risk Report October 2000.
7. Dimond BC. Legal aspects of radiography and radiology. Oxon: Blackwell Science; 2002.
8. Department of Health. A health service of all the talents: developing the NHS workforce. London: HMSO; 2000.
9. Lewis S. New angles on the radiographic examination of the hand – I. Radiography Today 1988; 54(617):44–45.
10. Lewis S. New angles on the radiographic examination of the hand – II. Radiography Today 1988; 54(618):29.
11. Lewis S. New angles on the radiographic examination of the hand – III. Radiography Today 1988; 54(619):47–48.
12. Eyres KS, Allen TR. Skyline view of the metacarpal head in the assessment of the human fight-bite injuries. Journal of Hand Surgery (British volume) 1993; 18(1):43–44.
13. Long BW, Rafaert JA. Orthopaedic radiography. Philadelphia: WB Saunders; 1995.
14. Swallow RA, et al. Clark's positioning in radiography. 11th edn. London: Heinemann; 1986.
15. Coyle GF. Radiographing immobile trauma patients. Denver: Multi-Media Publishing; 1980.
16. Garth WP, et al. Roentgenographic demonstration of instability of the shoulder: the apical oblique projection - a technical note. Journal of Bone and Joint Surgery 1984; 66A(9):1450–1453.
17. Wallace WA, Hellier M. Improving radiographs of the injured shoulder. Radiography 1983; 49(586):229–233.
18. Horsfield D, Murphy G. Stress views of the ankle joint in lateral ligament injury. Radiography 1985; 51(595):7–11.
19. Monks J, Yeoman L. Judet's views of the acetabulum: a demonstration of their importance. Radiography Today 1989; 55(628):18–21.
20. Foster LM, Barton ED. Managing pelvic fractures, part 2: physical and radiologic assessment. Journal of Critical Illness 2001; 16(5):255–256, 258.
21. Hunter JC, et al. Pelvic and acetabular trauma. In: El-Khoury GY. Imaging of orthopedic trauma. Radiologic Clinics of North America 1997; 35(3):ix,491–781.
22. Hardy M, Boynes S. Paediatric radiography. Oxon: Blackwell Science; 2003.
23. Royal College of Radiologists. Making the best use of a department of clinical radiology: guidelines for doctors. 5th edn. London: RCR; 2003.

24. Carver BJ, Roche D. An alternative technique for visualisation of the C7 T1 junction in trauma. Supplement to British Journal of Radiology 2000; 73:73.

25. Ireland AJ, et al. Do supine oblique views provide better imaging of the cervicothoracic junction than swimmer's views? Journal of Accident & Emergency Medicine1998; 15(3):151-154.

26. Daffner RH. Radiographic interpretation of cervical vertebral injuries. Topics in Emergency Medicine 1997; 19(3):11–25.

27. Ponsford A, Clements R. 1991 A modified view of the facial bones in the seriously injured. Radiography Today 1991; 57(646):10–12.

28. Carver BJ, Unett EM. The Aintree bucky. Journal of Diagnostic Radiography and Imaging 2001; 3(3):127–132.

29. National Institute for Clinical Excellence. Triage, assessment, investigation and early management of head injury in infants, children and adults. London: HMSO; 2003.

MAMMOGRAPHY: INTRODUCTION AND RATIONALE

Julie Burnage

Definitively, mammography is the radiographic imaging of the breast. The majority of mammograms are performed by women on women and for the purposes of this chapter it is be assumed that both patient and mammographer are female. It is not the intention of this chapter to present itself as a complete work on mammography – it is a brief introduction to a very specialised field.

Although mammography is the given name for this section, other methods of breast imaging are not ignored. A résumé of other methods for imaging is given at the end of this chapter and ultrasound of the breast is contained in a separate chapter within this section.

Historically, mammography has always been performed by radiographers; however, this is no longer the case and as radiographers take on other tasks as part of their professional development there has been a move towards the use of assistant practitioners. These practitioners are not radiographers but, due in part to the changes in the UK brought about by the ionising radiation regulations [IR(ME)R 2000],[1] they can now undertake mammography (once suitably trained and deemed competent) under the supervision of a state registered practitioner.[1] This new way of working is part of the proposed four tier model of the radiography profession, the four tiers being:

- Consultant/lead practitioner
- Advanced practitioner
- Practitioner
- Assistant practitioner

Mammography is widely used in both the investigation of symptomatic breast disease and is the modality used for breast screening. It has a sensitivity of 85–90%, but specificity is low.[2]

SYMPTOMATIC PATIENTS FOR MAMMOGRAPHY

Symptomatic patients are usually referred by a clinician and present with a potentially significant breast problem, i.e. they have symptoms such as a palpable lump, nipple discharge and pain, or a visual change such as skin tethering or puckering. Some women attend following screening mammography for follow-up assessment of an abnormality, or following check up after breast cancer treatment.

ASYMPTOMATIC PATIENTS

Asymptomatic patients are part of a screening programme such as the UK National Health Service Breast Screening Programme (NHSBSP), a research project or a family history trial.

Whatever a woman's reason for attending, there will always be common anxieties. The most significant concern is likely to be the outcome or fear of possible results following their investigation but, for many women, there are concerns about the procedure itself – is it painful, is it safe?

COMMUNICATION WITH PATIENTS UNDERGOING MAMMOGRAPHY

As for all interactions between patient and health professional, effective communication is vital during mammography and starts before the patient even attends for her mammogram. All patients should receive suitable, accurate and helpful written information prior to their appointment. This could include information about the procedure itself and, for breast screening patients, details about the risks and benefits, thus enabling them to make an informed decision. Any other information that may help to reduce the potential for anxiety should be incorporated, such as instructions on how to find the unit, waiting times and other tests that may be undertaken during their visit.

The majority of women attending for a mammogram will be given a 'normal' result and therefore will be likely to meet only one member of the breast team: the mammographer. With this in mind the mammographer has a vital role in ensuring that the patient receives all the information she requires and needs and that it is imparted in a compassionate and understandable way.

Essential communication stages for the patient:

- Before the mammogram, so that the patient knows what to expect and what is expected of her
- During the mammogram to ensure that she knows what is happening and to enable her to voice any concerns or indicate any discomfort she may be experiencing
- After the mammogram so that she knows when and how the results will be imparted

BREAST SCREENING

In 1957, The Commission of Chronic illness in the United States defined screening as 'the presumptive identification of unrecognised disease ... by the application of tests, examinations or other procedures which can be applied rapidly'[3]

No screening test can be considered perfect but the World Health Organisation's International Agency for Research on Cancer (IARC) concluded that there was sufficient evidence for the efficacy of breast screening of women between 50 and 69 years.[4] Examples of some essential considerations for a screening programme include:

- Is the disease an important health problem for the population?
- Can the population at risk be readily identified?
- Does early treatment lead to a better outcome?
- Are the benefits of screening greater than the harm caused?
- Does the screening identify the disease at a preclinical stage?
- Is treatment of the preclinical disease widely available?
- Is the screening modality acceptable to the target population?
- Is the method to be used cost effective?

Mammography has been the screening modality used for every randomised trial that has shown a significant population breast cancer mortality reduction.[5,6,7,8]

It has a high sensitivity in the detection of breast cancers, particularly invasive carcinomas and ductal carcinoma in situ (DCIS), but a lower specificity. The use of a multidisciplinary approach when women are recalled following their initial mammogram ensures that the screening process is specific. The assessments used are: further imaging, clinical examination and tissue sampling through biopsy.

Publication of the Forrest report[3] on breast screening and the subsequent implementation of the NHSBSP revolutionised mammography in the United Kingdom. The NHSBSP automatically offers mammograms to women between the ages of 50–70. Research to assess the efficacy of mammography in women between the ages of 40–49 is ongoing. This 'age trial' involves 65 000 women over 15 years and began in 1991 although it will be some years before the results are available. It is possible that the results will have great impact on workforce issues. The radiation benefit risk ratio will play an important part in the decision to recommend screening for younger women.

The Forrest report made numerous recommendations: projections that should be undertaken on each breast; the screening interval; interpretation of the mammograms; assessment and follow up of patients and implementation of quality assurance and quality control procedures at every step of the programme. Recommendation regarding setting up of an advisory committee then led to a report which gave guidance on quality issues, known as the Pritchard report.[9] Recommendations made in the Forrest and Pritchard reports do not only pertain to screening mammography services as they are pertinent wherever mammography is offered, thus ensuring equity of provision for all attending for mammography.

BREAST DISEASE

Benign breast disease

There are a number of benign breast conditions, which may manifest on mammograms, some examples are:

- *Benign breast change.* There is no evident disease process and changes are often brought about by hormonal variations. Conditions such as mastitis and fibroadenosis would come under this umbrella

- *Cysts.* Cystic changes in the breast are very common and, as with most benign breast conditions, tend to be bilateral
- *Fibroadenoma.* These are often found incidentally as they are usually too small to feel. Larger lesions occur in younger women. Fibroadenomas in postmenopausal women do not grow (except in women on hormone replacement therapy) and new lesions do not appear

Benign breast conditions and their mammographic appearances	
Cysts	Visualised as an increase in density – usually with smooth edges
Fibroadenoma	Has no specific characteristic features but is usually smooth, rounded, well defined and causes displacement of the surrounding tissues. When calcification occurs the lesion is said to have a 'popcorn' appearance

Breast cancer

United Kingdom breast cancer facts and statistics:[10]

- Breast cancer is the most common cancer in women
- The lifetime risk of getting cancer of the breast is 1 in 9
- 80% of breast cancers occur in postmenopausal women
- 5–10% of breast cancers are hereditary
- 90% of breast lumps are benign
- 1% of cases are adult male: 250 men are diagnosed in the UK each year, the majority being over the age of 60
- Breast cancer can be divided into two main types:
  - In situ carcinoma: this is contained within the breast ducts or lobules and has the potential to become invasive and threaten life
  - Invasive carcinoma: this spreads from the ducts or lobules into the surrounding breast tissue. It has the potential to metastasise, via the blood or lymphatic systems, to other parts of the body and may ultimately shorten the patient's life. Invasive cancers are often graded histologically, i.e. a high grade cancer has a high degree of pleomorphism, no tubule formation, is high in mitotic counts and thus has a poor prognosis. Low grade cancers show the opposite histologically and have a better prognosis

There are also some conditions for which mammography has a limited role in assessment as they often have no clearly recognisable features on mammograms. These conditions are recognised as being precancerous; some have little risk of progressing to malignancy whilst others have a significantly high risk, e.g. DCIS has a greater risk of developing into an invasive carcinoma than atypical lobular hyperplasia.

Cancer type and mammographic appearance	
Cancer type	*Appearance*
DCIS	Microcalcifications
Invasive ductal carcinoma	Usually spiculate mass but often has calcification and parenchymal distortion
Invasive lobular carcinoma	Similar to ductal carcinoma but microcalcification is less common

Mammography may often not distinguish between benign and malignant masses, which is why breast services do not stop at mammography but incorporate other imaging modalities such as ultrasound, magnetic resonance imaging (MRI), cytology, histology and clinical assessments. However it is possible to make some general observations from mammographic appearances:

- A spiculated mass with microcalcifications is highly suspicious and strongly indicates malignancy; any mass with distortion should be assumed to be malignant until proven otherwise
- Microcalcifications are difficult to evaluate but could represent DCIS
- Well-defined masses are likely to be benign

Dose implications for the breast undergoing mammography

It is important to remember that mammography uses radiation and there is therefore a potential to induce carcinoma by the biological effects of radiation.

The risk is considered to be low for the patient undergoing single mammogram because the dose is well below the threshold for deterministic effects and the reproductive cells are not exposed. Risks are highest in the youngest patients and are estimated to range from 9.1 fatal carcinomas induced per million per mGy in the 30–34 year age group, falling to 7.5 fatal carcinomas induced per million per mGy in the 45–49 year age group and 4.7 fatal carcinomas induced per million per mGy in the 60–64 year age group.[11]

For women of screening age (50–70 years) the risk of radiation-induced breast cancer is approximately 1 in 100 000 per mGy. Radiation dose for women attending the NHSBSP is taken to be on average 4.5 mGy per two view screening examination.

- The risk of radiation-induced cancer for a woman attending mammographic screening (two views) by the NHSBSP is about 1 in 20 000 per visit

- It is estimated that about 170 cancers are detected by the NHSBSP for every cancer induced[12]

ALTERNATIVE AND COMPLEMENTARY IMAGING TECHNIQUES

Magnetic resonance mammography (MRM)

MRM is increasingly used as an adjunct to mammography and ultrasound, although it currently does have drawbacks such as high cost, limited availability and several contraindications (patients with pacemakers, pregnant patients, those with claustrophobia and patients who are unable to lie in the required prone position which is necessary when using a breast coil). It is however particularly useful for:

- the assessment of implant leakages
- imaging dense, glandular breasts
- evaluation of indeterminate breast lesions[13]
- investigation of axilla nodal recurrence
- imaging suspected multicentric or multifocal lesions[14]
- differentiation of recurrent breast cancer from scar tissue[15]
- evaluation of the response of breast cancer to treatment[16]

Nuclear medicine

There are two main uses of nuclear medicine in breast imaging:

1. *Sentinel node biopsy.* This involves the use of Technecium labelled colloid to label the first axillary lymph node to drain the breast – the sentinel node. If this node is metastasis free then axillary clearance can be avoided. Sentinel node status is able to accurately predict axillary lymph node status in 97.5% of cases[17]
2. *Scintimammography.* This involves the use of Technecium labelled Sestamibi and, used as an adjunct to mammography, is comparable to MRM in both sensitivity and specificity in the demonstration of both palpable and impalpable tumours[18]

Ultrasound

Ultrasound of the breast has increased in recent years, due to the fact that it is a method that does not use ionising radiation on this radiosensitive area. It is a useful adjunct but is not a stand-alone method for imaging the breast. In any case, X-ray mammography does not have good specificity if not supplemented by other imaging methods. Since ultrasound of the breast is used more extensively than MRI, computed tomography (CT) and radionuclide

imaging (RNI), Chapter 30 is dedicated to this imaging method.

Computed tomography laser mammography (CTLM)

This is a recently developed breast-imaging device that uses laser technology instead of X-rays to scan the breast for abnormalities. The system uses computed algorithms to create cross-sectional and 3D images of the breast without the need for compression. Early designs of the system require the patient to lie prone, with their breast hanging through an opening in the table-top; the laser then rotates around the breast. The use of the term 'computed tomography' may be somewhat misleading as this device does not use ionising radiation. At the time of going to press, the system is undergoing clinical trials.

Dynamic optical breast imaging (DOBI) system

This is a non-ionising, non-invasive system which aims to diagnose carcinoma through the detection of vascular changes (angiogenesis) associated with malignant tumours at the earliest stages of its development. Infra-red light is transmitted through the compressed breast, and areas of increased vascularisation suggesting vascular supply to a tumour, are imaged in colour. Compression is less uncomfortable than with conventional mammography, since the unit uses inflation of a membrane over the breast to achieve compression. Images are easy to interpret as the area affected by pathology appears as distinctly different in colour to normal tissue areas. At the time of going to press, this system is undergoing clinical trials.

Both CTLM and DOBI systems are potentially exciting developments in the diagnosis of an insidious disease and final results of extensive clinical trials will prove interesting.

As can be seen from this introductory chapter, mammography is a highly specialised modality undertaken by a team of dedicated healthcare professionals who undergo rigorous training and continuing professional development to ensure that women in the UK are offered the best in breast health management.

References

1. The Ionising Radiation (Medical Exposure) Regulations 2000. London: HMSO.
2. Reaney S. Imaging of the breast: complimentary and alternative techniques. BMUS Bulletin 1999; 7(4).
3. Forrest AP. Breast cancer: the decision to screen. Journal of Public Health Medicine 1991; 13:2–12.
4. International Agency for Research on Cancer. Mammography screening can reduce deaths from breast cancer. Press release 139: 19 March 2002. Geneva: World Health Organisation.

5. Lee L, et al. Fundamentals of mammography. 2nd edn. London: Churchill Livingstone; 2003:143.

6. Bjurstram N, et al. The Gothenburg Breast Screening Trial. First results on mortality, incidence and mode of detection for women aged 39–49 years at randomisation. Cancer 1997; 80:2091–2099.

7. Nystrom L, et al. Breast cancer screening with mammography; overview of Swedish randomised trials. Lancet 1993; 341:973–978.

8. Shapiro S, et al. Periodic screening for breast cancer: the health insurance plan project and its sequelae, 1963–1986. London: John Hopkins University Press; 1988.

9. Pritchard J. Quality assurance guidelines for mammography. Report of a sub-committee of the Radiology Advisory Committee of the Chief Medical Officer. Oxford: NHSBSP Publications; 1990.

10. http://www.breastcancercare.org.uk/Breastcancer/Breastcancerfactsandstatistics

11. Law J. Risk and benefit associated with radiation dose in breast screening programmes: an update. British Journal of Radiology 1995; 68(812):870–876.

12. National Health Service Breast Screening Programme. Review of Radiation Risk in Breast Screening. 2003; Publication No 54:Feb.

13. Hickman PF, et al. The indeterminate breast mass: assessment using contrast enhanced magnetic resonance imaging. British Journal of Radiology 1994; 67:14–20.

14. Weinreb JC, Newstead G. MR imaging of the breast. Radiology 1995; 196:593–610.

15. Dao TH, et al. Tumour recurrence versus fibrosis in the irradiated breast: differentiation with dynamic gadolinium enhanced MR imaging. Radiology 1993: 187(3):751–755.

16. Gilles R, et al. Locally advanced breast cancer: contrast enhanced subtraction MR imaging of response to pre-operative chemotherapy. Radiology 1994; 191:633–638.

17. Vernosi U, et al. Sentinel node biopsy to avoid axillary dissection in breast cancer with clinically negative lymph nodes. Lancet 1997; 28; 349(9069):1864–1867.

18. Buscombe J, et al. Scintigraphic imaging of breast cancer: a review. Nuclear Medicine Communications 1997; 18(8):698–709.

MAMMOGRAPHY TECHNIQUE

Julie Burnage

EQUIPMENT

Purchase, commissioning and quality control of suitable equipment are essential for the provision of a quality mammography service.[1] Equipment must also be acceptable to both the operator (e.g. it must be light and easy to use) and the patient (e.g. there should be no sharp edges and there should be handles for support where required).

The machine simply consists of an X-ray tube connected to a breast support which houses the film cassette or imaging device on a C shaped arm, with a moveable compression paddle between the two (Fig. 29.1).

Functional requirements

- *High-voltage generator*. The generator must supply a near DC high voltage with ripple less than 5%
- *Kilovoltage (kVp) output*. Most modern mammography machines have automatic selection for kVp in order to optimise contrast. The generator provides a constant potential and the high voltage applied to the tube must be from 22 to 35 kVp in increments of 1 kVp
- *Focal spot size*. The focal spot should be as small as possible to ensure adequate resolution, e.g. 0.3 mm for general mammography and 0.1 mm (small focus) for magnification views
- *Tube current (mA)*. In order to keep exposure times to a minimum (and thus reduce the likelihood of movement unsharpness) the tube current should be as high as possible. At 28 kVp the current should be at least 100 mA on large focus
- *Grid*. A moving grid is essential and should have a grid factor of less than 2.5 at 30 kVp to ensure optimum image quality
- *AEC*. An automatic exposure control is essential because of the wide variation in breast sizes and compositions

(As there is a need for high radiographic contrast and consequently the system has low latitude there is little scope for error in the selection of mAs.)

Image recording

Currently the majority of mammography is still undertaken using traditional cassettes, intensifying screens and single emulsion film with dedicated processing. Processing parameters are strictly monitored and quality control and assurance programmes are vital to ensure that standards are not compromised, as reduction in film quality can lead to incorrect interpretation of images. However, digital mammography, like other areas in medical imaging, is poised to become the norm in the immediate future and there are already some digital mammography units in use in the UK.

Cassettes and film

The cassette contains a single intensifying screen and the film (usually green sensitive) has a single emulsion layer, both of which are required to give optimum resolution. The important physical factors of the film itself are its speed, latitude/contrast and characteristic curve. Mammography requires that the film has a high spatial resolution, enough speed to ensure that the dose is acceptable without being so fast that it causes visible quantum mottle and high contrast with enough latitude to show both dense glandular tissue and the skin edge.

Digital mammography

Digital mammography has some advantages over mammography using film. Chemical processing is not required and changeover of cassettes is unnecessary. This means that the examination time is cut and time between examining patients decreased. Markers are applied digitally and the images can be manipulated once produced. One of the main

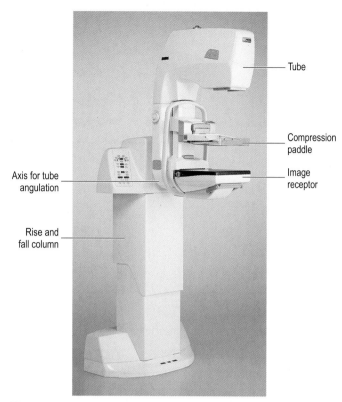

Figure 29.1 Mammography unit. Reproduced with permission from Xograph Imaging Systems

advantages of image manipulation is the ability to magnify the image with significantly less unsharpness than that associated with macro or magnification images that are sometimes required to demonstrate suspicious areas already seen on mammograms. An additional benefit of digital magnification is that it does not involve an additional exposure to radiation, which traditional magnification views require.

Viewing the images

It is recommended that craniocaudal (CC) images are viewed 'back-to-back' with the posterior aspect of the breasts touching, on the viewing box. Mediolateral obliques are viewed with the pectoral aspects touching. These strategies facilitate vital comparison of similar areas of each breast for each projection (Figs 29.2C and Fig. 29.3C).

A horizontal viewing box designed specifically for film mammograms provides the best viewing conditions. The height of the box is identical to the longest axis of the film but the width of the box can accommodate several images. Sections of the box can be switched off and the result offers the viewer a light box that fits the perimeter of the images; this ensures optimal viewing conditions.

Digital mammography does not require the viewer to assess images on a viewing box and light transmission through the image is not an issue. Images are still presented back-to-back on the screen since this is the most suitable method for comparison.

MAMMOGRAPHIC PROJECTIONS

Anatomical markers must be used on all projections undertaken and markers used in mammography usually incorporate legends, which identify the side under examination, the projection and orientation of the axilla.

■ Craniocaudal (CC) (Fig. 29.2A,B,C)

Positioning

• The mammography unit is positioned with the breast support table (image receptor holder) horizontal and the height adjusted to slightly above the level of the patient's inframammary angle

• The patient faces the machine, standing with their front approximately 5–6 cm back, feet facing the machine but her body rotated 15–20° away from the side under examination, so that the breast under examination is brought closer to the image receptor holder and aligned with the centre of it

• The patient's arms hang loosely by her side and her head is turned away from the side to be examined

• The breast is lifted gently up and away from the chest wall (the mammographer will use the left hand to raise the right breast and vice versa)

• With the mammographer supporting the breast, the height of the unit is adjusted so that the image receptor holder makes contact with the breast at the inframammary fold and the breast is at approximately 90° to the chest wall

• The breast is carefully placed in contact with the cassette; the mammographer removes her hand, whilst ensuring that no skin folds are created underneath the breast

• The arm of the side under examination is flexed at the elbow and the hand is placed on the patient's lower abdomen or relaxed at the side of the trunk; this relaxes the pectoral muscle. The shoulder is gently pressed down to bring the outer quadrant of the breast into contact with the image receptor

• The mammographer maintains slight pressure on the patient's back to ensure that she does not inadvertently pull back from the unit and cause some breast tissue to be lost from the resultant image

• The mammographer places her thumb on the medial aspect and middle finger on the superior aspect of the breast, pulling gently forwards towards the nipple while compression is applied slowly. The mammographer's other hand is placed on the shoulder of the side being examined to ensure that the shoulder stays relaxed

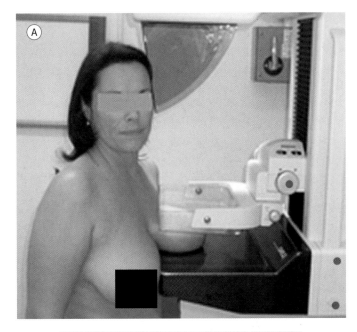

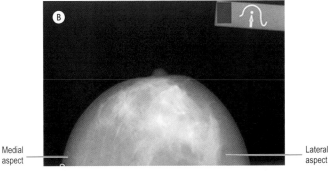

Medial aspect   Lateral aspect

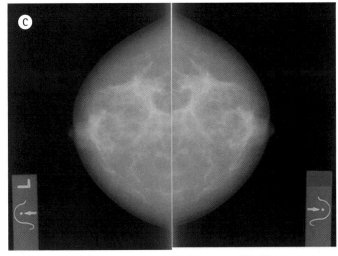

Figure 29.2 **(A)** CC projection; **(B)** CC image; **(C)** CC images are viewed back to back in order to make comparisons

- The light beam diaphragm can be used while compression is applied, to check that:
  (a) The nipple is in profile
  (b) All the breast is within the main beam
  (c) Both the medial and lateral margins are included

(d) There are no skin folds
(e) Compression of the breast is adequate*
(f) A CC marker with left or right identifier (relevant to the breast under examination) is positioned on the axillary edge of the cassette, within the primary beam
- The patient may need to press the breast not under examination laterally and against her body to avoid its inclusion on the film

*Compression is a vital component in achieving good mammographic images. It is also the part of the mammogram that causes the most concern to patients. If the mammographer explains the need for compression at the start of the examination the patient is less likely to find it uncomfortable and is more able to tolerate any possible discomfort when she knows that better quality images will be produced with the need for repeat examinations less likely.

Compression of the breast greatly improves image quality by:

- reducing the thickness of breast tissue irradiated, thereby reducing the superimposition of breast tissues and reducing the radiation dose to the breast
- reducing geometric unsharpness
- reducing movement unsharpness
- improving contrast (by reducing internal X-ray beam scatter)

Application of the right amount of compression certainly comes with experience although there are guidelines concerning the amount of pressure used. In the UK the maximum pressure allowed is 200 Newtons, however in practice, this amount of force is not necessary and most manufacturers limit their equipment to 160 Newtons.[1]

Criteria for assessing image quality
- The nipple is in profile and is pointing to the centre of the long axis of the film
- The majority of the medial and lateral breast tissue (with the exception of the axillary tail) is included
- Pectoral muscle is at the centre of the edge of the film; however, this is only seen on approximately 30% of individuals
- Exposure is determined by the AEC. mAs provides the adequate image density to demonstrate glandular tissue, fat and muscle
- The kVp must provide the optimum contrast between the different structures within the breast
- Image has been processed under quality assurance and quality control guidelines as indicated in the Pritchard report[2]
- Absence of artefact
- Absence of movement

Common errors	Possible reasons
Nipple is pointing downwards	1. Film holder may be too high – reduce height 2. Skin on the underside of the breast may be caught at the proximal edge of the cassette – reposition the breast by lifting it and gently pulling the underside of the breast forward 3. Excess loose skin on the superior surface of the breast? – apply tension to the skin surface, pulling it gently towards the thorax, and laterally and medially as compression is applied
Folds at the lateral aspect of the breast	1. There may be a pad of fat or skin above the upper outer quadrant – alter position of the arm 2. The patient may be leaning to the medial aspect – change patient position 3. The breast may be twisted – reposition the breast

45° Mediolateral oblique (MLO) left breast
(Fig. 29.3A,B,C)

Positioning

- The patient faces the unit with her feet pointing towards it
- From the position used for the CC projection, the unit is rotated through 45°, with the tube on the patient's right and the beam angled caudally, and the height is adjusted to bring the lower border of the cassette 2.5 cm below the inferior portion of the left breast. It may be necessary to further adjust the height during patient positioning
- The lateral edge of the left of the thorax is in line with the image receptor holder so that the left breast also lies next to it
- The mammographer stands behind and slightly to the right of the woman
- The patient raises her left arm and raises her chin (thus preventing superimposition of the mandible over the breast)
- The mammographer holds the left breast in her right hand and uses her left hand to hold the patient's right shoulder

- The patient is encouraged to lean forward into the machine and, with her feet still facing forwards, is asked to lean slightly laterally. The left axilla should lie over the corner of the image receptor that is nearest to the chest wall
- The mammographer stands behind the image receptor holder, takes the woman's left wrist in her left hand and uses her right thumb and fingers to lift the posterior skin edge of the left axilla to prevent skin folds occurring
- The mammographer gently pulls the patient's left arm across and behind the image receptor holder. The woman's elbow is flexed so that the forearm can be placed on the unit for support and the elbow is positioned so it hangs down comfortably behind the holder. The humeral head is gently pushed forwards. The corner of the image receptor lies in the axilla, anterior to the posterior fold
- The patient maintains this position while the mammographer goes to the tube side of the unit, i.e. to face the left breast
- The mammographer uses her right hand to ensure that there are no skin folds in the axilla or under the lateral aspect of the breast and to check for and remove any creases at the inframammary angle
- Holding the patient's left shoulder with the left hand, the left breast is lifted up and away from the chest wall with the right hand
- The right hand is now positioned with the thumb under the breast and fingers spread across the breast before compression is applied

45° MLO right breast

Positioning

- The patient faces the unit with her feet pointing towards it
- From the position used for the CC projection, the unit is rotated through 45°, with the tube on the patient's left and the beam angled caudally, and the height is adjusted to bring the lower border of the cassette 2.5 cm below the inferior portion of the right breast. It may be necessary to further adjust the height during patient positioning
- The lateral edge of the right of the thorax is in line with the image receptor holder so that the right breast also lies next to it
- The mammographer stands behind and slightly to the left of the woman
- The patient raises her right arm and raises her chin (thus preventing superimposition of the mandible over the breast)
- The mammographer holds the right breast in her left hand and uses her right hand to hold the patient's right shoulder

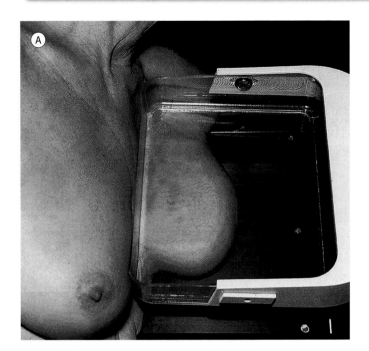

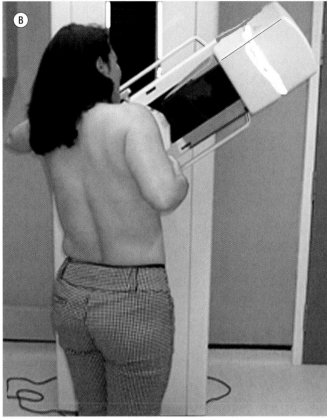

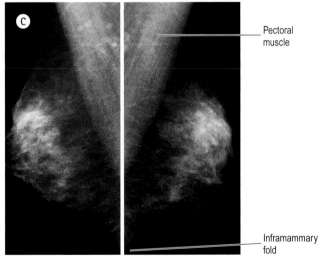

Pectoral
muscle

Inframammary
fold

Figure 29.3   (A) MLO projection (B) MLO position demonstrating
45° angle of unit; (C) MLO images. (A) and (C) Reproduced with
permission from Lee L, et al. Fundamentals of mammography.
2nd edn. London: Churchill Livingstone; 2003

- The patient is encouraged to lean forward into the machine and, with her feet still facing forwards, is asked to lean slightly laterally. The right axilla should lie over the corner of the image receptor that is nearest to the chest wall
- The mammographer stands behind the image receptor holder, takes the woman's right wrist in her right hand and uses her left thumb and fingers to lift the posterior skin edge of the right axilla to prevent skin folds occurring
- The mammographer gently pulls the patient's right arm across and behind the image receptor holder. The woman's elbow is flexed so that the forearm can be placed on the unit for support and the elbow is positioned so it hangs down comfortably behind the holder. The humeral head

is gently pushed forwards. The corner of the image receptor lies in the axilla, anterior to the posterior fold
- The patient maintains this position while the mammographer goes to the tube side of the unit, i.e. to face the right breast
- The mammographer uses her left hand to ensure that there are no skin folds in the axilla or under the lateral aspect of the breast and to check for and remove any creases at the inframammary angle
- Holding the patient's right shoulder with the right hand, the right breast is lifted up and away from the chest wall with the left hand
- The left hand is now positioned with the thumb under the breast and fingers spread across the breast before compression is applied

For both breasts

- The light beam diaphragm should be used to check that:
  - (a) the nipple is in profile
  - (b) the inframammary angle is clearly visible and included within the boundaries
  - (c) there are no skin folds
  - (d) the edge of the compression plate is adjacent to the thorax from immediately below the clavicle down to the inframammary angle
- Compression is applied slowly and evenly using the foot pedal whilst the mammographer maintains the breast in position, gradually moving her fingers forwards towards the nipple during compression application. The thumb maintains the lift of the breast until compression is complete and the breast is held in place by the compression paddle
- A marker is applied

Criteria for assessing image quality – both MLOs

- The entire breast and skin surface should be included
- The pectoral muscle should lie at the level of the nipple and at an angle of 20–35° from the vertical
- The nipple is in profile
- The inframammary angle is clearly demonstrated
- There are no skin folds
- The kVp must provide the optimum contrast between the different structures within the breast. mAs provides adequate image density to demonstrate glandular tissue, muscle and fat
- Correct processing
- Absence of artefact
- Absence of movement

Common errors	Possible reasons
Skin folds at axilla and/or inframammary angle	Film may be too high Overlap of the breast and abdominal wall – gently pull down the excess tissue between the lateral edge of the breast and the film holder and tuck it behind the film holder
Nipple is not in profile	Film may be too high The patient may have rotated her hips – reposition
Pectoral muscle not across the film	Film may be too high – adjust and reposition the shoulder

PGMI (PERFECT, GOOD, MODERATE, INADEQUATE) SYSTEM

The PGMI system was introduced in the UK in the early 1990s as a grading system and guide to performance criteria in the classification of oblique mammograms. It is still used in training centres and mammography departments (for ongoing development) as a means of evaluating mammograms; it is important to remember however that CC films, though not assessed by the PGMI system, must not be forgotten in performance evaluation.

As the PGMI system is subjective it is possible that individuals using it might grade the same films differently on separate occasions and this is the main reason for the validity of the system to be questioned. However, without a better system that utilises both the MLO and the CC projections for both training and continuing development, mammographers will continue to use it.

The PGMI system: summary[1]

P = perfect
To be graded as a 'perfect' image the following must apply.

1. *Whole breast imaged thus:*
   - Pectoral muscle to nipple level
   - Pectoral muscle at correct angle
   - Nipple in profile
   - Inframammary angle shown under the breast
2. *Correct annotations:*
   - Patient identification and examination date
   - Correct anatomical markers
   - Mammographer identification
3. *Correct exposure*
4. *Adequate compression*
5. *No movement unsharpness*
6. *Correct processing*
7. *Absence of processing and handling artefacts*
8. *Absence of skin folds*
9. *Symmetrical images*

G = good
To be graded 'good', both the oblique images must meet criteria 1–6 from the list above in the perfect section. Inadequacy in 7,8 and 9 can be accepted if shown in a minor degree.

M = moderate
'Moderate' images are considered acceptable for diagnostic purposes. Acceptable errors are:

- Pectoral muscle not level with the nipple or not at the correct angle but the back of the breast is adequately shown
- Nipple not in profile but the retroareolar area is well shown
- Inframammary angle is not clearly demonstrated but the breast is adequately shown
- Artefacts are present but the image is not obscured
- More severe skin folds but the breast image is not obscured – when other criteria are adequately fulfilled.

I = inadequate

- If part of the breast is not imaged
- Inadequate compression (inadequate compression will affect adequacy of exposure in that the image will appear underexposed. Inadequate compression will also cause image unsharpness and reduce contrast)
- Incorrect exposure
- Processing faults that interfere with image quality
- Artefacts or skin folds that cover the image of the breast
- Inadequate or incorrect identification or annotation of anatomical markers

SUPPLEMENTARY PROJECTIONS

There are a number of additional projections that can be utilised to supplement the basic CC and the MLO projections. They are used to gain further information when a lesion or possible lesion has been seen on the original films and often are all that is required to clarify any uncertainty.

These additional projections can also be used in situations where the patient has difficulty maintaining the original position thereby resulting in an inadequate examination, e.g. for those who are disabled, wheelchair bound, or those whose physical shape renders positioning difficult and/or painful.

Medially–rotated CC projection (extended CC)
(Fig. 29.4A,B)

This projection is useful to demonstrate more of the upper outer breast quadrant, towards the axillary tail. The equipment and the patient are positioned as for the CC projection but the patient then turns her feet 5–10° to the opposite side to that being examined and the patient is turned further to include the lateral aspect of the breast; the medial portion of the breast film will not be included on the image.

This projection will demonstrate lesions in the extreme lateral portion of the breast that are seen on the MLO but not on the CC image. It can also be used for women with large breasts who require more than one image film in the CC position.

Mediolateral projection (Fig. 29.5A,B)

This projection is used to assess the depth of lesions for localisation and is particularly useful after localisation. The majority of the breast tissue is demonstrated, with the exception of the axillary tail.

Positioning (left breast described)

- The breast support table is vertical
- The woman faces the machine with the lateral edge of the chest wall in line with the film holder

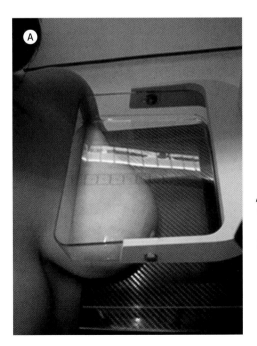

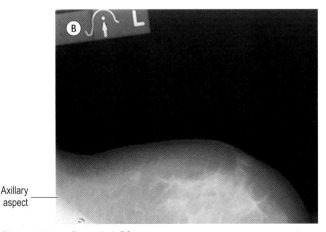

Axillary aspect

Figure 29.4   Extended CC

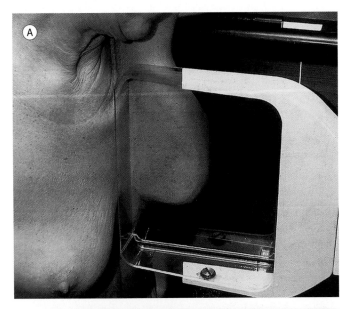

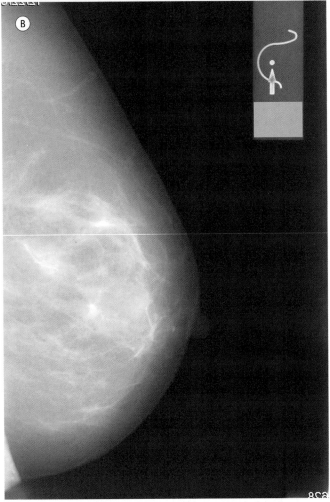

Figure 29.5 Mediolateral. (A) Reproduced with permission from Lee L, et al. Fundamentals of mammography. 2nd edn. London: Churchill Livingstone; 2003

- The left arm is raised and the patient is encouraged to hold the support handle. The breast should be in line with the centre of the cassette holder
- The mammographer uses her left hand to lift the patient's humerus and uses her right hand to lift the breast up and away from the chest wall. The woman is encouraged to lean into the machine and whilst keeping the nipple in profile and the inframammary angle in view the right hand is used to ease the patient's axilla onto the corner of the film by carefully pulling the upper portion of the pectoral muscle forward onto the film
- The woman's arm is rested on top of the machine and whilst supporting the breast with the right hand and maintaining the position of the left shoulder with the left hand, the mammographer applies compression ensuring that the nipple is in profile and the inframammary angle is clearly demonstrated prior to making the exposure

Criteria for assessing image quality
- Inframammary angle is included
- Nipple is in profile
- Inferior portion of pectoral is included

A *lateromedial* projection may also be undertaken if it is still necessary to demonstrate the inframammary fold. This essentially uses the opposite position of the mediolateral projection, with the patient initially standing with the vertical image receptor between the breasts; the medial aspect of the breast under examination is placed against the image receptor's surface and the breast elevated, positioned and compressed similarly to the mediolateral projection (Fig. 29.6).

Magnification (macro) views

These are used to magnify areas of suspicion seen on mammograms, usually areas of microcalcification which may well demonstrate their characteristics clearly when magnified. Communication and explanation is important, if the patient is aware of what is being done, why it is being done and what is required of her she will be able to assist the mammographer.

Adaptations to the equipment are required as follows:

- Fine focus
- Magnification table
- Compression paddles
- Film holder
- Full field diaphragm

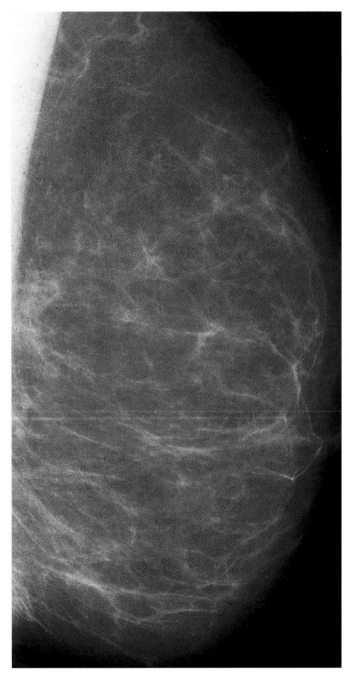

Figure 29.6 Lateromedial. Reproduced with permission from Lee L, et al. Fundamentals of mammography. 2nd edn. London: Churchill Livingstone; 2003

Units that use digital equipment do not require the use of magnification technique, since magnification of the image can be performed digitally with excellent detail of the area in question. The benefits of this include avoidance of a second exposure to radiation and reduction of examination time and discomfort for the patient.

Localised compression views (paddle views)

These are used to demonstrate if a lesion has clear or ill-defined borders and to demonstrate if a lesion is merely superimposition of tissues or is indeed a genuine lesion. A small compression paddle is attached to the compression unit and this is applied over the area of the lesion; it has the capacity to apply more effective and localised compression to a particular area of the breast.

Equipment requirements are:

- Fine focus (preferable)
- Small compression paddle
- Moving grid
- Full field diaphragm
- AEC selected at the chest wall

References
1. Lee L, et al. Fundamentals of mammography. 2nd edn. London: Churchill Livingstone; 2003.
2. Pritchard J. Quality assurance guidelines for mammography. Report of a Sub-committee of the Radiology Advisory Committee of the Chief Medical Officer. Oxford: NHSBSP Publications; 1990.

Further reading
Lee L, et al. Fundamentals of mammography. 2nd edn. London: Churchill Livingstone; 2003.

BREAST ULTRASOUND

Julie Burnage

Frequency of examination of the breast by ultrasound has increased in recent years, due in part to the fact that X-ray mammography does not have good specificity if not supplemented by other imaging methods. Open biopsy does supplement information but, of course, it is preferable for all if unnecessary and invasive procedures of this type can be avoided. As mentioned in Chapter 28, magnetic resonance imaging (MRI), ultrasound and radionuclide imaging (RNI) all have a role in identifying breast disease but recent developments in ultrasound mean that this imaging method can now offer high quality images that are most suitable for demonstrating both breast anatomy and any pathology which may affect it. When considering the dose implications of RNI, the range of contraindications for MRI and other comparable benefits, mainly in the areas of accessibility, speed of examination and equipment cost, it is clear as to why ultrasound has increased in use.[1]

The use of ultrasound in the diagnosis of breast disease, both on its own and as an adjunct to mammography, is well documented and there are numerous texts and articles devoted to it. This chapter aims to provide an overview of breast ultrasound rather than going into it in great depth.

COMMON PATHOLOGICAL APPEARANCES SEEN ON ULTRASOUND

Cysts

Cysts are a very common finding in women between the ages of 35 and 50 years but are rare in women under 25 and over 60 years.[1] They can be single or multiple and are often bilateral.

Generally they are:

- well marginated
- rounded or ovoid in shape
- anechoic
- compressible
- have a well-defined posterior wall with enhanced sound transmission

Complex cysts

These contain internal echoes, usually due to milk of calcium crystals, blood or pus and often occur following incomplete aspiration of a simple cyst.

Fibroadenoma

These appear as a solid, homogenous, hypoechoic nodule with an elongated shape and irregular borders.

Malignant lesions

Ultrasound is used in the diagnosis of breast cancer as an adjunct to mammography, which is the main diagnostic imaging tool. Appearances on ultrasound are often non-specific and there is frequently an overlap between benign and malignant lesions.

Generally, malignant lesions are hypoechoic, cause acoustic shadowing and have ill-defined/irregular margins and mixed internal echoes.

EQUIPMENT

Adequate ultrasound examination of any organ requires the use of appropriate equipment. Only high resolution instrumentation capable of producing high quality images should be used.[2]

The breast is a superficial structure which requires the use of high frequency, real time, hand held transducers (7.5–15 mHz) with a linear array configuration and a 'footprint' of approximately 4–7 cm.

A high frequency probe focussed in the near field may allow sufficient resolution to discern very subtle differences of acoustic impedance among soft tissues, as well as enhancing both spatial and contrast resolution.[3]

The use of Doppler analysis during an examination provides the clinician with an indication of blood flow to and from a lesion thus helping further with the formation of a diagnosis.

THE VALUE OF ULTRASOUND WITH MAMMOGRAPHY

Breast ultrasound as a complementary imaging modality is most often used in the following situations:

- Evaluation of a mass demonstrated with mammography: ultrasound is 100% sensitive when differentiating between solid and cystic lesions within the breast[1]
- Guidance of a needle during cyst aspiration or in the taking of a biopsy
- Evaluation of dense breast tissue: women most likely to have dense breasts are younger, premenopausal or on hormone replacement therapy (HRT). Where the breast tissue is dense it is often difficult to differentiate mass lesions on mammograms

As ultrasound and mammography are both vital in the diagnosis of breast disease it is important that the person performing the scan has an interest in, and a sound knowledge of, the anatomy and physiology of the breast and its diseases. Wherever possible the mammograms should be available to the sonographer to further aid the scan procedure.

SONOGRAPHY AS A STAND-ALONE DIAGNOSTIC TOOL

Ultrasound cannot be used to screen women for breast cancer. 'The use of ultrasound in population screening of asymptomatic women is associated with unacceptably high rates of both false positive and false negative outcomes.'[4] However, ultrasound is often used as the initial, and sometimes the only, imaging modality in the following situations:

- Determination of a palpable lump – solid or cystic
- Where the use of radiation may raise concern, e.g. pregnant patients, the patient under 30 years of age who is also likely to have dense breasts
- Patients who refuse mammograms
- Follow up for patients with fibrocystic disease
- To detect silicone leakage from breast implants

- In cases where the compression used in mammography would be intolerable to the patient, e.g. in acute breast conditions such as abscess or recent trauma

OVERVIEW OF BREAST ULTRASOUND TECHNIQUE

- The patient is undressed from the waist up and is (usually) in the supine or supine oblique position, thus reducing the breast thickness and therefore improving the visualisation of the deeper structures. Occasionally upper quadrant masses are better demonstrated in the erect position
- The arm of the side under examination is extended above the head to stretch the pectoralis muscle, thereby enabling better fixation and immobilisation of the breast and ensuring good visualisation of the lower quadrants and the inframammary fold
- When scanning, the transducer should be perpendicular to the skin surface with a gentle pressure applied to ensure complete contact. Compression is useful in reducing the thickness of the area to be examined and to assess changes in the shape of a lesion, e.g. flattening a cyst to confirm its nature. However, care must be taken that the compression does not inadvertently push lesions out of the scanning plane or deform structures within the parenchyma
- The whole of the breast and its adjacent tissues are examined, from the inframammary fold to the peripheral areas of the upper quadrants, and from the anterior midaxillary line and the axillary tail to the lateral aspect of the sternum
- Both longitudinal and transverse scans are undertaken along with radial scanning around the areola
- Whenever possible, both breasts are examined to enable contralateral comparison and the scanning procedure should involve overlap of scanning planes to ensuring a thorough examination
- Any lesions demonstrated should be described and measured. The position of any lesion is described as represented on a clock face, e.g. 1 o'clock, 9 o'clock, etc and the distance from the nipple given
- Correlation with mammographic and clinical findings should be undertaken when possible

ULTRASOUND IMAGES

It is common practice for hard copy images of the examination to be produced and incorporated into the patient's notes. The equipment used for this should be compatible with the ultrasound system and be serviced at the same time as the scanner, thereby ensuring good quality images are produced.

Quality assurance and quality control are of paramount importance for any imaging modality and the printer should be included when checks are undertaken.

NORMAL APPEARANCES

The skin surface is the superficial component of the breast and, when using high resolution probes, demonstrates a homogenous band which is more echogenic than the underlying fat tissue.

Coopers ligaments, the septa of connective tissue surrounding and supporting the glans from the dermis to the pectoral fascia, appear as hyperechoic, oblique lines going into the parenchyma. The breast parenchyma varies from woman to woman and with age.

A young breast is more glandular and therefore variably echogenic, whilst older breasts have more adipose tissue which presents as hypoechoic. Breast parenchyma is therefore not homogenous.

The parenchyma is seen to be triangular in shape with the apex towards the nipple.

The nipple is visualised as a well-defined, rounded nodule of medium echogenicity.

References

1. Ciatto S, et al. The contribution of ultrasonography to the differential diagnosis of breast cancer. Neoplasma 1994; 41(6):341–345.
2. NHSBSP Ultrasound Working Group. Review of the use of ultrasound scanners in the UK Breast Screening Programme. Publication 43 February 1999.
3. Solbiati L (ed). Ultrasound of superficial structures. London: Saunders; 1994.
4. Teh W, Wilson ARM. The role of ultrasound in breast cancer screening. A consensus statement by the European Group for breast cancer screening. European Journal of Cancer 1998; 34(4):449–450.

MAMMOGRAPHY LOCALISATION

Julie Burnage

If a patient is to undergo surgery to remove a lesion within the breast it is vital that the surgeon knows exactly where the lesion is, to ensure it and the surrounding tissues are removed completely with the best cosmetic result.

This 'localisation' involves the insertion of a needle and wire into the breast lesion under X-ray control using a stereotactic device. The lesion will have been previously diagnosed as significant enough to warrant surgical removal, usually having been diagnosed as malignant. The procedure to localise the lesion takes place immediately before surgery. The wire remains in the breast after the localisation, with its tip acting as a landmark for the surgeon who is to surgically remove the lesion in question. There are currently two types of 'stereo' device available, one involves the patient lying prone on a biopsy table and the other is an attachment to a mammography unit. A localisation needle is attached to this type of mammography unit, as shown in Figures 31.1A,B and 31.2. For the purposes of this chapter, the latter method will be described, as this is the most commonly encountered type in the UK.

The number of staff involved in the procedure should be kept to a minimum and yet there should be enough staff to ensure a high quality procedure. Consideration must be given to the fact that the patient must never be left alone. An ideal number of staff is three: the mammographer, localiser and a second mammographer or nurse.

Prior to bringing the patient into the room it is important to ensure that everything is ready for the procedure to begin, thereby minimising any anxiety and distress the patient may feel. The procedure is explained to the patient and she is seated in front of the machine. It is important to make sure that the patient is made comfortable; once positioned in the stereotactic device she will be required to stay still so as to reduce the margin of error when inserting the wire.

The position of the breast for localisation will have been determined using previous mammograms and assessing the location of the lesion from these. The patient is then appropriately positioned in the machine and the compression plate is applied. Once in position, the patient's comfort is ensured and maintained and the outline of the compression window is marked on her breast; if there is any subsequent movement of the breast this will then be seen easily and repositioning can be carried out. It is not easy for the patient to maintain her position as, in order to facilitate the swing of the X-ray tube, she may have to move her head. Two images are required of the breast, with tube shift between each one.

The first images are taken with the tube being moved in between each exposure and with the patient position supported during the tube movement. This first image is processed quickly (the processing time can be decreased) and checked to ensure that the abnormality is clearly demonstrated in the middle of each image. If necessary, the breast is repositioned and the image taken again. Once satisfactory stereo images have been obtained, the coordinates of the abnormality are determined (this and the needle and wire insertion are usually performed by a radiologist but radiographer role development is likely to see an increase in radiographer involvement in this stage of the procedure). The skin is cleansed and the needle inserted. The wire is then inserted into the breast and positioned just beyond the lesion; a further film is taken to check its position. It is important that mammograms are performed after the insertion of the wire(s) to check the position of the wire in relation to the lesion(s). The wire tip must be

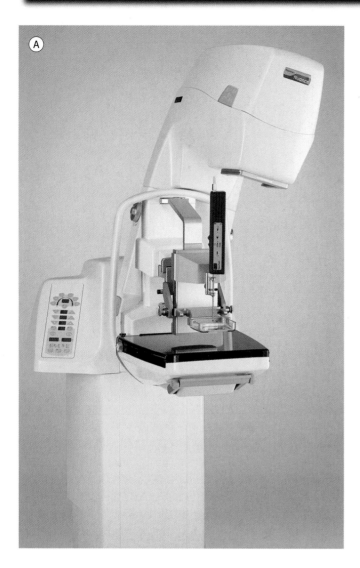

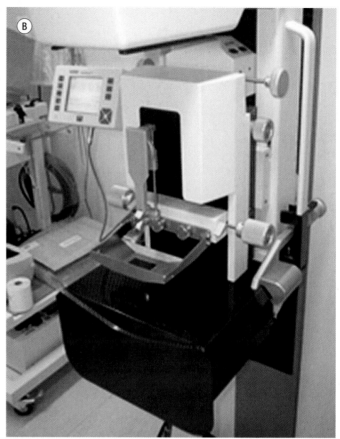

Figure 31.1 **(A)** Stereotactic unit. Reproduced with permission from Xograph Imaging Systems; **(B)** stereotactic unit. Note the similarities between the two units

positioned beyond the lesion because if it stops short of the abnormality, the surgeon may not be able to locate it.

Once the wire is deemed to be positioned satisfactorily the procedure is complete and sterile dry dressings are applied over the wire's entry site. The patient is then escorted back to the ward to await her surgery.

After surgery the excised lump is returned for X-ray assessment. The tissue (presented as the excised lump) is imaged and, following comparison with the presurgery mammograms, the surgeon is informed by imaging department personnel as to whether sufficient tissue has been removed or not.

This stereotactic procedure is also used to obtain core biopsies of the breast and aspiration of cells for histological assessment.

As an 'add on' to a conventional stereotactic unit, small field digital mammography (SFDM) is used in some departments and increases the accuracy and speed of the stereotactic procedure, thereby making it less distressing for the patient.

In addition it has also been shown to improve the sensitivity in the diagnosis of microcalcification.[1] In the absence of stereotactic equipment it is possible to obtain samples of breast tissue using modified compression plates or ultrasound.

Use of modified compression plates

There are two types of modified plates available, the perforated plate and the coordinated plate; these attach directly to the mammography unit by simply replacing the usual compression plate. The perforations or marked coordinates are displayed on the mammographic image and are visible on the skin surface, acting as a guide for needle insertion. These, however, are no longer widely used.

Ultrasound

Ultrasound guidance should be the method of choice for fine needle aspiration (FNA) and core biopsies.[2] If a lesion

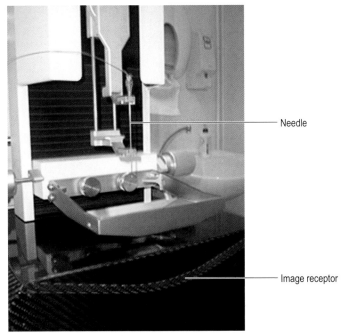

Needle

Image receptor

Figure 31.2 Localisation needle and guidewire positioned in stereotactic unit

can be seen on ultrasound it can be sampled relatively quickly and easily and is very accurate as the needle and its relationship to the lesion can be watched as the sample is taken. Ultrasound has some advantages over the stereotactic method for breast biopsy; for example, it is a faster procedure compared to conventional film mammography as there is no processing. Also, adjustments for movement or incorrect needle placement can be made immediately; it is more comfortable for the patient as she will be in the supine position and no compression is used. An important consideration is that further irradiation of the breast is avoided.

References

1. Whitlock JP, et al. Digital imaging improves upright stereotactic core biopsy of mammographic microcalcifications. Clinical Radiology 2000; 55(5):374-377.
2. NHSBSP Ultrasound Working Group. Review of the use of ultrasound scanners in the UK breast screening programme in 1998. NHSBSP Publication number 43 Feb 1999.

PAEDIATRIC IMAGING

PAEDIATRIC IMAGING

Tim Palarm, Michael Scriven, Elizabeth Carver

INTRODUCTION

Children presenting for radiographic examinations range from the newborn (neonates) to young adults. Each age group presents different challenges to the diagnostic radiographer. The authors have attempted to provide a succinct overview of the techniques used in paediatric radiography. This has been a challenge due to the range of anatomical areas to be included in one chapter, along with the myriad techniques suited to particular age groups. As such, some of the radiographic techniques described need to be cross-referenced with other chapters in this textbook, relating to radiography of adult patients, for more in-depth descriptions. The authors have chosen to include examinations that radiographers are most likely to routinely encounter in independent practice, rather than concentrating on specialised techniques which are more likely to be employed in specialised paediatric departments. Detail on invasive procedures and specialised examinations are therefore not included and the authors encourage readers to refer to specialist paediatric texts for in-depth information. This chapter is not meant to be definitive or exhaustive but provides an overview and background to the techniques, which from the authors' experience have been shown to work well. However, it is acknowledged that alternative methods may be used, which may also achieve similar results. It is also recommended that specialist paediatric medical imaging texts are studied for more intensive detail on paediatric imaging. In addition, diagnostic radiographers are encouraged to formulate collaborative practices through interprofessional working with other healthcare professionals. As well as being of direct benefit to patients this process forms part of a practitioner's continuing professional development.

SPECIAL CONSIDERATIONS WHEN IMAGING CHILDREN

A familiar phrase that applies to all radiographers, as well as other healthcare professionals, working with children is: '... to stand tall in this speciality is to get down on bended knees'. Earning a child's trust, in order that they may comply with the radiographic examination, is eminently preferable to 'old fashioned' immobilisation techniques. However, there will be times when this cannot be achieved, primarily in the younger age group. In infants, distraction techniques should be undertaken before immobilisation is actively considered. It is important to note that parental involvement in the examination gives the child a comfort factor through facilitating eye and/or physical contact. Similarly the presence of siblings, obviously located behind the protective screen, may also help to dispel fear. A radiographer who appears to be quietly confident and self-assured, and preferably not wearing a white coat, is more likely to achieve a higher success rate than less experienced colleagues. Forcing the child to adopt a particular position is likely to be less successful than gentle guidance interspersed with play. It is the authors' opinion that all undergraduate diagnostic radiographers, wherever possible, should be provided with learning opportunities in dedicated paediatric departments. The majority of radiographers will image children as early as during their first appointment, and certainly at some stage during their career, and the knowledge and skills obtained during such a student placement would be beneficial.

Ensuring that the physical environment is conducive to imaging children is another important factor, although the authors acknowledge that this may not always be possible. The Audit Commission (1993) recognise that the needs of children cannot be met without the appropriate facilities.[1] Child-friendly décor with toys and books can help to achieve this, and ideally in a different area from where adult patients wait. Good standards of personal hygiene, particularly in intensive care units, are essential to reduce the possibility of nosocomial infection. All efforts must be made to reduce heat losses from incubators.

Of course, with the vast range of size and capabilities of patients who are known as 'minors', the radiographer will need to adopt an equally vast range of approaches to each examination. Consider the rapid development of the human body in its size, appearance and intelligence from birth to the late teens; not only must the radiographer consider image receptor size and exposure factor selection but they must be capable of communicating successfully with babies, toddlers, children, adolescents and, very often, parents. This communication must be so skilled as to ensure compliance and concordance whilst displaying the empathy and understanding necessary to assure a stress-free examination for the child.

RADIATION PROTECTION AND DOSE REDUCTION

Radiation exposure in the first 10 years of life may have an attributable lifetime risk which is three to four times greater than that after the age of 30 years (CEC 1996).[2] As the life expectancy of children is longer than for adults there is a greater time period for any deleterious effects to become manifest. Ways radiographers can reduce the radiation dose to children are therefore of paramount importance.

The choice of radiographic exposures should be in accordance with the 1996 CEC guidelines,[2] varying according to the weight and size of the child. Information on exposure factors should be readily available throughout the department, as well as provided on mobile equipment. A common criticism is the tendency for radiographers to use disproportionably large X-ray field sizes, in order to ensure they 'capture' the area of interest even when immobilisation is difficult. Accessory equipment such as foam pads and sandbags help to ensure children maintain a certain position and reduce the possibility of repeat radiographs. This should provide the radiographer with the confidence to collimate more appropriately. Radiographers observing and recording dose area product (DAP) meter readings will encourage practitioners to adopt low-dose techniques.

In accordance with the Ionising Radiation (Medical Exposure) Regulations, [IR(ME)R] 2000, the policy is for radiographers to confirm the pregnancy status of all females of childbearing age before undergoing medical exposure.[3] The lower age limit for pregnancy status is generally considered to be 12 years, however some girls do commence menstruation as early as 10 years. When females of childbearing age present for radiographic examination where the primary beam is likely to irradiate the pelvic area, the procedure in some hospitals is to check if she has started to menstruate. If the answer is affirmative the radiographer needs to establish the likelihood of pregnancy and to officially record their status. This whole subject of ascertaining the pregnancy status of young children is recognised by the authors as being a complex issue, and must be treated delicately. An interesting viewpoint from McHugh, aptly entitled 'Teenage Pregnancy: Sex, Lies and Too Much Red Tape', alludes to the farcical nature of the process to confirm teenage pregnancy undertaken in X-ray departments.[4] The real challenge, according to this consultant paediatric radiologist, is to identify those girls who are truly at risk and target appropriate questioning effectively, but he concedes that the infrastructure and resources are not available within UK radiology departments.

Care should always be taken to minimise the radiation dose to persons assisting the radiographer in holding children for X-ray examinations. It is recommended that radiographers are never permitted to be involved in this activity. Parents or guardians are always the first option and other hospital personnel the second. Radiographers will provide these personnel with appropriate guidance in order to reduce the possibility of repeats due to poor handling techniques and advise them on fundamental radiation protection issues. Radiographers will first establish the possibility of pregnancy before women of childbearing capacity are asked to assist in the examination. Permanent records are kept on healthcare personnel who hold children for radiographic examinations.

RADIOGRAPHIC EXAMINATIONS COVERED IN THIS CHAPTER

Key examinations will be outlined in this chapter, covering the most common examinations that will be required on paediatric patients. This will provide the undergraduate and less experienced radiographer with basic, and hopefully useful, information required for a logical approach to these examinations. At times it is necessary to offer specific descriptions of techniques that may well differ in, at least part, of the approach for adult examination of that area. Other examinations may require only notes on possible differences; this is especially relevant to immobilisation strategies and positioning which requires a supine approach for the very young child or baby. Areas selected for inclusion are:

- chest (including ingested and inhaled foreign bodies)
- abdomen
- appendicular skeleton
  - upper limb: hands, arms, elbow, shoulder girdle
  - lower limb: feet, legs, knees, hips
- axial skeleton
  - pelvis, vertebral column, head
- skeletal survey requirements

COMPLIANCE, COOPERATION AND 'DISTRACTION' TECHNIQUES

Ensuring compliance by employing effective communication skills has already been briefly mentioned but, often, 'effective communication skills' are referred to vaguely without direct reference to useful techniques which actually *are* effective. One of the best ways to address the issue is to try to understand the child's experience from the child's point of view and before the examination begins. Think about these points:

- What is their age?
- How well are they feeling?
- What might be their level of understanding?
- What are their past and recent experiences in medical imaging or other hospital departments, if any?
- What might their fears be?
- What might their parents' fears be?

Environmental and privacy factors are also issues that must be considered in advance of the examination:

- How warm is the examination room?
- Will they have to take off some of their clothes and allow strangers to see their body?
- Will they have to place part of their body against something cold?
- How dim is the light?
- How noisy are tube and table movements?
- How noisy is the anode rotation?

The radiographer must take all of these into consideration; some factors may be immediately apparent but often the reluctant or fearful child may be feeling unwell, frightened because the last hospital department stuck a needle into their arm, and apprehensive because they are entering a dim room where a stranger is moving a piece of equipment which is making a rather scary rumbling noise. Talking to the child and/or parents in advance of the examination may seem to take valuable time but the

dividends are paid in the form of a stress-free and high quality examination. A list is provided below, which summarises some useful strategies for successful preparation:

- Prepare the room with the image receptor, immobilisation pads, X-ray tube and table in their correct position for the examination. This reduces the 'noise experience' provided by equipment movement during the examination. Movement of the X-ray tube can also cause light levels in the room to vary during this movement, as the ceiling mount passes under ceiling lights
- Select the approximate initial exposure factors for the first projection, preferably before the child enters the examination room. Collimate to the cassette, if used, and apply an anatomical marker; these will possibly require adjustment later
- Children clearly need a simple explanation of what to expect but, especially for very young children who require immobilisation by an accompanying adult, also explain the examination and its requirements to the adult. Acknowledge that you understand that they may be afraid of hurting the child but that you will show them an effective method that should not hurt or cause the child discomfort. Explain that immobilisation is important but so is maintenance of the position that you put their child in. We cannot expect non-radiographers to know this without telling them. This will help maximise the effectiveness of cooperation and assistance from the adult
- Talk to the child in the waiting area before inviting them in; ask them how they are today and if they know why they are visiting the department. Express sympathy if they say they are unwell or are in pain. Clearly the appropriateness of this relates to the child's age. Talking to the parents of babies whilst paying attention to the baby will establish a rapport amongst all involved
- At times, children will nestle under their parent's arm, refusing to communicate in any way with the radiographer. Time can be usefully spent sitting next to the parent and child, initially engaging in any sort of conversation and, eventually, bringing up the issue of the examination when the child becomes more used to the radiographer's presence. Presenting the child with a small soft toy, and *asking them to take care of it* often raises the child's morale by giving them this small responsibility. It also, more obviously, acts as a comforter
- A child with an appropriate level of understanding can be invited to look at the X-ray room before the start of the examination, with the radiographer pointing out one or two key pieces of equipment and using familiar language to identify them. This, to some extent, demystifies the procedure; as a bonus it may become apparent that the child has a scientific interest in the proceedings!

- Advance preparation through play has been described and discussed widely in paediatric and radiography journals;[5] this is also considered a valuable choice but may not be necessary for all examinations. It is especially useful for more invasive procedures

Once the preparatory stage has been completed the process continues with the actual examination. At this point the radiographer needs to position the child accurately and ensure this position is maintained. It has already been mentioned that the contribution of assisting adults will often be vital to success, and providing them with key information regarding their role is of paramount importance. Showing interest in the child and their accompanying adults shows everyone that their contribution is valued and interaction should include everyone. A second list for this section provides some tips on communication and ensuring compliance:

- If a child is upset, acknowledge that you notice this and that you do take this seriously. Act reassuringly. Do not belittle any of their apparent fears. Even the intended reassurance 'you will be fine' may seem dismissive to the child. Never forget the importance of eye contact as a mechanism to show you are interested in them and take them seriously – it will also hold their attention more effectively
- Demonstration of some positions may be more effective than description. This is especially relevant to examinations of limbs and extremities
- Asking the child to gaze at a specific target may maintain a required head position. One example of this is a toy positioned in front of and directly in line with the child's median sagittal plane (MSP); this could be supported on a chest stand for posteroanterior (PA) chest examinations
- Clicking the fingers above a child's head attracts their attention for an instant but not beyond; it is not effective for maintaining position
- Telling the child to keep watching the light beam diaphragm to see if the birdie comes out just is not on. You know it will not happen and the child will not appreciate your lies! If there is another exposure to be made do not expect any further compliance! In a similar vein, if a toy is used to help maintain head position by asking the child to gaze at it, do not say the toy might wink because it will not (this has been heard many times and the literal mind of the child does not appreciate it)
- A mobile toy which has been set in motion can be used over the head of a baby to attract visual attention and help maintain head position
- Even escorts who are effective immobilisers can distract children in their efforts to keep them still. Frequently parents will say 'keep still' at the last moment, causing the child to turn to look at them as they speak. Advance information on the perils of this will help the parent avoid such distractions
- Older children are less likely to need distraction techniques and are likely to respond well to the provision of adequate information required for their compliance. However, do not forget that a child of any age will not necessarily know that it is essential to keep still for their X-ray unless told to do so

THORAX AND ABDOMEN

CHEST

The chest X-ray is the most commonly requested radiographic examination for children. Depending on the child's age, someone, preferably a parent, is required to assist the radiographer with the examination. Similarly the child's age and physical condition will determine the level of cooperation the radiographer can expect to receive as far as breathing, etc is concerned. As for the adult patient, it is essential that the child is undressed to the waist and all potential artefacts removed. It may be standard practice to remove electrocardiogram (ECG) leads and pads prior to taking the radiograph but this must always be achieved in consultation with nursing or medical colleagues. It is imperative that no sheets or blankets, or other materials, are placed between the child and cassette as they may produce artefacts.

The PA erect chest, used for older and cooperative children, is not described as this does not significantly deviate in technique from the method used for adults.

■ Anteroposterior (AP) chest

The PA erect chest projection would ideally be preferred although in practice the AP projection is more readily performed in infants and young children, as they are more likely to cooperate with the examination. Clearly the decision relies rather heavily on the varying and individual capabilities of each child. It often, unfortunately, also relies on the confidence of the radiographer; the less capable radiographer may elect to use the AP projection when careful assessment and communication may have established that a PA projection may have been achievable. In some situations, particularly during the neonatal period, the AP projection is achieved with the child in a supine position. With this category of patient, insulating the cassette with a paper towel will assist in reducing heat loss as well as ensuring comfort.

Method 1: AP erect chest – seated and in imaging department

If cassettes are used, size and orientation will vary according to the size of the child.

Positioning
- A stool is placed in front of a chest stand. A rubberoid material e.g. Dycem™ can be placed on the seat to prevent the child slipping *or*
- A table-mounted erect paediatric chest stand is used on the table-top (Fig. 32.1)
- For digital receptors: the child sits on the stool, with their back to the erect image receptor
- Other receptors: the child sits on the stool or table, with their back to the erect chest stand and in contact with the cassette, which is placed with its upper border just above the shoulders
- A 15° radiolucent pad is placed between the child's back and the cassette, with the upper border at the level of the shoulders, in order to reduce the likelihood of acquiring a lordotic image
- Velcro™ can be utilised to safely secure the child for the examination
- The radiographer raises the child's arms to each side of their head and the assistant holds them together to ensure an optimum position

Beam direction and focus film distance (FFD)
From the horizontal angle 5–10° caudally
180–200 cm FFD

Centring point
In the midline between the sternal angle and the xiphisternum

Collimation
Apices, cardiophrenic sulci, costophrenic sulci, lateral margins of both lungs

> The radiographer observes the child's breathing and makes the exposure on full inspiration

Method 2: AP supine chest – on neonatal unit or in imaging department (Fig. 32.2)

The image receptor is placed horizontally on the table-top or in the incubator. If a digital receptor is used it must be of a size which will fit into the incubator. The incubator sides should be opened for the minimum time possible

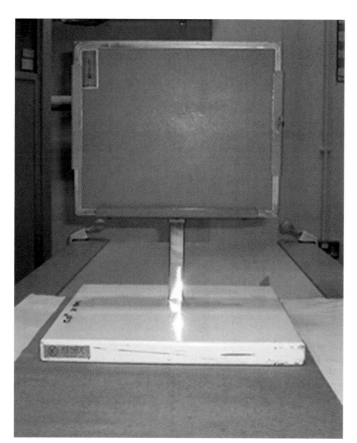

Figure 32.1   Paediatric chest stand used on a table-top

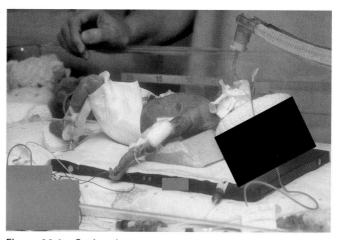

Figure 32.2   Supine chest

to avoid lowering the temperature of the neonate's environment.

Positioning

- A 15° radiolucent pad is placed towards the top of the image receptor, with the thicker end of the wedge also at the top
- Radiopaque objects are removed, e.g. ECG leads and electrodes
- The child is placed upon the cassette with their shoulders resting on the pad for the reasons described in method 1 and to assist in extending the neck to prevent superimposition of the chin and chest
- If possible, the arms are extended, abducted anteriorly, raised and held in position either side of the head. Most efficient immobilisation of the arms is met by holding the arms against the head by their elbows
- The assistant can place a hand on the child's pelvis to prevent rotation of the trunk. Immobilising the legs and knees will also prevent movement
- Lead rubber fenestration* can be placed on a perspex (polymethylmethacrylate) table-top, which is then positioned over the child, to facilitate 'shadow-shielding'; alternatively the lid of the incubator can be used. The sheets of lead rubber 'frame' the collimated area and act as additional field limitation

*Fenestration is not used for chest radiography in older children.

Radiation protection

- X-ray tube potentials between 60–65 kVp are recommended by the CEC (1996)[2]
- Employ 'shadow shielding' wherever practicable

Beam direction and FFD

From the vertical angle 5–10° caudally
100 cm FFD; ideally a larger FFD should be used if possible but supine chest radiography often precludes this due to incubator heights or limitations of available tube height. It is important that the distance is standardised for use by all radiographers; this distance may be higher than the 100 cm stated

Centring point

Babies: babies' lung fields occupy proportionally less space in the trunk than adults and older children. When employing a caudal angle as suggested, neonates will require a centring point over the midline of the sternal angle which seems rather high when compared to usual centring technique for the AP chest
Older children: as for adults

Collimation

T1 and T12, lung apices, cardiophrenic sulci, costophrenic sulci, lateral margins of both lungs

Note that the lower border of collimation on the neonate may appear to be rather high (it should fall approximately 2–3 cm below the nipples) but do not forget that the neonatal lungs are short in comparison with adults and children.

More tightly collimated radiographs, rather than including all of the former structures, may be undertaken to demonstrate specific devices, e.g. the position of endotracheal tubes in consultation with the referrer.

> The exposure is made on full inspiration, as outlined for AP erect chest

Criteria for assessing image quality (methods 1 and 2)

The same criteria are used for assessing paediatric films as for adult chest radiographs, with the following considerations:

- To ensure the thorax is not rotated the symmetry of the ribs is checked, as opposed to the clavicles in the adult chest radiograph. This is because the medial ends of the clavicles are cartilaginous (radiolucent) and overlie the segmented vertebrae, especially in the neonatal period
- To ensure the chest is not lordotically represented the ribs must take on a 'normal anatomical appearance'. In other words, they should travel obliquely down in the lateral direction from the spine (posterior aspect of ribs) and more obliquely down in a medial direction towards the sternum (anterior aspect of ribs)
- The mandible does not obscure the lung apices
- Sharp image of the lungs and heart
- Adequate penetration to demonstrate the retrocardiac area
- Ensure the image is relatively free from 'avoidable artefacts'
- T12 and L1 are included on the image

Common errors	Possible reasons
Dense circle appears on resultant image of chest undertaken on neonatal unit	The hole on the lid of the incubator (used to secure the position of ET tubes, etc) overlies the area of irradiation
Left to right asymmetry of anterior and posterior ribs	Child rotated

Common errors (*cont'd*)	Possible reasons (*cont'd*)
Posterior ribs do not follow normal anatomical appearance and appear 'flattened'	Child positioned lordotically, due to lack of caudal tube angulation and/or absence of pad under the shoulders
Ribs appear to be blurred	Voluntary or involuntary movement of subject e.g. crying. Also, the exposure time may be too long
Too large an X-ray field size	Overestimation of a child's anatomical proportions in relation to chronological age. A very common error is to include much upper abdominal tissue on the neonate's chest X-ray; the neonatal lungs finish at a level just below the nipples, higher than is usual in older children and adults

■ Lateral chest

Positioning

- Babies should be examined lying on their side on the image receptor with their head supported on a radiolucent support/pad
- Neonates in incubators may require the horizontal beam lateral position, while lying on a radiolucent support and with the image receptor supported vertically at their side
- Older children may be examined erect, as for adult technique
- Arms should be raised either side of the trunk, to clear from the field, with legs together and flexed at the knees – as for adult lateral thoracic spine projection

Beam direction and FFD

Horizontal or vertical, at 90° to the image receptor
FFD issues are as for AP chest but it is likely that 2 m FFD will be achievable for the older child who is examined erect

Centring point

Babies: midway between the anterior and posterior thoracic surfaces, at the level of the sternal angle
Older children: as for adults

Collimation

As for adults

Criteria for assessing image quality

As for adults

■ Ingested or inhaled foreign bodies

The ingestion of small foreign bodies (FBs) is fairly common, particularly in the inquisitive, wandering toddler. The radiographic examination of these patients may be useful to the clinician in some circumstances, although the use of procedures that do not involve the use of ionising radiation should be actively considered, e.g. use of a metal detector. Normally medical personnel will have taken an accurate history and excluded the concealment of the FB amongst the child's clothes, or in the nose or ear before being referred to the imaging department. However, it may be propitious for the radiographer to check that this activity has already been undertaken. If it is suspected that the FB has been inhaled a chest radiograph can be helpful on two counts. First, if the FB is radiopaque in nature then it is likely to be readily identifiable, thus enabling the clinician to arrange for its removal. In cases where the FB is non-opaque, a chest radiograph may be of value in identifying any associated collapse and/or consolidation of the lung, or possible air trapping. If it is suspected that the FB has been swallowed (as opposed to inhaled), a chest radiograph is performed, which is collimated to include the upper abdominal area. If the image of the chest is normal, an abdominal radiograph is only performed if the suspected FB is sharp or a 'watch-type' battery (leakage is dangerous). For these radiographs, an area of anatomical overlap is required. A lateral projection of the neck (lateral soft tissue neck) is only performed in cases where the child is demonstrating upper respiratory tract symptoms, e.g. gagging.

ABDOMEN

The abdominal radiograph is commonly performed in the radiography department as well as on the ward. In older children, mobile radiographs of the abdomen are not recommended unless absolutely necessary due to risks of the 'grid-cut-off' phenomenon, as well as the increased radiation hazard. Radiographic techniques such as the lateral or dorsal decubitus and erect abdomen are seldom undertaken, but may be justified in specific cases. The child is routinely undressed and potential artefacts removed from the radiation field. It is not uncommon for radiographs of the chest and abdomen to be requested at the same time, especially for referrals from neonatal intensive care. For reasons related to image quality, it is often standard practice to undertake two separate radiographs (one of the chest and another of the abdomen), except where the position of a line is required. The practice of undertaking two separate radiographs may be in contradiction to findings published in 2001, which advocate the use of a single exposure to demonstrate both anatomical regions on the same radiograph, as the effective dose was reported to be 5% less.[6]

AP abdomen

If used, the cassette is selected according to the child's size and positioned with its long axis coincident with the child's MSP. It is not necessary to use a scatter reduction device for babies and small children.

Positioning
- The child is positioned supine as for the adult abdominal radiograph
- For babies who do not require a secondary radiation reduction device, the child is placed in direct contact with the cassette
- For children who cannot remain immobile, the femora and upper torso are held by an assistant to prevent rotation and lateral flexion of the trunk
- Arms are raised onto the pillow to clear the long bones from scatter from the beam periphery
- For babies, an adult should maintain the arm position and hold the legs by gently gripping the knees
- If on the neonatal unit, an incubator lid can be used for the placement of lead rubber
- Avoidable artefacts should be removed wherever possible
- Ideally, the exposure is made during a period of arrested respiration

Radiation protection
- Employ X-ray tube potentials between 60–65 kVp with short exposure times (CEC 1996)[2]
- Employ 'shadow shielding' wherever practicable
- Consider radiation protection for assistants who may assist the radiographer in holding
- Do not use secondary radiation grids unless the child's size requires this

Beam direction and FFD
Perpendicular central ray
100 cm FFD

Centring point
In the midline at the level of the iliac crests. The umbilicus is a more reliable centring point during neonatal and infant periods of development

Collimation
To ensure the diaphragm is demonstrated, during neonatal and infant periods, the nipples must be included in the radiation field. The pubic symphysis is used as a palpable landmark so as to ensure the superior borders of the pubic rami are included on the resultant image. The lateral walls of the abdomen must also be included

Criteria for assessing image quality
- Diaphragm, superior border of pubic rami and lateral abdominal walls are demonstrated
- Symmetry of pelvic structures; spinous processes are demonstrated down the centre of the vertebral bodies
- Contrast between bone and soft tissues and soft tissues and bowel gas is demonstrated

Common errors	Possible reasons
Structures in the abdominal cavity appear to be blurred	Voluntary or involuntary movement of subject, e.g. crying. Also, the exposure time may be too long
Too large an X-ray field size	Overestimation of a child's anatomical proportions in relation to chronological age
Hemidiaphragms or superior borders of rami of pubic bones coned off	Radiographer underestimation of size in assessment of the child's anatomical proportions

APPENDICULAR SKELETON: UPPER LIMB

HANDS AND FINGERS

The same principles are applied here as with radiography of the hands and fingers of adults. The only differences relate to the variations in techniques due to the child's age and level of cooperation. The child may be examined in a supine position, or seated on an adult's lap for examina- tions of this type. When examining the infant's hand and fingers the greatest challenge is in ensuring the child maintains the correct position for the duration of the exposure. The use of adhesive tape or other radiolucent material to immobilise the fingers has been advocated. A sheet of clear perspex can also be placed over the hand and held in position by the child's escort. However, the authors believe that an assistant holding the child's hand in the desired position and removing this restraint immediately before the exposure is eminently successful and probably less traumatic for the child.

■ Dorsipalmar, obliques and lateral projections of the hand

General points on positioning
- If possible the child is positioned similarly to adults, but a supine position may facilitate easier positioning
- 'Avoidable' artefacts should be removed wherever possible
- Assistants may be required to assist in holding the affected limb; use of radiolucent pads for oblique projections is of utmost importance. Two radiolucent 45° pads may be placed with their vertical surfaces either side of the laterally positioned hand for immobilisation; the escort maintains the position of the sponges

Radiation protection
Radiation protection considerations include those for assistants who may assist in holding the child. It is important that the assistant's fingers or other body parts are not in the primary beam. If this is unavoidable, lead rubber gloves must be worn, or a radiolucent pad may be used to immobilise the part being radiographed

Beam direction, FFD, centring point, collimation and criteria for assessing image quality
This is as for adults (see the relevant chapter)

Common errors	Possible reasons
Images of assistant's fingers, or other body parts, in the region of interest	Extremities in the primary beam
Movement unsharpness or full area under examination not represented on the radiograph	Inadequate immobilisation technique employed

WRIST AND FOREARM

The amount of distal forearm required on the resultant radiograph will depend on the reason for the examination, although the inclusion of the distal third is the general rule. However, both wrist and elbow joints should be included on the same radiograph if a fractured forearm is suspected. Similar to when undertaking radiography of the hands and wrist, some children may be examined seated with an adult, or supine. Again, depending on the

age of the child and level of cooperation, an assistant may be required to help with immobilisation. Some of the general principles outlined in the paediatric elbow section can be used for radiography of the wrist and forearm.

■ AP and lateral projections of the forearm

General points on positioning
- If possible the child is positioned similarly to adults, but in some cases a supine position may be more easily achieved
- Avoidable artefacts should be removed wherever possible
- Assistants may be required to assist in holding the affected limb; holding the fingers and upper arm will keep the escort's hands clear of the radiation field (do not use this method if these areas are injured)

Radiation protection
Consider radiation protection for assistants who may assist in holding the child. It is important that the assistant's fingers or other body parts are not in the primary beam. If this is unavoidable lead rubber gloves must be worn

Beam direction, FFD, centring point, collimation and criteria for assessing image quality
This is as for adults (see the relevant chapter)

Common errors	Possible reasons
Images of assistant's fingers or other body parts are in the region of interest	Extremities in the primary beam
Movement unsharpness or full area under examination not represented on the radiograph	Inadequate immobilisation technique employed
The radius and ulna may not be superimposed on the lateral projection due to insufficient internal rotation	More often than not this is because of the excessive height of the X-ray table or poor immobilisation technique

ELBOW

In cases of trauma to the paediatric elbow, as with adults, under no circumstances should any force be applied to achieve the required projections. Volkmann's ischaemic contracture may result as the direct consequence of compressing the brachial artery through extreme ranges of movement. You may wish to review the lateral radiograph before progressing onto the AP. Radiographs of the paediatric elbow are notoriously difficult to interpret due to the presence of six centres of secondary ossification, which vary in appearance due to the chronological age of the child. As such, inexperienced medical practitioners, who are struggling to distinguish fractures from epiphyseal cartilage, may request projections of the unaffected side. This practice is seldom recommended and a radiologist should instead interpret the radiographs.[7]

The radiographic technique employed will depend on the age of the child, as well as their physical and mental condition, especially where trauma is involved. Neonates and young infants are likely to be examined whilst in a supine position whereas slightly older infants are often seated on the carer's lap (wearing a lead rubber apron), with their affected side adjacent to the end of the X-ray table. Although older children are usually seated unaccompanied, an assistant may be required to provide immobilisation in addition to more traditional methods, e.g. sandbags. As in adults, the projection that often presents the greatest challenge to the radiographer is the AP. Externally rotating the affected limb from the shoulder joint, in order to move the elbow into an AP position, is still advocated in children. However, with those who are less cooperative this may not always be successful. AP radiographs of the elbow should also be considered with the child in the erect standing position or supine with a horizontal beam. An axial projection of the flexed joint may be used as an alternative to the AP and the technique for this is outlined in the relevant adult section of this text (Ch. 27, 'Accident and Emergency'), which considers examination of the elbow in flexion. Height-adjustable X-ray tables, and accessory equipment such as sponge pads, are valuable aids to optimise patient positioning and comfort. Adaptation of the conventional radiographic technique is often required when examining the elbow. Supplementary projections are seldom required but should be discussed in advance with the referrer.

■ AP and lateral projections of the elbow

General points on positioning
- If possible the child is positioned similarly to adults, considering supine and erect standing positions as a possibility (see above)
- Avoidable artefacts should be removed wherever possible
- Assistants may be required to help with holding the affected limb

Radiation protection
If an assistant is used, it is important that their fingers or other body parts are not in the primary beam. If this is unavoidable, lead gloves must be worn

Common errors	Possible reasons
Images of assistant's fingers or other body parts are in the region of interest	Extremities in the primary beam
Movement unsharpness or full area under examination not represented on the radiograph	Inadequate immobilisation technique employed

Beam direction, FFD, centring point, collimation and criteria for assessing image quality
This is as for adults (see the relevant chapter)

SHOULDER GIRDLE AND HUMERUS

■ AP projections of the shoulder and humerus

General points on positioning
- Wherever possible, position in a similar fashion to adults
- Supine or erect (seated) positions may be adopted depending on the child's age and ability to cooperate
- The amount of the shoulder girdle and humerus to be included depends on the reason for the request
- For seated children, a stool can be placed in front of a chest stand and the rubberoid material (see information on AP erect chest in this chapter) used to prevent slipping
- Avoidable artefacts should be removed wherever possible
- A small radiolucent pad may be placed between the torso and limb to maintain the humerus in slight abduction and clear it from the trunk
- Another radiolucent pad may be placed under the shoulders of the non-affected side to assist in rotation of the trunk towards the contralateral limb
- The person accompanying the child may be required to provide some additional physical support
- Ideally, the exposure is made on arrested respiration

Beam direction, FFD and centring point
As for adults, but these may be modified to accommodate the clinical information

Collimation
For the humerus: as for adults
For the shoulder: the shoulder girdle and proximal third of the humerus. In some cases it may be necessary to demonstrate the full length of the humerus, including

the glenohumeral joint, and less of the shoulder girdle

Criteria for assessing image quality
See Chapters 6 and 7 on the adult shoulder and humerus

Common error	Possible reason
The shaft of the humerus cannot be fully visualised	The arm has not been sufficiently abducted, especially when presenting with a sling or collar and cuff

APPENDICULAR SKELETON: THE LOWER LIMB

Again, the same radiographic principles apply for children as in adult radiography. Any variations in technique are to accommodate the diversity of ages and levels of cooperation the radiographer may expect. Infants and babies are usually examined in a supine position on the X-ray couch or bed with an assisting escort present to help the child maintain the required position.

FEET AND TOES

As for adult radiography, dorsiplantar (DP) and oblique radiographs are routinely undertaken, but there may be cases where lateral projections are also required. When examining the foot the challenge is to ensure the child maintains the correct position for the duration of the exposure. Where possible, adhesive tape or other radiolucent material can be used to immobilise the extremity as for the hand and fingers. An escort can hold the child's lower leg to immobilise this region but the escort must wear suitable protective gloves. When examining toes an assistant holding the child's foot in the desired position, and removing this restraint immediately before the exposure, can be successful.

▇ DP, oblique and lateral projections of the foot and toes

General points on positioning
• Position as for adults
• Avoidable artefacts should be removed wherever possible
• The assistant may be required to hold the affected limb
• With babies it is suggested that they are seated on a small box or pillow so the mother can hold them with one arm while holding the affected limb with the other
• Adhesive tape can be used to keep the toes in contact with the cassette and reduce movement artefact
• Lateral projections are best achieved in babies with the trunk rotated towards the affected side and the baby possibly lying on that side

Radiation protection
Consider radiation protection for assistants who may help with holding the child. It is important that the assistant's fingers or other body parts are not in the primary beam. If this is unavoidable, lead rubber gloves must be worn

Beam direction, FFD, centring point, collimation and criteria for assessing image quality
This is as for adults (see the relevant chapter)

Common errors	Possible reasons
Images of assistant's fingers or other body parts are in the region of interest	Extremities in the primary beam
Movement unsharpness or full area under examination not represented on the radiograph	Inadequate immobilisation technique employed
Toes and metatarsals too superimposed in oblique projections	Over-inversion of foot
Phalanges over-blackened out and tarsus underexposed	Due to the differential in thickness between the two anatomical areas
Calcaneal apophysis mistakenly identified as a fracture	Inexperienced image interpreter

Suggested projections for conditions affecting the feet in children
Polydactyly
DP of the foot to check the number of metatarsals

Congenital talipes equino varus ('club foot')
DP and two lateral projections. One lateral in dorsiflexion and the other in extension

Additional projections
Although rare, where fractures of the calcanei are considered likely, e.g. landing on the heels from a height, axial

projections are justified. The reason for this request should be justified by the referrer

ANKLE JOINT, TIBIA AND FIBULA AND KNEE JOINT

It is regarded as poor practice to take one radiograph to include body parts from the knee down and another from the ankle up. If any fractures are present they may not be easily or accurately visualised with this technique. Unlike many adults, the majority of paediatric patients will have limbs that will easily fit on one image and the two projection approach should not be necessary.

■ AP and lateral projections of the ankle, tibia, fibula and knee

General points on positioning
- Position similarly to adults
- Consider horizontal-beam laterals for fat/fluid levels (lipohaemarthrosis)
- The assistant may be required to hold the affected limb
- Lateral projections are best achieved with the trunk rotated towards the affected side
- With babies the PA projection is purported to be more successful than the AP as the image of the lower leg is less likely to be rotated

Radiation protection
Consider radiation protection for assistants who may help with holding the child. It is important that the assistant's fingers or other body parts are not in the primary beam. If this is unavoidable, lead rubber gloves must be worn

Beam direction, FFD, centring point, collimation and criteria for assessing image quality
This is as for adults (see the relevant chapter)

Common errors	Possible reasons
AP projection of baby's lower limb appears oblique	Control over rotation of child's trunk has not been maintained
Lateral projections over- or under-rotated	Control over rotation of child's trunk has not been maintained
Bipartite patella can be mistaken for a fracture	Erroneous interpretation

Additional projections

Additional projections of the patella may be required, albeit infrequently, and in consultation with the referring senior clinician

Inferosuperior patella ('skyline')
Ossification of the patella starts at around 3–6 years of age, and is usually complete by the age of 8 years. This projection is therefore of limited value before the age of 8. If required, it is best achieved with the patient in a prone position, as is advised for the adult inferosuperior patella projection.

FEMUR

In younger children, the whole length of femur including the knee and hip joints, should be demonstrated on the AP radiograph. This requirement is not justified in older children as the site of interest should be apparent to the clinician.[8] 'Overlapping radiographs' are required, which should be taken at right-angles. With infants who cannot weight bear, inexperienced clinicians may request a radiograph of the contralateral side. Similarly to radiography of the elbow this practice is *not acceptable* and the radiograph should instead be reviewed by a radiologist.

■ AP and lateral projections of the femur

General points on positioning
- Position similarly to adults
- Lateral projections are best achieved with the trunk rotated towards the affected side, although horizontal beam laterals may be the most appropriate where trauma is involved
- Do not use lead rubber/gonad protection
- Do not apply any form of traction in order to achieve the required projections
- Avoidable artefacts should be removed wherever possible
- The assistant may be required to hold the affected limb

Radiation protection
Consider radiation protection for assistants who may hold the child. It is important that the assistant's fingers or other body parts are not in the primary beam. If this is unavoidable, lead rubber gloves must be worn. No secondary radiation grid is required for infants and small children

Beam direction, FFD, centring point, collimation and criteria for assessing image quality

This is as for adults (see the relevant chapter)

Common error	Possible reason
Gonad protection obscuring area of interest	Misplacement by radiographer or movement of child

AXIAL SKELETON: VERTEBRAL COLUMN

The newborn spine is straight when viewed from the lateral position. It is only when the child supports its head and weight bears that two secondary curvatures form ('S' type appearance). The spine will begin to resemble the shape of the adult skeleton. Children's spines are less likely to present with degenerative changes responsible for backache for which adults are frequently investigated. It is therefore rare to perform additional projections other than AP and lateral for the initial examination. In cases of trauma the radiographer must undertake the same preventative measures as in adult patients until fractures have been excluded.

CERVICAL SPINE

■ AP and lateral cervical spine

General points on positioning

- Position as for adults wherever practicable
- Remove artefacts from the area of interest wherever possible
- As for all examinations on small children, it must be remembered that anti-scatter grids are unnecessary.[7] For the AP projection of cervical spine a secondary radiation grid is never required, unless the child is very large (equivalent to large adult size)
- AP projection is best performed with the child supine as immobilisation is often difficult if erect
- Young children are best examined seated on a stool rather than standing for the lateral projection
- In young infants a supine position (horizontal beam) is best chosen to obtain the lateral projection
- 45° sponge pads may be placed either side the head and held by an assistant, for immobilisation
- AP projection of C1/C2 (peg projection) is routinely requested in cases of trauma

Beam direction, FFD, centring point, collimation and criteria for assessing image quality

This is as for adults (see the relevant chapter)

Conditions that may require special techniques

Torticollis
- AP (C3–C7/T1), AP (C1–C2) and lateral

Atlantooccipital subluxation
- Two laterals, one with the neck flexed and the other extended, albeit slightly. Neither movement should be forced

Fixed rotary subluxation
- Three AP projections of (C1–C2). One with the neck in a neutral position and the others with the head turned 15° to the left and then right

THORACIC SPINE

■ AP and lateral thoracic spine

General points on positioning

- Position as for adults wherever practicable
- Remove artefacts from the area of interest wherever possible
- As for all examinations on small children, it must be remembered that anti-scatter grids are often unnecessary[7]
- Lateral to be performed without using autotomography because of the risk of repeat exposure due to patient movement, therefore increasing radiation dose

Beam direction, FFD, centring point, collimation and criteria for assessing image quality

This is as for adults (see the relevant chapter)

LUMBAR SPINE

■ AP and lateral lumbar region

General points on positioning

- Position as for adults wherever practicable
- Remove artefacts from the area of interest wherever possible

- As for all examinations on small children, it must be remembered that anti-scatter grids are often unnecessary[7]
- Lumbosacral junction is not routinely performed

Beam direction, FFD, centring point, collimation and criteria for assessing image quality
This is as for adults (see the relevant chapter)

WHOLE SPINE EXAMINATION FOR SCOLIOSIS

Scoliosis is a lateral curvature of the spine. It is transient when postural in origin or structural where there is malformation of the vertebrae. The causes of scoliosis are varied and sometimes not obvious. They are usually grouped as congenital, neurological, muscular, thoracic and idiopathic or sometimes a combination of these causes. Once the diagnosis of scoliosis is made, it is important to keep the child under observation until growth ceases. The patient's spine is X-rayed periodically, and the frequency of this depends largely on the behaviour of the scoliosis. It is suggested that the initial image should include the lower cervical region down to the iliac crests to identify idiopathic scoliosis, with further images only on discussion with a radiologist.[7]

This initial examination is to ascertain if there are underlying pathological causes for the development of a scoliosis such as congenital hemivertebrae; if such a congenital abnormality is indicated by the initial AP, then additional projections of the hips and cervical spine may be indicated. Once the cause, if any, has been found, the child would usually be referred to an orthopaedic surgeon for management of the scoliosis. Follow-up images are required to monitor the scoliosis, which would result in a high radiation burden if separate AP and lateral projections of the thoracic and lumbar spine were taken each time. In these cases radiographs of the whole spine are performed, which allows a significant reduction in radiation dose.

AXIAL SKELETON: HIPS AND PELVIC GIRDLE

It is important to consider the range of normal anatomical variants, e.g. the ischiopubic synchrondroses, when evaluating images of the pelvis, although the details of these variants are beyond the scope of this chapter. The radiographic projections performed are governed by the reason for referral, namely for reasons relating to trauma or non-trauma, e.g. developmental dysplasia of the hip (DDH). Whilst many projections are described in literature, this text will focus on two, namely a variation on an AP pelvis projection (where the legs are not internally rotated), and the lateral hips projection which is known colloquially as the 'frog lateral'. Considering the potential deleterious effects of radiation, especially to children, many imaging departments have developed a strict protocol for the use of fenestration to shield radiosensitive structures, which are described below under the section on radiation protection. The shielding can be directly or remotely placed and Figures 32.3, 32.4, 32.5 and 32.6 illustrate the equipment used, their application and an example of an image produced using indirect fenestration.

■ Trauma to the pelvis

Although fracture/dislocations of the pelvis are rare, 80–90% of these patients will have multiple injuries to their head and/or abdominal viscera, where the likelihood of major blood loss is high.[8] These patients will be stabilised before presenting for X-ray. Computed tomography (CT) is widely regarded as a more effective imaging modality in the initial assessment of these patients. Where conventional radiographs are requested the following projection is required.

AP pelvis in trauma
Rarely are lateral projections (horizontal beam or turned lateral) of the hip required, as this region is seldom implicated in trauma. However, Salter Harris type fractures may not be readily identified on an AP projection alone.[8] The

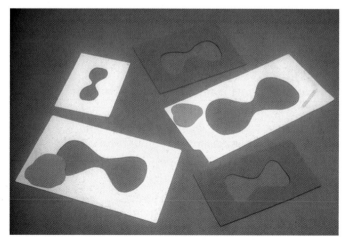

Figure 32.3 Fenestration

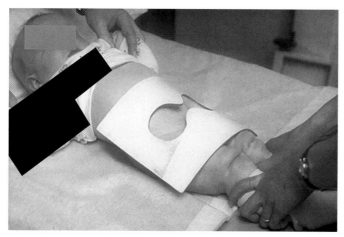

Figure 32.4   Direct fenestration technique for hips

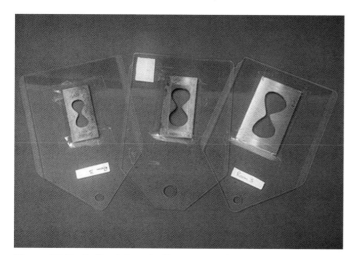

Figure 32.5   Indirect fenestration accessories

exclusion of this type of fracture is sufficient justification for a lateral radiograph.

Non-trauma pelvis

Plain radiographs of the hips are of limited value in children 6–9 months of age as the femoral head is primarily cartilaginous and therefore not radioopaque. In these cases diagnostic ultrasound is the imaging modality of choice, although exceptions to this would be suspicion of osteomyelitis and/or septic arthritis whereby an AP pelvis should be undertaken.

Developmental dysplasia of the hip

Congenital dislocation of the hip is an important condition affecting approximately 5 in 1000 babies at birth. This condition has recently been renamed DDH, rather than CDH (congenital dislocation of the hip) as it is thought this term more accurately describes the condition. A suggested imaging regime for this condition is given here:

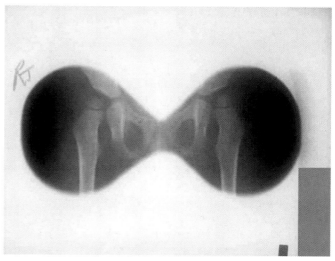

Figure 32.6   AP hips undertaken with indirect fenestration

- Until 12–18 months of age: diagnostic ultrasound
- Over 12–18 months of age: AP radiograph for the initial assessment and subsequent follow-up.[7] Additional views may be erect AP and/or Von Rosen projection

Irritable hip

This describes the acute onset of hip pain and stiffness. Radiographs of these children are often normal although it is not unusual for Perthes' disease, septic arthritis and osteomyelitis to present under the guise of 'irritable hip'. Ultrasound is often used for initial examination, with plain radiography undertaken for those with no abnormality noted with this modality. AP and a 'frog lateral projection' may be requested for this condition but radionuclide imaging will exclude Perthes' disease in those with chronic symptoms.[7]

AP pelvis and hips

Positioning

- The child is positioned in a similar fashion to the adult abdominal radiograph with their legs fully extended in a neutral position
- As for all examinations on small children, it must be remembered that anti-scatter grids are often unnecessary[7]
- The knees should be placed together but there is no need for the feet to be internally rotated
- Small children should be examined at the end of the X-ray table whereby the parent/carer can hold the legs in the correct position, and with relative ease

Radiation protection

Consider radiation protection for assistants who may help with holding the child. It is important that the assistant's fingers or other body parts are not in the primary beam. If this is unavoidable, lead rubber gloves must be worn

Beam Direction and FFD

Perpendicular central ray
100 cm FFD

Centring point

In the midline, level with the femoral pulses (as these lie directly over the femoral heads). Accurate location of this is described in the technique for AP of adult hips but sensible modification will be required for small children and babies since this technique uses a given measurement for location of the pulse. If the central ray passes though this level then accurate positioning of the hips is usually assured

Collimation

The complete pelvis: the iliac crests, hip joints, proximal femora

Criteria for assessing image quality

- No rotation of the pelvis; as for adults; the iliac wings must be symmetrical and of equal width at the level of the anterior superior iliac spines
- Obturator foramina must be symmetrical
- Greater trochanters should be in profile with no foreshortening of the femoral necks
- Periarticular soft tissue planes should be visible

▍Frog lateral hips

Positioning

- The child is supine on the couch with legs touching and initially extended
- The hips and knees are flexed equally and each is externally rotated until the lateral aspects of the femora are in contact with the table-top if possible
- After external rotation of the flexed limbs, the plantar aspects of both feet should be in contact. It may not be possible to fully abduct the affected hip, which may cause some degree of pelvic tilt. To overcome this, the legs should be adjusted so they are at equal angles to the pelvis. It may be necessary to place a radiolucent pad under one side of the pelvis (or even both) to help maintain symmetry of the position
- An image of an adult in this position is shown in Figure 10.6A

Beam Direction and FFD

Vertical central ray
100 cm FFD

Centring point

As for AP pelvis, as above

Collimation

The hip joints and proximal femora through the use of fenestration

Criteria for assessing image quality (Fig. 32.7)

- No rotation of the pelvis (see AP pelvis, above)
- Obturator foramina must be symmetrical
- Greater trochanters of the femora should preferably be symmetrical in appearance and not be foreshortened. If full external rotation cannot be achieved there should be symmetry of the trochanters and femoral necks
- Optimum demonstration of periarticular soft tissue

Radiation protection for pelvis and hip examinations

- Fenestration or other lead rubber protection should be used for all frog lateral projections, even as an initial examination
- No secondary radiation grids should be used for small children and infants
- Lead rubber gloves should be worn by an assistant if extremities are likely to be in the primary beam
- *No* lead protection is used on any projection following trauma
- *No* lead protection is used for initial radiographs in non-trauma AP pelvis
- Lead rubber *is* used for follow-up examinations relating to subsequent follow up of the same clinical condition
- There are radiation protection considerations for assistants who may assist in holding the child. It is important that the assistant's fingers or other body parts are not in the primary beam. If this is unavoidable, lead rubber gloves must be worn

Common errors	Possible reasons
Lead rubber obscuring area of interest	Misplacement by radiographer or movement of child
Assymetry of iliae and obturator foramina of the pelvis on all projections	Rotation
Assymetry of obturator foraminae, greater trochanters and femoral necks on frog laterals	May be due to over-abduction of one of the limbs, usually the non-affected side, resulting in the patient having an unstable platform
Translucent line of the growth-plate (physis) of the head of femur may be mistaken for a fracture	Erroneous image interpretation

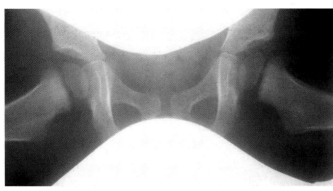

Figure 32.7 Frog lateral hips

- The legs are flexed at the knees and internally rotated
- A 90° block may be placed between the thighs to ensure that the thigh of each leg is 45° from the midline and that the legs are symmetrically positioned

FFD, centring point and collimation
As for AP hips

Criteria for assessing image quality
- As for AP hips but hips and femoral necks will be in internal rotation

▉ Von Rosen (AP with internal leg rotation)

Positioning
- From the supine AP position the legs are separated

AXIAL SKELETON: SKULL

CRANIAL VAULT

In cases of head injury the value of skull radiographs as a triaging tool is questionable because the absence of a fracture does not rule out an intracranial injury.[9] Abnormal neurological signs and symptoms are reported to be more reliable indicators of injury.[10,11] As such there is an increasing trend away from the use of skull radiography as CT possesses both a high sensitivity and specificity for the detection of intracranial bleeding. Back in 1990, Teasdale advocated the use of CT only when there is clinical evidence to justify the use of this modality[12] and other more up-to-date publications offer advice on the use of CT and plain film radiography of the head.[13,14] Conventional radiographs are still required in cases of suspected non-accidental injury where two projections are usually required. Where fractures are present their age can be assessed, which can be invaluable to the legal fraternity.

Radiography of the cranium can be performed using either isocentric or non-isocentric apparatus. The positioning guidelines for each type of equipment can be found in the relevant sections on radiography of the head in this text. Despite the increased radiation dose to the eyes, when using isocentric equipment it is often normal practice for frontooccipital (FO) as opposed to occipitofrontal (OF) radiographs to be undertaken, as young children are found to be less anxious if the cassette does not come close to their face. The area of the cranium under investigation informs the radiographer's choice of OF/FO projection (e.g. FO 30°/half-axial for the occiput or OF 20° for frontal

bone). A lateral projection is almost always performed in addition to the OF/FO. Skull radiographs are more easily acquired with the patient in a supine position, as is accepted practice in cases of trauma. If cassettes are used, either an 18 × 24 cm or 24 × 30 cm cassette is selected, depending on the size of the child's head. Other than considering the use of FO projections, the same procedures and set-ups should be followed as for adult skull radiography, apart from the considerations listed below.

▉ FO and lateral projections of the skull

Positioning
- For infants under 6 months of age a secondary radiation grid or anti-scatter device is not required
- Where compliance is not easily obtained, the upper limbs can be positioned adjacent to the chest and the torso of the infant wrapped in a blanket to assist in immobilisation
- For reasons relating to safety, and to assist in immobilisation, an assistant must accompany the child throughout the procedure
- Sponge pads can be used either side the head, as for the AP cervical spine projection, to assist with immobilisation. The chin may also be held but the assistant's fingers must not be included in the primary beam. Velcro straps may also be used for immobilisation
- Table-top or trolley technique: the image receptor should rest on a wedge-shaped support or sponge pad, which is of sufficient angle to ensure the orbitomeatal baseline (OMBL) is perpendicular to the cassette. It may be necessary to place the sponge over the cassette, with the child's

head resting upon the pad; this will cause some magnification unsharpness and further exaggerate distortion of the image and should be avoided if possible

- Isocentric technique: A pad may be used under the head to ensure that the anthropological baseline is perpendicular to the floor
- Beam limitation devices are essential so that the radiation field is not unnecessarily large

Radiation protection
- Consider radiation protection for assistants who may assist the radiographer by holding the child's head
- Ensure beam limiting devices are used effectively
- Older, cooperative children should have OF projections taken, as opposed to FO, wherever possible

Beam direction, FFD, centring point, collimation and criteria for assessing image quality

This is as for adults (see the relevant chapter). In addition to the criteria given in the chapter on adult skull radiographs:

- The fontanelles should be adequately demonstrated in babies

Common errors	Possible reasons
Especially in babies, the petrous part of the temporal bone is likely to be misaligned in relation to the orbits	Not actually radiographer error – craniofacial disproportion
Rotation, tilt and/or movement unsharpness of the resultant radiograph	The assistant may have difficulty in encouraging the child to maintain a constant position

PARANASAL SINUSES AND FACIAL BONES

Techniques to demonstrate these structures are seldom performed, but may be requested from time to time, especially in the older child. If radiographs of the sinuses of young children are requested, it is important to remember that this may not be a valid request, as these structures are not well demonstrated until the process of pneumatisation is complete. If plain radiography of the sinuses is justified, images are undertaken and evaluated as for adult radiographs of the region. Although plain radiography of the sinuses is deemed to be non-productive, lateral postnasal space may be undertaken in young children, to assess size of the adenoidal pad; this is also undertaken as for adults.

SKELETAL SURVEY

Skeletal surveys are most commonly undertaken in cases of suspected non-accidental injury (NAI) and for the investigation of skeletal dysphasia (non-trauma). Judging the alleged perpetrator is the role of the courts, and radiographers should assume the responsibility of managing the radiographic examination in a professional manner.

▮ Suspected non-accidental injury (NAI)

In these cases the purpose of a skeletal survey is to provide documentary evidence of an injury, which may be associated with a non-accidental mechanism. This examination can be performed on both living and deceased patients. It may not always be necessary to conduct a skeletal survey on every child with a suspected or proven bone injury. The radiographic examination should be undertaken in consultation with the referrer, and may be adjusted accordingly. It is recommended that departments undertaking NAI examinations should have a written protocol outlining the procedure from start to finish. Consideration needs to be

given to the following points, which should be included in the protocol.

- *Referral source.* Referrals are accepted from paediatricians and may have been initiated by the police or social services. Requests are generally not accepted from general practitioners or from personnel in A&E departments.
- *Prioritisation.* Skeletal surveys for NAI are not emergency procedures and should not routinely be performed outside normal working hours; however, in exceptional circumstances they may be required. For instance if a child is placed on a 48-hour protection order, the police and social services may need to know the length of time since injuries have been sustained.
- *Medico-legal issues.* It should be remembered that all skeletal surveys in cases of suspected NAI could be presented as evidence in a court of law. It is therefore important that all images are optimally centred, exposed, collimated and accurately labelled with the date, patient's demographic details and anatomical markers. The child

must be accompanied by an approved guardian (parent, medical staff or social worker). Two persons (health professionals) must be present during the examination and, post processing, the signatures of both persons in attendance should be included on all radiographs.[15] Identification and anatomical markers must not be added after the image has been produced, in order that such identifications cannot be brought into question; the primary radiographer who positions the child must ensure that these identifications are in place at the time of exposure.

- *Image quality.* Whole body images or multiple body areas on one image are not acceptable under any circumstances (these are frequently called 'babygrams' by radiographers) as this unnecessarily irradiates some body areas and does not provide adequate detail of all parts demonstrated.

Suggested projections for the NAI skeletal survey

A skeletal survey should normally include the following anatomical areas and projections:

Chest	AP, lateral and both posterior obliques (for lateral rib margins and clavicles)
Abdomen	AP to include both hip joints
Skull	FO/OF and lateral
Humeri and both forearms	AP
Femora and both tibiae/fibulae	AP
Hands	Dorsipalmar or DP oblique of both
Feet	Dorsiplantar of both
Spine	Lateral

Further projections of the limbs, e.g. lateral, may be undertaken if the radiographer identifies any areas of suspicion on the resultant film, e.g. a raised periosteum. Clearly less subtle appearances, such as fractures, will be more obvious but will still require additional projections. On completion of the study, the radiographs should be reviewed by a consultant radiologist and further projections undertaken if required. If there is no radiologist available at the time, the child should return to the ward and, if necessary, be recalled at a later date for further imaging.

Skeletal dysplasia

There are many hereditary disorders, some of which have a skeletal component (skeletal dysplasia), e.g. osteogenesis imperfecta (OI). Disorders may be trivial or associated with high mortality and morbidity rates. Diagnostic radiography can often play a major role in the diagnoses and subsequent classification of dysplasias.

Suggested projections for skeletal survey of skeletal dysplasias

Chest	AP/PA
Pelvis	AP
Skull	Lateral
Cervical, thoracic and lumbosacral spine	AP and laterals
Humerus and forearm*	Left limb – AP
Femur, tibia and fibula*	Left limb – AP
Hand	DP of left, to include wrist for bone age assessment, if required

*For any projections of long bones, it is important to ensure that both associated joints are demonstrated on the resultant radiographs.

Acknowledgements

The authors are grateful to Dr Joanne Fairhurst, Consultant Paediatric Radiologist, Southampton General Hospital, for her expert review of successive drafts. We wish to express our profound thanks to our colleagues in radiography and radiology, as well as our former teachers from both professional groups, who have helped us to learn the art and knowledge associated with paediatric radiography. Thanks also to Sheila Copeland, an inspirational role model when learning about communication techniques for adults working with children.

References

1. Audit Commission. Children first: a study of hospital services. London: HMSO; 1993.
2. European Guidelines on Quality Criteria for Diagnostic Radiographic Images in Paediatrics. The European Commission, EUR 16261 EN, CEC. Luxembourg; 1996.
3. The Ionising Radiation (Medical Exposure) Regulations 2000. London: HMSO; 2000.
4. McHugh K. Teenage pregnancy: sex, lies and too much 'red tape'. Radiology Now 2002; 19(3):2–4.
5. Hodgson J. Distraction techniques for use in micturating cysto-urethrograms. Synergy 2000; Jan:8–9.
6. Jones NF, et al. Neonatal chest and abdominal radiation dosimetry; a comparison of two radiographic techniques. British Journal of Radiology 2001; 74:920–925.
7. Cook JV, et al. Guidelines on best practice in the X-ray imaging of children: a manual for all departments. London: The St Helier NHS Trust and St George's Healthcare NHS Trust; 1998.
8. Thornton A, Gyll C. Children's fractures. London: Saunders; 1999.
9. Quayle KS, et al. Diagnostic testing for acute head injury in children: when are computed tomography and skull radiographs indicated? Paediatrics 1997; 99(5): E11.PMID 9113968 [PubMed indexed for MEDLINE]

10. Lloyd D, et al. Predictive value of skull radiography for intracranial injury in children with blunt head injury. The Lancet 1997; 349:821–824.

11. Glasgow JFT, McGovern SJ. Imaging the less seriously head injured child. Archives of Disease in Childhood; 2000 82:333.

12. Teasdale G, et al. Risks of acute traumatic intracranial haematoma in children and adults. British Medical Journal 1990; 300:363–367.

13. Head injury: Triage, assessment, investigation and early management of head injury in infants, children and adults. London: Guideline commissioned by the National Institute for Clinical Excellence; 2003.

14. Radiation Protection 118. Referral guidelines for imaging. Luxembourg: European Commission Directorate-General for the Environment; 2000.

15. College of Radiographers. Guidance for the provision of forensic radiography services. London: College of Radiographers; 1999.

CONTRAST STUDIES

CONTRAST MEDIA

Susan Cutler

Contrast media (also known as contrast agents) are substances used to highlight areas of the body in radiographic contrast to their surrounding tissues. Contrast media enhance the radioopacity and optical density of the area under investigation so that the tissue/structure absorption differentials are sufficient to produce adequate contrast with adjacent structures. There are numerous types of radiographic contrast media employed in medical imaging, which have different applications depending upon their chemical and physical properties. When used for imaging purposes contrast media can be administered by injection, insertion or ingestion.

HISTORY OF RADIOGRAPHIC CONTRAST MEDIA

Radiographic contrast has been used for over a century to enhance the contrast of radiographic images. In 1896, 1 year after X-rays were discovered, inspired air became the first recognised contrast agent in radiographic examinations of the chest. In 1898, the first contrast studies were carried out of the *upper gastrointestinal tract* using bismuth salts on a cat. These salts were very toxic and by 1910 barium sulphate and bismuth solutions were being used in conjunction with the fluoroscope, barium sulphate having been used with differing additives ever since for imaging of the gastrointestinal tract.

Images of the *urinary system* were achieved in the early 1920s. In the early 1920s, syphilis was treated with high doses of sodium iodide. During this treatment the urine in the bladder was observed to be radioopaque due to its iodine content. In 1923 the first *angiogram* and opacification of the urinary tract was performed using sodium iodide. Sodium iodide was too toxic for satisfactory intravenous

use, necessitating a need to find a less toxic iodinated compound.

The first *iodine based* contrast used was a derivative of the chemical ring pyridine, to which a single iodine atom could be bound in order to render it radioopaque. Iodine-based contrast media have been used ever since. These media, however, produced varying adverse reactions and it was realised that a contrast agent was needed that was both safe to administer and enhanced the contrast of the radiographic image. Modern ionic contrast agents were introduced in 1950 and were derivatives of tri-iodo benzoic acid; this structure enabled three atoms of iodine to be carried, rendering it more radioopaque. However, the contrast still caused adverse effects as they were still of high osmolarity, the term being explained as follows:

Ionic media dissociate in water; their injection into the blood plasma results in a great increase in the number of particles present in the plasma. This has the effect of displacing water. Water moves from an area of greater concentration to an area of lesser concentration by the process of osmosis, the physical process that occurs whenever there is a concentration difference across a membrane and the membrane is permeable to the diffusing substance. Osmolality (which is generally considered interchangeable with the term 'osmolarity') is defined as the number of solute particles, e.g. the contrast medium molecules, dissolved in 1 L (1000 g) of water. These media exert tremendous osmotic activity on the body. Normal human blood osmolality is given as around 290–300 mOsm/kg (milliosmoles per kilogram).

There remained a need to find a water-soluble, iodine-based contrast with reduced toxicity but that still produced satisfactory radioopacity on images. In the 1970s and 1980s, non-ionic low osmolality contrast media became widely available with the first non-ionic contrast medium being introduced in 1974, representing a major advancement in diagnostic imaging. Most recently the non-ionic dimers have emerged. These media are highly hydrophilic, resulting in lower chemotoxicity and they are isoosmolar with the respective body fluids, meaning they can be employed for examinations such as angiography and computed tomography (CT) arteriography which require high doses of contrast media to be administered, and where low toxicity is essential. At the time of going to press, only two compounds, iotrolan (Isovist) and iodixanol (Visipaque) are available.

REQUIREMENTS OF 'THE IDEAL' CONTRAST MEDIUM

Currently there is no contrast medium on the market that is considered to be ideal, but the ideal contrast medium should fulfil certain requirements for safe and effective application. It should be:

- easy to administer
- non-toxic
- a stable compound
- concentrated in the required area when injected
- rapidly eliminated when necessary
- non-carcinogenic
- of appropriate viscosity for administration
- tolerated by the patient
- cost effective

Contrast media are divided into two main categories. The first is *negative* contrast media which are radiolucent and of low atomic number, causing the part in which it is placed to be more readily penetrated by X-rays than the surrounding tissue; as they attenuate the X-ray beam less effectively than body tissue, they appear darker on the X-ray image. Gases are commonly used to produce negative contrast on radiographic images. The second type is *positive* contrast media; these are radioopaque and are of a high atomic number, causing the part in which it is placed to be less readily penetrated by X-rays than the surrounding tissue. Consequently this contrast agent-filled area appears denser than body tissue.

Barium and iodine based solutions are used in medical imaging to produce positive contrast. Both positive and negative contrast can be employed together in double contrast examinations to produce a radiographic image. Double contrast is used primarily in the alimentary tract but is also used in arthrography of joints. The positive contrast medium is used to coat the walls of the cavity and the negative contrast, in the form of a gas, is used to distend the area being imaged. Double contrast examinations permit optimum visualisation by producing a high inherent contrast whilst allowing adequate penetration of the area under examination. Use of a small amount of contrast agent in conjunction with the distended cavity allows coating of the structures in the cavity (or in the case of the alimentary tract, the mucosal lining) which provides better detail of the area when the thin coating is shown in contrast to the gas-filled area, rather than using large amounts which may be dense enough to mask important information.

NEGATIVE CONTRAST MEDIA

The following gases create negative radiographic contrast on images:

- *Air:* introduced by the patient during a radiographic examination, e.g. inspiration during chest radiography *or* can also be introduced by the radiographer as part of the examination in a double contrast barium enema
- *Oxygen:* introduced into cavities of the body for example in the knee when performing an arthrogram to demonstrate the knee joint
- *Carbon dioxide:* introduced into the gastrointestinal tract in conjunction with a barium sulphate solution to demonstrate the mucosal pattern, e.g. double contrast barium meal. For the barium meal it is formulated as effervescent powder (e.g. 'Carbex' granules) or ready mixed carbonated barium sulphate (e.g. 'Baritop'). Carbon dioxide can also be introduced into the colon when performing a double contrast barium enema. It has been recommended that carbon dioxide be used as the negative contrast agent in a double contrast barium enema, rather than air, as it causes less immediate abdominal pain[1] as well as less postprocedural pain and discomfort.[2] However, some studies have shown that carbon dioxide produces inferior distension and additional insufflations are required to maintain adequate quality distension.[3] Carbon dioxide can also be used as an alternative contrast to iodinated contrast for diagnostic angiography and vascular interventions in both the arterial and venous circulation. The gas produces negative contrast due to its low atomic number and low density compared with adjacent tissues

POSITIVE CONTRAST MEDIA

Barium and iodine solutions are used to create positive contrast on images.

Barium sulphate solutions (BaSO$_4$) used in gastrointestinal imaging

Barium solutions are the universal contrast media used for radiographic examinations of the gastrointestinal tract. The following characteristics of barium solutions make them suitable for imaging of the gastrointestinal tract:

- High atomic number (56) producing good radiographic contrast
- Insoluble
- Stable
- Relatively inexpensive
- Excellent coating properties of the gastrointestinal mucosa

Barium suspensions are composed from pure barium sulphate mixed with additives and dispersing agents, held in suspension in water. Compounds to stabilise the suspension are added; these act on the surface tension and increase solution viscosity. A dispersing agent to prevent sedimentation is added, ensuring an even distribution of particles within the suspension. Also added to the suspension is a defoaming agent, employed to prevent bubbles that may mimic pathology in the gastrointestinal tract. Flavourings are usually added to oral solutions, making them more palatable for patients.

The concentration of barium in the solution is normally stated as a percentage weight to volume ratio (w/v). A 100% w/v solution contains 1 g of barium sulphate per 100 mL of water; the density of the barium solution is therefore dependent upon the weight volume. There are many varieties of barium suspensions available and the type used is dependent upon the area of the gastrointestinal tract being imaged. It also depends greatly upon the individual preferences of the practitioner.

Patients rarely have allergic reactions to barium sulphate solutions but may react to the preservatives or additives in the solutions. Barium sulphate preparations are usually safe as long as the gastrointestinal tract is patent and intact. A severe inflammatory reaction may develop if it is extravasated outside the gastrointestinal tract; this is most likely to occur when there is a perforation of the tract. If barium sulphate escapes into the peritoneal cavity, inflammation and peritonitis may occur. Escaped barium in the peritoneum causes pain and hypovolaemic shock and, despite treatment which includes fluid replacement therapy, steroids and antibiotics, there is still a 50% mortality rate; of those who survive, 30% will develop peritoneal adhesions and granulomas.[4] Aspiration of barium solutions during upper gastrointestinal tract imaging is considered to be relatively harmless. It most frequently affects the elderly patient. Physiotherapy is usually required

in order to drain the aspirated barium and should be performed before the patient leaves the department.

Oral barium sulphate should not be administered in cases of obstruction as it may inspissate behind an obstruction, compounding the patient's problem. Sedated patients should not undergo examinations of the upper gastrointestinal tract as their swallowing reflex may be diminished.

When preparing the barium solutions for administration it is important to check expiry dates and ensure the packaging is intact. Solutions administered rectally should be administered at body temperature to improve patient tolerability and also reduce spasm of the colon. It is important that the administrator knows the patient's medical history and checks for any contraindications prior to administration. Barium sulphate solutions are contraindicated for the following pathologies:

- Suspected perforation
- Suspected fistula or to check an anastomosis site
- Suspected partial or complete stenosis
- Paralytic ileus
- Haemorrhage in the gastrointestinal tract
- Toxic megacolon
- Prior to surgery or endoscopy
- If the patient has had a recent gastrointestinal wide bore biopsy (usually within 3–5 days)

When barium sulphate solutions are contraindicated for gastrointestinal imaging, a water-soluble, iodine-based contrast medium (e.g. Gastrografin or Gastromiro) should be employed. These can be administered orally, rectally or mechanically, e.g. via stomas. The iodine concentration of Gastrografin = 370 mg/mL^{-1} and Gastromiro = 300 mg/mL^{-1}. When used for imaging the gastrointestinal tract, water-soluble contrast produces a lower contrast image than barium due to its lower atomic number.

The patient's consent must be given prior to the administration of barium contrast solutions. The patient should be reassured about the examination and given the opportunity to ask questions. It is important when using barium sulphate solutions that associated pharmacological agents such as buscopan and glucagon are fully understood and the indications and contraindications adhered to ensuring their safe application.

Iodine-based contrast media used in medical imaging

The largest group of contrast media used in imaging departments are the water-soluble organic preparations in which molecules of iodine are the opaque agent. These compounds contain iodine atoms (iodine has an atomic number of 53), bound to a carrier molecule. This holds the iodine in a stable compound and carries it to the organ under examination. The carrier molecules are organic, containing carbon, and are of low toxicity and high stability. Iodine is used as it is relatively safe and the K edge = 32 keV (binding edge of Iodine K-shell electron) and is therefore close to the mean energy of diagnostic X-rays. The selection of kVp used for imaging examinations utilising iodine-based contrast plays a part in providing optimum attenuation. The absorption edge of iodine (35 keV) predicts that 63–77 kVp is the optimal range. The iodine-based compounds are divided into four groups (Fig. 33.1) depending upon their molecular structure; the four groups are:

1. Ionic monomers
2. Ionic dimers
3. Non-ionic monomers
4. Non-ionic dimers

Ionic monomers – high osmolar contrast media (HOCM) (Fig. 33.2)

The basic molecule of all water-soluble, iodine-containing contrast media is the benzene ring. Benzene itself is not water soluble; to make it soluble, carboxyl acid (COOH) is added. Three of the hydrogens in this molecule are replaced by iodine, rendering it radiopaque, but it still remains quite toxic. The remaining two hydrogens (R$_1$ and R$_2$ in Fig. 33.2) are replaced by a short chain of hydrocarbons, making the compound less toxic, and more acceptable to the body. The exact nature of these compounds differ between different contrast media but are usually prepared as sodium or meglumine salts as these help to provide solubility.

Ionic compounds dissociate (dissolve) into charged particles when entering a solution. They dissociate into positively charged cations and negatively charged anions. For every three iodine molecules present in ionic media, one cation and one anion are produced when it enters a solution. Their 'effect' ratio is therefore 3:2. These solutions are highly hypertonic with an osmolality approximately five times higher than human plasma (1500–2000 mOsm/kg H$_2$O compared with 300 mOsm/kg H$_2$O for plasma).

Ionic dimers – low osmolar contrast media (LOCM) (Fig. 33.3)

A contrast medium was therefore needed with reduced osmotic effects. As already stated, the higher the 'effect' ratio, the lower the osmolarity of the contrast media. An attempt was made to increase the 'effect' ratio and produce a contrast medium with lower osmolarity. This was achieved by linking together two conventional ionic contrast media molecules. The resulting dimeric ionic contrast medium was an improvement on the HOCM. Reduced osmolality (600 mOsm/kg H$_2$O) made the contrast more tolerable for patients. The ionic molecule still dissociated into two particles, a positive cation and a negative anion. However, there are now twice as many particles in solution with twice the osmolarity. Each molecule now carried six iodines (as opposed to three in the HOCM), hence there is an iodine atom to particle ratio of 6:2; so to achieve the same iodine concentration, only half the number of molecules are needed.

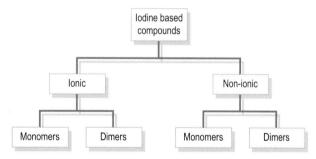

Figure 33.1 Classification of ionic contrast media

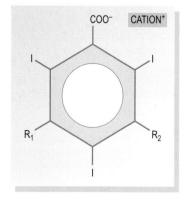

Figure 33.2 Molecular structure of an ionic monomer (HOCM)

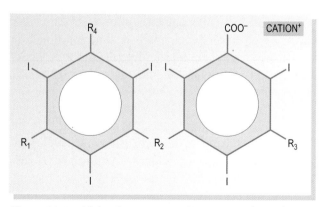

Figure 33.3 Molecular structure of ionic dimer (LOCM)

Non-ionic monomers (LOCM) (Fig. 33.4)

These are low osmolar agents and do not dissociate into two particles in a solution, making them more tolerable and safer to use than ionic contrast. For every three iodine molecules in a non-ionic solution, one neutral molecule is produced. Non-ionic contrast media are referred to as 3:1 compounds. They substitute the sodium and meglumine side chains with non-ionising radicals $(OH)n$. Two major advantages arise through the change in chemical structure: the first being that the negative carboxyl group is eliminated, decreasing the neurotoxicity and, the second, the elimination of the positive ion reduces osmolality to 600–700 mOsm/kg H_2O. Non-ionic LOCM are used for intrathecal and vascular procedures.

Non-ionic dimers (isotonic) (Fig. 33.5)

These are dimeric non-dissociating molecules; for every one molecule there are six iodine atoms. The ratio is therefore 6:1, double the non-ionic monomers. They are isotonic, i.e. the contrast solution has similar osmolality to blood plasma (approximately 300 mOsm/kg H_2O). Their isoosmolality, combined with a slower diffusion of the larger molecules across vessel walls from the vascular space, plays a significant role in imaging venous phase images following arterial injections (and arterial phase images following venous injections). These compounds represent a gold standard, water-soluble, iodine contrast medium.

■ The percentage solution

The percentage solution indicates the amount of solute in the solvent. The percentage solution does not indicate the percentage iodine content as demonstrated in the following table.

| | Percentage iodine content in contrast media | |
Contrast media	Percentage solution	Iodine concentration of solution
Urografin 150	30%	146 mg/mL^{-1}
Urografin 370	76%	370 mg/mL^{-1}
Gastrografin	76%	370 mg/mL^{-1}
Niopam 370	75.5%	370 mg/mL^{-1}

The solvent affects viscosity of the contrast agent. Viscosity is the resistance to flow of a contrast medium and relates to the concentration, molecular size and the temperature of the contrast. The volume and density of contrast used is dependent upon the examination being undertaken, the pathology being investigated, the age of the patient and the patient's medical status.

■ Essential criteria for the 'ideal' intravenous contrast agent

- Water soluble
- Heat/chemical/storage stability
- Non-antigenic
- Available at the right viscosity and density
- Low viscosity – making them easy to administer
- Persistent enough in the area of interest to allow its visualisation
- Selective excretion by the patient when the examination is complete
- Lower or the same osmolarity compared to plasma
- Non-toxic, both locally and systemically
- Low cost

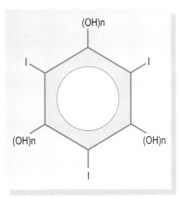

Figure 33.4 Molecular structure of non-ionic monomer

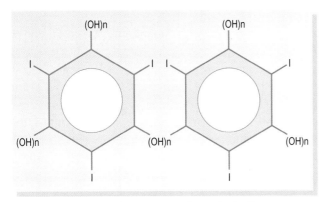

Figure 33.5 Molecular structure of non-ionic dimer

POSSIBLE SIDE-EFFECTS OF IONIC-BASED CONTRAST MEDIA

Any water-soluble ionic contrast introduced into the vascular system can cause potential physiological adverse effects. These effects are caused by the high osmolarity and chemotoxic effects of the medium. Although both ionic and non-ionic iodine media have physiological effects on the body, ionic media are of higher osmolarity and potentially cause more side-effects in the patient. An ionic contrast has approximately five times the osmolarity of human plasma (i.e. it is hyperosmolar). Water-soluble organic iodine contrast media have two effects: the desirable primary effect of attenuating X-rays and providing the radiographic image with adequate contrast and the unwanted secondary effect of inducing potential side-effects in patients.

Primary effect – image contrast

Optimum attenuation is achieved by selecting the appropriate concentration of iodine in solution for the examination undertaken. Two solutions with the same iodine content should provide the same iodine concentration in blood after intravenous injection. This is not the case and the concentration may be affected by small molecules diffusing out of the blood vessel lumen, or by solutions of high concentration within the blood vessel drawing water out of adjacent cells by osmosis (therefore diluting the solution), as mentioned in the introduction to this chapter. To illustrate this, remembering that osmolality is defined as the number of solute particles (e.g. the contrast media molecules) dissolved in 1 L (1000 g) of water, a comparison between normal blood plasma osmolality and different contrast agents is shown:

- Normal blood plasma ~ 300 mOsm/kg water
- Ionic monomer ~ 1200–2400 mOsm/kg water, making it very hypertonic
- Ionic dimers, and non-ionic monomers and dimers (LOCM) are still hypertonic but to a much lesser degree, reducing the osmotic activity, however they are more expensive. Isotonic Iodixanol (Visipaque) has approximately a third the osmolality of the non-ionic media and a sixth that of the monomeric ionic media of equi-iodine concentration (i.e. 290 mOsm/kg water vs 844 and 1800 mOsm/kg water respectively)

When comparing two contrast media of the same iodine concentration, a higher venous concentration of iodine is obtained when diffusion of contrast medium is slowed down by using large molecules (dimers) and osmotic effects are decreased by decreasing the number of molecules/ions in solution (monomers).

Secondary effect – adverse events

Contrast media are specifically designed to minimise secondary effect or adverse reaction. The 'perfect' contrast agent would cause no adverse affects at all. Acute adverse reactions do occur, however, and are defined as reactions that occur within 1 hour after administration of a contrast medium. Adverse reactions to contrast media or drugs are generally classified into two categories:

- Idiosyncratic reactions which are dose dependent and unpredictable, having a prevalence of 1–2% (0.04–0.22% severe) and are fatal in 1 in 170 000.[5]
- Non-idiosyncratic reactions are divided into chemotoxic and osmotoxic reactions. They are predictable and more likely to occur in debilitated patients or patients in poor medical health. They are dose dependent and are caused primarily by osmotic effects causing shifts in fluids from the intracellular to extracellular structures, causing cell dehydration and dysfunction.

The onset of reactions is variable; 70% of reactions occur within 5 minutes of injection, 16% occur more than 5 minutes after the injection and the remaining 14% within 15 minutes of the injection. It is advisable that a suitably qualified staff member remains with the patient for at least 15 minutes post injection. Contrast media affect specific organs or systems of the body; the following are a summary of some of the major systemic effects of contrast media.

Cardiovascular toxicity

Pain can occur at the injection site during intravascular contrast administration. Thrombus formation and endothelial damage may occur and contrast may impair platelet aggregation and blood clotting and it may provoke a painful sickle cell crisis. Osmotic effects of the contrast media can also cause vasodilatation with associated hot flushing. Fluid shifts, as already discussed, can produce an intravascular hypervolemic state, systemic hypertension and pulmonary oedema. Contrast media can lower the ventricular arrhythmia threshold and precipitate cardiac arrhythmias or cause an angina attack. In rare cases, this may lead to cardiac arrest, necessitating urgent medical intervention.

Nephrological toxicity

Ionic contrast may affect renal output, causing renal impairment; this is usually a temporary impairment. Contrast medium nephrotoxicity is defined as an impairment in renal function (an increase in serum creatinine by more than 25% or 44 mmol/L) following the intravascular administration of a contrast medium in the absence of an alternative aetiology. The following conditions may increase the incidence of nephrotoxicity in patients who receive an intravascular contrast medium:

- Pre-existing kidney disease
- Diabetes mellitus
- Multiple myeloma
- Dehydration
- Large volume of contrast injected
- Age of patient

In patients with renal impairment it may be necessary to consider alternative imaging strategies, which do not require the administration of iodinated contrast media. Nephrotoxic effects can be minimised by ensuring that the patient is well hydrated and by using low or isoosmolar contrast media. This has implications for patient preparation for the intravenous urogram (IVU); in the past, practitioners have sometimes requested that patients restrict fluid intake prior to the IVU, intending to maximise concentration of the contrast agent in the urine produced. However, modern contrast agents do provide satisfactory concentration in the urine without fluid restriction and this practice should be discouraged for the IVU examination.

Special consideration must be given to diabetic patients on oral metformin (Glucophage). These patients often have associated renal impairment and are more prone to developing lactic acidosis if iodine based contrast media is administered. However, this rare complication occurs only if the contrast medium causes renal failure, and the patient continues to take metformin in the presence of renal failure. Continued intake of metformin after the onset of renal failure results in a toxic accumulation of this drug and subsequent lactic acidosis. To avoid this complication, metformin must be withheld after the administration of the contrast media for 48 hours, during which the contrast induced renal failure becomes clinically apparent. If renal function is normal after 48 hours, metformin intake can be reestablished.

Neurotoxicity

The incidence of serious neurotoxic effects is low following the administration of intravascular contrast media; neurotoxicity of contrast media is related to the osmolality of the solution. Entry of contrast media into the central nervous system is normally limited but may be increased by the osmotic opening of the blood–brain barrier. The blood–brain barrier gives protection for the brain by acting as a selective barrier; it regulates the amount and composition of the brain's cerebrospinal fluid, in order that exchanges across the barrier between the blood and cerebrospinal fluid, which would harm the brain, are reduced, whilst exchanges of essential substances are facilitated. Ionic media are hyperosmolar with respect to human plasma and they may dehydrate the cerebral endothelial cells, causing them to dysfunction and breach the barrier, resulting in depolarisation of cerebral neurons and leading to possible seizures. Seizures are more likely to occur in patients with brain tumours, abscesses and other processes that disrupt the blood–brain barrier. Convulsions may also occur secondary to cerebral hypoxia (caused by hypotension), cardiac arrest or anaphylaxis, which may be induced after administration of a contrast medium. Neurotoxicity can be reduced by employing a low contrast (concentration) osmolar contrast media as they are less likely to breach the blood–brain barrier.

What happens during a reaction and how reactions may be prevented

Improvements in the chemical structure of contrast medium molecules have resulted in a significant reduction in the number of acute reactions. Severe reactions are a rare occurrence and previous allergic reactions to contrast material, asthma, and known allergies are factors associated with an increased risk of developing a reaction. An injection of contrast medium causes the release of histamine from the basophils and mast cells in the blood. Some patients release more histamine than others and the reason for this is still not fully understood. Another possible mechanism for reactions to contrast media is thought to be the inhibition of enzymes, e.g. cholinesterase, which deactivates and hydrolyses acetylcholine, causing symptoms of vagal overstimulation resulting in bronchospasm and cardiovascular collapse.

Patients must be assessed and past medical history ascertained before any contrast medium is administered. Any patient with a medical history that raises concern can be given prophylactic treatment before administration of contrast material, to prevent potential reactions. Injection of hydrocortisone may be given before the contrast agent to suppress inflammatory and allergic responses. This treatment decreases the chance of allergic reactions, including anaphylaxis, renal failure or a possible life-threatening emergency. Prophylactic drugs should be administered in a separate syringe as they may cause crystallisation when they come into contact with contrast media. Serious reactions still occur, and awareness and treatment of the different types of reaction is paramount for any staff member involved in intravenous administration of contrast media.

Non-ionic versus ionic contrast media

As already discussed, ionic media dissociate in solution and alter the sodium balance in the body, whereas non-ionic media, which are made of compounds, do not dissociate in solution. Non-ionic contrast agents do not give the extra ion load that ionic contrast media do and are therefore more 'in tune' with body homeostasis and physiology. Non-ionic contrast media are usually safer to administer and better tolerated by patients. Ionic contrast is less expensive and is usually used for examination such as cystograms when contrast is introduced into a body cavity and not directly into the circulatory system. Non-ionic contrast is used primarily in examinations where the contrast is administered directly into the circulatory system. Advantages of non-ionic contrast medium include:

- reduction in the number of side-effects; reactions prove to be 3–10 times lower with non-ionic contrast, due to the fact that it stimulates less histamine release
- decreased vasodilatation, producing less alteration in the body haemodynamics and causing less damage to the vessel endothelium
- less effect on the blood–brain barrier
- improved tolerability for the patient

ADMINISTRATION OF INTRAVENOUS CONTRAST MEDIA

All personnel employed in the imaging department must be aware of the legal and professional regulations relating to the administration of contrast media as part of a radiological examination. All staff employed should have the appropriate training and hospital trusts and departments should have protocols and procedures in place to ensure a safe and effective procedure for all parties concerned.

Whenever possible, LOCM should be administered to all patients but especially:

- infants
- the elderly
- those with cardiac or renal impairment
- diabetics
- patients with a history of asthma or severe allergy
- patients with a history of a previous reaction to contrast media

If a patient presents with a history of a previous reaction to a contrast agent, there is a serious danger of producing a severe and possibly fatal reaction if the examination is undertaken. Allergic patients who have previously tolerated an injection of contrast media may have become sensitised, and great care must be taken on any subsequent examination. The referrer should evaluate the risk involved against information to be gained from the examination being undertaken and alternative imaging modalities employed if deemed more appropriate.

Precautions taken before administration of contrast media

Reactions from the administration of a contrast medium are not predictable and all patients should be monitored closely during the procedure. The importance of assessing the patient before the procedure cannot be over-emphasised. This will give the radiographer a baseline value from which to measure the patient's condition throughout the procedure. The radiographer should be familiar with the symptoms of the various adverse events that may occur. The following is a summary of general advice and precautions to be taken before, during and after the administration of an intravenous contrast media.

Before injection:

- Know the patient and their medical history
- Reassure the patient and gain the patient's consent
- If the patient is a high-risk patient, consider the administration of a low osmolar contrast medium
- Consider the following high risk factors which are associated with the administration of intravenous contrast medium:
  - A previous severe adverse reaction to contrast medium
  - Asthma or a significant allergic history
  - Proven or suspected hypersensitivity to iodine
  - Severe renal or hepatic impairment
  - Severe cardiovascular disease
  - Epilepsy
  - Hyperthyroidism
  - Multiple myeloma
  - Pre-existing thyrotoxic symptoms
  - Severe respiratory disease
  - Diabetes
  - Sickle-cell anaemia
- Check the batch number and expiry date of the contrast
- Ensure the contrast agent is at body temperature
- Check the sterility of the packaging
- Know the procedure, indications and contraindications and be aware of the possible adverse effects that might occur
- Check emergency equipment and be familiar with its application
- Obtain a positive identification check on the patient
- Check the correct contrast volume, dose and strength for the procedure being undertaken

During the injection

- Know where the radiologist/administering doctor may be reached

- Evaluate the patient's vital signs and observe respiration, pulse, blood pressure, patient colour, and level of consciousness

After the injection

- Remain with the patient for at least 15 minutes
- Correct completion of all relevant documentation regarding the contrast agent used should be undertaken upon completion of any contrast administration. All relevant information regarding the contrast agent and its administration must be included in the patient's permanent medical record:
  - contrast medium used
  - volume administered
  - density
  - batch number
  - who performed the injection
  - any adverse effects and any treatment or drug therapy given
- Any adverse reactions should be reported to the manufacturing company to coordinate worldwide data collection on reactions, and ensure a global perspective
- When the examination is complete check that the patient is fit to travel home and do not allow them to leave if there is any doubt. If any concerns are identified the patient should be checked by a medic prior to leaving

Radiographers performing intravenous administration

In the imaging department it is now common practice for radiographers to administer intravenous contrast media. Radiographers are actively involved in clinical procedures where performing intravenous injections are entirely within the role development framework outlined by the College of Radiographers. It is paramount that radiographers undertaking this role are adequately trained and aware of the professional issues. They must operate under an agreed protocol and a written scheme of work. The employing authority should be informed in writing and be assured of the competency of any radiographer undertaking this role; it is recommended that this should be via a nationally recognised and transferable qualification. Before performing any intravenous administration it is important that the radiographer is aware of the:

- related anatomy, physiology and pathology
- correct choice and disposal of any equipment used
- criteria for choosing the vein
- indications and contraindications for any contrast media used
- potential problems that may arise

Aseptic technique must be maintained throughout the procedure. The circulation is a closed sterile system, and venepuncture can provide a method of entry of commensals into the system. Intravenous related infection is a major cause of mortality and morbidity in hospitalised patients. The reasons for minimisation of infections is obvious and a reduction in hospital-acquired infections is at the forefront of government policy, since the majority of these infections are both preventable and an expensive drain on finances. Patients with cannulae in situ are prone to developing a nosocomial infection and, as the majority of acute patients in hospital are cannulated, the potential to develop an infection is high if careful technique and protocols are not observed. Any intravenous cannulation can potentially cause infection to the patient. Commensals can be transmitted from contaminated equipment used, such as the distal tip of the needle or venflon, hubs or connectors or from the healthcare worker's hands. All departments have a hand washing policy that must be adhered to in order to minimise risks, since bacteria can invade the site where the needle is inserted and local infection may develop in the skin around the needle. Bacteria can also enter the blood through the vein and cause a generalised systemic infection.

Prevention of these potential harmful infections can be reduced by:

- being aware of touch contamination of equipment
- ensuring all packaging is intact before opening
- checking expiry dates
- choosing insertion sites carefully
- minimal manipulation of connections
- application of hand washing procedures
- investigating mild pyrexias that may develop and treating immediately
- observing and recording intravenous (IV) sites regularly

Health and safety issues

Because of the increase of blood-borne viruses it is necessary for the professional administering the contrast medium to protect themselves from any potential blood spills. Good quality gloves should be worn when performing venepuncture; these will protect from blood spillage but will not prevent a needlestick injury, which are hazardous for healthcare workers. Needlestick injuries account for a high number of accidents to staff in hospitals. Hepatitis B is more easily transmitted than human immunodeficiency virus (HIV), so any healthcare professional working with body fluids and performing intravenous injections should be vaccinated for Hepatitis B and have their antibody levels checked as recommended. The impact for staff who suffer a needlestick injury can be devastating in terms of health effects and the waiting period for results of blood tests following an exposure can be psychologically traumatic.

Needlestick injuries usually occur when:

- the needle misses the cap (sheath) and accidentally enters the hand holding it
- the needle pierces the cap and enters the hand holding it
- the poorly fitting cap slips off of a recapped needle and the needle stabs the hand

Recapping can account for 25 to 30% of all needlestick injuries amongst nursing and laboratory staff. There is no substitute for careful technique when performing any venepuncture procedure. Used needles should be discarded directly into a sharps container without being resheathed.

Treatment of needlestick injuries

Recent campaigns have targeted improved infection control, better management and staff training to reduce exposure to blood-borne pathogens. However, whilst these methods can remove human error, they cannot remove the primary risk – the needle or sharp itself.

If a needlestick injury occurs, departmental safety policy should be followed and, in any case, the following steps should immediately be followed:

- Bleed the puncture site immediately
- Wash the needlestick injury site under running cold water
- Report the incident to your supervisor and occupational health department
- Seek medical treatment if necessary

Vein choice

The choice of vein is vital when performing an intravenous contrast injection. Painful, sore or bruised sites should be avoided as these may be irritated as a result of previous use, or they may be sclerosed. Always use veins with the largest diameter possible, these are easily palpable with good capillary refill. If at all possible, use veins on the non-dominant side; veins that cross joints or bony prominences or have little skin cover (e.g. the wrist) ought to be avoided. The area selected should have no broken skin, infection, lymphoedema, arteriovenous shunts or fistulas. There are also some practical considerations to consider, for example, the purpose of the cannulation and the length of time the needle is to remain in situ. Always choose the injection device after assessing the condition and accessibility of the individual patient's veins. The sites of choice on the upper limb are branches of the basilic, cephalic or median cubital vein. Preference should be given to veins that are patent and healthy and are easily detectable visually or by palpitation as already discussed.

Arterial administration of contrast media

In arteriography, a contrast medium is introduced via a catheter into an artery, rendering the lumen of the vessel opaque to X-rays. As the contrast is delivered as a bolus under high pressure, a pressure injector is employed in the administration. The femoral artery is the most frequent approach to the arterial system in angiography using the Seldinger technique. Low osmolar contrast is employed for all angiographic studies. Isotonic contrast is recommended for use as it has improved tolerability for patients when high doses are administered. The quantity and strength of the contrast used is dependent upon the area of the vascular system being investigated.

Magnetic resonance angiography (MRA) studies blood vessels, utilising magnetic resonance imaging (MRI) technology to detect, diagnose and aid the treatment of heart disorders, stroke, and blood vessel diseases. MRA provides detailed images of blood vessels without using any contrast material, although contrast is usually given to enhance the MRI images.

Preparation of injection site

Care should be taken in preparing the site for injection. Asepsis is vital, as the skin is being broken and a foreign device introduced into the sterile circulatory system. The two major sources of microbial contamination are:

- cross infection from the practitioner to patient
- skin flora of the patient

Good hand washing and drying techniques are essential, and gloves must be worn for each patient. The skin around the injection site should be cleaned with a preparation such as isopropyl alcohol or 1% iodine. In practice, alcohol swabs are usually used. To reduce the risk from the patient's own flora, the area should be cleaned for at least 30 seconds and it is important the area is swabbed in one direction only. Once the site is swabbed it should not be touched again and it should be allowed to dry for approximately 30 seconds before insertion of the needle to facilitate coagulation of organisms ensuring disinfection. Allowing the area to dry also prevents stinging.

Needle insertion technique for administration of an intravenous contrast injection (for IVU)

- Ensure all the equipment required is ready and available prior to commencement of the injection procedure

- Approach the patient in a confident manner and explain the procedure
- Gain consent
- Ascertain medical history and check allergies
- Allow the patient to ask questions
- Support the chosen limb on a pad
- Apply the tourniquet to the upper arm on the chosen side to assess the injection site. (Tourniquets and pads used are potentially a mechanism for cross infection that staff need to be aware of.) The patient may assist by clenching and unclenching their fist
- Select a vein using the criteria already discussed
- Wash and dry hands
- Put on gloves
- Clean the skin carefully for at least 30 seconds using the appropriate preparation. Do not palpate the vein or touch the skin
- Anchor the vein by applying manual traction to the skin a few centimetres below the chosen injection site
- Insert the needle smoothly at an approximately 30° angle
- Release the tourniquet
- When administering contrast a butterfly needle is used. To eliminate air from the system and to ensure accurate positioning in the vein, it is common practice to withdraw blood into the syringe. However, use of a 'closed system' should be considered, where the syringe is connected to the butterfly and flushed with contrast medium. This is because it has been shown that thrombus formation may occur if blood mixes with the contrast agent[10]
- Inject the contrast medium
- Place a sterile cotton wool ball over the site
- Remove the needle
- Apply pressure to the site after the needle has been removed and continue to apply pressure until bleeding has stopped, for approximately 1 minute
- Ensure the patient has no allergies to plasters. Inspect the injection site before firmly applying a dressing
- Discard waste in the correct manner
- Remove gloves and wash hands

Treatment of adverse reactions to contrast medium

It has already been stated that all patients must be kept under constant observation during and after contrast media administration, and emergency drugs and oxygen should be readily available if required. All staff working in the area should be trained in cardiopulmonary resuscitation and know how to initiate an emergency call. Contrast media should be administered at body temperature and the manufacturer's optimum doses should not be exceeded. This minimises the risk of an adverse reaction. Before initiating any treatment, the severity of the event should be carefully evaluated; this ensures the appropriate treatment can be given. Reactions to intravenous administration of contrast media can be classified into three categories:

- Mild reaction
- Moderate reaction
- Severe reaction

Mild reaction

Mild reactions simply require careful observation of the patient. Most of the symptoms will pass within a few minutes post administration. Some schools of thought have postulated that a great many mild adverse effects are the result of the patient's fear and apprehension.[5] Mild adverse reactions are encountered in as many as 15% of patients after administration of intravenous ionic high-osmolar contrast media and up to 3% of patients after non-ionic, low-osmolar contrast media.[6] Signs and symptoms of a mild reaction include:

- nausea
- a warm feeling that may be associated with hot flushing
- sneezing
- rhinorrhoea
- a metallic taste in the mouth
- headache
- pallor
- pruritis (itching) and diaphoresis (sweating)

Treatment of mild reactions usually only involves observation of the patient and reassurance. Usually no medical treatment is required and the reaction does not interfere significantly with the examination procedure being undertaken.

Moderate reaction

This is a more severe reaction in which medical treatment is necessary and/or where the examination procedure is delayed or otherwise affected. Signs and symptoms of a moderate reaction include:

- erythema
- urticaria
- pruritis
- chest pain
- abdominal pain
- vasovagal syncope
- facial swelling caused by oedema

Treatment of a moderate reaction may vary. Compression and tight clothing should be released and the patient reassured. The patient will need to be seen by a medic and the adverse reaction requires information to be entered in the patient's permanent medical record. All documentation should be completed according to department protocols. Drug therapy may be required, such as administration of antihistamine (e.g. Piriton 10 mg) intravenously, or adrenaline (epinephrine) 0.5 mL 1 : 1000 solution subcutaneously, to reduce the symptoms.

Severe reaction

Seek medical advice immediately; medical treatment with hospitalisation is necessary. The examination is terminated. The management of severe adverse reactions, including drug treatments, should be handled by the resuscitation team.[7] Signs, symptoms and effects of a severe reaction may include:

- paralysis
- seizures
- pulmonary oedema
- bronchospasm
- laryngeal oedema
- anaphylactic shock
- respiratory arrest
- cardiac arrest

It is important that the radiographer recognises the significance of certain signs:

- *Pulmonary oedema* – dyspnoea and cyanosis; the patient develops a cough with white frothy sputum, accompanied with dyspnoea
- *Anaphylactic shock* – dramatic onset; pallor, sweating, nausea, syncope. A weak pulse due to hypotension, bradycardia or tachycardia may be observed. In severe cases, cardiac arrest may occur
- *Cardiac arrest* – dramatic onset; absence of palpable pulse, dilated pupils, pallor, cyanosis
- *Respiratory arrest* – abrupt onset of cyanosis with cessation of breathing
- *Cerebral oedema* – leading to convulsions and possible coma

Administration of oxygen by mask (6-10 L/m) is vital and should be administered as soon as possible, as hypoxia may occur.

Severe reactions require immediate recognition and evaluation of the patient's cardiopulmonary status. Cardiopulmonary resuscitation (CPR) equipment should be readily available in any area where contrast media are used. The radiographer should be trained in the techniques of CPR. Treatment of a severe reaction should follow the 'ABCD system':

- Airway open
- Breathing restored
- Circulation maintained
- Drug and definitive therapy

Contrast media should never be injected by anyone unfamiliar with resuscitation procedures. Radiology staff and management should continually review departmental protocols to ensure all staff are aware and are able to accomplish their roles should an event occur.

■ Potential complications for the patient after IV cannulation

Any patient who undergoes an intravenous cannulation has the potential to develop any of the following complications. Some are preventable, others are not:

- Infection
- Phlebitis and thrombophlebitis
- Emboli
- Vasovagal response
- Pain
- Haematoma/haemorrhage
- Extravasation
- Unintended arterial cannulation
- Allergy

Tissue damage from extravasation of contrast material is caused by the direct toxic effect of the agent. This is usually absorbed fairly quickly, cream such as Lasonil which is anti-inflammatory can be applied to the injection site to facilitate this. Compartment syndrome may occur if enough contrast material leaks into surrounding tissue. Compartment syndrome occurs when swelling takes place within a compartment of a limb and increases pressure on arteries, veins, and nerves. In addition to causing extreme pain, this slows circulation to the muscles and nerves and may cause permanent damage to these tissues. This may lead to impaired blood flow and muscle and nerve damage. A compartment syndrome is a medical emergency requiring immediate treatment to prevent tissue death and permanent dysfunction.

CONTRAST MEDIA USED IN BILIARY AND HEPATIC IMAGING

Contrast examinations of the biliary system have been superseded by cross-sectional imaging such as CT and ultrasound. The molecule of biliary contrast media features two vacant binding sites that encourage it to bind with serum albumin to form a molecule that is too large to be filtered by the kidneys. Biliary contrast media are tri-iodo benzoic acid derivatives. The oral contrast media have a single benzene ring (Biloptin) whilst the intravenous medium (Biliscopin) is a dimer with a polymethylene chain connecting the two rings.

Oral cholecystography

This examination is very rarely undertaken in a modern imaging department. For its success it requires the contrast medium, usually sodium ipodate (Biloptin) to be absorbed from the gut. It is then bound to albumen and transported to the liver via the portal vein. The contrast is then excreted from the liver with the bile and concentrates in the gall bladder. The usual dose of contrast for this examination is six capsules of Biloptin, each containing 500 mg of sodium ipodate. Imaging of the gall bladder takes place 10–12 hours after the contrast has been administered. Oral contrast media are then excreted in the stool.

Intravenous cholangiogram (IVC)

This examination has been superseded by other imaging modalities such as ultrasound, CT and endoscopic retrograde cholangiopancreatography (ERCP).

The examination requires an infusion of meglumine iotroxate (Biliscopin) and conventional tomography for imaging.

ENDOSCOPIC RETROGRADE CHOLANGIOPANCREATOGRAPHY

This examination is a collaborative technique undertaken by an endoscopist but requires radiological screening and imaging. After the endoscope has been introduced, the ampulla of Vater is located and the contrast introduced. Low density water-soluble contrast is used to prevent obscuring any calculi that may be present.

Other biliary examinations requiring contrast media are listed in Table 33.1.

IODISED OILS AS A CONTRAST MEDIUM

These are very infrequently used in the imaging department today. The examinations employing these contrast media have in the main been superseded by cross-sectional imaging modalities. They are employed in examinations where water-soluble agents are contraindicated or where a viscous compound is required:

- Sialography 0.5 to 2 mL of Lipiodol per side
- Dacrocystography 0.5 to 2 mL of Lipiodol per side.

These contrast agents are not easily absorbed and in some cases may carry a risk of oil embolus.

CONTRAST MEDIA USED IN OTHER RADIOGRAPHIC EXAMINATIONS

Table 33.2 highlights other radiographic examinations undertaken in the imaging department that employ contrast media to enhance the images.

CONTRAST MEDIA USED IN ULTRASOUND

Contrast agents can improve the image quality of sonography, either by decreasing the reflectivity of undesired interfaces or by increasing the back scattered echoes from the desired regions. Use of contrast media in ultrasound has been well established for cardiac imaging since the 1980s, for example, air was used to demonstrate atrial septal defects. Blood was taken from the patient, shaken to introduce air bubbles and then re-injected and then

Table 33.1 Contrast media used in the biliary system

Examination	Contrast media	Rationale for use
Preoperative cholangiography	HOCM or LOCM 150 5 mL and then 20 mL usually used	Low iodine content to avoid obscuring any stones
Postoperative cholangiography (T-tube)	HOCM or LOCM 150 Approx. 20–30 mL	Low iodine content to avoid obscuring any stones
Percutaneous transhepatic cholangiography (PTC)	LOCM 150 20–60 mL	Low iodine content to avoid obscuring any stones
Biliary drainage	LOCM 200 20–60 mL	Low iodine content to avoid obscuring any stones

Table 33.2 Contrast media used in other examinations

Examination	Contrast media, dose, strength and volume	Comments
Hysterosalpingography (HSG)	HOCM or LOCM 10–20 mL	LOCM has no advantage. Using non-ionic dimers is associated with decreased procedural and delayed pain[8]
Contrast venography	Approx. 30 mL LOCM	Use to image possible DVT's. It is invasive and is dependent upon cannulation of a vein often in a swollen foot
Arthrography	4–10 mL HOCM or LOCM Air or oxygen can also be used to create a double contrast image	Volume of contrast used dependent upon joint under investigation
Cystography and micturating cystourethrography	HOCM or LOCM can be used	Volume used dependent upon the size of the structure and also patient tolerance
Renal imaging including retrogrades, nephrostomy, percutaneous nephrolithotomy	LOCM is frequently used	IVU: 50 mL 370 mg/mL^{-1} standard for adult[4] Other areas: volume dependent upon anatomical area HOCM can be employed dependent upon radiologist

imaged. The problem encountered with this technique was the reproducibility and homogeneity of the contrast effect due to variation in bubble size. This led to the development and manufacture of specialised products, e.g. Echovist – an echo-rich, microbubble, microparticle suspension. The gas microbubbles almost totally reflect ultrasound, the reflectivity of the microbubbles is high, resulting in a strong echo enhancement. The use of contrast media in abdominal ultrasound is still in its infancy; it is particularly useful in demonstrating portal vein thrombosis, alleviating the need for conventional, more invasive, angiography examinations. Also, intravenous vascular contrast agents can aid the imaging of malignant tumours in the liver, kidney, ovary, pancreas, prostate, and breast.[9] Tumour angiogenesis and doppler signals from small tumour vessels may be detectable after an injection of contrast medium. However, these contrast media can cause adverse reactions, as already discussed.

Simple solutions of water or saline can also be used to outline gastrointestinal structures, enabling adjacent structures to be visualised.

CONTRAST MEDIA USED IN MRI

Contrast enhancement plays a major role in MRI. MRI generates high natural contrast in images but contrast media are still employed to improve tissue characterisation. Contrast media in MRI improve the potential for examining the function of systems and structures. MRI contrast is used to improve the detection of disease and increase the sensitivity of diagnosis. In some brain pathology, little difference exists in signal intensity between healthy and diseased tissue, hence the need for the equivalent of an iodinated contrast agent in MRI, for image enhancement. Gadolinium is most frequently used. Gadolinium is a rare earth metal, is paramagnetic and provides contrast between the lesion or pathology and the surrounding tissue by shortening the T1 relaxation time. Gadolinium has to be chelated with diethylenetriamine penta-acetic acid (DTPA), as free gadolinium ions are toxic. It is hydrophilic, having very low lipid solubility and so does not cross the blood–brain barrier. There are several categories of MRI contrast agents available on the market today and the choice is dependent upon the pathology being investigated.

Clinical indications for MRI contrast use:

- Central nervous system tumours
- Spinal imaging
- Brain abscess, in which MRI will demonstrate ring enhancement
- Assessment of the blood–brain barrier to see if it is intact
- Demyelinating diseases
- Staging disease progression in multiple sclerosis and malignant disease
- More accurate delineation of tumour margins from oedema
- Cardiac/aortic imaging

CONTRAST MEDIA USED IN CT

Contrast media are used to enhance the image quality of images produced during CT examinations. The contraindications, which have already been discussed, apply to the employment of contrast in these examinations. Contrast media for CT examinations are administered in four different ways:

- Intravenous injection
- Oral administration
- Rectal administration
- Inhalation - this is a relatively uncommon procedure in which xenon gas is inhaled for a highly specialised form of lung or brain imaging. The technique, xenon CT, is only available at a small number of locations worldwide and is used only for rare cases

Almost all CT examinations of the abdomen and pelvis require the administration of oral contrast agents to opacify the gastrointestinal tract. Good bowel opacification helps differentiate between the lymph nodes, tumour masses and unopacified loops of bowel. Contrast enhancement in CT scanning of the abdomen and pelvis necessitate drinking oral contrast medium, which is usually a water-soluble, iodine-based contrast medium (however, dilute barium sulphate solutions can be used). Scanning is usually performed 1 hour after drinking the contrast to allow time for it to pass into the intestine. While this may seem an inconvenience, the oral contrast makes an essential improvement in quality of the CT study, and results in a more accurate diagnosis by providing delineation of low contrast structures. Contrast can be administered rectally to help distinguish anatomical areas in the lower abdomen.

Water can be used as a negative agent, which is useful for assessment of carcinoma of the stomach. Another approach to negative contrast is, when scanning a female pelvis, to place a tampon in the vagina, which allows radiolucent air to distend the vagina, creating additional contrast between the reproductive organs. Air is used in CT for virtual colonoscopy for contrast purposes and to distend the bowel to unfold the mucosa. This procedure of the large bowel produces 3D images of the entire colonic mucosa similar to those obtained during colonoscopy. Patients undergo full bowel preparation, an intravenous smooth muscle relaxant is administered, and the colon is then insufflated with room air until it is fully distended. Once satisfactory distension has been achieved, spiral CT is performed to image the entire colon. The procedure is also referred to as a spiral CT pneumocolon. There has been mention of the use of CO_2 in this chapter, relating to double contrast barium enemas, which has the advantage of improved tolerance compared to air but the disadvantage of requirement of reinsufflation during the procedure. Reinsufflation renders use of CO_2 inappropriate for some CT scanners but rapid multislice scanners are likely to be fast enough to allow the use of CO_2 for virtual colonoscopy.

Non-ionic, water-soluble, isotonic contrast agents are employed in CT to highlight blood vessels and to enhance the tissue structure of various organs such as the brain, spine, liver and kidneys. CT angiography has developed rapidly and increased greatly since the early to mid-1990s and many UK imaging departments undertake CT angiography as an adjunct to axial scanning. With CT contrast examinations, the ability to time image acquisition to coincide with peak contrast enhancement has been, in the past, a challenge for practitioners working in this imaging modality. The use of a pressure injector, coupled with CT software, addresses this issue whilst ensuring that the radiographer is distanced from the CT scanner during exposure.

References

1. Farrow R, Stevenson GW. In: Armstrong P, Wastie ML, eds. A concise textbook of radiology. London: Arnold; 2001.
2. Farrow R, et al. Air versus carbon dioxide insufflation in double contrast barium enemas: the role of active gaseous drainage. British Journal of Radiology 1995; 68:838–840.
3. Holemans JA. A comparison of air, carbon dioxide and air/carbon dioxide mixture as insufflation agents for double contrast barium enemas. European Radiology 1988; 8:274–276.
4. Chapman S, Nakielny R. A guide to radiological procedures. 4th edn. London: WB Saunders; 2002.
5. Lalli AF. Urographic contrast media reactions and anxiety. Radiology 1974; 112:267–271.
6. Thomsen HS, Morcos SK. Management of acute adverse reactions to contrast media. European Radiology 2004; 14(3):476–481.
7. O'Neil JM, Bride KDM. Cardiopulmonary resuscitation and contrast media reactions in a radiology department. Clinical Radiology 2001; 56(4):321–325.
8. Goldberg BB. Ultrasound contrast agents. London: Martin Dunitz; 1997.
9. Brokensha C, Whitehouse G. A comparison between iotrolan, non-ionic dimer, and a hyperosmolar contrast medium, Urografin, in hystersalpingography. British Journal of Radiology 1991; 64:587–590.
10. Robertson H. Blood clot formation in angiographic syringes containing non-ionic contrast media. Radiology 1987; 162:621–622.

GASTROINTESTINAL TRACT

Joanne Rudd, Darren Wood

The gastrointestinal tract (GI tract) has traditionally been examined using X-radiography, barium sulphate and gas as a double contrast agent. Accessory organs of the tract (Ch. 35) have traditionally been examined using iodine-based contrast agents. However, the rapidly changing field of medical imaging now sees the tract examined by a variety of methods, some of which supersede conventional contrast radiography.

Besides examination of the tract itself, other contrast enhanced X-ray imaging procedures provide studies of the abdominal region; namely, these are angiography and arteriography. Angiography is an injectable contrast agent based technique, used to provide a 'road map' which shows the arterial or venous supply to the entire abdominal cavity. Arteriography is mainly used to assess tumour respectability or demonstrate suspected gastrointestinal haemorrhage. The superior mesenteric artery, inferior mesenteric artery and ceoliac axis are filled with contrast agent, in order to show the entire region. Venography is used in assessment of the portal venous system and is generally used for presurgical demonstration of varices. In particular, the use of computed tomography (CT) and magnetic resonance (MR) angiography is reducing the need for these procedures.

NOTES ON POSITION TERMINOLOGY FOR FLUOROSCOPIC EXAMINATION

Positioning terminology used in the UK tends to describe positions in relation to the image receptor. This concept is generally easily understood when the traditional position of the image receptor is described (e.g. under the examination table) but can become confusing when over-couch image receptors are used; fluoroscopic units often fall into this category. Further confusion occurs when it is realised that fluoroscopy units may have over- or under-couch image receptors; this then makes it even more difficult for an author to ensure that their readers fully understand position descriptions.

For example, if a patient is initially supine on a *conventional radiography examination table (over-couch *tube, **under-couch** *image receptor)* with their right side raised, then the position is described as a left posterior oblique (LPO) since the patient is oblique with the posterior aspect of their trunk still in contact with the table-top (Fig. 34.1); on a *fluoroscopy table with* **under-couch** *tube and* **over-couch** *receptor*, this same body position is usually described as a right anterior oblique (RAO) as the right anterior aspect of the body is nearest the image receptor. Simpler projections such as anteroposterior (AP) change to posteroanterior (PA) with over-couch receptors and under-couch tube. Students, in particular, become very confused by this and many radiographers resort to describing the positions as 'right side raised' or 'left side raised' to avoid confusion.

For the purpose of this chapter and to avoid this confusion, the authors have decided to use the *traditional under-couch receptor and over-couch tube descriptor*, identical to that used for general under-couch image receptor over-couch tube radiography. Figure 34.1 identifies the positions in full. We hope that this proves less confusing than using the traditional fluoroscopy description technique.

Figure 34.1 Positioning descriptions for use in this chapter

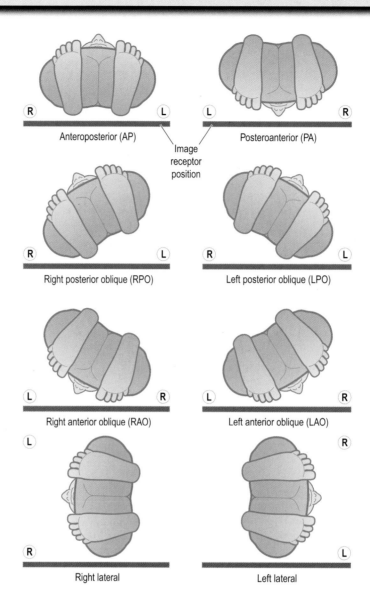

Anteroposterior (AP)

Image receptor position

Posteroanterior (PA)

Right posterior oblique (RPO)

Left posterior oblique (LPO)

Right anterior oblique (RAO)

Left anterior oblique (LAO)

Right lateral

Left lateral

UPPER GI TRACT

The upper GI tract consists of the oropharynx, hypopharynx, oesophagus, stomach and first part of the duodenum (for a general appraisal of the layout of this part of the GI tract see Fig. 34.2A and B). The aim of a contrast examination is to outline these structures in single and/or double contrast to obtain optimum visualisation. The most common contrast agent used is a barium sulphate suspension, although ionic and non-ionic contrast agents can be used.

Most patients who have upper GI symptoms are primarily referred for oesophagogastric duodenoscopy (OGD) but this may be used in conjunction with other tests in order that a 'gold standard' approach has been applied.[1] For some symptoms there is, as yet, no acknowledged stand-alone gold standard.[2] There are, however, sometimes reasons why contrast enhanced X-ray studies are required, usually those when patients cannot always tolerate an OGD due to medical constraints. They may also simply refuse the procedure or their symptoms may persist after a normal result of the OGD examination.

REFERRAL CRITERIA FOR EXAMINATION OF THE UPPER GI TRACT

- Anaemia
- Dysphagia
- Dyspepsia
- Epigastric discomfort/upper abdominal mass
- Gastrooesophageal reflux (GOR)

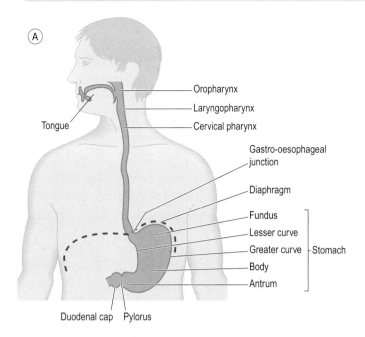

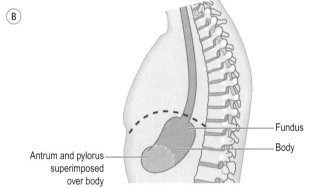

Figure 34.2 **(A)** Upper GI tract – diagrammatic representation from AP view; **(B)** position of stomach – lateral view from left

- Carcinoma
- Assessment of oesophageal perforation (water soluble contrast must be used)

PATIENT PREPARATION – ALL EXAMINATIONS OF THE UPPER TRACT

- The patient should be starved for at least 6 hours before the examination[3] but 5 hours is considered adequate by some.[4] It is suggested that this should be the case even if only a barium swallow is indicated, in case views of the stomach are found to be required; this avoids the patient having to return for a second examination
- All jewellery or artefacts (e.g. hearing aids) should be removed
- Patient clothing should be removed and a patient gown should be worn

- The patient should then be informed of the procedure (they should have received information with their appointment prior to attending) so they can give their consent
- Compliance with instructions on the starvation period should be checked

BARIUM SWALLOW AND MEAL

Historically, this examination has been carried out on patients as a complete examination. With the development of radiographer-led procedures there is a move towards giving a direct answer to a set of clinical indications and questions and so tailoring the examination to fit this need. The barium swallow and meal can therefore reasonably be split into a number of 'subexaminations' when the clinical picture has a definite direction.

Upper ('high') barium swallow

This examination is used for patients who have high dysphagia or definite oesophageal symptoms, or have quite often had a normal OGD but are still symptomatic; quite often a motility disorder may be the cause.

Contraindications
- Known aspiration during ingestion (although this can be overcome by using non-ionic water soluble contrast)

Contrast agent
- Barium sulphate suspension 250% w/v[3,4] *or* water soluble contrast medium

Additional equipment
- Disposable cup
- Tissues

Technique
If there is any query that the patient may aspirate, the initial swallow is best carried out using a water-soluble contrast medium, although aspiration of barium has been considered by some to be relatively harmless.[3] Aspiration may not be suspected but unsuspected 'silent aspiration' may be found. Otherwise use the following technique (ensure that you have understood the notes on fluoroscopic examination positioning descriptors earlier in this chapter before considering technique descriptors):

- The patient is asked to stand erect in the AP position on the fluoroscopic table and hold the cup of barium in their hand, usually the left, as further turning of the patient is usually to the left. The arm will then lie clear of the trunk, without the patient having to negotiate its movement around the intensifying screen carriage. The patient is turned into a lateral position in order to commence with routine assessment of possible aspiration; if this is the case the examination should be terminated immediately

- They are asked to take a 'normal' sized (for them) mouthful of the liquid and hold it in their mouth until asked to swallow. This is to give the operator a chance to centre on the area of interest and optimise the collimation
- If the radiographic equipment allows, a frame rate of 3 per second is suggested as an initial choice; modern digital equipment can allow recording of the screened image. This offers a radiation dose reduction by allowing retrospective and repeated study of the patient's swallowing action without returning to rescreen missed actions, and also allows a more real time assessment to take place
- The patient is then asked to swallow and the exposure is initiated. Real time recording (exposure) is terminated when the barium bolus passes beyond the screened image or point of interest
- The AP view is the optimum for hypopharyngeal anatomy;[5] it will be seen in single and double contrast images (Fig. 34.3). This view can then be repeated at least once more to ensure there is consistency in the images, making it easier to definitively identify pathology

- The patient is then turned into the lateral position and the same procedure of taking a mouthful and swallowing on request is imaged. This view allows the posterior wall to be optimally viewed (Fig. 34.4)

The most common abnormalities shown are persistent cricopharyngeal impressions or diverticulae, the most common diverticulum type being Zenker's; this occurs in the mid-hypopharynx and is more common in the older population. They are quite often termed hypopharyngeal pouches.[5] The pouches can become quite large, often causing patients to be referred due to regurgitation of undigested food some time after they have eaten. They are also often difficult to endoscope as the scope enters the pouch and cannot be passed further; the barium swallow can thus quite often be the most appropriate test for confirming the presence and extent of this pathology.

Oesophageal webs are also best seen on the lateral projection, shown on the anterior wall, although they are best viewed with rapid imaging sequences; they have been noted in 1–5% of asymptomatic patients and 12-15% of dysphagia patients.[5]

◼ Barium swallow and reflux assessment

Patients for this type of study often present with clinical symptoms of GOR. They often have a feeling of retrosternal discomfort and no other symptoms. Although pH moni-

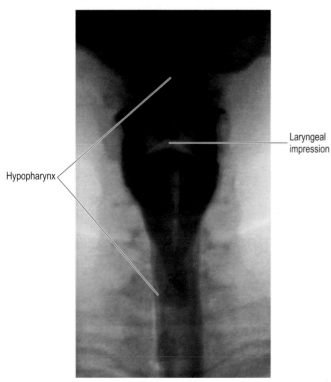

Figure 34.3　AP barium swallow showing normal hypopharyngeal anatomy

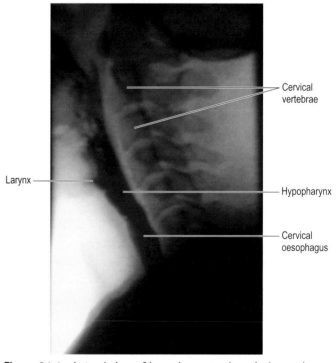

Figure 34.4　Lateral view of hypopharynx and cervical oesophagus

toring is an effective way of evaluating GOR, there is not as yet a gold standard test.[2] The barium study can still be useful as an adjunct to other tests, as some GOR patients may have small hiatus hernias that are not seen on endoscopy. These patients often have mucosal changes in the distal third of the oesophagus, so the swallow is used to view the region closely and observe the fundus to check for herniation.

Patient preparation

Patient preparation and contraindications are as for the upper swallow

Contrast agent and pharmaceutical aids
- 250% w/v barium sulphate suspension
- An effervescent agent will be required, e.g. a combination of sodium bicarbonate and citric acid, to produce carbon dioxide to distend the stomach. This will also act as double contrast against the barium, to enhance visualisation of the mucosa[4]

Additional equipment
- Disposable cup
- Small cup for effervescent agent
- Tissues
- A straw may be required for ingestion of barium when the table is horizontal (if needed)

Technique
(Ensure that you have understood the notes on fluoroscopic examination positioning descriptors earlier in this chapter before considering technique descriptors.)

- AP and lateral projections can be taken of the oesophagus as previously described for the barium swallow
- A more useful view of the distal third of the oesophagus is provided by the erect left posterior oblique, taken after the patient is asked to swallow. The barium bolus is imaged as a column and spot films taken to show the distal third of the oesophagus. This allows mucosal rings and peptic strictures to be shown well.[5] As the column passes and the mucosa relaxes, spot films can be taken; this often shows oesophagitis
- The patient is then asked to take the effervescent granules (either dry or mixed with a small amount of water if dry is too difficult) or other effervescent aid, followed by the citric acid. It is important to impress on the patient that these will produce gas in the stomach and may give them the feeling that they need to belch; it is imperative they do not succumb to temptation and the best way to avoid this is to tell them to keep swallowing. Advance explanation of this, giving reasons for its importance, will maximise compliance

- The patient is then asked to swallow another mouthful of barium whilst in the LPO position (Fig. 34.5) and images can be taken of the lower oesophagus (either spot image recording or 1 frame per second is likely to be adequate). This will give a double contrast examination of the oesophagus, allowing a good look at mucosal detail
- To detect signs of a hiatus hernia (if one has not been noted so far) or GOR, the fluoroscopic couch is then placed horizontally and the patient turned to their right to assess reflux. Spot images of the area are taken
- The patient is then asked to rotate through 360° at their own pace; this will ensure coating of all aspects of the gastric mucosa ready for assessment of the stomach. Whilst they are performing this movement it is best to screen periodically in case any additional lower oesophageal pathology is noted so that a spot image of the lower oesophagus and gastroesophageal junction can be taken. On completing this manoeuvre, further images of the stomach are taken at key stages:
  1. the patient is asked to turn to their left (LPO) where a spot image is taken
  2. turned back to supine (AP)
  3. turned to their right (RPO)
  4. the patient is returned to the erect position, turned slightly to their left and an erect (LPO) film is taken to show the distal oesophagus and the fundus of the stomach

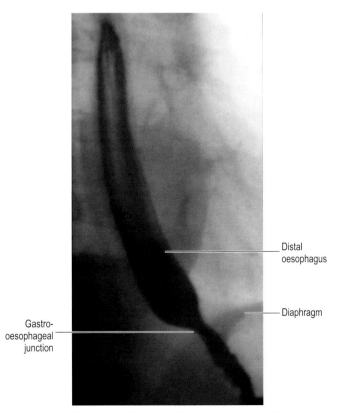

Distal oesophagus

Diaphragm

Gastro-oesophageal junction

Figure 34.5 Distal oesophagus and gastrooesophageal junction (GOJ) (LPO)

- To show reflux actually occurring, the patient can be tilted head downwards (Trendelenburg position) as this mimics stress reflux but, as this is an artificial position, it may have limited bearing on the accuracy estimation of the true extent of reflux
- If reflux is demonstrated the freedom with which it occurs and the level it attains should be noted (e.g. free reflux to the cervical region) as this will be an aid to the clinician in the assessment of the patient. It is noted, however, that reflux may only occur in about a third of symptomatic patients[5]

Barium meal

This examination is performed to show the stomach and duodenum. It is becoming a less frequently requested test with the increase in the use of endoscopy as the front-line test and, indeed it is recommended for use in a very limited number of circumstances. These include: if endoscopy proves negative and symptoms persist, or after (healed) surgery to assess afferent loop, narrowed anastamoses, and closed loops or internal hernias.[6] It therefore can be seen that the barium meal can still be useful for those people who are not considered fit for, or refuse, OGD.

Patient preparation
Patient preparation is as for all upper tract examinations

Contraindications
- Complete large bowel obstruction[3]

Contrast agents and pharmaceutical aids for the examination
- Barium sulphate suspension 250% w/v
- Effervescent granules and citric acid, or other gas producing agent
- An anti-spasmodic agent such as Hyoscine-N-butyl bromide (Buscopan) may be used intravenously. These help to reduce peristalsis in the stomach and prevent rapid progress of the barium into the small bowel[3]

Additional equipment
- Disposable cup
- Small cup for effervescent agent
- Tissues

Technique
(Ensure that you have understood the notes on fluoroscopic examination positioning descriptors earlier in this chapter before considering technique descriptors.)

If required the patient may given the antispasmodic pharmaceutical immediately prior to commencing the examination, although administration during the examination may also be required.

- The patient is asked to stand on the step of the fluoroscopic couch and then the procedure for ingesting the gas producing agents is explained. The importance of keeping the gas in the stomach is emphasised, and an explanation of a strategy to prevent belching (dry swallowing) is given
- The patient is given the effervescent agent (dry, or mixed with a small amount of water if this is more tolerable for the patient); they are then asked to drink the citric acid, to produce carbon dioxide and distend the stomach
- The patient is turned slightly to their left and asked to swallow a mouthful of the barium; the barium column is screened and spot images are taken of the distal oesophagus with single and double contrast
- After 3 or 4 reasonable mouthfuls of barium have been ingested, the table is tilted horizontally and the patient asked to rotate (at least once) through 360° to enable the barium to coat the stomach mucosa. Periodic screening during this movement allows for images to be taken if the radiographer feels it is necessary, especially if a small hiatus hernia or GOR are noted. This also enables the operator to note which positions show the anatomy most effectively, in preparation for other spot images. Quite often the most difficult region to image well can be the duodenal cap, due to the peristaltic action of the small bowel (which can occur even after administration of intravenous muscle relaxant); therefore, if the duodenal cap is well visualised during the patient's initial movements, there may be an opportunity to obtain the spot images required
- Once the patient has completed their rotation and good mucosal coating and distension of the stomach have been noted, it is possible to obtain the spot images. If coating is poor, give the patient more barium or ask them to perform another 360° rotation; if distension is inadequate then repeat the dose of effervescent agent. Because this is a dynamic investigation it is best to take the spot images as quickly as possible and if the chance arises and an area is well shown whilst moving the patient, take the opportunity
- The following positions are a general guideline to how best to show the anatomy of the stomach and duodenum in double contrast:
  1. The patient with their right side raised (LPO) demonstrates the antrum and the greater curve (Fig. 34.6)
  2. If the patient is supine this demonstrates the antrum and the body of the stomach and also the lesser curve (Fig. 34.7A,B)

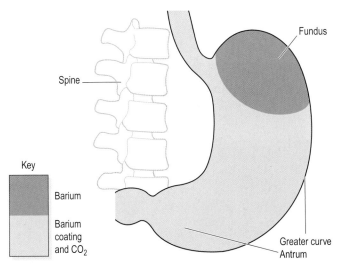

Figure 34.6 LPO position for antrum and greater curve. The stomach is turned to the left: the barium drops into the fundus and obscures it; CO_2 rises into the body and antrum to act as double contrast for good visualisation of these areas. The greater curve is also visualised

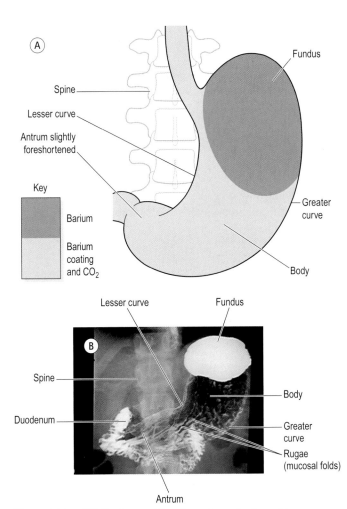

Figure 34.7 **(A)** Supine position for antrum, body and lesser curve – barium pools in the lowest point which is the fundus in the supine position, allowing CO_2 to rise into the body and antrum which are coated with barium; **(B)** supine stomach

3. Turning the patient into the RPO position demonstrates the lesser curve en face (Fig. 34.8)
4. Moving the patient into the right lateral position with head tilted up shows the fundus (Fig. 34.9A,B)

- A combination of the following positions will help to best demonstrate the duodenal loop and duodenal cap. It may be necessary to use magnification at this point to optimise the view:
  1. LPO (Fig. 34.10)
  2. Supine
  3. RPO, centred on and collimated to the duodenal loop
  4. Prone

- The patient can then be tilted erect and turned slightly to the left to show the fundus (Fig. 34.11). If visualisation of the duodenal cap has been poor during the earlier (table horizontal) stages of the examination, turning the patient in both directions (whilst they are standing) may provide better views of the duodenal cap

Aftercare

- The patient should be informed that their stools will be paler or white for a few days, and to keep their fluid intake up to reduce any chance of constipation
- If a muscle relaxant is used the patient must remain in the department, if there is any blurring of their vision, until this has passed

Possible complications

- Leakage of barium from an unsuspected perforation
- Aspiration of barium
- Partial bowel obstruction becoming complete obstruction due to barium impaction[3]

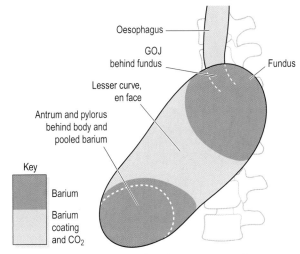

Figure 34.8 RPO position to show lesser curve en face. Obliquity moves the lesser curve to turn it from profile to an en face position; it is seen through the CO_2 filled body. Barium will pool in the fundus and antrum as these are the lowest points of the stomach in this position

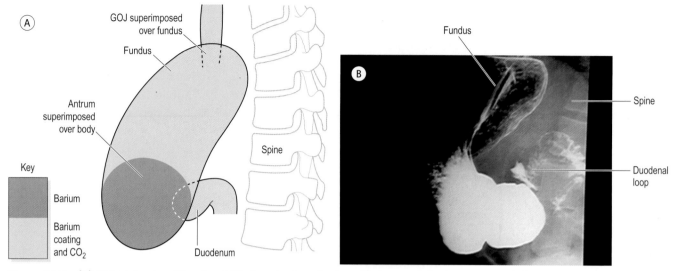

Figure 34.9 **(A)** Right lateral position, head tilted up, to show fundus – barium pools in the antrum as it is now the lowest positioned part of the stomach and CO_2 rises to the fundus; **(B)** Right lateral, head tilted up

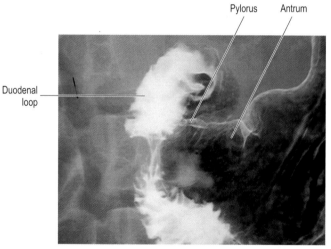

Figure 34.10 LPO: antrum and duodenal loop

Supplementary techniques

For patients with dysphagia it may be necessary to undertake the swallowing section of the examination using an imitation 'food bolus', as liquid may show no abnormality. Common examples of imitation food bolus are marshmallow coated in barium or pieces of fresh bread coated in barium. If a patient is unable to ingest the barium rapidly the relaxing effect of adding ice to the barium could be used.[5]

Video fluoroscopy

This is often undertaken in conjunction with speech therapists. Recording may be made on video but digital record-ing at several frames per second (e.g. 4–6) is now very valuable. Its aim is to assess patients who have swallowing dysfunction due to mechanical or neuromuscular problems, with the result that they are at increased risk of aspiration and inevitable associated chest problems.

Most referrals are for patients who have suffered:

- cerebrovascular accident
- motor neurone disease
- multiple sclerosis
- Parkinson's disease

The technique requires the patient to swallow small amounts of liquid, semi-solids and solids in order to ascertain

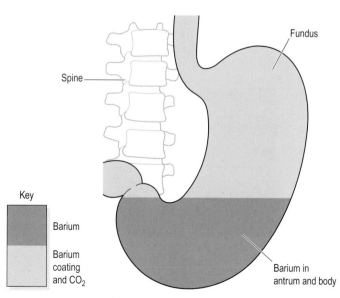

Figure 34.11 Erect (slight RPO) position to show fundus. Barium sits in the antrum and body; CO_2 rises into the fundus

the safety of the patient eating and drinking after discharge from hospital. The patient is screened as they swallow the various consistencies and the process is recorded on video to allow close examination of the process. As well as demonstrating aspiration at different consistencies, videofluoroscopy allows coping strategies to be tried; for example, using a chin tuck on swallowing or turning the head to one side may prevent aspiration. The aim of the process is to decide on the best strategy, which is compatible with nutrition, to help the patient cope with their problem.

SMALL BOWEL

The small bowel (from the duodenojejunal flexure to the ileocaecal valve) can be examined by one of two methods – the barium follow through (Ba FT) or the small bowel enema (SBE). The aim is to produce a continuous column of barium suspension outlining the small bowel.[3]

Referral criteria

- Anaemia
- Diarrhoea
- Persistent pain
- Crohn's disease
- Meckel's diverticulum

Ba FT

During this examination the patient has to drink a volume of barium sulphate suspension and images (fluoroscopy and/or permanent image recording) are taken as the small bowel fills. The examination frequently takes 2 hours and can take most of the day in some instances.[8]

Contraindications
- Suspected perforation
- Complete obstruction

Patient preparation
Patient preparation is usually the same for both follow through and small bowel enema and imaging department protocols do vary. Generally the patient is not allowed to eat or drink for 5–6 hours prior to the examination. Some centres may give the patient a mild laxative and/or a clear fluid diet the day prior to the examination

Contrast agent
- At least 300 mL 100% w/v barium sulphate suspension is required for an adult Ba FT.[3] The constituents of the drink are:

1. Barium sulphate suspension
2. Effervescent agent (may be carbonated barium sulphate suspension)
3. Water
4. Accelerator, e.g. Gastrografin or metoclopramide hydrochloride (Maxalon)

Additional equipment
- Disposable cup
- Small cup for effervescent agent
- Tissues

Technique
- The patient is asked to drink the barium sulphate suspension steadily. Drinking too quickly can cause nausea; drinking too slowly causes the barium suspension to flocculate and the small bowel does not distend adequately to obtain diagnostic images
- The imaging technique used depends on the equipment available, preference of the practitioner, or local imaging department protocol. The actual timing of imaging depends on each individual patient and motility speed of the bowel. Transit of barium through the proximal bowel (jejunum) is usually rapid whereas transit through the distal bowel (ileum) is often less rapid[8]
- A series of over-couch abdominal radiographs (see Ch. 36 for prone positioning) may be taken at predetermined time intervals, e.g. every 30 minutes, or alternatively each radiograph is individually assessed in order to determine the timing of the subsequent radiograph. The radiographs are often taken prone as the pressure on the abdomen helps to separate the bowel loops.[3] The first image is usually taken 15–20 minutes after drinking commenced. When the barium has been seen to reach the terminal ileum, fluoroscopy is used to image the ileocaecal area, although over-couch images can be taken if necessary (Fig. 34.12)

The terminal ileum will be shown on a prone image of the abdomen. The patient lies prone and a radiolucent pad is placed in their right iliac fossa; to correctly insert the pad the patient lies on their left side and the pad is placed and held firmly in the right iliac fossa. The patient then rolls prone to prevent small bowel falling back against the caecum and obscuring the terminal ileum. Prone positioning then follows as for the prone abdomen/KUB as described in Chapter 36, Figure 36.9A, with collimation to include the whole of the small bowel.

Alternatively, fluoroscopy may be used to image the small bowel at the necessary intervals. Using fluoroscopy the proximal jejunum is often imaged supine or in the RPO position. All the other loops are usually imaged supine until the terminal ileum is reached.

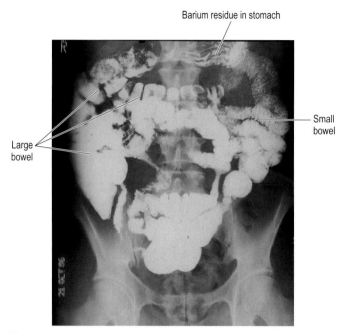

Barium residue in stomach

Small bowel

Large bowel

Figure 34.12   Prone abdomen: Ba FT

- Regardless of imaging modality, all bowel loops should be palpated (using lead rubber gloves with hands outside the primary beam) or the abdominal wall compressed with a radiolucent pad, during imaging. Barium does not move into areas of adhesions, which are difficult to spot anyway as they are often subtle in nature and can be obscured by overlapped loops of barium-filled bowel
- Fluoroscopy of the terminal ileum frequently requires an LPO position but sometimes will be more satisfactorily seen with RPO or prone positions

    An erect abdominal view may be required to show fluid levels, usually required when jejunal diverticulosis is present.[3] This is usually imaged with fluoroscopy but an over-couch image may be taken.

Complications
- Constipation
- Abdominal pain
- Transient diarrhoea (due to a large volume of fluid)

Patient aftercare
- Ask the patient to increase their fluid intake over the next 48 hours to prevent constipation
- Warn the patient about white stools

    There are certain criteria and common errors that relate to all small bowel barium studies – see below.

Criteria for assessing image quality
- All barium-filled loops of bowel (area of interest) are included on the film
- Sharp image clearly demonstrating valvulae conniventes
- Adequate penetration to demonstrate detail in the contrast-filled bowel

Common errors – Ba FT	Possible reasons and strategies to overcome these
Image is pale and valvulae conniventes are not demonstrated	Image is under-penetrated. Increase the kVp. A high kVp technique increases the range of densities visualised (as well as reducing exposure time and radiation dose)[4]
Slow barium transit of the proximal bowel	Ask the patient to lie in the right lateral decubitus position to promote gastric emptying[8]
Slow barium transit of the distal bowel	Give the patient a hot drink. If the patient has been in the department for a long time, a small snack can be given to try to encourage small bowel movement[3]
Overlying loops of bowel	If the overlying loops of bowel are deep within the pelvis ask the patient to avoid micturition, as a full bladder may push up and separate the loops of bowel. If the bladder is already full and the bowel loops are overlapping ask the patient to empty their bladder. Alternatively the patient can lie prone over a radiolucent pad to displace the loops[3]

Small bowel enema (Fig. 34.13A,B)

During a small bowel enema the duodenum is intubated and a contrast agent is introduced. This is arguably the ideal method for imaging the small bowel as it results in improved visualisation of the bowel loops.[3,4] This is because the infusion of contrast agent avoids segmentation of the barium column and the small bowel is unobstructed by the overlying barium-filled stomach and duodenum. This

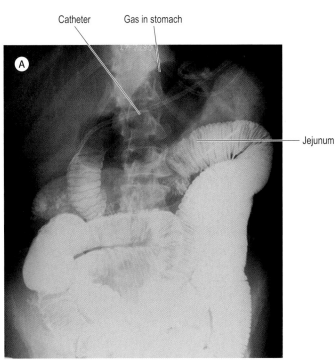
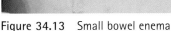
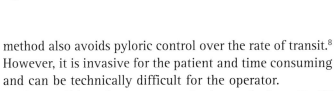
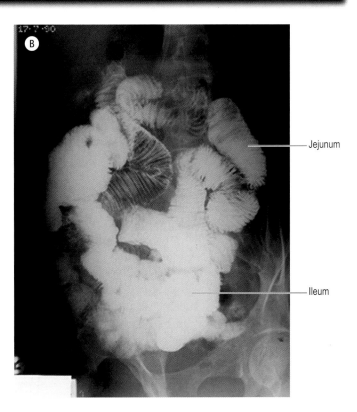

Figure 34.13   Small bowel enema

method also avoids pyloric control over the rate of transit.[8] However, it is invasive for the patient and time consuming and can be technically difficult for the operator.

The small bowel enema may also be used after a Ba FT to localise a lesion or examine a particular section of small bowel.[3]

Contraindications
- Facial surgery or trauma
- The patient is prone to nose bleeds
- Active Crohn's disease (especially of the duodenum)
- Severe gastrooesophageal reflux/hiatus hernia
- Suspected perforation
- Complete obstruction

Patient preparation
- As for Ba FT
- Explanation of the procedure must be carefully delivered as this procedure is often difficult for the patient to tolerate[3]

Contrast agent
For single contrast, typically, 1000 mL of fluid is used.[4] The mixture comprises barium sulphate suspension and water; the ratio of barium to water tends to vary according to the preferences of the examining radiographer or radiologist. For double contrast examination, 150–200 mL barium sulphate suspension is followed by up to 2 L methylcellulose 0.5%.[4]

Additional equipment
- Nasogastric or duodenal catheter
- Lubricating jelly for the tube
- Anaesthetic spray
- Tissues
- Sterile gloves
- Swabs to wipe the tube after removal

Technique
- The patient lies supine and, under fluoroscopic control, the duodenal or nasogastric catheter is inserted until the tip of the catheter is shown in the duodenojejunal flexure. The anaesthetic spray may be used to numb the throat but the use of this prevents the examination continuing by follow through if the intubation is unsuccessful
- The guidewire within the catheter acts as a stiffener to prevent coiling and enables manipulation into the correct position
- The barium solution is infused by gravity or by an enteroclysis pump
- Imaging is usually by fluoroscopy but spot films can be taken as well. The terminal ileum may need prone imaging as for Ba FT
- For a double contrast study methylcellulose solution is infused after the barium suspension until the terminal ileum is demonstrated in double contrast

- During a single contrast examination air may be introduced at the end of the examination to demonstrate the terminal ileum in double contrast. Air may be introduced via the duodenal catheter or by a rectal catheter

- All the loops of bowel are usually imaged supine until the terminal ileum is reached and oblique views may be needed

Potential complications and postprocedure care
- As for Ba FT

LOWER GI TRACT

LARGE BOWEL

The large bowel comprises the colon, rectum and caecum and is usually examined by the double contrast barium enema. Virtual colonoscopy may supersede the examination in the future but at the time of publication this is not the mainstream examination for colon disease.

Referral criteria

- Change in bowel habit
- Iron deficiency anaemia
- Rectal bleeding
- Tenesmus
- Left iliac fossa pain
- Palpable mass
- Documented cancer on endoscopy: to exclude synchronous lesions

Double contrast barium enema (DCBE)

The aim of this examination is to image the entire large bowel in double contrast, using gas (CO_2 or air) to distend the bowel, facilitate a fine coating of barium on the bowel mucosa and to act in extreme contrast with the dense barium.

Contraindications
- Biopsy via rigid sigmoidoscope within 7 days[3]
- Toxic megacolon
- Incomplete bowel preparation
- Suspected perforation
- Obstruction

Patient preparation
- There are various preparations available but the most commonly used method is to instruct the patient to follow a low residue diet and take laxatives 48 and/or 24 hours before the examination. However, cleansing enemas can be given and some centres also restrict fluids for 4–6 hours prior to the examination. Fluid restriction does exacerbate the dehydrating effects of the laxative, which is potentially dangerous for all patients. In certain cases, laxative use is contraindicated (ileostomy, currently clinically active inflammatory bowel disease) or should be used with caution, as in patients with a colostomy
- Elbow pads may be provided immediately prior to the examination to reduce the risk of skin damage in the frail or elderly

Contrast agents
- Barium sulphate suspension. Warm water is added to the barium powder/liquid to ensure a high density and low viscosity suspension. The powder is usually supplied in an enema bag
- Air or carbon dioxide

Additional equipment/pharmaceuticals
- Funnel to fill enema bag with water or barium
- Additional clamp (although rare, clamps supplied on enema bags may fail)
- Rectal catheter with additional gas insufflation line
- Drip stand for barium bag
- Air or CO_2 insufflation device
- Lubricating jelly
- Gauze swabs for application of lubricant to catheter
- Wide adhesive tape to help maintain position of catheter
- Latex or vinyl gloves
- Muscle relaxant, needle and syringe

Technique
(Ensure that you have understood the notes on fluoroscopic examination positioning descriptors earlier in this chapter before considering technique descriptors.)

As the aim of the examination is to provide clear images of the whole bowel, the natural variations in bowel orientation will necessitate selection of a method of barium coating and patient positioning which varies. Selection of the most suitable technique may rest solely upon the individual but may also be based on variations around an agreed protocol. The routine presented here is one option only:

- The patient lies on their left side with their knees and hips flexed and a lubricated catheter is inserted into the rectum. The catheter is then taped in place. A hypotonic agent (also known as a smooth muscle relaxant), e.g. Buscopan or Glucagon is frequently given at this point to reduce bowel spasm. Contraindications for Buscopan include cardiovascular disease and glaucoma so Glucagon may be given instead[8]

- The bag or bottle of barium suspension is suspended on the drip stand about 1 metre higher than the patient. The patient remains on their left side and the table is tilted slightly (with the patient's head down); the clamp on the barium solution is released and the fluid is slowly run into the colon

- The first phase of the study is to introduce enough barium and air to coat the bowel mucosa. Introduction of too much barium increases the likelihood of barium reaching the caecum and refluxing into the terminal ileum where it will obscure sigmoid loops before spot images of the sigmoid can be recorded. Not enough barium will mean that the entire length of the colon will not be coated. Under fluoroscopic assessment, flow of the barium is monitored

- When the barium suspension reaches the splenic flexure the patient turns prone until the barium suspension has filled half of the transverse colon. At this point the patient turns back onto their left side and the bag/bottle of barium suspension is placed on the floor to enable excess fluid to drain back out of the patient

- Air or carbon dioxide is then gently insufflated into the rectum and the imaging sequence begins. The gas is insufflated throughout the examination as required to ensure double contrast throughout; as CO_2 is absorbed by the colon, it is more likely to require additional insufflation than air

- It can be difficult to move barium and air around the bowel and some strategies are available to achieve this:

  1. Tipping the patient head down (supine position) – clears barium from the caecum
  2. Lying the patient on their left side, turning them to prone then back to the left side also clears the caecum. However, if the ascending colon is long, and the caecum lies in the midline or left of the midline it may be necessary to turn the patient from supine to lie on their right side and then back to supine
  3. Turning the patient 360° to coat the mucosa effectively. This will only work if enough barium is in the region of interest and may require additional barium to be run into the region, or rotation of the patient to bring barium to the area

- Once the bowel is coated and adequately gas-filled, projections are taken and may include:

  1. LPO of the rectum and sigmoid (Fig. 34.14)
  2. RAO of the rectum and sigmoid (any areas obscured by barium suspension in the LPO view should now be outlined with air)

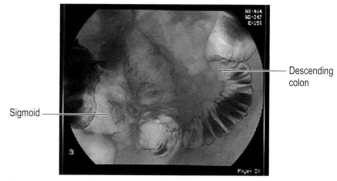

Figure 34.14   LPO rectosigmoid region

3. Prone rectum
4. Lateral rectum (Fig. 34.15)
5. RPO descending colon
6. Supine and erect (Fig. 34.16) transverse colon
7. Erect RPO splenic flexure (Fig. 34.17)
8. Erect LPO hepatic flexure (Fig. 34.18)
9. LPO ascending colon and caecum
10. Slight RPO and supine caecum with palpation. The table may be tilted slightly head down for these views
11. Left lateral decubitus (positioned with left side down and right side raised). This view demonstrates the medial wall of the rectum, sigmoid, descending colon; the superior and inferior wall of the transverse colon; the lateral wall of the caecum, ascending colon and hepatic flexure (Fig. 34.19)
12. Right lateral decubitus (right side down). This view demonstrates: the lateral wall of the rectum, sigmoid and descending colon; the superior and inferior walls of the transverse colon; the medial wall of the caecum and ascending colon

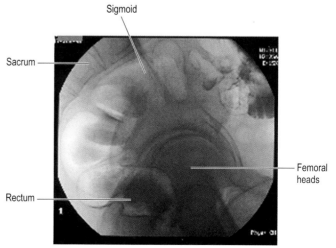

Figure 34.15   Lateral rectum

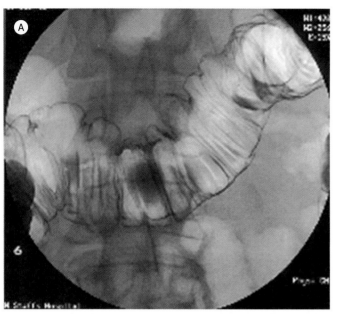

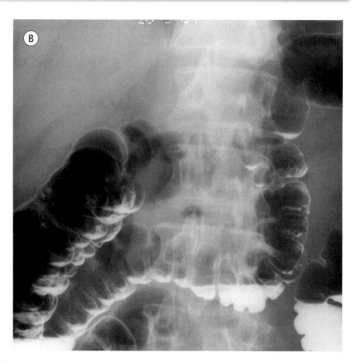

Figure 34.16 **(A)** Supine transverse colon; **(B)** erect transverse colon

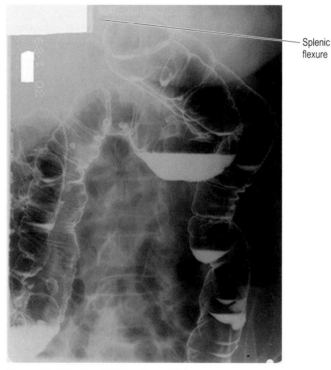

Splenic flexure

Figure 34.17 Erect RPO splenic flexure

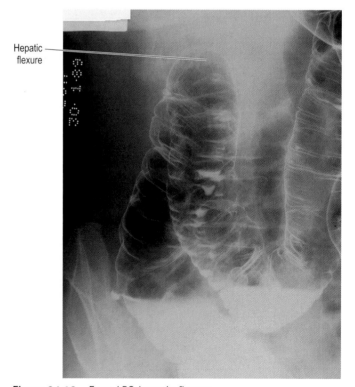

Hepatic flexure

Figure 34.18 Erect LPO hepatic flexure

13. When the rectum is included on lateral decubitus views it is not always possible to include the splenic flexure. It is preferred that the rectum is included in preference to the splenic flexure, which should have been included on spot images

14. For additional information on the distal descending colon and sigmoid, employ the prone 30–35° projec-tion (described later in this section and shown in Figures 34.21 and 34.22)

15. The examination is not complete until the appendix and ileocaecal junction are adequately demon-strated.

Lateral decubitus (Fig. 34.19, 34.20)

The lateral decubitus projection is most frequently employed as part of the barium enema examination. The patient is examined on both sides for barium enema, the projection affording demonstration of lateral aspects of the large bowel mucosa. The raised side ensures air rises above barium, showing mucosal detail.

Unfortunately, some confusion can arise when describing the decubitus projections; the right side raised will demonstrate the right side of the bowel and is often incorrectly referred to as a 'right lateral decubitus' because of this. Since the patient is lying on their left side for this the correct term is actually 'left lateral decubitus'. And vice versa for the left side raised position, which is the 'right lateral decubitus'.

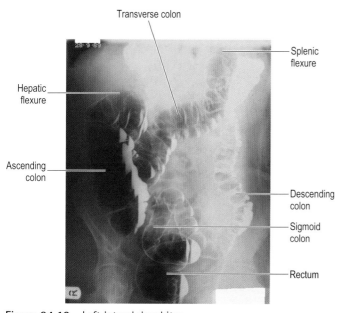

Figure 34.19 Left lateral decubitus

(Labels on Figure 34.19: Transverse colon, Splenic flexure, Hepatic flexure, Ascending colon, Descending colon, Sigmoid colon, Rectum)

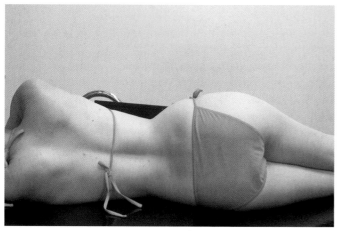

Figure 34.20 Left lateral decubitus (positioning)

If used, a 35 × 43 cm cassette with grid, or gridded cassette, is selected for this examination and placed in an erect cassette holder at the side of the patient.

Positioning
- The patient lies on a thick radiolucent pad, on the table-top and turns to a lateral position with their back to the radiographer, with the right or left side raised. The arms are raised onto a pillow and the knees flexed to aid stability
- The image receptor is positioned vertically with its tube side in contact with the patient's abdomen and its long axis coincident with the median sagittal plane (MSP). The MSP is perpendicular to the cassette
- A PA anatomical marker is applied within the primary beam

The radiolucent pad will bring the spine to a position where it will be more likely to be coincident with the midline of the cassette. Difficulties do arise when trying to insert the pad under the patient, in addition to asking the patient to lie on their side. The concept is somewhat alien to patients and the complications of catheter retention and barium/air retention only compromise cooperation. Instructions should be given clearly, and also step by step, only moving to the next instruction once an action has been completed successfully. It is vital that the catheter remains in place during positioning, as last minute reinsufflation may be required to ensure optimum image quality.

Beam direction and focus film distance (FFD)
Horizontal, 90° to the image receptor
100–120 cm FFD

Centring
Over the 4th lumbar vertebra, in the midline at the level of the iliac crests

Collimation
Symphysis pubis, as much upper abdomen as possible, lateral soft tissue or bowel outlines

Note that no AP positioning has been described above. Although it is common practice to undertake the lateral decubitus images for barium enema by turning the patient first AP and then PA (or vice versa), it is actually advantageous to position both in the PA position, by moving the patient's head to the opposite end of the table. These advantages are:

1. The large bowel is positioned relatively anteriorly in the peritoneal cavity and magnification of this is reduced on both projections to ensure maximum coverage of bowel area with minimum number of exposures made to demonstrate the whole of the large bowel

2. Since radiosensitive organs are generally positioned more anteriorly, the PA projection affords some dose reduction to these organs as the posterior tissue attenuates a proportion of beam energy
3. The abdominal tissue can be compressed gently against the cassette, allowing a reduction in exposure factors in the PA position and reduction of scatter

Unfortunately the suggested procedure is somewhat difficult for the patient with rectal catheterisation, especially as the typical barium enema patient is over 45 years old, but careful consideration for assistance and instruction may result in success.

Variation in abdominal tissue thickness over the area of interest ('belly sag')

Adipose tissue in the abdomen has a tendency to sag towards the table-top, creating a variation in tissue thickness which is thicker on the side nearer to the table-top and thinner on the raised side. Undertaking both projections in the PA position is likely to partially address this by compressing the tissue against the cassette.

Other methods for compensation of this variation in density include use of a high kVp to reduce the range of densities on the image, or application of a wedge filter over the light beam diaphragm (LBD).[4] However, since the recommended kVp for fluoroscopic examination using barium is a minimum of 100, it is likely that kVp in use will already be relatively high. The wedge filter is positioned coincident with the raised side of the patient, the tapering edge pointing towards the table-top. It is tempting to position the top of the wedge level with the superior edge of the LBD but, in fact, this will often place the useful wedge thickness above the bowel. For this reason the radiographer should ensure the thickest part of the wedge lies level with the thinnest part of the patient; in practice this often means that the wedge appears to be in a relatively low position on the LBD housing.

AP lateral decubitus

If AP positioning *is* required, the MSP is still positioned as perpendicular to the cassette and centring is as for the AP abdomen, using a horizontal beam and AP marker. The centring point is in the midline, level with the iliac crests. The beam is horizontal and at 100–120 cm FFD.

Criteria for assessing image quality: all lateral decubitus positions

- Rectum, descending colon, splenic and hepatic flexures, ascending colon and caecum are included on the image

- Spinous processes of vertebrae are seen coincident with the midline of the image and centralised and aligned down the middle of the vertebral bodies
- Sharp image demonstrating air in the bowel and in contrast with barium-coated mucosa

> **Expose on arrested respiration**

Common errors (lateral decubitus)	Possible reasons
Region/s of bowel omitted from field	Large patient *or* AP rather than PA position has been used; may need additional examination of missed area *or* undertake in PA position. If a radiolucent pad is not used, the lateral portion of the bowel on the lowered side is also likely to be omitted from the field
Over-penetrated/ overexposed, air-filled area on raised side, possibly under-penetrated/underexposed on area nearest table-top	Wedge filter not used, or not used correctly (see paragraphs relating to varied tissue thickness, above)
Grid 'cut-off'	If a cassette is used, it will produce grid cut-off if it is allowed to tilt from its vertical position

◼ Prone 30–35° to demonstrate the sigmoid colon: Hampton's projection (Fig. 34.21, 34.22)

Notes on cassette selection (if used)

In the case of the barium enema examination, if additional information on the *sigmoid colon* is required, the Hampton's projection may be used.

A 35 × 35 cm cassette is placed in the table bucky for this projection. It has been noticed that this projection has sometimes been undertaken using a 35 × 43 cm cassette which is placed longitudinally in the table bucky tray and this irradiates the whole abdomen and even the upper femora. Since the projection is specifically intended to demonstrate the sigmoid colon, rectum, rectosigmoid junction and distal descending colon, only these areas should be included within the field of radiation.

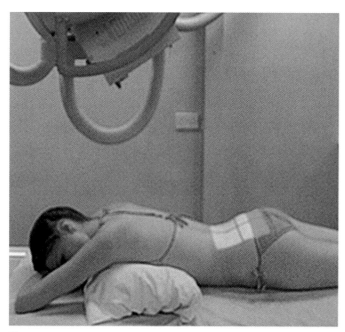

Figure 34.21   Prone 30–35°

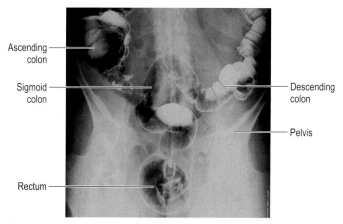

Ascending colon
Sigmoid colon
Descending colon
Pelvis
Rectum

Figure 34.22   Prone 35° sigmoid colon

Positioning
- The patient is prone, head turned to the side and arms raised onto the pillow for stability and comfort
- The MSP is coincident with the long axis of the table
- For males, lead rubber or lead gonad protection is applied below the buttocks to protect the male gonads
- ASIS are equidistant from the table-top

Beam direction and FFD
A vertical central ray is angled 30–35° caudally
100 cm FFD

The image receptor is displaced until its centre is coincident with the central ray.

Centring
Over a point in the midline, at the level of the 1st sacral segment

Collimation
Rectum, sigmoid colon

Criteria for assessing image quality
- Rectum and sigmoid colon are included on the image
- Spinous process of upper sacral segments seen coincident with the midline of the image and centralised and aligned down the middle of the sacrum

> **Expose on arrested respiration?**
> At the level of the sigmoid, the abdominal organs are less likely to be affected by diaphragmatic movement and exposure need not be made after expiration. In fact, it is likely that the image may not show movement unsharpness even if exposure was to be made during gentle respiration.

- Sigmoid colon is no longer superimposed upon itself in a craniocaudal direction, but 'opened out' along its length by the effect of caudal angulation
- Sharp image demonstrating air in the bowel and in contrast with barium-coated mucosa

Common error	Possible reason
Sigmoid not demonstrated centrally on the image	Inaccurate centring of beam or centring of image receptor to central ray

Patient aftercare
The examination is not complete until the ileocaecal junction is adequately demonstrated

- Remove the catheter and escort the patient to the toilet
- Warn the patient about constipation and encourage a high fibre diet and plenty of fluids over the next 48 hours
- Warn the patient about white stools
- Ensure the patient knows how to obtain results
- If a muscle relaxant has been used, warn of the possibility of blurred vision and ensure that the patient does not leave the department until any blurring of vision has resolved

Complications
- Constipation
- Impaction
- Obstruction
- Barium appendicitis

Modifications to the barium enema

- A water-soluble contrast agent may be used to demonstrate a recent bowel anastomosis or in cases of suspected bowel perforation
- Patients with an ileostomy or colostomy may require a barium examination to examine their proximal bowel. A soft Foley catheter is gently inserted into the stoma and the barium sulphate solution is slowly infused into the colon

References

1. Chua TS, et al. Validation of ^{13}C-urea breath test for the diagnosis of helicobacter pylori infection in the Singapore population. Singapore Medical Journal 2002; 43(8):55–57.
2. Moayyedi P, et al. New approaches to enhance the accuracy of the diagnosis of reflux disease. Gut 2004; 53:55–57.
3. Chapman S, Nakielny R. A guide to radiological procedures. 4th edn. Edinburgh: Saunders; 2001.
4. Whitley AS, et al. Clark's special procedures in diagnostic imaging. Oxford: Butterworth Heinemann; 1999.
5. Ott DJ. In: Sutton D, Young WR, eds. A short textbook of clinical imaging. St Louis: Mosby; 1995.
6. RCR Working Party. Making the best use of a Department of radiology: guidelines for doctors. 5th edn. London: The Royal College of Radiologists; 2003.
7. Grainger RG, Allison DJ. Diagnostic radiology: an Anglo-American textbook of imaging. London: Churchill Livingstone; 1996.
8. Bryan G. Diagnostic radiography: a concise practical manual. 4th edn. Edinburgh: Churchill Livingstone; 1987.

ACCESSORY ORGANS OF THE GASTROINTESTINAL TRACT

Darren Wood, Elizabeth Carver

SALIVARY GLANDS

Contrast examination usually involves the parotid or submandibular glands, as it is considered very difficult to introduce contrast agent into the sublingual duct. Plain radiographic examination can be undertaken of the sublingual area, using submental occlusal dental radiography (see Ch. 22) to show radiopaque calculi. Contrast enhanced computed tomography (CT) is useful for assessing tumours arising from or involving salivary glands, and contrast enhanced or non-contrast magnetic resonance imaging (MRI) is also useful in the investigation of malignancy. Radionuclide imaging (RNI) can assess gland function and duct patency[1] and ultrasound also may have a role in imaging the area.[2]

Referral criteria
- Pain
- Swelling

Both symptoms are often noted on or after eating.

Contraindications

Acute infection or inflammation[2,3]

Contrast agent
- High or low osmolar water soluble contrast agent 240–300 mgI/mL *or* oily contrast agent (480 mgI/mL). Neither contrast agent appears to be more advantageous than the other

Additional equipment
- Small syringe (2 mL)
- Filling cannula

- Lacrimal dilator (sterile)
- 18 G blunt needle with catheter (sterile)
- Sterile gloves
- Gauze swabs
- Sialogogue (used to stimulate salivation and help dilate the salivary duct for cannulisation). This may be in the form of lemon juice, a citrus-flavoured sweet or sherbet
- Wooden spatula
- Mouthwash and disposable cup

Patient preparation
- Removal of artefacts, including false teeth
- After plain radiography has been undertaken, the sialogogue is administered to promote salivation and maximise visualisation of the salivary duct
- Explain to the patient that it will be necessary for them to indicate when the salivary duct feels full of contrast agent. Arrange for a distinctive sign to be given by the patient (e.g. raising a hand) when the relevant area feels tight or full. It is important that the patient understands the process before the procedure starts, as explanation whilst undergoing cannulation often proves ineffective
- Explain to the patient that it will be necessary for them to keep their lips closed gently over the cannula, to ensure it stays in place in the duct

For all areas, control images are taken prior to administration of the contrast agent; basic information on head positioning can be found in corresponding position descriptors in relevant chapters on radiography of the head or teeth (Chs 16,18,19,22), although centring and collimation differ for sialography; some slight modifications from basic head positions are outlined, if relevant, in this chapter. If cassettes are used, 18 × 24 cm are of sufficient size (for all except occlusal images), orientated horizontally or vertically in the bucky, according to size and orientation of the area under examination, and projection.

Parotid glands

Control images required:

1. *Anteroposterior (AP) (frontooccipital (FO) position)* projection with the head rotated 5° away from the side under investigation. Centre midway between the symphysis menti and the angle of the mandible on the side under examination. Collimate to include soft tissues of the neck and face, symphysis menti and zygoma on the side under examination. Figure 35.1 shows an AP projection (of the right submandibular gland) after contrast injection
2. *Lateral*, centred to the angle of mandible. Collimate to include soft tissues of the neck and under the chin, external auditory meatus (EAM), zygoma and to level with the ala of the nose anteriorly. Figure 35.2 shows a lateral projection (of the right parotid gland) after contrast injection
3. *Lateral oblique* with the patient's head tilted 15° towards the side under investigation. Tube angle of 10–15° cranially, centre midway between the angles of mandible. Figure 35.3 shows a lateral oblique projection (of the right submandibular gland) after contrast injection

Technique

- If the gland is not visible, the sialogogue may be used to promote salivation
- Saliva is blotted away from the duct area, using a gauze swab and the duct is dilated with a lacrimal dilator
- The duct is cannulated, using the blunt-ended sialographic needle/catheter apparatus
- Post cannulation, up to 2 mL of contrast is injected until the patient indicates that the gland feels 'full' (see the preparation section with regard to a signal for this)
- The catheter tubing is taped to the skin surface, away from the duct and gland area
- The precontrast images are repeated

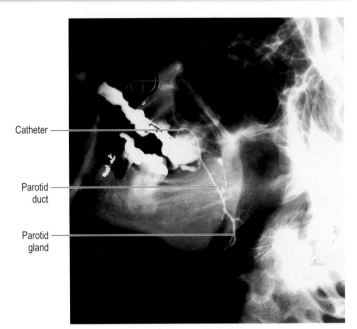

Catheter
Parotid duct
Parotid gland

Figure 35.2 Lateral parotid gland. From Ryan S, et al. Anatomy for diagnostic imaging. 2nd edn. Edinburgh: Saunders; 2004.

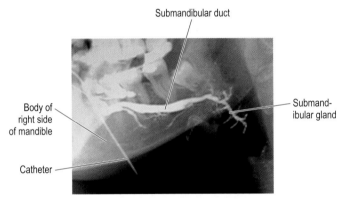

Submandibular duct
Body of right side of mandible
Catheter
Submandibular gland

Figure 35.3 Lateral oblique submandibular gland

- After the images have been taken the patient is given a mouthwash to promote saliva secretion and a lateral view can then be taken to demonstrate drainage of the duct and any sialectasis if present

Submandibular gland

Control images required:

1. A *lower occlusal* image, with the image receptor possibly displaced over to the side in question
2. *Lateral*, as for the parotid gland, centred to the angle of mandible with the floor of the mouth depressed by a wooden spatula
3. *Lateral oblique*, as for the parotid gland

Technique

- The procedure then follows that described for the parotid gland but the occlusal film is not required post-contrast

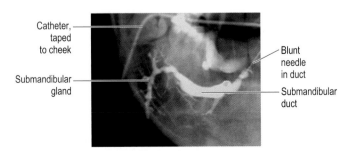

Catheter, taped to cheek
Submandibular gland
Blunt needle in duct
Submandibular duct

Figure 35.1 AP submandibular gland

introduction and it is not necessary to use a spatula in the lateral projection. A post-sialogogue lateral film is required

The control films for both these examinations can be taken using conventional radiographic equipment or, if a C-arm image intensifier is used, recorded directly on the unit.

Aftercare: parotid and submandibular glands
- Provide further mouthwash, if the patient requires it
- Advise your patient that they may experience an unusual taste (which may occur intermittently) until the contrast has fully drained

Possible complications: parotid and submandibular glands
- Infection
- Duct orifice damage
- Duct rupture

Supplementary techniques

Digital subtraction sialography
This technique is undertaken as previously described but the final images are recorded on digital units at 1–2 frames per second, as for arterial angiography, producing a subtracted image that will show only the contrast agent within the duct. There is, however, an increase in patient dose in relationship to that of the conventional technique. The benefits of image quality versus dose implications should be considered.

Magnetic resonance sialography
This is a non-invasive technique and is therefore not dependent on duct cannulation; it compares favourably to digital subtraction sialography but is not as readily available as conventional technique.[4]

CT
With duct cannulation and contrast enhancement, this is also becoming a useful technique. It is also useful for imaging without contrast for tumour enhancement. Dose plays an important factor, especially compared to all other techniques, but image quality is high.

Ultrasound
This is particularly useful for assessing solid mass salivary gland pathology, and also effective in conjunction with fine needle aspiration due to the high resolution that can be attained. It has also been advocated as a quick and simple process to use in assisting fine needle aspiration of tumours.[5]

GALL BLADDER AND BILIARY TREE

Oral cholecystography

Oral cholecystography remains an excellent method of gallstone detection, but its role has diminished due to the advantages of ultrasound.[6] Despite a huge reduction in the number of referrals, it is still undertaken in some centres due to its accuracy.

The examination has three phases:

1. Control plain radiography
2. Contrast images
3. Contrast plus gall bladder drainage images (after fatty meal or AFM)

Referral criteria
- Suspected gall bladder pathology

Contraindications
- Hepatorenal disease
- Serum bilirubin levels in excess of 34 $\mu mol/L^{-1}$
- Acute cholecystitis
- Dehydration
- Previous cholecystectomy

Contrast agent
- There are a number of agents on the market all producing the required result. The most common are sodium iopodate (Biloptin) and iopanoic acid (Telepaque)

First stage of the examination and patient preparation
- Prior to the examination a *control film* is taken. Its use is advocated by Twomey et al, who estimate that it could aid in the diagnosis of up to 5% of calculi.[7] The projection used for this is the 20° left anterior oblique (LAO) described in the second stage examination procedure and positioning technique
- An information sheet and contrast agent are given to the patient to take home; this provides instructions on appointment time for the second stage of the examination, contrast agent and dietary preparation
- The patient is instructed to follow a light, fat-free diet on the day before the examination and to fast from 6 p.m. the night before their cholecystogram appointment.[2] They are encouraged to drink water to ensure hydration
- They are then instructed to take the contrast agent 12 hours prior to their appointment. They are asked not to smoke

Second stage: examination procedure and positioning technique
On arrival in the imaging department, a combination of the following images may be produced. If used, a 24 × 30 cm

cassette is usually large enough for oral cholecystography, although 30 × 40 cm is appropriate for large patients. The cassette is placed in the table bucky or erect bucky, depending on whether the patient is erect or supine.

Prone 20° LAO to show the fundus (Figs 35.4, 35.5)
- From the prone position, the right side is raised 20° and radiolucent pads are used to support the abdomen
- The right arm is placed on the pillow and the left knee flexed, to aid immobilisation

Central ray and focus film distance (FFD)
Vertical central ray
100 cm FFD

Centring
Level with the spinous process of L1, midway between the spine and the right flank
It is acknowledged that patient build will affect centring quite significantly. Slim patients will require centring to fall lower, closer to the spine, and well-built patients will require centring to lie higher and further from the midline (closer to the flank).[8]

Collimation
Collimate to include the soft tissue on the right of the abdomen, spine, 11th rib, iliac crest

For second 20° LAO after ingestion of contrast agent
- Mark the posterior abdominal wall over the point used for centring, to aid positioning later in the examination

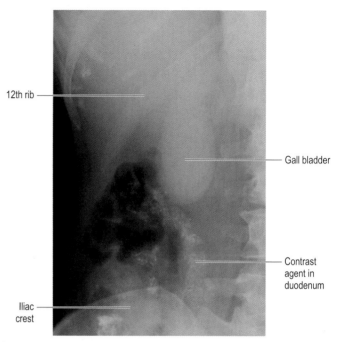

Figure 35.5 LAO gall bladder. The position and shape of the gall bladder will vary according to patient build. This example is of an 'average build' patient. In hypersthenic patients the gall bladder shape will be rounder and sits higher in the abdomen; it will also tend to lie more obliquely towards the lateral abdominal wall, or even horizontally. In asthenic patients the gall bladder will be longer and lie lower in the abdomen; it is also likely to lie closer to the spine. As a result, centring should be modified according to patient build[8]

> **Expose on arrested expiration**
> Exposing after full expiration will ensure that the gall bladder always lies in the same position in the abdomen for every exposure.

Supine 20° right posterior oblique (RPO) to show the gall bladder neck (Fig. 35.6)
- From the supine abdomen position, the patient is rotated 20° to their right
- The left side is supported on radiolucent pads

This projection may also clear appearances of faeces or bowel gas, which can obscure detail over the gall bladder.

Central ray and FFD
Vertical central ray
100 cm FFD

Centring
In the right midclavicular line, approximately 5 cm above the lower costal margin (but possibly varying with patient build)

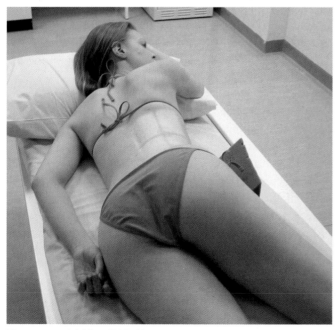

Figure 35.4 LAO gall bladder

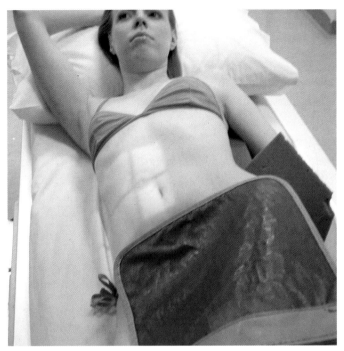

Figure 35.6   Supine RPO gall bladder

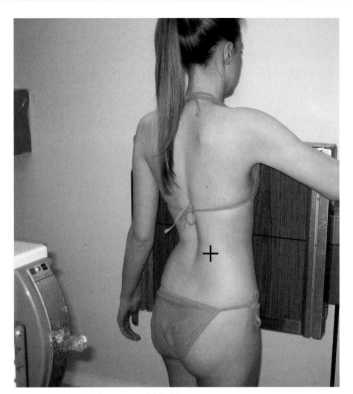

Figure 35.7   LAO erect gall bladder

Collimation
Collimate to include the soft tissue on the right of the abdomen, spine, 11th rib, iliac crest

Expose on arrested expiration

Erect 20° LAO (Figs 35.7, 35.8) for possible floating gallstones
- From the erect posteroanterior (PA) position, the right side is turned 20° away from the bucky
- The right arm is placed on top of the bucky apparatus

Central ray and FFD
Horizontal central ray
100 cm FFD

Centring
Using the centring mark made after the prone 20° projection, centre 2–3 cm below and 2–3 cm medially to the mark. This allows for the change in gall bladder position that the erect position causes

Collimation
Collimate to include the soft tissue on the right of the abdomen, spine, 12th rib, iliac crest
If there are any overlying bowel shadows, fluoroscopic assessment may be made whilst the patient's trunk is rotated to clear the image of the gas from the gall bladder. If this method fails, conventional tomography may be required.

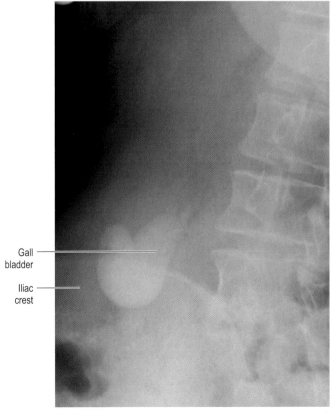

Gall bladder

Iliac crest

Figure 35.8   LAO erect gall bladder. Note how much lower the gall bladder is in this position when compared to the prone LAO image in Figure 35.5

Third stage: AFM

The images for this stage should show that the gall bladder is emptying satisfactorily, and is not obstructed by calculi. After satisfactory contrast images have shown the gall bladder, the patient is given a fatty meal (e.g. chocolate bar or a fat emulsion drink).

At this stage the images may be more strictly collimated, as the second stage images can be studied to ascertain the exact gall bladder position; the radiographer uses the marks made over the second phase centring points, adjusting the third phase centring if the gall bladder has not been shown in the centre of the radiation field at the second phase. The gall bladder will also have contracted. As a result, it is possible to select an 18 × 24 cm cassette (if cassettes are used).

30 minutes after ingestion of the fatty food, a prone 20° LAO image is taken (Fig. 35.9). It may be necessary to also repeat the 20° erect LAO and/or the supine RPO.

Rare complications[2]
- Nausea
- Diarrhoea in up to 50% of patients
- Headache
- Urticaria

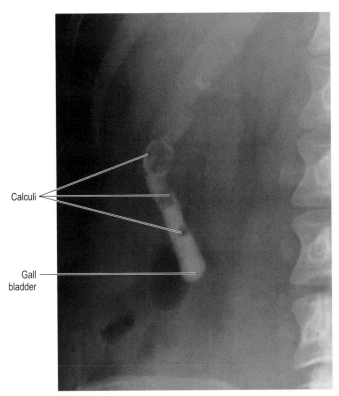

Figure 35.9 Calculi in the contracting gall bladder (prone 20° LAO) AFM

▮ Other diagnostic techniques for the gall bladder

Ultrasound

Ultrasound has a high degree of accuracy for the diagnosis of gallstones, similar to that of oral cholecystography with a number of significant advantages. It is also an excellent method of evaluating the common bile duct and common hepatic ducts without the use of contrast. Advantages of ultrasound are:

- Patients only have to fast for 6 hours
- No contraindications
- Pain on scanning can be related to acute cholecystitis (Murphy's sign)
- No complications
- No use of ionising radiation
- Less time consuming for the operator and patient
- Other structures can be imaged at the same time (e.g. the bile duct, liver, pancreas)

RNI

Cholescintigraphy is possibly the best way to determine acute cholecystitis because a normal 99 m Tc-IDA scan excludes the diagnosis as it provides a direct assessment of the cystic duct patency.

CT

CT can be used to visualise this region but is not always as accurate as ultrasound in the diagnosis of gallstones, and has additional risks associated with the use of ionising radiation. CT can be useful in the very obese patient, as these patients prove difficult to ultrasound.

With later generation CT scanners, patients can be scanned without contrast to show a dilated bile duct system. Infusion of contrast agent before the scan will produce a CT cholangiogram.

MRI

This technique is constantly finding new applications as technology and expertise continues to grow within the field; the most common examination used is the magnetic resonance cholangiopancreatogram (MRCP), which will be mentioned in more detail later in comparison with endoscopic retrograde cholangiopancreatography.

Intravenous cholangiography (IVC)

This examination is almost never undertaken in the 21st century thanks to safer imaging via ultrasound, endoscopic retrograde cholangiopancreatography (ERCP) and MRCP.[2]

Operative cholangiography

The radiographer undertakes this examination under sterile conditions in the operating theatre.

Referral criteria

- During cholecystectomy and/or bile duct surgery, if there is concern that calculi remain in the biliary tract

Contraindications

- There are no contraindications

Contrast agent

- Low iodine content, e.g. Niopam 150

Technique

- This is a sterile procedure performed in the operating theatre. The surgeon will cannulate the cystic duct and introduce approximately 20 mL of the contrast agent. The aim is to show contrast flow into the duodenum and outline the length of the common bile duct (CBD) with minimal filling of the intrahepatic ducts (Fig. 35.10). Images of the area are taken using a mobile X-ray machine or, more frequently, using a mobile image intensifier (this can negate the need for further injections and reduces the risk of missing the information required by taking subsequent plain films). Sterile towels will cover the abdomen and the surgeon generally indicates the region of interest by pointing or putting a spot of sterile water on the towel to aid correct centring. No radiographic positioning is necessary. The area is viewed and/or images are taken after 10 mL of contrast agent have been injected and then exposure is repeated after a further 10 mL has been injected

Complications

- If the biliary tract is obstructed there is a risk that injection of contrast under pressure could cause septicaemia

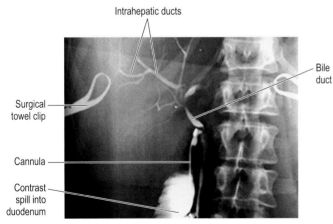

Figure 35.10 Operative cholangiography

Postoperative (T-tube) cholangiography

Referral criteria

- To demonstrate or exclude calculi in the biliary tract if it is suspected that calculi remain in the tract after gall bladder surgery

Contraindications

- There are no contraindications

Contrast agent

- As for operative cholangiography

Additional equipment

- Syringe and needle
- Filling cannula
- Antiseptic
- Gauze swabs
- Sterile gloves
- Clamp

Technique

- The examination is carried out using fluoroscopy, generally at 7–10 days post operation
- The patient lies supine on the fluoroscopic couch and a fluoroscopic spot control film may be taken to show the position of the internal drain
- The external drainage tube is cleaned with antiseptic and clamped. A needle is inserted into the tube, between the clamp and the skin surface. Contrast agent is then injected until the ducts are demonstrated fluoroscopically
- Images are then taken, as required, after turning the patient until optimum visualisation of the area is achieved. Alternatively, if a C-arm intensifier is used, the tube may be rotated to achieve the same effect. It may be necessary to elevate the patient's head, shoulders and trunk (using table tilt) to assess duct drainage

Complications

- As for operative cholangiography

Percutaneous transhepatic cholangiography (PTC)

This technique involves introduction of contrast agent into the hepatobiliary system via a needle technique, through the lateral abdominal wall and into the liver. Needle insertion takes place using spot fluoroscopy for guidance.

Referral criteria

- Jaundice – to check for hepatic bile duct obstruction
- Prior to interventional procedures, e.g. biliary drainage or stenting

Contraindications

- Tendency towards bleeding, platelets less than 100 000 or prothrombin time more than twice the control figure
- Infection of the biliary tract
- Hydatid disease

Contrast agent

- High or low osmolar contrast media with a concentration of 150–300 mgI/mL

Additional equipment

- 22 G flexible, long needle
- Small syringe and needle for administration of local anaesthetic
- Local anaesthetic
- Sterile gloves
- Antiseptic skin wash
- Gauze swabs
- Filling cannula
- Suturing equipment or skin sealant spray and skin dressing for after the procedure

Patient preparation

- Results of blood results must be available and checked to ensure they are within acceptable limits, due to the risks associated with bleeding
- The patient should also be given prophylactic antibiotics prior to the procedure (and also post) to reduce the risk of infection
- Dietary preparation should include 'nil by mouth' to reduce the chance of nausea and/or vomiting
- It is recommended that the patient be given sedative premedication as the procedure can be uncomfortable
- As this is an invasive procedure and there are risks associated with it, written informed consent should be obtained

Technique

- The patient is positioned supine on the fluoroscopic couch. If a C-arm intensifier is being used, their right arm can be placed on an arm board and extended out to allow for the lateral C-arm movement and so that the lateral projection can be taken more easily. Using a C-arm intensifier means that the patient will not be required to turn during the procedure
- Initial screening of the region with the patient in full inspiration and expiration will allow the clinician to make a decision as to the best point to enter the liver
- Using aseptic technique, the area is cleansed and local anaesthesia given
- The flexible needle is inserted through the skin and into the liver with the patient on arrested respiration. The patient is then asked to breathe in a more shallow fashion to reduce needle movement and therefore discomfort. The needle is advanced into the centre of the liver
- Contrast agent can then be injected into the liver as the needle is slowly withdrawn; this process can be repeated whilst moving the needle tip in any direction until the ducts begin to fill with contrast. The more dilated the ducts are, the easier cannulation will be. When the hepatic duct system is filled the needle can be withdrawn, unless access is still required for a therapeutic procedure

- Images taken may vary but often include:
  - Supine
  - 45° lateromedial angle (from left and right); this will require 45° rotation of the patient in each direction if the C-arm is not available
  - right lateral
- Because contrast is heavier than bile it may be necessary to tilt the patient head down (Trendelenburg position) to ensure filling of the system. The patient can then be tilted more erect to check for obstruction or to see if contrast flows into the duodenum

Aftercare

- After withdrawal of the needle, the area is sealed (or sutured) and a clean dressing is applied
- After the procedure, pulse and blood pressure should be taken every 15 minutes for the first hour and then half hourly for 5 hours
- The wound site is monitored
- Abdomen size is monitored

Complications
(Morbidity is approximately 4%)

- Pyrexia
- Pancreatitis
- Perforation of the T tube[2]

ERCP (Figs 35.11, 35.12)
Referral criteria
- Extrahepatic biliary obstruction
- Jaundice
- Post-cholecystectomy patients who remain symptomatic
- Pancreatic disease
- Other diffuse biliary tract diseases

Contraindications
- HIV/AIDS
- Australia antigen positive

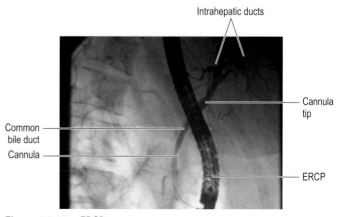

Figure 35.11   ERCP

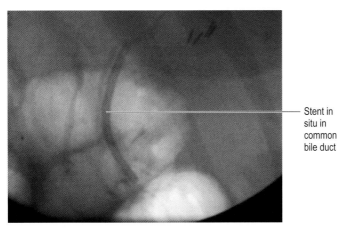

Stent in situ in common bile duct

Figure 35.12 ERCP – post-stent insertion

- Previous gastric surgery (affects the normal anatomy)
- Acute pancreatitis
- Severe cardiorespiratory disease

Contrast agent
- Low osmolar contrast with an iodine concentration of 240–300 mgI/mL is considered optimum. This is generally diluted to half strength with saline when cannulation has been confirmed to reduce the risk of obscuring any calculi and decrease the possibility of pancreatitis

Patient preparation
- Nil by mouth for 4–6 hours prior to the procedure
- Antibiotic cover to reduce any infection risk
- As this is an invasive procedure which may need further therapeutic intervention, written informed consent must be obtained. Advance explanation is important as the patient will be sedated imminently before the examination

Technique
In the past, this procedure has generally been carried out by surgeons or gastroenterologists under fluoroscopic control, within a medical imaging department. Although this remains the more usual scenario, radiographers and nurses are increasingly carrying out this procedure.

- The patient's pharynx is anaesthetised using anaesthetic spray (to aid in the passage of the endoscope); an intravenous sedative (e.g. diazepam or hypnoval) is administered
- The patient is then asked to lie down on their front with their right side raised 30–45° and radiolucent pads are used to support the right side; the endoscope is then introduced
- During the procedure the patient is monitored for pulse and oxygen saturation to ensure their safety
- The endoscopist passes the scope into the duodenum and locates the ampulla of Vater (the bile duct orifice). Once located, a small catheter is positioned in the entrance and contrast agent introduced and viewed under fluoroscopic

control. It is possible at this point for the endoscopist to cannulate the pancreas and obtain images, although repeated cannulation and introduction of contrast is to be avoided due to an increase in the risk of pancreatitis
- As contrast agent begins to fill the common bile duct, images can be taken which will demonstrate any calculi that might be present
- As for the PTC, the patient may be tilted (a) into the Trendelenburg position to fill the intrahepatic ducts and (b) semi-erect to fill the distal end of the CBD and gall bladder
- If there is no need to progress to a therapeutic procedure, or a sphincterotomy has been performed (thereby aiding in the ease of recannulation of the duct), the scope may be removed; this will allow a better view of the duct, over which the scope may have been lying

Aftercare
- The patient should continue to starve until sensation in their throat has returned
- The patient should have their pulse, temperature and blood pressure monitored half hourly for 4–6 hours
- If pancreatitis is suspected, serum amylase tests should be undertaken

Complications
- Damage caused by the endoscope (e.g. to the ampulla, distal ducts and the oesophagus)
- Acute pancreatitis 0.7–7.4%[2]

Comparing the last two procedures, ERCP has three main advantages over PTC which are that:[9]

- ERCP enables visualisation of the ampulla, which can be the site of a tumour, and allows for biopsy during the procedure
- ERCP can demonstrate both the biliary tree and the pancreatic duct
- there are better therapeutic possibilities via ERCP, e.g. sphincterotomy, removal of stones via basket or balloon, drain or stent insertion

However, these do not negate the PTC, which:

- has a growing role as a precursor for interventional procedures that cannot be achieved via ERCP
- generally shows the intrahepatic ducts better than ERCP, although the use of balloon catheters during ERCP means the endoscopist can improve their view of the area

Supplementary techniques for the gall bladder and biliary tree

Ultrasound
Whilst the PTC may have been a primary investigation for obstructive jaundice in the past, ultrasound has now estab-

lished itself in that role; it is non-invasive, involves no radiation and has no complications. Ultrasound has become very accurate in assessment of level and cause of biliary obstruction; even early studies showed that the level of biliary obstruction was correctly noted in 95% and the cause correctly noted in 88% of cases,[10] and ultrasound equipment and techniques have improved significantly since this time.

CT

This has also proved itself as an appropriate modality for the diagnosis of obstructive jaundice. Studies have shown multislice CT to have a useful role in assessment of cholangiocarcinoma although MRI is also considered useful.[11]

MRI

MRI has become increasingly useful for assessment of the biliary tree with the MRCP (Fig. 35.13). Compared to endoscopy this is a non-invasive technique that negates the need for contrast injection. A recent study showed that MRCP had a high accuracy rate in evaluating common bile duct stones (choledocholithiasis).[12] It did, however, infer that patients with a high probability of disease should undergo ERCP, as some form of therapeutic procedure might be required. The conclusion must be that in low-risk patients or failed ERCP, MRCP will become an increasingly important imaging modality.

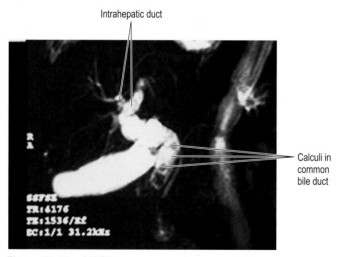

Figure 35.13 MRCP

PANCREAS

In X-radiography, the pancreas is only visualised via ERCP, with direct injection of contrast, but if a patient is suffering acute pancreatitis this is contraindicated. Ultrasound, CT and MRI are the best methods for imaging the pancreas as they are non-invasive and also have the bonus of being able to show the involvement of surrounding structures.

References

1. Pilbrow WJ, et al. Salivary gland scintigraphy – a suitable substitute for sialography? British Journal of Radiology 1990; 63(747):190–196.
2. Chapman S, Nakielny R. A guide to radiological procedures. 4th edn. Edinburgh: Saunders; 2001.
3. Whitley AS, et al. Clark's special procedures in diagnostic imaging. Oxford: Butterworth Heinemann; 1999.
4. Marburg D. MR sialography initial experience using T2 weighted TSE sequence in comparison with digital subtraction sialography. Presentation 1028. Vienna: Proceedings of the European Congress of Radiology; 1999.
5. Daneva S, et al. Ultrasound and fine needle aspiration of the salivary glands. ECR presentations; 1999: lecture ref 8–008.
6. Gregory A, et al. Gallbladder stones: imaging and intervention. Radiographics 2000; 20:751–766.
7. Twomey B, et al. The plain radiograph in oral cholecystography: should it be abandoned? British Journal of Radiology 1983; 56(662):99–100.
8. Unett EM, Royle AJ. Radiographic techniques and image evaluation. London: Chapman & Hall; 1997.
9. Summerfield JA. Biliary obstruction is best managed by endoscopists. Gut 1988; 29:741–745.
10. Gibson RN, et al. Bile duct obstruction radiologic evaluation of level cause and tumour respectability. Radiology 1986; 160:43–47.
11. Schima W. Biliary malignancies: multi-slice CT or MRI? Cancer Imaging 2003; 3(2):75–78.
12. Calvo MM, et al. Role of MRCP in patients with suspected choledocholiathiasis. Clinical Proceedings 2002; 77:422–428.

INVESTIGATIONS OF THE GENITOURINARY TRACT

Elizabeth Carver, Catherine Williams

URINARY TRACT

As outlined in Chapter 33, contrast enhanced imaging of the urinary tract was originally developed in the early 1920s, when suitable contrast agents were first used. For the most part of the 20th century, contrast conventional radiography was the only option for imaging of the tract but all complementary imaging methods, and especially ultrasound (US), now offer a significant contribution to imaging the area. The most commonly used investigation in the past has been intravenous urography (IVU) but numbers of requests for this examination have dropped steadily since the late 1980s.

CLINICAL INDICATIONS FOR IMAGING OF THE URINARY SYSTEM

Patients with suspected urinary pathology can present with a range of symptoms and varying degrees of pain or discomfort. They often complain of feeling generally unwell, at times with some loss of appetite, but acute cases may present with severe symptoms. The more common acute signs and symptoms are:

- severe single-sided loin pain
- anterior abdominal pain extending to the groin (renal colic)
- vomiting
- nausea
- pyrexia
- dysuria
- nocturia

- haematuria
- cystitis
- frequency of micturition
- poor stream of urine
- cloudy and/or foul smelling urine
- passing clots in urine
- recurrent urinary tract infection (UTI)
- collapse

Some patients present with little or no signs or symptoms, but have other clinical indications for possible renal disease such as microscopic haematuria, incidental finding of calculi during another investigation, and raised calcium levels.

COMMON PATHOLOGIES AFFECTING THE SYSTEM

Please note that the following is not an exhaustive list, and covers pathologies which are *most commonly encountered*.

Calculus/calculi

A typical IVU request is: '*Severe left-sided loin pain, vomiting and haematuria ?Renal calculi...*' Calculi (or renal stones) form when salts in the urine solidify into insoluble clumps which, if small enough (<4 mm), can pass unnoticed out of the urinary system via the urethra. Larger calculi are likely to lodge in the ureter and, due to their uneven surface, they cause severe pain (renal colic) and, possibly, haematuria. The peristaltic action of the ureter exacerbates the pain.

Constituents of calculi vary but the most common are calcium oxalate and calcium phosphate. Calculi are often radiopaque and will attenuate ionising radiation, forming a visible image on a radiograph. These clumps of salts are not as dense as bone and therefore will not attenuate to the same extent; they appear as very small opacities within the urinary system, superimposed by other anatomical structures that might obscure their position. An IVU is often used to demonstrate such calculi, non-contrast images being taken to identify any visible calculi prior to the administration of contrast, which may obscure them later. Post-contrast IVU films will identify any obstruction caused by calculi within the renal pelviureteric junction or ureter, and it is at this point that the site of obstruction by radiolucent calculus may become apparent. In the first part of the 21st century, computed tomography (CT) is being used more often in the assessment of patients with renal colic and current UK guidelines suggest unenhanced CT as the investigation of choice, with IVU as a 'suitable alternative'.[1]

On radiographic images the site of ureteric obstruction by a calculus that is still situated in the ureter will be seen as a blunt end at that obstruction site (although the stone itself may not be shown). However, a calculus may have actually passed from the urinary system yet still cause obstruction in the ureter. Trauma to the walls of the ureter may lead to inflammation and swelling, causing the swollen ureter walls to obstruct the lumen of the ureter. In these cases the obstruction site will appear as a tapering of the contrast agent in the ureter. This type of obstruction usually clears as the swelling subsides. In many cases the ureter may also appear distended above the obstruction, possibly accompanied by blunting and/or enlargement of renal calyces and delayed contrast concentration; this is known as *hydronephrosis* (Fig. 36.1).

Large radiopaque calculi may occupy the space within the pelvicalyceal system, filling it in almost exactly the same shape as the system; these are known as staghorn calculi (Fig. 36.2) and can mimic the appearance of a contrast-filled pelvicalyceal system. They can be an incidental finding, seen on abdomen or kidneys, ureter and bladder (KUB) control images.

Radiopaque calculi in the bladder are most often seen on the control radiograph, but will be obscured once the bladder fills with contrast.

Benign prostatic hyperplasia/hypertrophy (BPH)

A large proportion of men over 60 years old will have an asymptomatic enlarged prostate known as BPH.[2] Symptoms of an enlarged prostate include frequency of micturition, poor stream of urine and dysuria. Extreme forms can cause bladder outlet obstruction.

A prostate mass (benign or malignant) can appear as a slightly opaque sphere in the inferior pelvis on the pre-contrast control KUB image and an area of decreased density in the lower third to half of the bladder on contrast images; extensive prostatic enlargement can cause the bladder to have a mushroom-shaped appearance on the contrast image. However, US is more effective in its differentiation between malignant and benign tissue. It is also useful in assessment of bladder residual volume, which contrast radiography cannot address. US should be the first examination when investigating BPH and the extent of its effect, and contrast radiography is not indicated for this condition.[2]

Carcinoma

The renal system can produce several different types of carcinoma because it is composed of many different

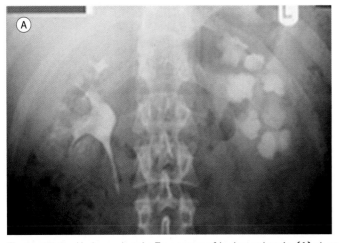

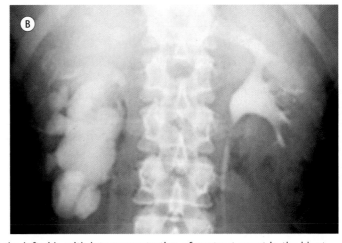

Figure 36.1 Hydronephrosis. Two cases of hydronephrosis, **(A)** shows the left side with late concentration of contrast agent in the blunt calyces and **(B)** shows the affected right side but in this case the distended renal pelvis is also seen. Compare the hydronephrotic kidney in both cases with the normal kidney on the opposite side

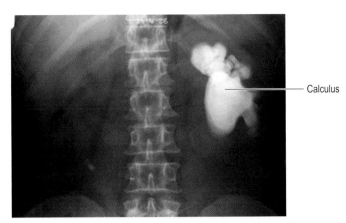

Figure 36.2 *Staghorn calculus on control image. The radiopaque calculus has filled the pelvicalyceal system, almost mimicking a hydronephrotic kidney filled with contrast agent*

Calculus

types of cells. The most common type is bladder carcinoma or transitional cell carcinoma, which is often visualised postcontrast as an irregular structure either protruding into the bladder or causing an irregular filling defect along the bladder wall with contrast radiography (IVU and cystography). However, contrast radiography is less efficient than US for provision of information regarding the anterior or posterior bladder walls. Epithelial cell tumours also affect the renal tract and are demonstrated with IVU and CT. The IVU was considered to be superior to CT for demonstration of these tumours but recent advances in multislice CT technology have led to a change in opinion.[3]

The kidney can produce three main tumour types: nephroblastoma (Wilm's tumour) – a paediatric condition developing during fetal growth, renal cell adenocarcinoma, and transitional cell carcinoma. Wilm's tumour tends to present at around 3 years of age and is dealt with aggressively. Renal cell adenocarcinoma and transitional cell carcinoma will appear as either space occupying lesions causing distortion of the renal capsule, or as narrowing and constriction of renal vessels on IVU[4,5] and can also be detected with CT.

One of the most common cancers occurs in men and involves the prostate gland found at the base of the bladder.[6] Adenocarcinoma comprises 95% of tumours in this gland, and mainly affects men over 55 years of age. Although the prostate is not strictly speaking part of the urinary system, it is connected to that system by the seminal vesicles and vas deferens; therefore a prostatic tumour quite often spreads by direct extension into the bladder and urethra. US is the most efficient method for differentiation between benign and malignant prostatic tissue types.

Duplex system

There is a duplication of part or parts of the urinary system, involving the kidney and ureter. The most extensive form presents as a single kidney which has two sets of calyces, two renal pelvi and two ureters (Fig. 36.3); this may be unilateral or bilateral. Less extensive forms of the variant may show as two renal pelvi entering a single ureter or two pelvi entering two ureters, which later fuse before entering the bladder. The variant is usually an incidental finding but is monitored in children due to its relationship to recurrent UTI.

Ectopic kidney

The kidney is found in an area away from the usual site, sometimes on the opposite side to where it should lie (crossed ectopia).

Floating kidney

The kidney may appear to be in a normal position, which changes in later images in an IVU series, or poses as a fixed ectopic kidney which moves as an examination progresses.

Horseshoe kidney

A fairly rare variant. The two kidneys are joined at their upper or lower poles, the latter being by far the most common. Each kidney has its own ureter and the contrast images show the calyces to appear similar to the appearance of a 'normal' kidney which has been placed in an oblique position if the kidneys are joined at their lower pole (Fig. 36.4). In these cases the ureters cannot leave the

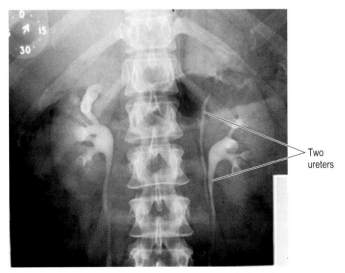

Two ureters

Figure 36.3 *Duplex system. In this case the pelvicalyceal systems are duplicated but most duplex systems are not so extensive*

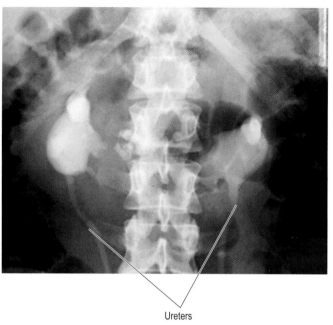

Ureters

Figure 36.4 Horseshoe kidney

kidney pelvis and hilum medially as in the normal kidney, and travel forwards and over the adjoined lower poles.

'Reflux' and pyelonephritis

Ureteric or vesicoureteric reflux and reflux nephropathy. Reflux, in these cases, refers to tracking back of urine from the bladder into the ureter and possibly to the kidney due to failure of the vesicoureteric valve in the bladder. This condition can lead to infection in the kidney (pyelonephritis), causing dysfunction, malformation, scarring and ultimately renal failure if left untreated. Vesicoureteric reflux can be assessed using micturating cystography and radionuclide imaging (RNI), which does provide a non-invasive approach to diagnosis.

RADIOGRAPHIC EXAMINATION OF THE URINARY SYSTEM

IVU

The aim of this examination is to *demonstrate the renal cortex, calyceal size and shape, renal pelvis, pyeloureteric junction (PUJ), ureteric drainage and the bladder* (although demonstration of the bladder may not be required). Contrast agent is administered intravenously, usually via the median cubital vein, and images of the kidney are obtained through various stages of contrast synthesis.

A range of projections are used for the IVU, in various combinations to demonstrate the system, and appropriate selection of this combination will be discussed later in this section. Projections used are taken from the following list:

- Full-length KUB
- Prone KUB
- Cross-renal, collimated to the kidneys and upper ureters
- Oblique single kidney
- Bladder anteroposterior (AP) with caudal angle of approximately 15° to clear the bladder from the upper border of symphysis pubis
- Oblique bladder

Contrast agent can be seen almost immediately after injection of contrast agent, shown as a 'blush' of contrast agent in the renal cortex and known as a 'nephrogram' (Fig. 36.5). This shows glomerular filtration of the contrast

agent, before it reaches the calyceal systems. It is important to see the renal outlines as changes in the smooth outline may indicate presence of tumours, cysts or cortical scarring. It also provides early information on renal size. It is possible to see appearances of renal blush for some time after injection and it is not always considered necessary to show the first blush immediately after injection of contrast agent, since renal outlines can be assessed along with the calyceal systems at later stages in the examination.

Around 5 minutes after injection the calyces should be seen to fill with contrast agent (Fig. 36.6), which then passes down the ureters to fill the bladder. In some cases the calyces empty quickly, preventing adequate demonstration of the

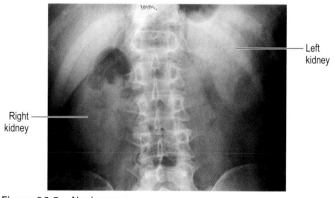

Right kidney

Left kidney

Figure 36.5 Nephrogram

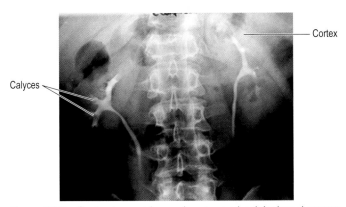

Calyces

Cortex

Figure 36.6 Contrast agent in renal cortex and pelvicalyceal system

calyces and renal pelvis. To counteract this, external compression of the umbilical region of the abdomen is required, which restricts the flow of excreted contrast down the ureters. This, therefore, retains contrast agent within the kidney for a longer period of time to ensure adequate imaging of the collecting systems. Compression is usually left in place for around 5 minutes before an image of the kidneys is taken and it must be noted that excessive and prolonged compression may cause the calyces to appear slightly blunted and distended (imitating early hydronephrosis). It is recognised that compression is applied routinely, often 5 minutes after injection, to ensure that there is optimisation of contrast build up in the calyces but there are contraindications for the use of compression which must be considered. These include:

- renal colic
- known renal calculi
- abdominal tenderness
- recent abdominal surgery
- recent pregnancy
- renal transplant (since the transplanted kidney will be located in the right iliac fossa)

In addition to fast drainage, there may be other reasons for failure to demonstrate the cortex or calyces and these are related to pathology or overlying bowel gas and faeces. Additional or supplementary projections/techniques may be necessary to improve visualisation in these situations. These include:

- images on the opposite phase of suspended respiration to potentially change the position of overlying appearances such as bowel gas, faeces or radiopacities
- zonography to clear images of bowel gas and faeces
- tomography to provide more detailed information after calyceal and renal pelvis images suggest or cannot exclude filling defects. Tomography (and zonography) should not be used routinely

Once the calyceal system has been demonstrated it is necessary to provide information of the ureters and bladder, with evidence of ureteric drainage being especially important. Ideally a KUB examination at this point (around 15–20 minutes after injection) will show renal outlines, calyceal systems, renal pelvis, ureteric length and some bladder information (Fig. 36.7). If the use of compression has been necessary it must be released in order to allow kidney drainage and, in practice, the renal outline is often ill defined as a result since the kidney responds to the removal of compression by vigorous excretion of urine and contrast. However, if the renal area has been adequately demonstrated previously, this may not be an issue. In any case, whether compression has been applied or not, sections of the ureters may not be visible on the KUB, due to the fact that urine is transported down these structures by peristalsis (the contraction of external muscle layers forcing fluid along its length). If the exposure is made at a point of contraction, portions of the ureters will be constricted and that portion of the ureter will not be visible on the image. This in itself does not really pose a problem; if the ureter is obstructed then there should be other evidence to suggest this, including distended or blunted calyces, hydronephrosis (seen initially as delayed concentration of contrast agent and later as distended and club-shaped calyces), distended ureters (or even megaureter) and failure of contrast to pass the obstructed area on prone KUB or oblique bladder images. The prone KUB is particularly useful to show the ureteric obstruction site: the kidneys lie in the retroperitoneal abdomen upon the posterior abdominal wall and the ureters extend from the kidneys anteriorly until they are approximately level with L4/L5 and then towards the bladder, which is situated in the anterior pelvis. Therefore, in the supine patient, urine is moving 'uphill' for the first section of the ureter; turning the patient prone (after sitting the patient upright for 5 minutes to allow urine drainage) reverses this and allows the urine to pool 'downhill' towards the site of obstruction.

But what is considered to be a conventional series of projections? Most series will include a control non-contrast KUB, cross renal view/s, KUB with contrast, and a post-micturition bladder projection (although this is not always indicated). Texts describing excretion urography do vary on the suggested standard or routine 'protocol' for the examination,[7,8,9] and the matter of most appropriate IVU series is certainly still open for discussion. Perhaps an increase in radiographers who take full responsibility for the IVU series may help address this, as it did when radiographers began undertaking barium enemas and they needed standardisation of this series when providing images for radiologist report? When we look at the IVU situation in recent years, radiographers have had varying

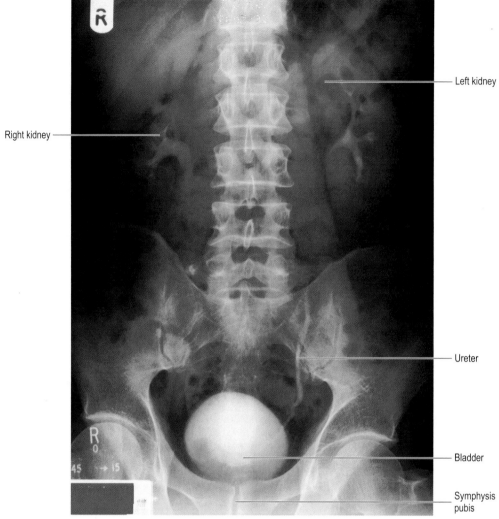

Figure 36.7   KUB with contrast. The bladder appears to sit above the symphysis pubis, although its lower portion lies behind it in the pelvic cavity. The appearance is a result of oblique rays at the lower periphery of the beam, which project the symphysis clear of the bladder

input into the series of images used for IVU, ranging from the radiographer who is required to show almost every image at every stage to a radiologist, to one who uses their knowledge of the examination requirements to produce clear evidence of the condition of the renal system. Over the past 10 years it has been acknowledged that there is a shortage of radiologists in the UK and there is now a need to promote and develop radiographer roles, although this is already evident in urinary imaging.[10,11]

So, we must accept that at the moment it does seem that a 'conventional' or ideal IVU series may not be believed to exist, and that the 'routine' IVU series varies dramatically in different imaging departments. When radiologists control the series, that series will even vary between radiologists in the same department.[12] This variation illustrates how difficult it is to arrive at a satisfactory conclu-

sion on a 'routine' series and it is clear that this 'routine' must also change when pathology becomes apparent. Some imaging departments have already responded to the situation by introducing standardisation of the IVU through a set protocol, describing a series that has been agreed between the radiologists (as often happened in the early days of radiographer involvement in barium enemas). This means that protocols may still vary between hospitals, with some having as few as three set images and others having as many as seven or more. This issue must be governed by two principles: the need to reduce the dose to the patient to a level as low as reasonably practical (ALARP) as stated in current regulations and guidelines,[1,13,14,15] and the need to adapt the series effectively to achieve the best possible diagnostic images for each individual patient and their clinical history (or the appearances found as the examination progresses).

So, considering the range of projections available, strategies to improve visualisation of key areas and effects of pathology on appearances of the system, it is difficult to present a set of instructions that are guaranteed to work every time for every patient. The most important point is that, even if a set 'protocol' is agreed, it is essential that radiographers carrying out IVU examinations must have a thorough understanding of the aims of the examination plus anatomy, physiology, pathology, and radiographic principles involved, in order to ensure that those aims are met. Indeed, some imaging departments who consider and agree on set protocols do produce more than one protocol: one for the 'routine' (if such a thing exists) category patient, plus others for renal colic (which should only require a limited series), haematuria, trauma or follow up after previous known presence of calculi. A suggested 'routine' technique follows:

1. Control KUB on inspiration for assessment of gross anatomy and presence of obvious pathology such as radiopaque calculi
2. Position the patient for a cross-renal image
3. Injection of the contrast agent
4. Cross renal 5 minutes after injection, to assess renal outlines and calyces and taken on arrested expiration. If calyces are not well demonstrated, apply compression if this is not contraindicated and repeat the cross renal 5 minutes later. If there is suspected pathology, or gas or faeces impair detail, undertake zonography or tomography of the renal area. Fulcrum heights selected for this will vary according to patient build but three 'cuts' are usually taken from a range between 7–11 cm
5. If compression has not been applied, 15–20 minute KUB with contrast, taken on inspiration. If compression has been applied, release compression and undertake KUB after calyces have been adequately demonstrated
6. Collimated AP 15° caudal angle bladder image, taken after micturition

Variations in this routine should be made with regard to clinical history, ongoing findings during the examination and patient condition:

Hydronephrosis

This may be known to preexist or may manifest itself during the examination as:

- failure to demonstrate the calyces (especially easy to note when one kidney appears as normal in comparison to a non-apparent kidney on the other side in the early stages of the examination). This is due to excessive urine, which dilutes the contrast agent, remaining in the kidney. Often there is concentration of the contrast agent later in the examination but sometimes not for several hours. The cause of the hydronephrosis is impairment or obstruction of drainage at some point, from the pelviureteric junction down to the bladder, usually due to calculus or tumour. It can also be caused by bladder outlet obstruction
- blunted and distended calyces
- chronic hydronephrosis is likely to be accompanied by loss of renal cortex

Simple modification involves ensuring that there are delayed images of the affected kidney, initiated at around 20 minutes after injection, to allow for more contrast agent to mix with the urine and improve image contrast over the calyces and pelvis. Tomography may be useful, especially if gas and faeces make visualisation even more difficult. If the other kidney appears to be functioning, the rest of the 'routine' aspect of the examination may continue, with further delayed images of the affected kidney being supplied at intervals (related to how quickly concentration of contrast agent appears to be progressing). Micturition is delayed until adequate demonstration of both kidneys has been achieved, unless several hours pass and this is not possible.

Ureteric obstruction

Hydronephrosis will manifest itself as a result of obstruction, and the radiographer will therefore initiate modification for hydronephrosis, followed by methods to show the site of obstruction. These include:

- sitting the patient for 5 minutes (or 10–15 minutes if the hydronephrosis is severe) and then undertaking a prone KUB image
- tilting the patient (if a tilt facility is available) with their head up for 5–15 minutes and undertaking a cross-renal image in this position
- when the suspected site of obstruction is at or near the vesicoureteric junction, (where the lower ureter lies behind the contrast filled bladder): oblique bladder, with affected side raised
- at post-micturition stage, undertaking a KUB image to show contrast and urine remaining in the ureter above the site of obstruction

Renal colic

(If CT is unavailable) confirmation or exclusion of calculus is essential and the acutely ill patient will present in the emergency situation. It is possible to keep radiation exposures to a minimum and a limited series is possible, suggested as:

1. Control KUB
2. Administration of contrast agent
3. KUB 15 minutes after injection

Renal transplant patients

Although RN1 is most suitable for assessment of function of the transplanted kidney, IVU may be still be used in centres with limited or no access to this facility, or if it is suspected that the kidney is being compressed by abdominal or pelvic pathology. Transplant patients will have one functioning kidney, the transplanted one, attached to a short ureter and placed in the right iliac fossa. This negates the use of compression and affects the projections taken. Full length KUB is not appropriate, nor is cross-renal positioning, and images should be confined to the pelvic region. If cassettes are used, a 35^2 or 30×40 cm cassette (placed transversely in the table bucky) are most appropriate, with centring as for an AP pelvis projection and including the bladder and anterior superior iliac spine (ASIS) in collimation. The method is as follows:

1. A control image of the area is taken, as described above
2. Contrast agent is injected
3. 5 minutes after injection of contrast agent, another image of the area is taken
4. 15–20 minutes after injection, another image of the area is taken
5. A post-micturition image of the area is taken

Clearly, any pathology or renal failure in the transplanted kidney will affect this routine in the same way as the other effects considered previously in this chapter.

Radiation protection and the IVU

Protection is afforded as for the AP abdomen for the AP supine kidneys, ureters and bladder projection; the supine or oblique projections of renal outlines require placement of lead rubber over the lower abdomen. Since the edge of collimation for cross-renal, oblique and KUB projections falls next to breast tissue in the adult female, it is recommended that lead rubber is also placed over the breasts for these images. The upper abdomen can be protected during the oblique bladder projection.

RADIOGRAPHIC PROJECTIONS FOR THE IVU

Kidneys, ureters and bladder (KUB) (Fig. 36.8)

This projection may be undertaken as a 'control' image for the IVU examination (Fig. 36.8) or as a stand-alone projection to assess position of existing radiopaque calculi. Discussion on the AP abdomen in Chapter 24 carries many points which are also relevant to the KUB projection.

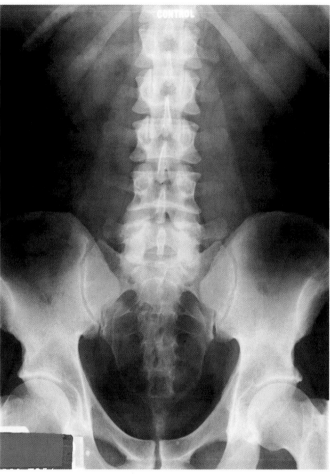

Figure 36.8 KUB control

Positioning
• The patient is initially positioned as for the supine abdomen (see Ch. 26, Fig. 26.1)

Beam direction and focus film distance (FFD)
Vertical
100–115 cm or higher in tall patients

Centring
In the midline at the level of the iliac crests

Collimation
Symphysis pubis, upper poles of kidneys

Lateral borders of collimation can be brought in to coincide with the ASISs, as information on the whole of the abdomen will not be needed for IVU unless additional general information on the abdomen is required. This will avoid unnecessary irradiation of lateral areas of the abdomen.

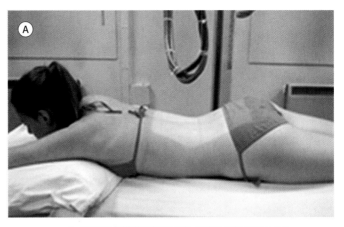

Expose on arrested respiration

In the discussion on arrested respiration for the AP abdomen (Ch. 26) comments are made on the phase of arrested respiration during exposure. These are also relevant to the KUB projection and exposure on suspended inspiration is recommended, to ensure the whole of the system is included on this image.

Criteria for assessing image quality

- Symphysis pubis and renal outlines are included on the image
- Spinous processes of the vertebrae are seen coincident with the midline of the image and centralised and aligned down the middle of the vertebral bodies
- Symmetry of the iliac crests
- Sharp image demonstrating soft tissue of the kidneys in contrast with bowel gas and bony structures

Common errors	Possible reasons
Symphysis pubis not included on the image	Inaccurate centring/ positioning *Or tall patient?* It may be necessary to undertake two projections to cover the area. It is suggested that these are (a) an image with symphysis pubis and as much upper tissue as possible is included and (b) a cross-renal image. Excessive overlap of irradiated areas should be avoided
Upper abdomen not included; symphysis pubis is well above the lower edge of the film	May have been centred using the lateral borders of iliac crest rather than the highest point of crests at the back
Vertebral column is not coincident with the midline of the film	Xiphisternum to symphysis line is inaccurately positioned *or* scoliotic patient
Spinous processes are not demonstrated in the midline of vertebral bodies	MSP not perpendicular to table-top; palpate ASIS to ensure it is equidistant from the table *or* patient is scoliosed

Prone KUB (Fig. 36.9A,B)

This projection is used to demonstrate the site of ureteric obstruction, draining the affected kidney so that contrast

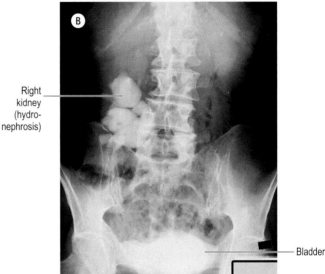

Right kidney (hydro-nephrosis)

Bladder

Figure 36.9 Prone KUB. **(B)** is a prone image which shows hydronephrosis on the right side. Note how the position affects appearances of the pelvis and bladder when compared to the supine KUB in Figure 36.7. The iliac crests appear flattened and much of the bladder now appears to lie behind the symphysis pubis (rather than above it as in the supine KUB). These differences are the result of the effects of oblique rays and change in position of the structures

and urine lie at the lowest possible point (the site of obstruction). The patient should be asked to sit up for around 5 minutes, to encourage kidney drainage, before turning them prone for positioning. If the patient is unable to sit, their trunk can be propped up into a semirecumbent position using pillows and sponges.

If used, a 35 × 43 cm cassette is placed in the table bucky.

Positioning

- The patient is prone, head turned to the side and arms raised onto the pillow for stability and comfort. Care must be taken to ensure that any needle in situ is not moved
- The median sagittal plane (MSP) is coincident with the long axis of the table

- For males, lead rubber or lead gonad protection is applied, below the buttocks, to protect the male gonads
- ASISs are equidistant from the table-top

Beam direction and FFD
Vertical
100–115 cm FFD or higher in tall patients

Centring
Over the spine, level with the iliac crests

Collimation
Symphysis pubis, renal outlines

> Expose on arrested inspiration

Criteria for assessing image quality
- Symphysis pubis and renal outlines are included on the image. However, as this projection is intended to identify the location of ureteric obstruction, it may not be necessary to insist that all of the bladder and upper renal outlines are included
- Spinous processes of vertebrae seen coincident with the midline of the image and centralised and aligned down the middle of the vertebral bodies
- Symmetry of iliac crests, which appear flattened out when compared to their appearances on the supine AP image
- The symphysis pubis should appear to be deeper and the obturator foramina more open than in the AP projection
- Sharp image demonstrating contrast filled structures in contrast with bowel gas and bony structures

Common error	Possible reason
Rotation, demonstrated by asymmetry of the iliac crests and spinous processes not seen in the midline of the vertebral column	Trunk has been turned to one side as the patient turns their head for comfort. Often this is addressed by simply turning the patient's head the opposite way

▓ Supine AP kidneys ('cross renal', 'cross kidney')
(Figs 36.5, 36.10)

If used, a cassette is placed transversely in the table bucky. Note that a specific cassette size is not stated here; each patient's size must be assessed individually for suitable cassette size. It has been noted that a 30 × 40 cm cassette

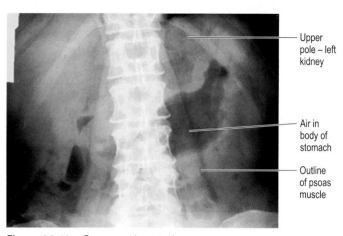

Figure 36.10 Cross-renal control

Labels: Upper pole – left kidney; Air in body of stomach; Outline of psoas muscle

is often unnecessarily selected for this projection, reasons for this being given as 'we can show four borders of collimation' or that 'all male patients are too large for a 24 × 30 cm cassette'. If it is not clear which size of cassette is most suitable, a 30 × 40 cm cassette can be selected for the initial exposure and subsequent cross-renal images can be undertaken on the appropriate size once the first image has been assessed. A positioning image is not provided as this projection is an adaptation of the supine abdomen and KUB, with variation of the centring point only.

Positioning
- The patient is positioned as for the supine AP abdomen

Beam direction and FFD
Vertical
100 cm FFD

Centring
In the midline, at a point found between the xiphisternum and the level of the lower costal margins

Collimation
Renal outlines
   The lateral borders of collimation can be left as those used for the KUB projection, or modified after the KUB has been viewed.

> Expose on arrested respiration
> Exposure should be made on arrested expiration so that the renal shadows lie in a consistent position when exposures of the area are made at later stages in the examination.

Criteria for assessing image quality
- Renal outlines are shown on the image
- Spinous processes of vertebrae are seen coincident with the midline of the image and centralised and aligned down the middle of the vertebral bodies
- Sharp image demonstrating renal outlines tissue in contrast with bowel gas and bony structures for this projection when undertaken without contrast enhancement. After injection of contrast agent, image contrast will be enhanced further and the renal outlines should still show in good contrast to other soft tissue; calyces and renal pelvis should also be seen in contrast with the renal cortex

Common errors	Possible reasons
Vertebral column not coincident with the midline of the film	Xiphisternum to symphysis line is inaccurately positioned *or* scoliotic patient. Severe scoliosis may significantly alter the kidneys' positions and necessitate less stringent lateral collimation
Spinous processes not demonstrated in the midline of vertebral bodies	MSP is not perpendicular to the table-top; palpate ASIS to ensure it is equidistant from the table *or* patient is scoliosed
Vertebral column not coincident with the midline of the film	Xiphisternum to symphysis line inaccurately positioned *or* scoliotic patient

Oblique kidney (Fig. 36.11A,B)

This projection is used at the control stage, to ascertain the position of radiopacities that appear to lie over the renal outline, or after injection of contrast to clear appearances of bowel gas or faecal matter from the renal image.

If used, an 18 × 24 cm cassette is placed longitudinally in the table bucky.

Positioning
- From the supine AP position, the patient's trunk is rotated 30° *towards* the side under examination. Radiolucent pads are placed under the trunk to aid immobilisation and the arm on the lowered side is raised onto the pillow for comfort

Beam direction and FFD
Vertical
100 cm FFD

Centring
In the midline, midway between the xiphisternum and level of the lower costal margins

As the renal outlines generally lie with the left kidney slightly higher than the right, previous cross-renal images can be assessed to ascertain the exact kidney position before centring the beam for the oblique kidney projection. Note that centring is recommended as over the midline and not in the midclavicular line (sometimes erroneously quoted by students); this is due to the posterior position of the kidneys in the abdominal cavity – as the trunk rotates, the image of the kidney moves closer to the midline.

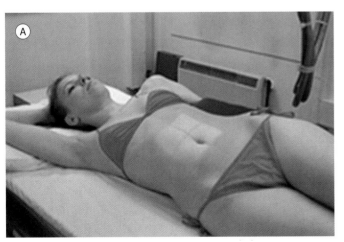

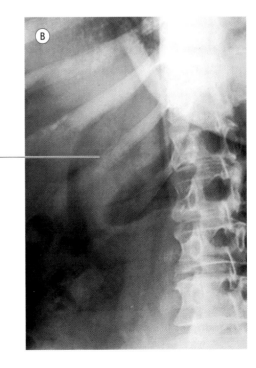

Right kidney

Figure 36.11 Oblique kidney. **(A)** Note that the central ray is in the midline, not in the midclavicular line (which is sometimes believed to be the centring plane for this projection); **(B)** the oblique kidney projection is often used before injection of contrast agent (as in this case) to provide further information on position of opacities which overlie the kidney on supine images. It can also be used after injection of contrast agent, at any stage thereafter

Collimation
Kidney under examination

Criteria for assessing image quality
- Kidney under examination is seen on image
- If contrast agent has been injected the calyces and renal pelvis should appear shortened in a lateromedial direction

Common error	Possible reason
Medial aspect of the kidney is omitted from the image	Centring over the midclavicular line rather than over the midline of the patient

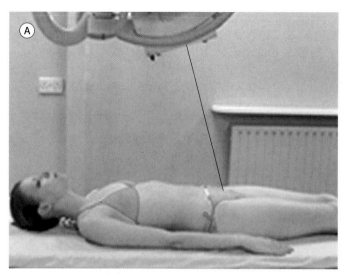

Bladder: supine AP 15° caudal angle (Fig. 36.12A,B)

If used, a 24 × 30 cm or 18 × 24 cm cassette is placed longitudinally in the table bucky. Longitudinal orientation is suggested as this will allow for inclusion of the lower ureters on the image. Transverse orientation reduces the amount of receptor space for ureters and the increased lateral film space lies over the pelvis (ischium) and therefore does not cover the more centrally positioned bladder and ureters.

Positioning
- The patient is positioned as for the supine abdomen (KUB)

Beam direction and FFD
Initially vertical, angled 15° caudally
100 cm FFD

Centring
In the midline, midway between the upper border of the symphysis pubis and the level of the ASIS. The emergent beam should coincide with the image receptor; cassettes will require displacement to facilitate this

Collimation
Symphysis pubis, bladder, lower ureters

Criteria for assessing image quality
- Symphysis pubis, bladder and lower ureters are shown on the image
- Symphysis pubis is seen below and clear of the bladder
- Sharp image demonstrating the bladder in contrast with the surrounding soft tissue, if contrast has been used. This projection is less likely to be produced without contrast agent but is sometimes used as an additional control

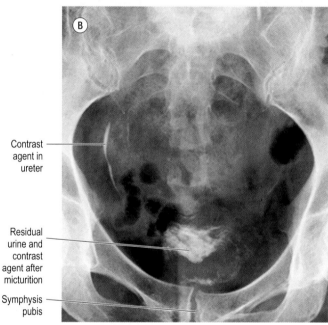

Contrast agent in ureter

Residual urine and contrast agent after micturition

Symphysis pubis

Figure 36.12   15° bladder

film if the lower abdomen has not been demonstrated on the KUB

Common errors	Possible reasons
Top of bladder is close to the top of the image, or outside collimation/boundaries of the film	Centring too low, often found to be over the symphysis pubis or Cassette was not displaced correctly (too low)
Base of bladder is omitted from the boundaries of the film	Centring too high or Cassette was not displaced correctly (too high)

Posterior oblique bladder (Fig. 36.13A,B)

This projection is usually employed to demonstrate the lower end of the ureter as it enters the bladder posteriorly and inferiorly. To achieve this the area is brought into profile by raising the side of interest; note that this is opposite obliquity to that required for the oblique kidney. Caudal angulation is not vital as the area of interest is the vesicoureteric junction, which is not superimposed over the pubis in an AP direction. However, angulation may reveal more information if it is required.

If used, a 24 × 30 cm cassette is placed longitudinally or transversely in the table bucky.

Positioning
- The patient is initially positioned as for the supine AP KUB
- The affected side is raised 30° and the trunk is supported and immobilised with radiolucent pads
- The arm on the lowered side is placed on the pillow for support

Beam direction and FFD
Vertical or caudally angled 15°
100 cm FFD

Centring
Midway between the middle of the upper border of the symphysis pubis and the ASIS on the raised side. Cassette displacement is required if an angle is used

Collimation
Symphysis pubis, bladder

Criteria for assessing image quality
- Symphysis pubis and bladder are seen on the image
- Contrast-filled ureter on the raised side is seen at its site of entry into the bladder

Common error	Possible reason
Ischium of raised side is superimposed over lower ureter and bladder	Too much obliquity

BLADDER AND URETHRA: CYSTOGRAPHY AND URETHROGRAPHY

It must be mentioned that US offers high quality information on the bladder and prostate, especially due to its ability to differentiate between benign and malignant prostatic disease. It is also more efficient in its representation of disease affecting anterior and posterior bladder walls. It has largely replaced cystography in the adult but cystography may still have a place in the assessment of vesicoureteric reflux, which is especially relevant in patients with recurrent UTI. This condition is most frequently assessed in children.

Cystography involves administration of contrast agent via the urethra and into the bladder. The examination is undertaken using fluoroscopic control, and bladder emptying and the urethra are also monitored, whilst the patient micturates. This is termed *micturating cystourethrography* (MCU). Its potential as an embarrassing examination is clear and the radiographer has the usual responsibilities

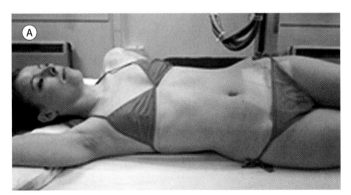
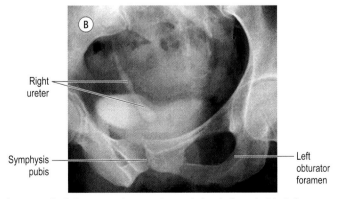

Figure 36.13 Oblique bladder. The oblique projection aims to raise the lower end of the ureter in question to bring it from behind the bladder. In this case the intention was to show the lower end of the left ureter, which has failed to be demonstrated as there does not appear to be contrast agent in this lower portion (possibly because there is actually no obstruction at this point). The right ureter is seen, however, projected behind the contrast filled bladder. There does appear to be some distension in this ureter and an oblique with the right side raised will help confirm or exclude obstruction

for respecting the patient's privacy and dignity during the procedure. In addition to this respect, the radiographer must clearly convey that they know this is important for the patient. The opportunity for this lies in clear explanation of the procedure, before the examination.

MCU (Fig. 36.14)

Referral criteria
- Stress incontinence
- Suspected vesicoureteric reflux
- Assessment of the urethra in micturition

Contraindications
- Cystitis or other UTI infection
- Urethral stricture

Contrast agent
- High or low osmolar contrast agent – up to 300 mL of 150 mgI/mL

Additional equipment
- Sterile towels
- Drip stand
- Saline
- Clamp
- Sterile gloves
- Gauze swabs
- Antiseptic skin wash and sterile receptacle
- Foley catheter
- Sterile anaesthetic jelly
- Incontinence pads
- Receptacle for receiving urine

Patient preparation
- Explanation of the procedure, particularly paying attention to the fact that patient privacy is taken most seriously. Requirement for micturition during the examination should also be explained and that it will be necessary for the patient to let staff know when their bladder feels full. The patient will also need to effect the action of 'straining' without passing urine and this must also be explained in advance
- Micturition immediately prior to the examination

Technique
- The area around the urethral opening is cleansed and the urethra is catheterised
- The bladder is drained of any remaining urine via the catheter

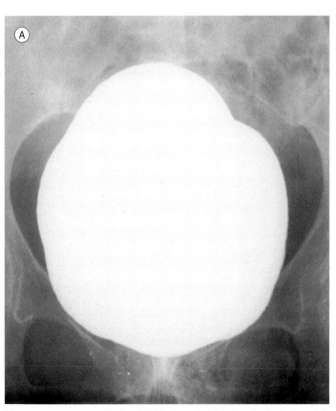

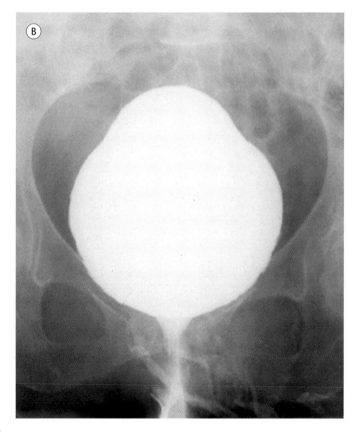

Figure 36.14 **(A)** MCU – full bladder; **(B)** MCU – during micturition

- After connecting the contrast agent to the catheter, the contrast agent vessel is hooked onto a drip stand and contrast agent is allowed to run into the bladder; the flow should be controlled initially to allow early filling to be assessed fluoroscopically (to ensure that the catheter is positioned in the bladder and not in the vagina or ureter)
- Contrast agent is followed by saline, until the patient indicates that their bladder feels very full; it may be necessary to tilt the patient's head down slightly to ensure that the bladder fills completely
- Spot images are recorded in a variation of positions which include:
  - any position where vesicoureteric reflux is seen
  - AP
  - right posterior oblique (RPO) and left posterior oblique (LPO) (following normal positioning descriptor as outlined in Ch. 34 and in Fig. 34.1) which will show distal ureters
  - lateral to demonstrate a fistula
- Additional images are taken with the patient 'straining'. The lateral is considered to be useful as well as an AP – male patients may be able to use a urine receptacle in the lateral decubitus position. For females, sitting erect will allow the patient to sit on a bedpan. This may require special equipment such as a high platform to be used, which is placed against the erect fluoroscopy unit that has had the step removed
- The catheter is removed and further images taken during micturition

Patient aftercare
- The urethral area is wiped with a gauze swab
- The patient may wish to micturate further after the examination is complete
- The patient may wish to wash the genital area and facilities should be available for this
- Antibiotic cover should be given to patients who have demonstrated vesicoureteric reflux

Possible complications
- Urinary tract infection
- (Rarely) reaction to contrast agent
- Perforation of the tract by the catheter

Urethrography

The male urethra only is examined by this method.

Referral criteria
- Urethral fistula
- Congenital abnormality

- Urethral stricture

Contraindications
- UTI
- Recent cystoscopy or catheterisation

Contrast agent
- 5–20 mL high osmolar contrast media (HOCM) or low osmolar contrast media (LOCM), 200–280 mgI/mL

Additional equipment
- Sterile towels
- 20 mL syringe
- Filling tube for contrast agent
- Knuttson's (penile) clamp or urethral catheter with balloon
- Sterile water if a balloon catheter used
- 2 mL syringe for pushing water into the balloon
- Sterile gloves
- Gauze swabs
- Antiseptic skin wash and sterile receptacle
- Sterile anaesthetic jelly
- Incontinence pads
- Receptacle for receiving urine

Patient preparation
- Explanation of the procedure
- Empty bladder

Technique
- The area is cleansed with antiseptic and anaesthetic jelly inserted into the urethra
- The penile clamp is applied to the tip of the urethra *or* the catheter inserted into the fossa navicularis. If the catheter is used it is also necessary to expand its balloon using 1 or 2 mL of water
- Approximately 5–10 mL of contrast agent is injected into the urethra and checked by fluoroscopic control. Further administration of contrast agent may be required to fill the long urethra or filling defects
- Spot images in RPO, LPO and AP positions are taken (following normal positioning descriptor as outlined in Ch. 34 and in Fig. 34.1), plus additional images if they provide useful information
- Further contrast filling may be necessary in order to allow the patient to micturate enough contrast agent to show the urethra during bladder voiding. Spot images may also be recorded during this action

Patient aftercare
- Cleanse the area and allow the patient to micturate further if they wish

Possible complications
- Urinary tract infection
- Urethral tear

Other methods for imaging the urinary system

US and CT
In the late 1970s, US technology advanced and improved with the introduction of B-mode scanning.[16] This enabled the clinician to investigate gross pathology of the kidney prior to IVU and established US as a 'safe' imaging tool, since it does not employ ionising radiation. It has replaced contrast radiography as a first line examination for the urinary system in many cases but the IVU is still used to confirm some features such as the site of ureteric obstruction or calculus size. In short, the US plus IVU approach remains for some circumstances but CT, as a stand-alone investigation, has certainly galloped ahead in others, especially in the acute situation.[3,17]

There is no doubt that as US technology improves, particularly with the introduction of microbubble contrast agents,[18] its place in urinary imaging is assured. Yet the picture constantly changes in light of advances in technology. Another study compared US and non-contrast helical CT in the diagnosis of renal calculi.[19] It was found that both types of investigation were equally excellent at detecting renal stones, but CT was also able to demonstrate more conclusively alternative pathology such as acute appendicitis. It was recommended therefore that all patients should have US in the first instance and those with inconclusive diagnoses or without access to US, should continue to have CT. However, support for the idea of CT becoming the investigation of choice in urinary imaging is evident in later work.[3] Much of the work published since 2000 compares either unenhanced helical CT or CT urography with conventional IVU, with the emphasis of the different studies most often related to image quality (diagnosis) and/or comparison of effective doses.[3,19,20,21] Studies mentioned agree that CT and IVU will both demonstrate calculi within the urinary system equally well, that CT will also demonstrate incidental but crucial pathology such as extraurinary malignant lesions not seen on IVU, and that effective dose is almost impossible to compare accurately between the two modalities.[21] This last point is the cause of much confusion and difficulty, due to the vagaries of patient size and shape, and the variances in technique in both IVU and CT protocols. Some researchers refer to the fact they are using low-dose non-enhanced helical CT, in an attempt to reduce patient dose.[22] However, it should be noted that in one study there was a reported increase in dose to the patient undergoing CT urography of three times that received during IVU.[23]

Until an accurate method of dose comparison is found, clinicians will still be aware of and concerned about the increase in dose to the patient during CT examination. This concern is always offset by the benefit to the patient, particularly if a CT procedure could highlight previously unsuspected life-threatening pathology or differential diagnosis, and so the responsibility in justification lies with the referring clinician and the imaging department. Recent developments in CT are helping this imaging modality provide information on aspects of the urinary system that it was previously unable to provide. Indeed it has been suggested that it is becoming more of a contender for the 'single renal imaging test' and is likely to replace IVU 'within the next several years' although radiation dose still remains an issue.[3]

There *are* other advantages of using CT over IVU, the most obvious one being the ability to produce diagnostic images without contrast agent (unenhanced CT) and its associated risks. One of the biggest attractions of CT urography has to be the exciting 3D image reconstructions now available. Advances in medical software mean that information gained through coronal sectional imaging can be digitally reconfigured to produce accurate anatomy/pathology that can be viewed from any angle on a computer screen.

Magnetic resonance imaging (MRI)
The role of MRI should not be forgotten in this debate, particularly regarding the concern of associated risk of radiation dose to the patient. MRI is a relative newcomer in urinary imaging and has been used to demonstrate ureteric dilatation and obstruction.[24] It is not as accurate as other modalities in the diagnosis of small calculi due to the bright signal received from urine, which can obscure tiny stones. The place of MRI in this type of investigation is governed mainly by the patient and their suitability, or unsuitability, for other techniques. If the use of contrast agent or ionising radiation is contraindicated (e.g. in children or pregnant women), MRI is a possible alternative although not all patients can tolerate the procedure if they are claustrophobic;[25] it is also contraindicated in the early stages of pregnancy.

RNI
Renal function is effectively assessed by use of radionuclide imaging, this probably being the most appropriate imaging technique for this. It can differentiate between obstructive uropathy and non-obstructive dilation of the renal pelvis, delineate areas of renal scarring due to infection and can localise ectopic kidneys after US fails to find its location. Its ability to assess function is useful in the assessment of transplanted kidneys. It can also assess vesicoureteric reflux, providing a less invasive and less

traumatic diagnostic tool than cystography since it does not involve urethral catheterisation.

UTERUS AND UTERINE TUBES (FALLOPIAN TUBES)

Hysterosalpingography (HSG)

This is assessment of the anatomy of the uterus and uterine (fallopian) tubes, undertaken under fluoroscopic control. Spot images are recorded.

Referral criteria
- Infertility – to check for patency of uterine (fallopian) tubes
- Recurrent spontaneous abortion (miscarriage)
- To assess patency of uterine tubes after reversal of female sterilisation
- It is possible that the procedure may have a therapeutic effect and clear obstructed uterine tubes

Contraindications
- Known or possible pregnancy
- Recent surgery
- Recent miscarriage
- Recent infection such as pelvic inflammataory disease or salpingitis

Contrast agent
- Approximately 20 mL HOCM or LOCM 280–300mgI/mL

Additional equipment
- Sterile towels
- 20 mL syringe
- Filling tube for contrast agent
- Sterile gloves
- Gauze swabs
- Antiseptic skin wash and sterile receptacle
- Vaginal speculum
- Vulsellum forceps
- Uterine cannula or Foley catheter
- Incontinence pads
- A portable anglepoise light will help with visualisation of the cervix
- Sanitary pad

Patient preparation
- Prior to attending for the examination the patient is advised to use contraception from their last period and up to the examination, or abstain from sexual intercourse. Alternatively, the '10-day rule' is applied and the patient is only examined in this 10-day safe period after menstruation. However, some practitioners are reluctant to undertake the examination close to menstruation (within 4 days of menstruation), to avoid the risk of extravasation or intravasation of contrast agent via the uterine endometrium.[9] If the 10-day rule is to be employed in conjunction with this second rule, the patient can only be examined during days 5 to 10 of their menstrual cycle, providing a very narrow window of time for this examination. On arrival, the radiographer should ascertain that information on pregnancy status is correct
- The patient may feel more comfortable if they micturate before the examination
- The procedure is explained, stressing that staff will observe privacy rights of the patient. It will also be helpful to indicate that the procedure may be uncomfortable, rather than painful

Technique
- The area is cleansed and the speculum inserted to allow for location of the cervix
- The vagina and cervix are cleansed
- It may be necessary to stabilise the position of the cervix with the vulsellum forceps before using the cannula. The cannula or catheter is inserted into the external os of the cervix and the contrast agent injected into the uterus. The speculum is removed, although sometimes it may be left in place if secure cannulisation of the cervix is at risk
- Filling of the uterine cavity is observed under pulsed or intermittent fluoroscopy
- Spot images are recorded in the AP position; when the contrast agent is seen to reach the uterine cornua, when it starts to fill the fallopian (uterine) tubes, and then when the contrast agent has filled the tubes, spilling into the peritoneal cavity (Fig. 36.15)
- The cannula or catheter is removed and the area is wiped with gauze swabs

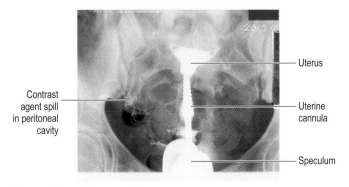

Contrast agent spill in peritoneal cavity — Uterus — Uterine cannula — Speculum

Figure 36.15   Hysterosalpingogram

Patient aftercare

- Give advice on using analgesia if she has low abdominal discomfort or slight cramps; advise that slight aching is not a matter for concern
- Provide the patient with a sanitary pad
- Explain that slight bleeding is possible and may last for a few days
- Advise that heavy bleeding or clotting is not normal and medcial help should be sought if these occur

Possible complications

- Trauma to the vagina or cervix
- Severe abdominal cramps
- Extravasation/intravasation of contrast agent via the endometrium to the uterine veins; this creates the risk of embolus
- Infection

References

1. RCR Working Party. Making the best use of a department of radiology: guidelines for doctors. 5th edn. London: The Royal College of Radiologists; 2003.
2. Prezioso D, et al. Lifestyle in patients with LUTS suggestive of BPH. European Urology 2001; 40(suppl 1): 9–12.
3. Noroozian M, et al. Multislice CT urography: state of the art. British Journal of Radiology 2004; 77:74–86.
4. Harvey C, et al. Renal imaging. Medicine 2003; 31(5):18–29.
5. Hellstrom, et al. Clinical and radiological renal characteristics of patients with terminal uraemia. Scandinavian Journal of Urology and Nephrology 2002; 36(6):455–463.
6. Irani J, et al. Obesity in relation to prostate cancer: risk comparison with a population having benign prostatic hyperplasia. BJU International 2003; 90(6):482–483.
7. Unett EM, Royle AJ Radiographic techniques and image evaluation. London: Chapman & Hall; 1997.
8. Whitley AS, et al. Clark's special procedures in diagnostic imaging. Oxford: Butterworth Heinemann; 1999.
9. Chapman S, Nakielny R. A guide to radiological procedures. 4th edn. Edinburgh: Saunders; 2001.
10. White P, McKay JC. The specialist radiographer – does the role justify the title? Radiography 2004; 10(3):217–227.
11. Freeman C. Role development revisited. London: The College of Radiographers; 2003.
12. Smith T, et al. Comparison of radiation dose from intravenous urology and $^{99}Tc^{m}$ DMSA scintigraphy in children. British Journal of Radiology 1998; 71:314–319.
13. The Ionising Radiation (Medical Exposure) Regulations 2000. London: HMSO.
14. Statutory Instrument 1999 No. 3232. The Ionising Radiations Regulations 1999. HMSO: United Kingdom.
15. European Commission Directorate-General for the Environment 2000. Referral guidelines for imaging. Radiation protection 118.
16. Goldman S, Sandler C. Genitourinary imaging: the past 40 years. Radiology 2000; 215:313–324.
17. Collins MC, Rosario DJ. Emergency uroradiology. Imaging 2001; 13:100–111.
18. Blomley MJK, et al. Microbubble contrast agents: a new era in ultrasound. British Medical Journal 2001; 322:1222–1225.
19. Patlas M. Ultrasound vs CT for the detection of ureteric stones in patients with renal colic. British Journal of Radiology 2001; 74:901–904.
20. Cadili E, et al. Urinary tract abnormalities: initial experiences with multidetector row CT urography. Radiology 2002; 222:353–360.
21. Ng CS, et al. Evaluation of early abdominopelvic computed tomography in patients with acute abdominal pain of unknown cause: prospective randomised study. British Medical Journal 2002; 325:1387.
22. Liu W, et al. Low dose nonenhanced helical CT of renal colic: assessment of ureteric stone detection and measurement of effective dose equivalent. Radiology 2000; 215:51–54.
23. Rimondini M, et al. Effective dose in X ray examinations: comparison between unenhanced helical CT (UHCT) and intravenous urography (IVU) in the evaluation of renal colic. European College of Radiology; proceedings of ECR 2002: presentation C 0732.
24. Sudah M, et al. Patients with acute flank pain: comparison of MR urography with unenhanced helical CT. Radiology 2002; 223:98–105.
25. Maher MM. Spinal dysraphism at MR urography: initial experience. Radiology 2000; 216:237-241.

CARDIOVASCULAR SYSTEM

Mark Cowling, Colin Monaghan

INTRODUCTION

This chapter will consider diagnostic angiography and venography. There are now several non-invasive methods available for evaluation of the cardiovascular system such as doppler ultrasound, computed tomography angiography (CTA) and magnetic resonance angiography (MRA). However, intraarterial angiography, occasionally intravenous digital subtraction angiography, and venography remain important diagnostic tools, which are likely to remain in clinical use for some years to come. Indeed, although it is invasive, intraarterial angiography has the benefit of being able to proceed directly to intervention should that be appropriate.

EQUIPMENT

Digital subtraction angiography (DSA) has been available for over 15 years, and in the UK almost all hospitals undertaking this kind of work have acquired such systems. However, it is noteworthy that in the recent NCEPOD (National Confidential Enquiry into Perioperative Deaths)[1] report on interventional vascular radiology, it was reported that 8% of hospitals in the UK were still undertaking vascular work on barium screening systems. It is not clear how many of these lack DSA, but it is likely that a number do.

All dedicated DSA units now have the X-ray tube and image intensifier mounted on a 'C-arm', allowing oblique views to be obtained easily without moving the patient. When angiographic images are acquired (often referred to as an angiographic run), a number of images are obtained before the injection of contrast intraarterially; these are used as mask images. Contrast is then injected and the arteries are opacified. The mask image is then subtracted from the contrast images. All detail on the mask, such as

bone, is thus removed from subsequent images leaving only the contrast opacifying the vessels on the image. Although the spatial resolution of this technique is a little less than that for traditional film-based angiography, this is more than compensated for by the much greater contrast resolution. In other words, the finer detail is not obscured by overlying structures such as bone. Digital acquisition of the image data means that the subtraction process is performed by computer, and the subtracted images are available in real time.

In general DSA is an excellent technique, but there can be problems with image quality, particularly caused by patient movement. One method of dealing with this is to use a facility termed pixel shifting. This involves using the computer to move the mask and contrast images relative to one another such that they are properly aligned, removing misregistration artefact (Fig. 37.1). This method of image processing is most suited to movement in relatively simple anatomical structures such as a limb, and also in situations where movement has only been slight. More extreme movements can be very difficult, if not impossible, to correct by pixel shifting. This is because pixel shifting involves a simple translation of image data in two dimensions, whereas patient movement actually occurs in three dimensions, often involving a degree of rotation, rather than pure translation.

Further degradation of image quality can be encountered due to the patient breathing during an acquisition, and due to bowel peristalsis. The former can be problematic in both the chest and the abdomen, and pixel shifting is of little value. It may prove necessary to perform the angiographic run again, but if a patient is very ill (the most common reason for being unable to suspend respiration adequately) it is often more helpful to acquire a larger number of masks than normal while the patient is breathing gently and 're-mask' each image to improve the diagnostic quality. This involves changing to a different mask whilst looking at a

Figure 37.1
(A) Digital subtraction arteriogram of distal calf showing misregistration artefact due to patient movement; (B) after pixel shifting the image quality is much improved

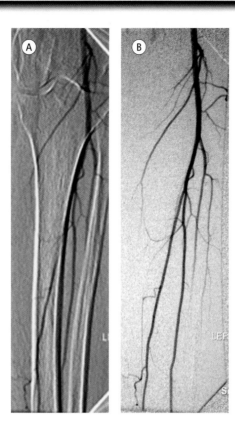

single contrast image. The mask giving the least degree of misregistration artefact is chosen.

Misregistration due to bowel movement can cause marked degradation of images of the abdominal aorta and its branches, as well as the iliac arteries. In addition, it is nearly impossible to obtain images of diagnostic quality when undertaking mesenteric arteriography for gastrointestinal bleeding. Misregistration caused by gut peristalsis can be largely prevented by administering buscopan (hyoscine-N-butylbromide) 20 mg either intravenously or through the arteriography catheter. This abolishes peristalsis for about 15 minutes, improving the quality of arteriographic images in the abdomen and pelvis. With regard to images obtained during mesenteric angiography for acute gastrointestinal bleeding, misregistration of bowel loops can give the impression of contrast extravasation into the lumen where there is none. Buscopan can be very helpful and should be administered, but overall it is also best to review the images without subtraction in order to avoid misdiagnosis.

Other techniques have been used previously to try to avoid problems with gut misregistration. For example, compression of the abdomen with a balloon between the patient and the image intensifier could be used to displace bowel loops laterally. However, such methods can no longer be employed because of the presence of proximity sensors within the equipment that prevent it from moving if in contact with the patient or any other object.

TECHNIQUE

Points of access for arteriography

Arteriography is most commonly performed by introducing a catheter through the common femoral artery in the groin. If this is not possible, the preferred route is to use the brachial artery at the level of the elbow joint. Alternatives include the radial artery, high brachial and axillary routes. Translumbar aortography, involving direct puncture of the abdominal aorta is no longer practised in the UK.

The transfemoral approach

This involves administration of local anaesthetic to the skin and deeper tissues, followed by the insertion of an arterial puncture needle. A suitable guidewire is introduced through the needle into the vessel. It is usual to observe the passage of the wire superiorly through the iliac arteries into the abdominal aorta with fluoroscopy. This is helpful because it is possible for the guidewire to enter the inferior epigastric artery rather than the external iliac artery. This problem is immediately obvious if observed on fluoroscopy, and can be corrected. It should be noted, however, that as operators become more experienced and used to the 'feel' of the guidewire in the vessel, they may undertake little or no screening during this part of the procedure unless they encounter resistance to the passage of the guidewire.

The guidewire may fail to advance satisfactorily for a variety of reasons. Sometimes this can be resolved simply by repositioning the needle tip so that backflow of blood is improved, indicating that the needle tip has been positioned more ideally within the vessel lumen. However, on other occasions it may be necessary to screen over the needle tip while the operator is manipulating the puncture needle, and possibly even injecting contrast. At such times the primary beam is very near the operator's hands. It is important that, and very helpful if, the screening radiographer remains vigilant and collimates as closely as possible to the needle tip to reduce the chances of the operator's hands entering the primary beam.

Once the guidewire has been correctly introduced into the aorta, the needle is removed, leaving the guidewire in place, and a suitable catheter or sheath is introduced over the guidewire. The next stage in the procedure will depend very much on the examination to be performed, and will be dealt with below.

Complications of the transfemoral route are minimal during diagnostic arteriography, though the recommended upper limit for complications is as high as 3%.[2]

The transbrachial route

This route is very useful if the femoral pulses are impalpable. The complication rate associated with this route of access is in fact quite low, and it would be quite reasonable to use it routinely, and may even have advantages for outpatient or day case angiography. However, it is used much less frequently than the transfemoral route, probably because it is technically more demanding and therefore a little more time consuming, and also because of concerns about placing a catheter across the origin of the left vertebral artery. The technique is very similar to that described above for the transfemoral route. However, a vascular sheath is used to facilitate administration of antispasmodic and anticoagulant drugs during the procedure, as these are considered to reduce the incidence of brachial artery occlusion.

Most arterial territories can be examined using the transbrachial route, although the manipulations required are often more difficult because the catheters tend to be longer. In general the left brachial approach will be used wherever possible, as this avoids placing the catheter across the origins of the great vessels, with the associated potential for formation of pericatheter thrombus and consequent embolic stroke. Most frequently the femoral arteries will be examined, and this involves placing the catheter inferiorly into the descending thoracic aorta and distally into the abdominal aorta. Although the initial brachial puncture and vascular sheath insertion can usually be achieved without fluoroscopy, when passing a pigtail catheter proximally into the brachial and subsequently axillary artery it is not at all uncommon for the catheter and guidewire to enter branches such as the circumflex humeral arteries. It is therefore necessary to use fluoroscopy to follow the passage of the catheter and guidewire.

It can be difficult to screen sufficiently laterally, and careful positioning of the patient before the start of the procedure is important. The more modern angiographic tables are able to pivot laterally; moving the table in this way can be very helpful. Once the catheter and guidewire have reached the origin of the subclavian artery, the operator will manipulate the catheter into the descending aorta. Depending on the tortuosity of the vessels this may be relatively difficult. One of the issues is the proximity of aerated lung to the aortic arch, which can make the catheter very difficult to see. Use of filters, collimators and sometimes magnification can be very helpful in improving visibility. In addition, on modern angiographic units with pulsed fluoroscopy, it can occasionally be helpful to raise the pulse rate which will often improve image quality.

Complications of brachial puncture for diagnostic arteriography are also said to be low, with a rate of up to 0.3% requiring surgery being reported.[3] Minor complications not requiring surgery and resolving spontaneously have been reported as 8–15%.[3,4]

Other routes of access

Other routes of access are now much less commonly used. The axillary and high brachial routes were associated with a relatively high incidence of haematoma formation and occasional consequent nerve damage (up to 2.4%),[5,6] due to difficulty in achieving adequate compression. The translumbar route is no longer used in the UK, because of the high incidence of retroperitoneal bleeding, need for general anaesthetic and lack of flexibility for performing selective arteriography. Of the other routes mentioned at the beginning of this section, the transradial approach has found favour with many cardiologists. However, although radiologists have used this approach for arteriography, it has not entered widespread use.[7]

Intravenous DSA

This involves injection of a large bolus of contrast, typically 50 mL, into a catheter placed directly into the right atrium. Performing multiple runs, for example during a femoral arteriogram can therefore involve giving very large volumes of contrast. In addition, in the presence of poor cardiac function the images are frequently suboptimal. In general the images are of less good quality than those obtained using a direct arterial injection, but when DSA first entered clinical use this method represented a less invasive alternative to using arterial access.

However, non-invasive vascular imaging is now so improved, that intravenous DSA is rarely required. Where arteriography is required to supplement non-invasive vascular imaging, the quality of intravenous DSA is usually inadequate for the purpose and adds little to the information already available.

ARTERIAL TERRITORIES EXAMINED

A variety of arterial territories can be examined, and the indications for each vary slightly. This section will discuss the approach to the examination of the various different territories, and where relevant, will describe differences in technique according to the indication for the examination.

Femoral arteriography

This describes examination of the abdominal aorta, iliac arteries and arteries of the lower limbs. This procedure is almost exclusively undertaken to demonstrate arterial stenoses and/or occlusions causing intermittent claudication or critical lower limb ischaemia (Fig. 37.2). It is the most commonly performed peripheral arteriogram at the time of writing.

The patient lies supine on the angiographic table, and their legs are placed as close together as possible. Some angiographic systems required the placement of lead rubber filters between and lateral to the legs. This reduces the variability in exposure across the field and will help to diminish flare. The filters also help to support the lower limbs and keep them still during acquisitions. Other devices for providing limb support, such as bean bags, are also available.

Having gained arterial access, the catheter, typically a pigtail, is positioned within the abdominal aorta. Contrast is then introduced using a pressure injector. Exact protocols for injection vary. A typical protocol is to administer 25 mL of a non-ionic, iodine-based contrast medium, 300 mg I mL^{-1}, at 10 mL per second. The pressure is set at 750 psi with a rise time of 0.5 seconds.

With many angiographic systems it is necessary to image the lower limb vessels in sections. Thus an abdominal aortogram will be performed, followed by a pelvic view to image the iliac vessels and so on until the entire lower limb down to the foot has been imaged.

This is a disadvantage over the traditional film changer systems, where a bolus of contrast was administered, a series of views taken in one position, the table then automati-

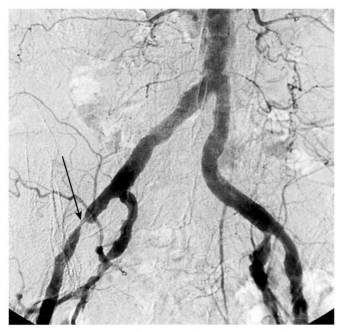

Figure 37.2 Pelvic view from a digital subtraction arteriogram showing a severe focal stenosis of the right external iliac artery (arrow)

cally moved to the next position, another set of films exposed and so on until the whole lower limb was imaged. This allowed only about 70 mL of contrast to be used, rather than approximately 150 mL for an equivalent DSA examination acquiring images at individual levels.

Of course, the traditional non-subtracted, film-based systems did not allow imaging in real time, meaning that if there were a significant difference in flow rates down the two lower limbs, only the vessels in one of them might successfully be imaged. In addition it is possible to dilute the contrast used in a DSA examination, making the doses similar.

Newer systems have attempted to address this issue with 'bolus chasing'. Precise protocols vary between manufacturers, but the principle involves obtaining mask images along the entire length of both legs and then injecting a single bolus of contrast and following this as it flows distally along the lower limb vessels. The flow of contrast can be monitored in real time, meaning that the table movement can be slowed or hastened appropriately. Some systems also allow the speed of table movement to be set up automatically, depending on the time taken for a test bolus of contrast to reach the popliteal artery. Regardless of the method used, however, the system will provide subtracted images along the entire length of the lower limbs.

Although this facility is useful, the image quality is less good than that provided by static images, examining a single area at a time, because the signal to noise ratio is reduced. However, by using bolus chasing to perform an overall 'survey' of the lower limb vasculature, followed by static images over areas of concern, it is possible to reduce the overall contrast dose.

The C-arm allows appropriate oblique views to be performed. This can be most useful in the iliac arteries where either the PA view has shown no abnormality when a lesion is suspected clinically, or where there is a suspicion of a stenosis on the PA view and confirmation of its location and severity is required. If the right iliac arteries are to be imaged then a left anterior oblique (LAO) projection is used, and if the left iliac arteries are to be examined a right anterior oblique (RAO) projection is used. An angulation of approximately 30° produces the best results.

Another area that is often shown poorly on the standard PA images is the origin of the profunda femoris artery. In this instance, LAO is used for the left side and RAO for the right side, with an angulation of 25–30%.

Renal arteriography

The renal arteries arise from the abdominal aorta. Their positions and number are variable, though they most frequently arise at the level of the L1/L2 vertebral bodies, and there is usually a single artery to each kidney. However, it is not at all unusual for a kidney to be supplied by two arteries, and they may be even more numerous than this. Furthermore, when the aorta is considered in cross-section, each artery may arise either from the anterior or posterior quadrant. The most common arrangement is for the left renal artery to arise from the left posterior quadrant, and the right renal artery to originate from the right anterior quadrant. However, this is also very variable.

Such anatomical variability requires scrupulous angiographic technique to ensure that every part of every renal artery is imaged. The most common indication for renal arteriography is to search for possible renal artery stenosis. In the majority of patients the cause for this is atheroma, and such lesions are most frequently located at the origin of the renal artery. Therefore, flush aortography is used at least initially, and there may be no need to go on to selective arteriography for diagnosis.

The pigtail catheter is positioned in the abdominal aorta at about the level of the L1 vertebral body. The image is centred such that the entire abdominal aorta is imaged. Around 30 mL of a non-ionic, iodine-based contrast medium, 300 mgI mL^{-1}, is administered at 15 mL/second, and images are acquired at two or three frames per second (Fig. 37.3). The first acquisition allows the number of

renal arteries to be assessed, and may provide some information regarding the presence of stenoses. However, stenosis cannot be excluded until the renal artery origins have been satisfactorily visualised, and this almost always requires oblique views; magnification is also often helpful. Both LAO and RAO images centred on the renal arteries are obtained. Typically an angulation of 15° may be used, however sometimes different angulations are required.

If selective arteriography is required, for example in the event of doubt about the presence of stenosis especially if fibromuscular dysplasia is suspected, or because of bleeding from the kidney, a selective catheter will be introduced into the vessel origin, and having centred on the individual artery, contrast is injected by hand while images are acquired.

Mesenteric arteriography (Fig. 37.4)

This is most commonly performed to identify a bleeding source, but may also be undertaken to identify stenoses or occlusions in the mesenteric vessels of patients suspected of suffering from gut ischaemia. In the case of the latter, an abdominal aortogram is performed in the same way as for the renal arteries, but a lateral view is performed to profile the mesenteric vessel origins.

In the case of mesenteric arteriography performed for gastrointestinal bleeding, selective arteriograms are performed on each individual vessel. Injection into the coeliac axis and the superior mesenteric artery is best performed with a pump, delivering around 20 mL of contrast media at 6 mL per second. The inferior mesenteric artery is generally a smaller vessel, and is imaged using a hand injection. The operator may well advance the catheter more distally into the vessel to perform superselective injections. These will also be performed by hand, and will require magnified views.

Cardiac arteriography

This is the radiological demonstration of not only the heart's structure but also its function. Routinely only the left ventricle, ascending aorta and both coronary arteries are studied. In order to reduce complications and risks, cardiac studies require constant monitoring of arterial pressures and ECG waveforms.[8,9] This often requires the presence of electrocardiogram (ECG) technicians and it is quite common for these examinations to be performed by cardiologists.

High quality fluoroscopic imaging equipment is essential, preferably using a biplane system. Biplane systems can reduce procedural times and the amount of contrast used. However, rotational or 'spin' angiographic techniques can also be effective.[10] High acquisition frame rates are essential, with all major equipment manufacturers offering cardiac

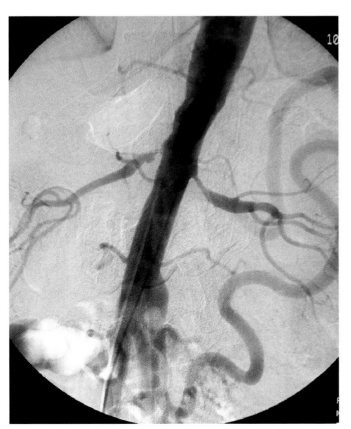

Figure 37.3 Frontal view from a digital subtraction abdominal aortagram showing severe bilateral renal artery stenosis

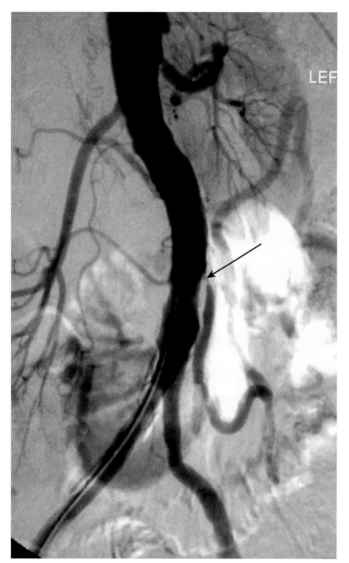

Figure 37.4 RAO view (70°) of the abdominal aorta showing a severe stenosis of the inferior mesenteric artery. The coeliac axis and superior mesenteric artery were occluded, and the patient was suffering from symptoms of mesenteric ischaemia

units with exposure rates between 10–50 frames per second. Arterial access is traditionally via the femoral approach although radial approaches are not uncommon.

Ventriculography

A pigtail catheter is guided through the aortic valve and positioned midchamber in the left ventricle. Correct positioning is essential to avoid complications (tachycardia or myocardiac staining) or misleading results (forced mitral valve regurgitation).

Ventriculography is usually limited to two projections. RAO 30° and LAO 60° will demonstrate ventricular wall motion. A lateral projection is more useful in assessing mitral valve regurgitation.

A pressure injector should be used to deliver a bolus of contrast agent. 30 mL at 10 mL per second is sufficient to assess ventricular function.

Aortography

The same pigtail catheter can be withdrawn and positioned just above the aortic valve in order to perform an aortogram. Aortography is also usually limited to two projections.

LAO 60° or lateral projections are useful for demonstrating ascending aortic dissections. Both projections offer an open view of the aortic arch and the position of the neck vessels. RAO 30° is also helpful in delineating aortic dissections but can also demonstrate more of the descending thoracic aorta.

Two projections will also allow assessment of any aneurysmal dilatations and the competency of the aortic valve.

A pressure injection of contrast agent should be used. Parameters of 40 mL of contrast at 20 mL per second are not uncommon.

Coronary arteriography

The coronary arteries are cannulated using separate selective catheters. The positioning of the catheters is crucial to avoid occluding the artery or mimicking and/or camouflaging osteal diseases.[9]

The non-linear and oblique courses of the coronary arteries necessitate a number of different angiographic projections. The number of projections will vary from patient to patient. The following projections are commonly used and will adequately demonstrate the coronary anatomy:

- Left coronary artery: PA, lateral, RAO 30°, LAO 60°. RAO 30° with caudal 30°, LAO 60° with cranial 30°
- Right coronary artery: RAO 30°, LAO 60°, PA, lateral

Power injections of contrast can be used and are as safe as hand injections. However, hand injections offer advantages and flexibility for rapid repeat injections.

5–10 mL at 3–4 mL per second are commonly used.

Upper limb arteriography

This is infrequently required, as arterial pathology in the upper limb is much less frequent than in the lower limb. However, conditions such as subclavian steal (due to subclavian arterial occlusion), damage to the vessel because of trauma from cervical ribs or peripheral embolus may require arteriography. The examination will start with an arch aortogram, followed by selective catheterisation of the relevant subclavian artery, with views obtained along the length of the arm.

Venography

Until the 1990s, venography was most commonly performed in the lower limb for diagnosis of deep vein thrombosis (DVT). DVT can now almost always be diagnosed or excluded on the basis of Doppler ultrasound, and venography is only rarely required. Once a vein on the dorsum of the foot has been cannulated, and tourniquets applied just above the ankle and just above the knee, contrast is injected and images of the calf obtained in PA, RAO and LAO views. Then the knee tourniquet is removed and views of the popliteal, femoral and iliac veins are obtained. It is also possible to perform arm venography and superior vena-cavography using similar techniques (Fig. 37.5).

FUTURE DEVELOPMENTS

As mentioned in the introduction to this chapter, there have been major developments in non-invasive vascular imaging in recent years. Doppler ultrasound provides a non-invasive and relatively cheap method of assessing the vasculature. However it does not produce an anatomical map for the surgeon or interventional radiologist who will subsequently undertake treatment. CTA and MRA have

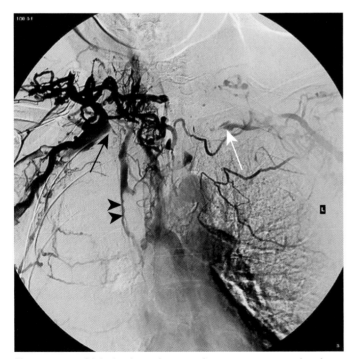

Figure 37.5 Digital subtraction superior vena cavagram showing occlusion of the right (black arrow) and left (white arrow) brachiocephalic veins. The superior vena cava is narrow and contains thrombus (double arrowheads). The underlying diagnosis was bronchogenic carcinoma

improved considerably in recent years, and may supplant purely diagnostic angiography in the near future.

With the advent of multislice technology, CTA can be undertaken over large anatomical areas, such as the entire thorax abdomen and pelvis, in a single breathold. Therefore, CTA has considerable advantages over DSA such as being non-invasive, using a lower overall contrast dose when assessing large areas, and also demonstrating information about structures beyond the lumen of the vessel. Thus, in the assessment of aneurysmal disease, the wall of the vessel and the true size of the aneurysm can be assessed. DSA can be misleading in this situation, as the presence of intramural thrombus can give a misleading impression of the size of the aneurysm. In addition, although CTA has the disadvantage over MRA of using ionising radiation, it has the advantage of being usable where MRI is contraindicated, e.g. if a patient has a pacemaker, and is less likely to cause claustrophobia. In addition, multislice CTA tends to be faster than MRA.

SUMMARY

Intraarterial angiography is a well-established and relatively safe technique for imaging the arterial tree. Where there has been evidence of substantial risk either locally, such as in the case of axillary artery puncture, or in the territory to be examined, such as the carotid arteries, other techniques or approaches have been employed.

The current mainstay of carotid artery imaging is Doppler ultrasound. However, this technique requires regular auditing to ensure that there is minimal inter- and intraobserver variation. Such audit becomes difficult to undertake if, as in many centres, carotid arteriography is no longer performed and surgeons are prepared to operate on duplex findings alone. This approach has the benefit of removing the potential stroke risk associated with carotid angiography for an individual patient but the hidden consequence is that if Doppler ultrasound results are inaccurate, some individuals may be treated inappropriately, and some requiring treatment may not receive it.

Despite progress in non-invasive vascular imaging techniques such as MRA, a large number of invasive arteriograms are still carried out in the UK. This is at least on the surface undesirable, as the costs in terms of bed days of this strategy are relatively high. However, a significant number of patients will be unsuitable for imaging on MRI, for example due to having cardiac pacemakers, claustrophobia or other contraindications. Furthermore, MRA lends itself very much to planned outpatient type work, such as may be undertaken in patients with intermittent claudication.

However, many such patients do not require imaging at all, as there is little evidence to support treatment in this group unless their exercise tolerance is less than 100 metres. Patients with acute or chronic critical limb ischaemia require either urgent or, at the very least, prompt imaging and management to prevent limb loss. Due to the availability of MRA in the UK most centres would find it difficult to provide such a non-invasive service on this basis. In addition, due to its tendency to overestimate the severity of vascular lesions, there may be confusion between severe stenosis or occlusion in a vessel. Such a distinction can be critical in deciding whether to employ open surgical or endovascular therapy.

Using intraarterial angiography in this clinical situation has the advantages of better distinction of stenosis versus occlusion, though it can still prove difficult to identify distal vessels, and of being able to proceed directly to endovascular therapy if that is appropriate.

One area in which MRA has proved invaluable is in the evaluation of patients suspected of having atheromatous renal artery stenosis. This avoids catheter manipulations in the aorta and the potentially nephrotoxic contrast administration of intraarterial angiography. Non-invasive imaging is very attractive in evaluation of the renal arteries, as there are no reliable clinical or biochemical tests for exclusion of atheromatous renal artery stenosis. However, one of the dangers of having access to a safe and reliable imaging technique such as this is a marked increase in demand.

References

1. Callum K, Whimster F. Interventional vascular radiology and interventional neurovascular radiology. A Report of the National Confidential Enquiry into Perioperative Deaths. November 2000.
2. Royal College of Radiologists. Standards in Vascular Radiology 1999. Ref BFCR(99)9.
3. Gritter K, et al. Complications of outpatient transbrachial intra-arterial digital subtraction angiography. Work in progress. Radiology 1987; 162:125–127.
4. Heenan S, et al. Transbrachial arteriography: indications and complications. Clinical Radiology 1996; 51:205–209.
5. Chitwood R, et al. Surgical complications of transaxillary arteriography: a case control study. Journal of Vascular Surgery 1996; 23:844–849.
6. McIvor J, Rhymer J. 245 transaxillary arteriograms in arteriopathic patients: success rate and complications. Clinical Radiology 1992; 45:390–394.
7. Cowling M, et al. The role of transradial diagnostic angiography. Cardiovascular and Interventional Radiology 1997; 20:103–106.
8. Noto T, et al. Cardiac catheterisation 1990: a report of the Registry of the Society for Cardiac Angiography and Interventions. Catheterization and Cardiovascular Diagnosis 1991; 24:75–83.
9. Kern M. Cardiac catheterization handbook. St Louis: Mosby; 1999.
10. Raman S, et al. Rotational X-ray coronary angiography. Catheterization and Cardiovascular Interventions 2004; 63(2):201–207.

INTERVENTIONAL AND THERAPEUTIC PROCEDURES

Mark Cowling

INTRODUCTION

Interventional and therapeutic procedures undertaken in the medical imaging department accurately locate body structures before intervention and assess the progress and accuracy of the procedure to follow. Interventional procedures often use a contrast radiology approach (hence the inclusion in the contrast studies section of this text) but almost equally often use computed tomography (CT) or ultrasound (US). Use of magnetic resonance imaging (MRI) is also being initiated or considered as a medium for vascular intervention. Interventional and therapeutic procedures involve angioplasty, embolisation, dilation, stent or filter insertion, stone removal, and biopsy.

Peripheral angioplasty was first carried out in the femoral artery by Charles Dotter in the USA in 1964. He used coaxial catheters of progressively increasing sizes to widen the lumen of the vessel. Initial results were not as good as would be expected today; however the equipment available has progressively developed such that results of angioplasty are now vastly improved and a number of other techniques are available for treatment of vascular lesions.

In addition to angioplasty, other interventional vascular procedures available include embolisation in various arterial or venous territories and stent grafting for aneurysms.

VASCULAR INTERVENTIONAL PROCEDURES

Indications

The most common indication for interventional vascular procedures is limb ischaemia, usually of the lower limb.

This can present in a variety of ways, such as intermittent claudication (pain in the limb on exercise and relieved by rest), chronic critical limb ischaemia (e.g. causing ulcers) or acute limb ischaemia (causing pallor, coldness and numbness of the limb). The common feature is the presence of stenoses or occlusions within the arteries supplying blood to the limb. In general, the greater the severity of the vascular disease, the greater the severity of the symptoms. Limb ischaemia considered suitable for management by interventional radiological techniques can be treated in a variety of ways such as angioplasty, stent insertion and thrombolysis.

Embolisation, on the other hand, may be undertaken for a variety of reasons. First, there may be uncontrolled bleeding: for example, from the gastrointestinal tract, tumours in various sites and from the kidney, liver or other solid organs after trauma or biopsy. Embolisation is also useful in the treatment of some aneurysms. This is particularly true of aneurysms in the cerebral circulation, where coil embolisation may be used as an alternative to surgical aneurysm clipping to prevent recurrence of subarachnoid haemorrhage. Other indications include treatment of arteriovenous malformations and embolisation of the testicular vein for varicocoele. Uterine artery embolisation can be used for the treatment of uterine fibroids.

Stent grafting is used in the treatment of aneurysms. A true aneurysm of a vessel describes a situation where the vessel is abnormally dilated because of expansion of all three layers of the vessel wall, making it prone to rupture. When such an aneurysm is present in the abdominal aorta, rupture causes bleeding and is usually fatal without emergency surgery. Therefore, if an abdominal aortic aneurysm measuring 5.5 cm or greater in diameter is identified, it is usual for surgical aneurysm repair to be undertaken to remove the risk of rupture. From the 1990s on, stent grafts have been and continue to be developed, which may provide an alternative to open surgical repair, particularly in patients who are at high risk from open surgery. True aneurysms may also arise at other sites such as the thoracic aorta and iliac arteries, and may also be amenable to treatment by stent grafting.

A false aneurysm is not surrounded by normal vessel wall. Instead it represents the persistent leak of blood into a cavity surrounded by haematoma. They are most commonly seen as a result of trauma to the vessel, often due to iatrogenic injury, though may also arise due to erosion by tumours or due to the presence of infection in the vessel wall. Stent grafting may also be useful in the treatment of false aneurysms. However, if infection is thought likely to be present then a stent graft should not be implanted, as being of a foreign material its presence would make the infection impossible to eradicate. In deciding whether or not to use a stent graft the site of the false aneurysm should also be considered. For example, a false aneurysm arising from the common femoral artery (CFA) after arterial puncture is positioned directly over the hip joint: a stent graft implanted at this site would be subject to repeated stress and would eventually fail. False aneurysms at this site are therefore better treated with US guided injection of thrombin, which thromboses the false aneurysm.

ANGIOPLASTY

The basic principles of angioplasty are the same in whichever vascular territory they are to be applied. These will be described first, followed by important caveats with respect to different arterial territories.

Once an arterial stenosis requiring treatment has been identified, it is traversed with a suitable guidewire and catheter combination. In very narrow stenoses, which can be very difficult to cross, it can be extremely helpful to use the 'roadmap' facility available on modern digital subtraction angiography (DSA) equipment. This allows contrast to be injected whilst screening, and the image of the vessels to be retained on the monitor. When the screening pedal is next depressed, the image of the vessel remains superimposed over the real time image of the catheter and guidewire as they are being manipulated.

Once the lesion has been crossed it is an important principle that either a guidewire or a catheter should remain across it at all times until the procedure has been completed. When an angioplasty is undertaken, complications such as vessel dissection, occlusion due to acute thrombosis or distal embolisation, or even vessel rupture may occur. If a guidewire has been left across the lesion it is a comparatively simple matter to go on to manage the complication appropriately. If the guidewire has been removed from

across the lesion it may be possible to cross again, but this is often highly complex, is not always successful and may result in vessel dissection and irretrievable occlusion.

Angioplasty itself is undertaken using a balloon catheter designed for the purpose. Balloons are available in a wide variety of diameters and lengths to suit the vessel and lesion being treated. The majority of balloons have radioopaque markers at each end to facilitate the correct positioning of the device in relation to the stenosis (some have a marker in the middle). The balloon catheter is inserted through the vascular sheath over the guidewire, and advanced into the correct position. This can be done using the roadmap, or bony landmarks may be chosen to facilitate positioning. The balloon is then inflated to the correct pressure for 30 seconds in the first instance. It is then removed, leaving the guidewire in place, and an angiogram is performed to demonstrate the response. If the result of the angioplasty has been satisfactory, the guidewire can be safely removed. If the result is unsatisfactory, further balloon inflations may be undertaken, perhaps to a greater diameter or for a longer period of time, or, depending on the site a vascular stent may be inserted.

Iliac angioplasty

The results of iliac angioplasty are generally very good, with a low complication rate.[1,2] The procedure is sufficiently safe and successful and in many centres it is offered to patients who have intermittent claudication occurring after 100 m walking or less. It may also be of great value as an adjunct to surgery.[3] For example, if a lower limb bypass graft is to be undertaken, iliac angioplasty to a stenosis above the proposed site of the proximal anastomosis will improve the inflow of blood, making a successful bypass more likely and reducing the extent of the surgery required.

When undertaking an iliac angioplasty it is often possible to choose whether to approach the lesion ipsilaterally and retrogradely or contralaterally and antegradely. An ipsilateral approach, puncturing the artery on the side to be treated followed by crossing the stenosis in a retrograde fashion, offers an advantage: should a vessel dissection occur it is unlikely to lead to vessel occlusion, as the blood flow distally along the vessel will tend to close the intimal flap. The alternative, which involves puncturing the contralateral femoral artery, crossing the aortic bifurcation and then traversing the lesion is technically more demanding and if a dissection occurs the blood flow will tend to cause the intimal flap to extend potentially causing vessel occlusion.

Superficial femoral artery (SFA) angioplasty

This procedure is most commonly undertaken for the management of critical lower limb ischaemia or short distance intermittent claudication. Such ischaemia is most likely to be caused by SFA occlusion, rather than a simple stenosis; thus to perform an angioplasty one must first cross the occlusion with a guidewire. This can be difficult but the use of a hydrophilic guidewire, such as that produced by the Terumo Corporation of Tokyo, will facilitate successful crossing in the vast majority of cases, with a growing number of operators electing to pass the guidewire subintimally. SFA angioplasty is less commonly performed for treatment of intermittent claudication, as generally the results are inferior to those of iliac angioplasty,[4,5] and two randomised studies have shown that the results are no better over the long term than those observed after a supervised exercise programme.[6,7]

As with iliac angioplasty, SFA lesions can be approached either contralaterally or ipsilaterally. The contralateral approach is the same in technical terms as that used for the iliac vessels. However, the ipsilateral approach to the SFA is technically more difficult, as an antegrade puncture of the CFA is required. To perform an antegrade puncture, the femoral head is first identified under fluoroscopy and its position marked on the skin surface with a metal marker. Local anaesthetic is infiltrated into the skin over the femoral pulse as it is palpated at this level. A puncture needle is introduced first and a guidewire is then introduced along the SFA. It is possible that the guidewire may pass into the profunda femoris, and for this reason it is important to observe its progress under fluoroscopic control. If it proves difficult to enter the SFA, it may be necessary to screen over the needle tip whilst manipulating it into different positions to facilitate guidewire advancement. When doing this it is very easy for the operator to put their hands into

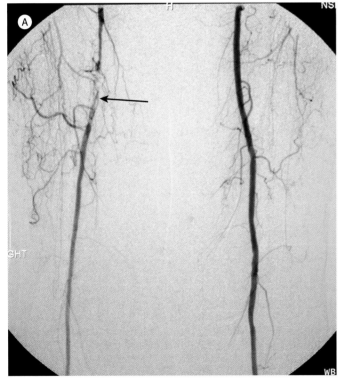
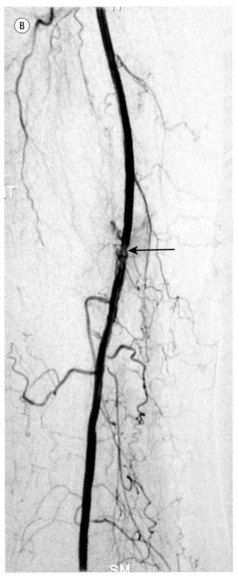

Figure 38.1 **(A)** Digital subtraction angiography (DSA) of superficial femoral and popliteal arteries – this image shows occlusion at the right adductor canal level (arrow) in a patient with critical ischaemia of the right foot. **(B)** angioplasty – the occlusion seen in (A) was crossed easily and there was a good result from angioplasty (arrow)

Continued

Figure 38.1 cont'd **(C)** embolus in the peroneal artery – best practice involves obtaining views of the distal vessels to look for any possible complication. This image shows an embolus occluding the peroneal artery and projecting across the origin of the posterior tibial artery (arrow). **(D)** peroneal artery post embolectomy – after aspiration embolectomy much of the embolus seen in (C) was removed. The posterior tibial artery is now patent, though it was not possible to clear the peroneal artery completely

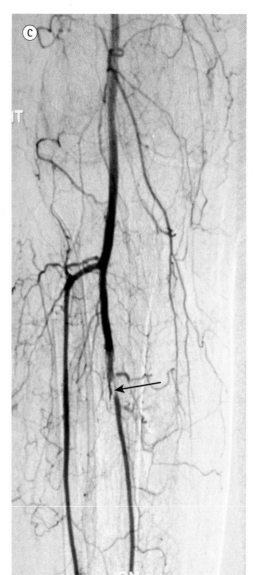
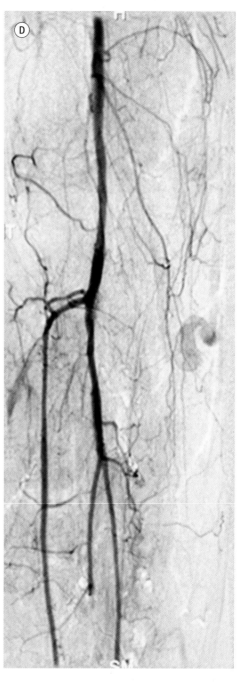

the X-ray beam without realising. The radiographer can prevent or minimise this by centring only on the very tip of the needle, rather than its whole length, and using the collimators appropriately. Antegrade puncture is often employed because the distance from the puncture site to the angioplasty site is short, avoiding the need to use very long guidewires. It also avoids any problems associated with catheter manipulation when dealing with tortuous iliac arteries or an acutely angled aortic bifurcation; in the event of a complication occurring, the subsequent management, e.g. aspiration embolectomy, is much more straightforward (Fig. 38.1C,D).

Popliteal artery and the tibial vessels

Lesions in these vessels will only be treated with angioplasty in the presence of critical lower limb ischaemia or short distance claudication (Fig. 38.2A,B). The potential benefit of angioplasty at these sites in patients with uncomplicated intermittent claudication would be completely outweighed by the potential risk and of the likely recurrence rate in the future.[8] Technically there is very little difference between angioplasty performed here or elsewhere in the lower limb. Smaller diameter balloons are used, and some operators prefer to use finer guidewires.

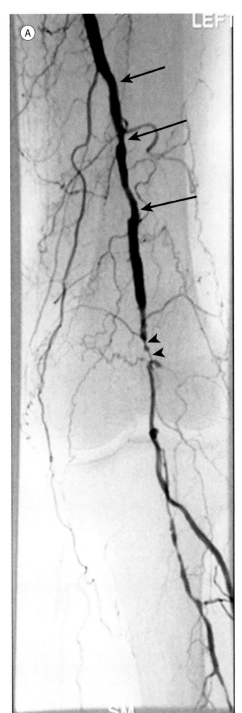

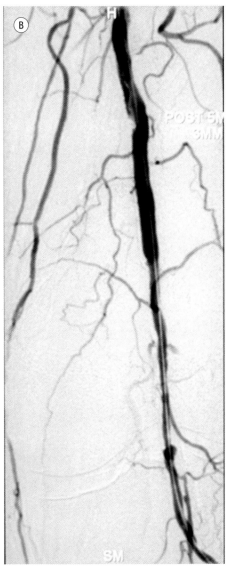

Figure 38.2   **(A)** Stenosis of popliteal artery – arteriogram demonstrating a stenotic segment of above knee popliteal artery (arrows) and a tight stenosis at the origin of the anterior tibial artery (arrowheads), which has an abnormally high take-off. **(B)** arteriogram post angioplasty – a good technical result after angioplasty in the case shown in (A)

VASCULAR STENT INSERTION

The term 'stent' describes a device designed to keep a passage or conduit open. Vascular stents have become accepted as devices that are extremely helpful both in maintaining patency where the result of angioplasty alone has been suboptimal, and in certain locations where they provide such markedly superior benefits in comparison with angioplasty alone, that they are considered to be the first line of treatment.

Vascular stents are metallic, commonly made either of stainless steel or nitinol. Nitinol is a nickel-titanium alloy which has great elasticity and 'shape memory' which allows it to return to its original state even after significant manipulation and bending. Stents of either kind may be self expanding or balloon expandable. Prior to deployment, stents are compressed onto a delivery catheter; each end of the stent either has radioopaque markers on the device itself or on the catheter, to facilitate correct positioning.

The technique used for deployment of a stent is much the same as that described for angioplasty, with the obvious difference that instead of performing simple balloon dilation, a stent is deployed instead. It will often prove necessary to perform angioplasty prior to stent deployment, and further angioplasty after deployment may be required to ensure that the stent is fully expanded.

Stents are used commonly in the iliac, renal and subclavian arteries. They are being used increasingly in the carotid arteries, although this remains experimental. In the UK, stents have only been employed in the SFA as a 'bail out' if angioplasty has resulted in vessel occlusion. However, stents have been used much more freely in the SFA elsewhere and evidence is starting to show, at least with more modern stent designs, that concerns about low long-term patency rates of stents in the SFA (when compared to those of angioplasty alone) may be unfounded. Stents are generally not used in the popliteal or tibial vessels.

Stenting the iliac artery (Fig. 38.3A,B)

It has been shown that if iliac angioplasty is technically successful, there is no advantage in terms of clinical outcome in adding a stent.[9,10,11] However, in about 50% of cases the outcome from angioplasty is suboptimal, due perhaps to elastic recoil of the vessel wall or dissection causing flow limitation. Many professionals would now add to this and comment on the failure to reduce the intra-arterial pressure gradient across the lesion to less than 10 mmHg.

The exception to this is the treatment of iliac artery occlusions where, if angioplasty alone is used, there is an incidence of up to 50% of peripheral embolisation.[9] For this reason, primary stenting is undertaken when treating iliac occlusions endovascularly. Thus, a self-expanding stent is first deployed across the occlusion, and is subsequently dilated using an angioplasty balloon.

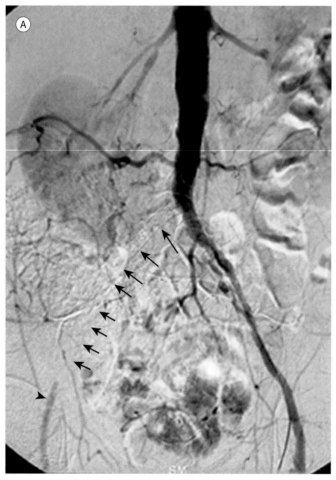
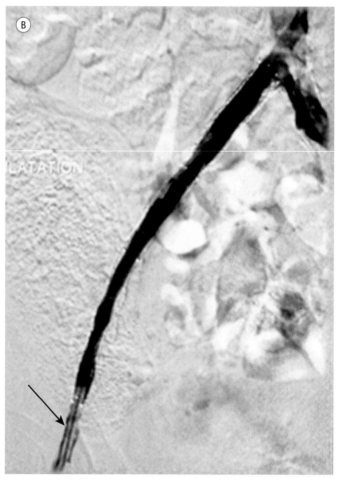

Figure 38.3 **(A)** Occluded common iliac artery – patient with rest pain in the right foot. A previous right common iliac stent is now occluded, along with the external iliac artery (arrows). There is reconstitution of the common femoral artery distally (arrowhead). **(B)** stenting the occlusion – The patient in (A) was considered a very poor risk for surgery. Therefore, the occlusion was successfully stented despite the fact that there was concern that the distal end of the stent would be very near the hip joint and might be damaged during hip flexion. There is a filling defect distally caused by the vascular sheath (arrow)

Stenting the renal artery (Fig. 38.4A,B)

Renal artery stenosis is generally caused by one of two pathologies – either fibromuscular hyperplasia or atheroma. Fibromuscular hyperplasia is an uncommon cause of uncontrollable hypertension, and responds well to angioplasty alone. Atheromatous renal artery stenosis (ARAS), when it requires treatment, responds very poorly to angioplasty alone, and it has clearly been demonstrated that primary stenting is superior both in the short and the longer term.[12] This happens because the vast majority of ARAS occurs at the origin of the vessel and is caused by aortic atheroma rather than true atheroma of the renal artery. Therefore, an expansile force applied to the stenosis causes shear stresses within the aortic plaque, rather than an expansile force within the renal artery lumen. Once the angioplasty balloon is removed the stenosis will frequently recur as the aortic plaque moves back into position.

Balloon expandable stents are favoured for the treatment of ARAS. In order to avoid the stent being compressed by the aortic plaques, it is necessary to position the stent so that it projects 2–3 mm into the aortic lumen. Such precision is much easier to achieve with balloon expandable stents, as they do not shorten when they are deployed. Although much improved over older designs, even modern self-expanding stents show some shortening.

Subclavian stenting

Although stenoses or occlusions can occur in the subclavian arteries at any point, by far the commonest site of disease is the origin of the left subclavian artery. The majority of these lesions are asymptomatic. However, where there are symptoms of arm claudication or subclavian steal syndrome, intervention may be indicated. Stents are frequently employed at this site, especially in the presence of arterial occlusion. However, there is little reliable published data in this area to allow firm conclusions to be drawn.

If there is occlusion at the origin of the left subclavian artery, it is usually very difficult indeed to cross the lesion using a catheter inserted via the groin. It is therefore often helpful to use a transbrachial approach. This may require a surgical cut-down onto the vessel, as sheaths of seven or eight French in size are required. Many angiography rooms in UK X-ray departments are not equipped to operating theatre standard, so careful attention needs to be paid to the area around the patient's arm to ensure that the conditions remain sterile in order to diminish the risk of wound infection.

VASCULAR STENT GRAFTS

As mentioned previously, stent grafts are used in the treatment of true or false aneurysms. The technology

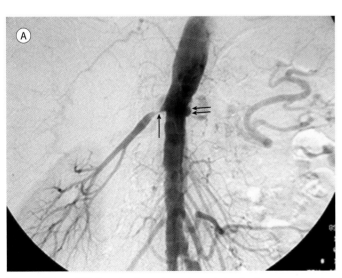

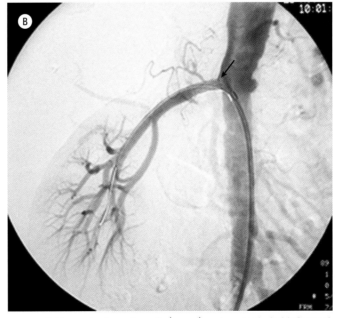

Figure 38.4 **(A)** Renal artery stenosis – abdominal aortogram showing severe right renal artery stenosis (arrow) and an occluded left renal artery (double arrow). **(B)** renal artery stent – the patient was experiencing episodes of flash pulmonary oedema and had deteriorating renal function and right renal artery stent was inserted (arrow) with good technical and clinical results, with improvement in cardiac failure and greatly improved renal function

continues to evolve, and it is not possible to say at this point in time whether stent grafting will replace open surgery in the treatment of aneurysmal disease. However, there is growing evidence to support the use of stent grafts in the treatment of thoracic aortic aneurysms, where the risks of surgery are considerably greater than the open surgical risks for abdominal aneurysms.[13] Furthermore, there is some evidence to suggest that stent grafting may be of value in patients who would be at greater than average risk for abdominal surgery, for example if they have renal failure.[14,15,16]

When used for aortic aneurysms, stent graft delivery systems are large, and require surgical exposure of one or both common femoral arteries. Smaller aneurysms, such as in the iliac arteries, can be treated without surgical exposure of vessels (Fig. 38.5A,B) Therefore, aortic stent graft procedures are frequently performed in the operating theatre with a mobile image intensifier. A better alternative, which is becoming increasingly available, is to use an angiographic suite that has been constructed to operating theatre standard. This provides a sufficiently sterile environment with a high standard of imaging.

Prior to the stent graft procedure the aneurysm is assessed for the diameter of the proximal and distal landing zones, as well as the overall length of the device. A number of 'off the shelf' devices are available on the market, and several manufacturers are able to supply custom made stent grafts for more complex cases.

Angiographic 'runs' are performed to ensure precise positioning of the device. For example, in the case of stent grafting of abdominal aortic aneurysms it is clearly vital to avoid covering (and therefore occluding) the renal arteries with graft material. However, there are devices that have a bare stent at the proximal end which is designed to lie over the renal arteries. Once an image has been selected as the reference image for the deployment of the device it is vital that the C-arm is not moved. Even slight movement can cause errors due to parallax, which could cause misplacement of the stent graft.

EMBOLISATION

Commonly used embolisation agents include gelatin sponge (for temporary embolisation), polyvinyl alcohol particles and coils (for permanent vessel occlusion). The full range of embolic materials available for clinical use is vast, complex and includes materials that would require a whole chapter to describe and explain in detail. Embolisation procedures are often complex and time consuming. They may require the use of superselective coaxial catheter systems, and multiple magnified views of the area are needed.

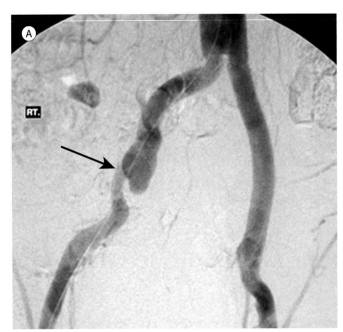

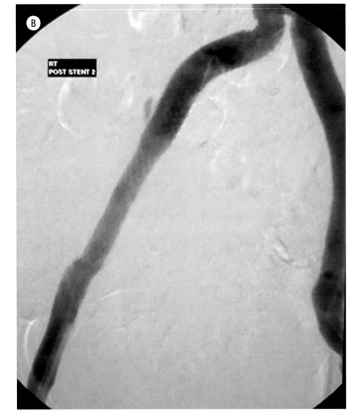

Figure 38.5 **(A)** External iliac aneurysm – this arteriogram shows a 3 cm diameter external iliac aneurysm arising at the distal end of an aorto-bi-iliac graft. **(B)** treating the aneurysm with stent graphs – the aneurysm seen in (A) was successfully treated with two balloon expandable stent grafts

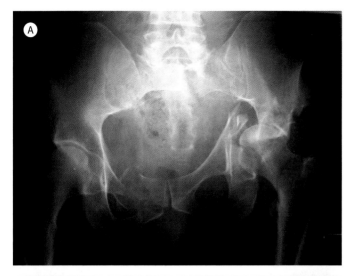

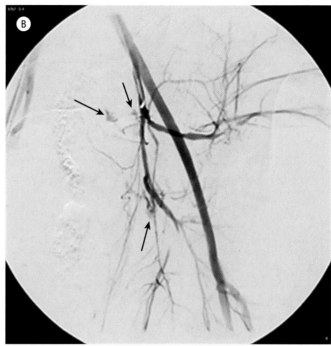

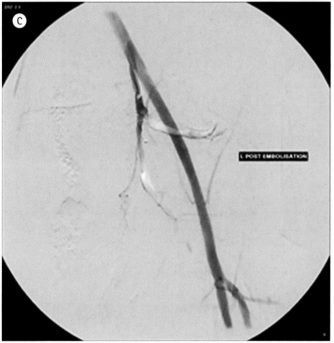

Figure 38.6 **(A)** Plain film showing very obvious pelvic fracture involving the left acetabulum and the pubic rami on the right. Pelvic fractures can be associated with severe bleeding, as was the case here, and angiography with a view to embolisation was performed. **(B)** iliac arteriogram after pelvic fracture – selective left internal iliac arteriogram showing at least three bleeding points (arrows) on the case seen in (A). Appearances were similar on the right side as well. **(C)** embolisation after trauma to internal iliac artery – the case seen in (A) and (B) after embolisation with gelatin sponge; no further bleeding is seen

The basic principle of embolisation is to identify the target vessel and place the catheter tip in the correct location prior to introducing the embolic material. Generally one would wish to place the catheter as far distally as possible to avoid embolisation of normal tissue. In addition, when delivering particulate materials it is important to avoid reflux of emboli. It is important, therefore, to use continuous fluoroscopy when injecting such materials.

Some embolisation procedures are relatively simple, such as treatment of varicocoeles. Varicocoeles normally affect the left testis, and occur because the valve at the confluence of the left testicular and renal veins is incompetent, allowing reflux of blood at systemic venous pressure into the venous drainage of the testis. Treatment involves embolisation of the left testicular vein. One example involves placing a catheter in the left renal vein and injecting contrast whilst screening and also saving the fluoroscopic image. Once valve incompetence has been confirmed, and the anatomy has been demonstrated, the testicular vein is entered and embolisation coils are placed along its length. Generally patients requiring embolisation of the testicular vein are young, and it is clearly important to minimise radiation dose during this procedure.

Other procedures are more complex, such as embolisation for gastrointestinal bleeding (Fig. 38.7A,B,C), and require a more flexible approach to determine the precise anatomy and demonstrate the bleeding point accurately, followed by therapy. Highly complex situations, such as therapy for arteriovenous malformations may be better referred to centres with a specialist interest in this area.

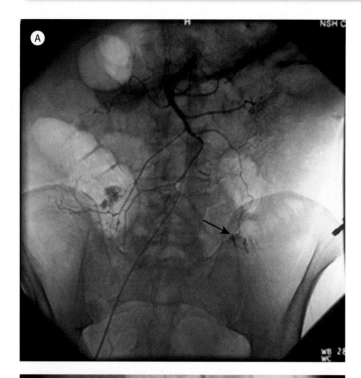

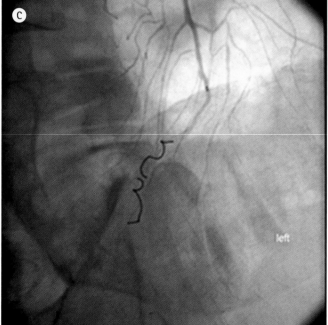

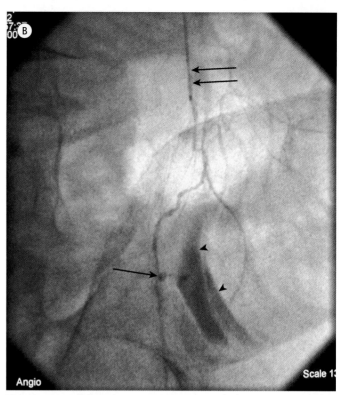

Figure 38.7 **(A)** Mesenteric arteriogram – (without subtraction) showing a bleeding point in the distal ileum (arrow). There is also a calcified lymph node on the right side, which should not be confused with a bleeding point. **(B)** superselective arteriogram – on the case seen in (A), using a microcatheter (double arrow) showing a bleeding point (arrow) which is allowing extravasation of contrast material into the bowel lumen (arrowheads). **(C)** embolisation – the bleeding vessel seen in (A) and (B) was successfully embolised using two microcoils

VENOUS INTERVENTIONS

Commonly undertaken venous interventions include placement of tunnelled venous lines and inferior vena cava (IVC) filter insertion. Stents are also used in the venous system; however, the techniques used are very similar to those employed in arteries so it is not necessary to describe them in any greater detail.

Tunnelled central venous lines

Tunnelled central venous lines are used for a variety of purposes including administration of chemotherapy, total parenteral nutrition (TPN) and temporary haemodialysis access. The line is tunnelled subcutaneously; near the point where the tunnel exits, the skin has a Dacron cuff attached to it which becomes incorporated into the tissues, making accidental dislodgement much more difficult than for non-tunnelled lines. There are also port systems available in which the entire device can be placed subcutaneously and be accessed percutaneously with a needle for drug administration.

The most commonly accessed vessels are probably the internal jugular veins, followed by the subclavian veins. On occasion, these vessels are occluded; this is particularly the case for patients who have had multiple central lines placed in the past, e.g. for haemodialysis. In these instances it may prove necessary to use alternative vessels such as the external jugular vein or even direct puncture of the IVC to provide venous access.

A useful method of guiding the vessel puncture is US, which has the clear benefit of avoiding the use of ionising radiation, although some professionals prefer to opacify the target vein with contrast, and guide the puncture in this way. Fluoroscopy is used to identify the catheter tip when positioning it in the superior vena cava (SVC). The first choice of vein for puncture is the right internal jugular. This vein follows an almost straight course into the right brachiocephalic vein and subsequently the SVC, meaning that there is little potential for kinking of the introducer sheath during insertion. Use of the left internal jugular and subclavian veins is usually straightforward, whereas the use of the right subclavian vein can be difficult, as kinking of the introducer sheath can be a major problem here.

The procedure is performed using local anaesthetic, often with light sedation. The target vein is punctured, using US or contrast-aided fluoroscopy as guidance, and the guidewire introduced; passage of the guidewire through the heart into the IVC confirms that a venous puncture has been achieved. A short incision is made at the puncture point, and a tunnel measuring approximately 6 cm in length is formed on the anterior chest wall. A specific tunnelling device is used for the purpose, and the catheter is then dragged through the tunnel and inserted through a peel away sheath into the vein. The catheter tip is visualised on fluoroscopy and positioned in the lower part of the SVC. By using image guidance for the insertion of tunnelled central venous catheters, complications should be minimised. For example, pneumothorax rates with image guided vein puncture have been reported as being as low as 0% compared with a rate of 5% for blind puncture.[17]

IVC filters

IVC filters can be permanent or removable, and are designed to prevent the passage of thrombus from the lower limbs, as prophylaxis against pulmonary embolism, which can be fatal. The standard treatment for deep vein thrombosis (DVT) is anticoagulation with heparin and subsequently warfarin. IVC filters are therefore only used in certain situations, such as when anticoagulation is contraindicated, when pulmonary embolism has occurred despite anticoagulation, and on occasion as prophylaxis against pulmonary embolism during surgery for pelvic trauma. Although these are accepted by many as standard indications, the evidence surrounding the use of IVC filters is very weak,[18] and practice varies widely around the world.

Many types of IVC filter are available, and insertion via the internal jugular or femoral routes is possible. There is currently one design of retrievable filter on the market, though it is very likely that there will soon be others. The principles of filter insertion are relatively simple. Access to the venous system is achieved and an inferior venacavagram is obtained to document the size of the IVC and the location of the renal veins. Assuming that the IVC is not of an abnormally large diameter, the filter is deployed below the level of the renal veins. Although it is occasionally necessary to deploy above the renal veins, this is to be avoided wherever possible so that in the event of IVC thrombosis the renal veins do not also thrombose.

IVC filters have been shown to be effective at preventing pulmonary emboli,[19] and have replaced the previous treatment of surgical ligation of the IVC. However, in the longer term, IVC filters do not prevent recurrence of DVT. The complication rate of IVC filter insertion is low, but includes potential migration of the device, IVC thrombosis and IVC perforation.

FUTURE DEVELOPMENTS AND CURRENT IMPACT OF INTERVENTIONAL VASCULAR PROCEDURES

There has been a massive impact of these minimally invasive procedures in the management of patients with vascular disease. For example, iliac angioplasty or stent insertion has now replaced surgery for many patients with iliac artery disease who require treatment. In addition, where open surgery is required, adjunctive angioplasty or stent insertion can be of great value in reducing the complexity of surgery undertaken. This chapter has necessarily concentrated on the better established techniques or devices. However, there is constant development in the devices industry, and there is little doubt that solutions will be found for some of the problems encountered with current technology. Perhaps one of the best publicised examples in the arena is the development of drug eluting stents. The stent surface is coated with a drug that inhibits endothelial cell growth, preventing in-stent stenosis or occlusion by neo-intimal hyperplasia.[20,21]

There is also work progressing on the use of MRI for guidance when performing these procedures. Interventional MRI is becoming fairly well established in some areas, such as biopsy or image guided surgery. However, the situation with vascular procedures is more complex, in that device movement needs to be monitored in real time. Work is being undertaken to allow catheter tracking to this end.[22]

REFLECTION ON ENDOVASCULAR THERAPY

The evidence around the use of endovascular therapy in the management of intermittent claudication is fairly clear. However, in the management of critical limb ischaemia the issues are more complex. The argument that is frequently advanced is that attempting an endovascular procedure does not preclude the subsequent use of surgery, which is usually true. However, consumables for these procedures are relatively expensive and if, to take an extreme, they were rarely successful, endovascular therapy in this arena would be highly wasteful of resources. The evidence for their use is often conflicting. The patients being treated in the various studies are, of course, a heterogeneous group, and the endpoints used are often different, making direct comparisons between studies very difficult.

In the 'real world' endovascular therapy is used by many as the first line, with surgery being held in reserve. Surgery for critical limb ischaemia, which will usually involve some form of distal bypass, is complex and may not be possible if there is no good vein available for use as a graft. Furthermore, wounds from open surgery may become infected, which in an already compromised limb can be disastrous, especially if infection is due to a multi-resistant organism. If revascularisation fails, amputation will inevitably follow. Not only is this expensive in terms of resources for rehabilitation, but many patients in fact never manage to use their prosthetic limb, and the mortality from amputation is also very high. Therefore there is a need for pragmatism in this area. Even if patency rates from endovascular therapy for critical limb ischaemia are far from perfect, avoiding amputation can only be regarded as a good thing.

With regard to stent grafts, the picture is still evolving. There is really very little doubt that anatomically suitable thoracic aortic aneurysms should be treated by stent grafting, as the mortality and morbidity from open surgery is so high. With regard to the abdominal aorta, we must await the outcome of randomised trials in order to know who should be treated with this technology. There is however little doubt that, as technology improves to allow treatment of larger numbers of patients with challenging anatomy and to improve the durability of devices, use of abdominal aortic stent grafting is likely to increase.

What of the future for conventional open vascular surgery? There has been much talk in the UK of the development of a single specialist with skills in both open and endovascular surgery. However, it has become apparent more recently that the shortage of people wanting to enter both vascular surgery and interventional radiology requires that both groups of specialists remain at the present time. In addition, it is unlikely that there is sufficient time available in the training years to become competent in both. Elsewhere in Europe and the USA many vascular surgeons have adopted endovascular techniques. However, it is almost certainly true that individuals tend to concentrate on one or the other, as it is very difficult to remain highly skilled at both. For the foreseeable future there will be a continued need to use open surgical techniques, but as technology improves, endovascular therapy is likely to be usable in ever increasing numbers of patients.

NON-VASCULAR INTERVENTIONAL PROCEDURES OR THERAPIES

This sphere of interventional radiology is often referred to as non-vascular interventional radiology, and encompasses techniques in the gastrointestinal tract, liver and biliary system, the urogenital system, the musculoskeletal system and the airways. Before considering the interventional techniques employed in specific systems, it is worth examining the subjects of biopsy and drainage, which are very commonly used techniques that do not fit within a systems categorisation as they are employed in many organs and cavities.

Image-guided biopsy

This term refers to any procedure conducted under image guidance that yields tissue for histological or cytological examination. Although not strictly a therapeutic procedure, it is a common invasive procedure that is frequently a prerequisite to some form of therapy. The principles for fine needle aspiration (FNA) where cells are sampled with a narrow gauge needle for cytological examination, and core biopsy, where a larger core of tissue is obtained for histological examination, are the same. However, if FNA is to be undertaken the diagnostic yield is greatly enhanced by a technician or cytologist being present at the time of biopsy to ensure that the sample is diagnostic. If that is not possible, experience shows that it is better, wherever feasible, to obtain a core of tissue for formal histological examination. This applies even in the lung, where one might imagine that a thinner needle may produce lower complication rates.

Biopsies are perhaps most commonly performed under either US or CT guidance. Some biopsies, particularly in the lung, are performed using fluoroscopy, though there has been an increasing move towards the use of CT because of its better resolution in the lung. It is also possible, using non-ferromagnetic needles, to perform biopsies using interventional MRI scanners. The principles governing image-guided biopsies are very similar, with CT and fluoroscopy requiring additional considerations regarding use of ionising radiation.

Having chosen the most suitable modality for performing a biopsy, and ensured that there are no contraindications such as abnormal blood clotting, the first decision concerns what position the patient should be placed in. This will be based on where the skin entry point needs to be, not only to allow the needle to follow the shortest path to the lesion, but also in order to avoid important structures such as vessels. Patient comfort and stability are important issues in order to assure safe execution of the procedure. Supine or prone positions are commonly used, having the advantage of being fairly stable, meaning that patient movement during the procedure is rarely a problem. Some older patients do have problems with lying prone for prolonged periods, especially if they have arthritis of their cervical spine, which may give neck pain during the procedure. Lying patients on their side may sometimes be necessary, and if so it is important that suitable support is provided to eliminate movement during the procedure.

One must be cautious when performing a biopsy in a different position from that of the diagnostic imaging, as the relationships of various structures can be altered. A good example is in performing CT guided adrenal gland biopsy. When a patient has a CT scan in the supine position, the upper abdominal organs and diaphragm tend to fall backwards, obliterating much of the posterior costophrenic recess, giving an apparently straightforward path to the adrenal glands. However, the adrenal glands are in the retroperitoneum and it is necessary to perform a biopsy with the patient in the prone position. This causes the organs of the upper abdomen and the diaphragm to displace anteriorly, widening the posterior costophrenic recess and extending it caudally. In the majority of patients this means that aerated lung will now lie between the target adrenal gland and the nearest skin entry point. It is therefore necessary to insert the biopsy needle with a cranial angulation in order to travel upwards towards the adrenal gland whilst avoiding the lung. The advent of CT fluoroscopy makes such manoeuvres more easily achievable as the needle can be viewed in real time.

In some situations there may be no immediately obvious path available. A good example is that of lesions in the chest positioned behind the heart. Clearly there is no path from the anterior chest wall, and trying to reach the lesion from a lateral approach would involve crossing a great deal of lung parenchyma with the consequent risk of pneumothorax or even bleeding. It is possible to use a posterior approach by injecting normal saline paraspinally to produce a window through which the biopsy needle can pass. This avoids crossing lung parenchyma and any potential pneumothorax.

Percutaneous drainage procedures

A large number of drainage procedures are undertaken to treat abdominal or pelvic abscesses, for even in the antibiotic era, if pus is not drained from an abdominal or pelvic abscess cavity, the mortality rate remains high. Abdominal and pelvic abscesses may arise from a variety of causes, including as a complication of surgery, diverticular disease, Crohn's disease and pancreatitis. Pancreatitis may also cause pseudocysts in the pancreas itself, and abscesses may develop in the liver and occasionally spleen. Drainage procedures are also increasingly being undertaken in the thorax, both for simple pleural effusions, and for empyemas.

A variety of drains are available, varying from 6 French (2 mm) to 16 French (5.3 mm) in diameter. In general, the more viscous the material to be drained the wider the catheter required. If initial drainage with a catheter fails, it may be worth exchanging it for a larger one.

Drains can be inserted using US, CT, fluoroscopy or MRI for guidance. Clearly there are issues for MRI-guided procedures, related to the requirement for using non-ferrous materials.

The fluid collection or abscess is first identified via the chosen diagnostic imaging procedure and then the optimal position for intervention is decided upon in much the same way as for percutaneous biopsy. If a collection is relatively large and superficial it may be straightforward to insert a drain directly into it on a trochar, without the use of a guidewire. If this is to be done, it may be helpful to insert a narrow gauge Chiba needle first and check its position, to provide an idea of the direction in which the larger drain needs to be inserted.

If the procedure is particularly complex it is often effective to insert an 18G Chiba needle under CT guidance and, having checked that the needle tip lies within the collection, insert a guidewire over which the drain can be inserted. There is less chance of kinking the guidewire if the procedure is visualised in real time so CT fluoroscopy is again useful. If CT fluoroscopy is not available, it may be advantageous, once the Chiba needle has been inserted, to move the patient into a fluoroscopy suite for guidewire insertion and drain introduction, but as long as the procedure is undertaken with extreme care, insertion of the guidewire and drain without fluoroscopy ought not to cause problems.

When draining pancreatic abscesses or pseudocysts, one must take particular care to prevent formation of a fistula between the pancreas and the skin. This is best achieved by using a transgastric approach; thus if a fistula does form after drain removal, it will be between the pancreatic duct and the stomach, rather than the skin. Pancreatic secretions will therefore pass harmlessly into the stomach. Although it is possible to puncture the stomach under US guidance, the greater degree of confidence is given by using CT. Having entered the pseudocyst, a drain is inserted as for a normal collection. However, it should be noted that the fluid from pancreatic collections is often quite thick, and larger drains are often required.

NON-VASCULAR INTERVENTIONAL TECHNIQUES: GASTROINTESTINAL TRACT

Oesophagus

Interventional techniques in the oesophagus are most commonly employed in the relief of obstruction which causes dysphagia, although treatment is sometimes required for oesophageal fistulae or perforations. Oesophageal obstruction may be due to benign causes such as peptic strictures caused by chronic reflux oesophagitis, achalasia, radiotherapy or ingestion of caustic substances. Alternatively, the cause may be malignancy, due to oesophageal carcinoma or extrinsic compression from malignant lymph nodes.

Oesophageal dilation

Oesophageal dilation, when performed under fluoroscopy alone, is achieved using balloon dilators. It appears that many endoscopists are also switching to use balloons rather than bougies (a series of flexible dilators of increasing thickness). Dilation alone is suitable only for treating benign lesions of the oesophagus (as in Fig. 38.8a,b, when dilation is required due to resection after surgery for malignancy, rather than due to the original malignancy); when used in an attempt to relieve malignant dysphagia the results are usually only very short lived, and there is up to a 10% incidence of oesophageal perforation.

At the start of the procedure the patient is placed on the fluoroscopic table in the left lateral position. The throat is anaesthetised with xylocaine spray, and the patient is sedated. A suitable catheter and guidewire are used through a per oral approach to cross the stricture, and the catheter is exchanged for a balloon. The size of balloon used varies according to the type of lesion being treated. Thus fibrotic lesions such as those caused by radiotherapy or ingestion of caustic substances need to be treated initially with small angioplasty balloons, with diameters of 8–10 mm, as there is a high incidence of perforation. Over a number of treatments, progressively larger balloons are used, with the aim of reaching a final diameter of 20 mm. Strictures resulting from chronic reflux oesophagitis can normally be treated with 20 mm balloons immediately, whereas in achalasia, where the aim is to tear muscle fibres, larger balloons of 30–40 mm in diameter are required.

Generally, technical success rates of around 95% are quoted.[23,24,25] These results are as good as if not better than those of bougienage, and avoid the morbidity and mortality associated with surgery. Stricture recurrence can be a problem, but up to 70% of patients remain asymptomatic at 2 years. Recurrent dysphagia can usually be successfully treated with repeat dilation. The main potential complication of oesophageal dilation is perforation. Overall, the perforation rate does appear to be very low, with some workers reporting no incidence of this; when taking consent from patients, quotation of a perforation rate of less than 1% can be supported.[23,24,25] However, there are important exceptions to this; for example the perforation rate for dilation of caustic strictures has been quoted as being as high as 25%. One would expect the situation to be similar for strictures induced by radiotherapy.

Oesophageal stent insertion

At the time of presentation 50–60% of patients with oesophageal carcinoma have lesions that are not amenable to surgical resection. However, they all have or will develop dysphagia that requires palliation. Available treatments include surgery, chemotherapy, radiotherapy, laser therapy, rigid plastic tubes and self-expanding metallic oesophageal stents. There is now wide experience in the use of oesophageal stents, and they form an important part of the palliation of malignant oesophageal obstruction.

The technique of insertion is very similar to that for oesophageal dilation. However, once the stricture has been crossed with a guidewire, it is predilated to 15 mm in diameter. Using a balloon of a smaller diameter than the stent diminishes the risk of over-dilating the oesophagus, which would increase the risk of stent migration. Some workers do not dilate the oesophagus prior to deploying a stent; however, in some cases this may mean that the stent expands insufficiently to allow removal of the delivery system through it. Once the stent has been deployed the delivery system is removed and contrast medium injected to ensure patency and that there has been no perforation.

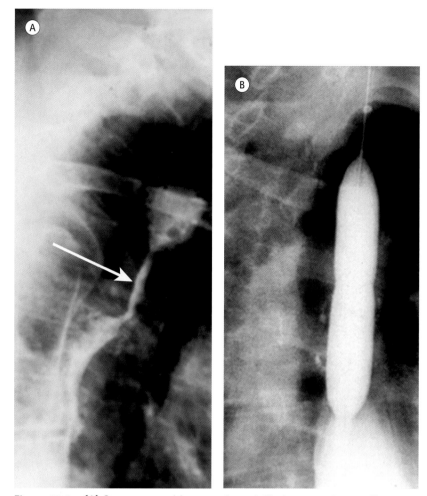

Figure 38.8 **(A)** Structure requiring oesophageal dilation – contrast swallow showing a tight stricture at the anastomosis between the upper oesophagus and a gastric pull-up after resection of an oesophageal carcinoma (arrow). **(B)** oesophageal dilation – 20 mm oesophageal balloon fully inflated across the stricture

After the patient has recovered from the sedation they are allowed initially to take sips of fluid, and over the next few hours to take increasing volumes.

The results of oesophageal stenting are generally good, with improvement or complete relief of dysphagia in 83–100% of patients.[26,27,28] Complications include: perforation, for which insertion of a covered stent is the treatment anyway, stent migration, pain, upper gastrointestinal haemorrhage, aspiration pneumonia and fistula formation. The results of stenting are better than those reported for palliative surgery,[29] chemotherapy and radiotherapy,[30,31] both in terms of success in the relief of dysphagia and the complications encountered. Results of a randomised study have in addition shown stent insertion to be superior to the use of laser therapy.[32] Covered stents are also highly successful in sealing leaks and fistulae to the airways caused by malignant tumours (Fig. 38.9A,B).[33]

Stomach and duodenum

The two main interventional radiological procedures undertaken in this anatomical location are percutaneous gastrostomy and stent insertion. Balloon dilation is occasionally undertaken for strictures involving surgical anastomoses or due to pyloric dysfunction after gastric pull-up operations performed for oesophageal carcinoma. However, such balloon dilation differs little from that performed in the oesophagus, and will not be described in further detail here.

Percutaneous gastrostomy

In many hospitals in the UK fluoroscopically guided gastrostomy insertion is only undertaken if the endoscopic approach has failed. Gastrostomy is performed most commonly to provide enteral nutrition if there is an anatomical or

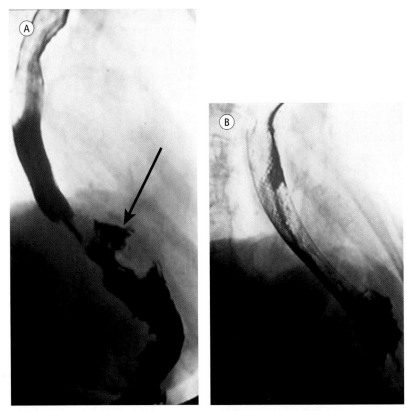

Figure 38.9 **(A)** Oesophageal malignancy and endoscopic perforation – carcinoma of the oesophagogastric junction causing obstruction and associated with perforation after endoscopy (arrow). **(B)** using a covered stent to treat a stricture and seal perforation – the stricture has been successfully treated and the perforation sealed with a covered oesophageal stent

functional difficulty in swallowing. It is also sometimes undertaken to decompress the stomach. Over the last few years fewer gastrostomies have been required in cases of oesophageal carcinoma because of the advent of oesophageal stents. One of the commonest reasons, if not the most common, for gastrostomy insertion is stroke.

Prior to gastrostomy a nasogastric tube needs to be inserted, preferably the day before, to drain gastric contents. A US scan is performed to identify the left lobe of the liver, and this is marked on the skin. In addition, some radiologists advocate the administration of barium the night before to opacify the transverse colon. Both of these are aimed at preventing inadvertent puncture of adjacent organs. The stomach is then fully inflated with air introduced via the nasogastric tube; this displaces the colon inferiorly and brings the anterior gastric wall as close as possible to the anterior abdominal wall. A suitable pathway to the stomach is identified under fluoroscopy and the skin is infiltrated with local anaesthetic. A needle is then passed into the stomach; either the stomach can be fixed to the anterior abdominal wall with 'T' fasteners, or a guidewire can be inserted, followed by proceeding directly to gastrostomy tube insertion.

The technical success of the procedure is reported as being 99–100%.[34,35,36] Potential complications include reflux of the enteral feed into the oesophagus, with the risk of causing aspiration pneumonia. If such reflux occurs, the gastrostomy can be converted to a gastrojejunostomy, which usually solves the problem. Further major complications of the procedure include severe bleeding, peritonitis and sepsis, and have been reported in 1.4–6.0% of cases. Minor complications include peritoneal irritation, local infection and tube migration or displacement.[34,35,36]

Gastric and duodenal stenting

Stents are used in the stomach and duodenum in the management of strictures, which are usually caused by malignant tumours of the stomach or the pancreas. They are occasionally required for the treatment of pyloric dysfunction after gastric pull-up operations if balloon dilation is unsuccessful;[37] peptic strictures are becoming increasingly uncommon with improved treatment for peptic ulcer disease.

Often insertion of gastric or duodenal stents for malignancy is only requested if patients are considered unfit for surgery. However, as experience grows, it would appear that stents are being used for these indications more commonly as an alternative to surgery in fit patients.

Stent procedures in the stomach and duodenum are technically more complex than those in the oesophagus. The reasons for this are that the large size and distensibility of the stomach allows space for loops of guidewire and catheter to form, and the fact that greater catheter and delivery system lengths are required, both making manipulation across strictures more difficult. For these reasons many workers advocate the use of endoscopy in conjunction with fluoroscopy; whilst not always required, endoscopic assistance can be very helpful in difficult cases.

Prior to the availability of dedicated stents, 16-mm diameter vascular wall stents were employed (Fig. 38.10A,B), as the standard oesophageal stents were not available on a sufficiently long delivery system. However, there are now specific stents available for use in the stomach, duodenum and colon, e.g. the enteral wall stent and the memotherm (a nitinol stent). The procedure is very similar to that for oesophageal stent insertion, other than for the different anatomical location, so it will not be described in any further detail. Success rates of 80–100% have been reported.[38,39,40,41] The only reported complication is aspiration of gastric contents into the airways, and this is infrequent. Although perforation of the stomach or the duodenum is a theoretical possibility it has not been reported.

Colon

Colonic stents

Colonic stents were originally intended for temporary use in patients presenting with acute large bowel obstruction secondary to colonic carcinoma. This allows bowel preparation to be given and a primary bowel anastomosis to be formed at the time of tumour resection, rather than having to perform a defunctioning colostomy and return some weeks later to rejoin the bowel loops. However, more recently, colonic stents have been used as the sole treatment for obstruction for patients who will only receive palliative therapy. As such they are used not only in the management of irresectable colon tumours, but also in the management of other extensive pelvic tumours causing colonic obstruction.

The details of the available stents are given in the above section. The technique involves gaining access to the colon

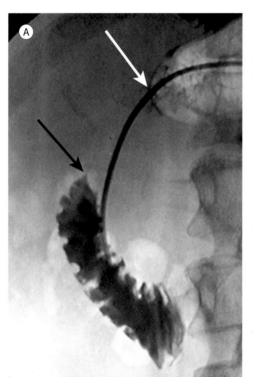
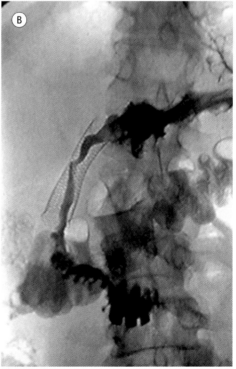

Figure 38.10 **(A)** Gastric outlet obstruction – this patient had gastric outlet obstruction due to carcinoma of the pancreas. A catheter is positioned across the obstruction, the limits of which are defined by air in the stomach proximally and contrast in the duodenum distally (arrows).
(B) relieving gastric outlet obstruction – a contrast study performed on the day after stent deployment shows full stent expansion and complete relief of gastric outlet obstruction

through a per rectal approach and traversing the stricture with guidewire and catheter techniques (Fig. 38.11A). As the colon is tortuous and the haustra can make catheter and guidewire manipulation difficult, it may be helpful to use either a supporting sheath or a colonoscope to provide additional support. Once the stricture has been crossed the stent is deployed (Fig. 38.11B); post deployment, balloon dilation is occasionally required, though if possible it is the author's practice to avoid this and rely on gradual stent expansion over 24 hours or so in order to minimise the risk of bowel perforation.

Around 70% of colonic carcinomas are on the left side of the large bowel. Clinical success rates of 64–100% are reported, with right-sided lesions being much more difficult to reach and treat.[42,43,44] In addition, cost reductions of around 28% have been reported when using stents rather than the conventional approach of defunctioning colostomy. Complications of colonic perforation, stent displacement and obstruction have been reported. More minor complications include rectal bleeding, tenesmus, transient anorectal pain and faecal impaction.[42,43,44]

NON-VASCULAR INTERVENTIONAL TECHNIQUES: THE BILIARY TREE

It should be noted that the majority of interventions in the biliary tree are undertaken at the time of endoscopic retrograde cholangiopancreatography (ERCP). This is generally performed by gastroenterologists or surgeons, with only a few radiologists involved in this field. However, if ERCP fails for any reason the percutaneous approach to the biliary tree is required. The most common procedure undertaken by interventional radiologists in the biliary tree is stent insertion. Biliary drainage is also frequently carried out, usually prior to stenting, and there is occasionally a call to dilate benign biliary strictures. Biliary drainage will be described first, as access to the biliary tree is an essential component to all of these procedures.

Indications for intervention in the biliary tree include palliation of unresectable primary or metastatic malignancy, benign biliary strictures, sepsis accompanying biliary obstruction, and preoperative decompression. ERCP is also frequently used in the treatment of calculi in the bile ducts and percutaneous biliary intervention may be required where the bile ducts have been opacified at ERCP but it has not been possible to secure drainage with a stent; if obstructed bile ducts are left undrained in this situation there is a significant risk of cholangitis.

ERCP

ERCP is now, in most centres, the first line in imaging and intervention for the biliary tree, and technical success rates of 75–98% are reported.[45] The procedure involves using a side-viewing endoscope to visualise and then cannulate the ampulla of Vater in the second part of the duodenum. Contrast is then injected through the cannula, and the biliary

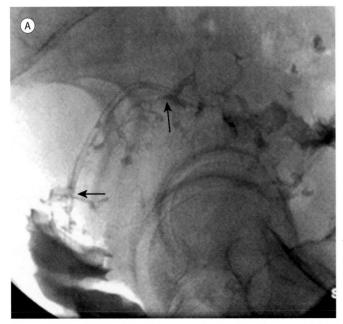
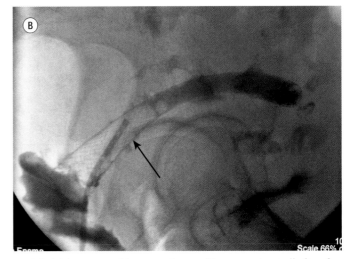

Figure 38.11   (A) Rectal stricture – catheter placed across a fairly long rectal stricture caused by a carcinoma. The approximate limits of the stricture are shown by the arrows. (B) relieving rectal obstruction – the obstruction has been relieved by deployment of an enteral wall stent

tree and pancreatic duct are opacified. Having made a diagnosis, appropriate therapy can often be delivered at the same sitting. Thus, in cases of obstruction, a sphincterotomy is first performed; essentially this involves making a cut at the lower end of the common bile duct to allow instruments to pass. If obstruction is being caused by gallstones in the common bile duct, sphincterotomy alone occasionally allows a stone to drop out of the duct; more frequently it proves necessary to trawl the duct with baskets or balloons to extract the calculi. If there is a benign biliary stricture this can be balloon dilated, whereas malignant strictures require stent insertion.

ERCP is also of value if the biliary tree is not dilated. One example of this is in patients who have experienced bile duct trauma at the time of laparoscopic cholecystectomy and have a resultant biliary leak. Placement of a plastic biliary stent for around 6 weeks to divert the flow of bile away from the area of leakage into the duodenum will usually result in sealing of the leak. After 6 weeks the stent can be removed.

A further example is that of primary biliary sclerosis, where there is widespread narrowing of bile ducts. In this situation it is sometimes possible to identify a 'dominant stricture' which can be dilated with the relief of some or all of the patient's symptoms.

Potential complications of ERCP include death, sepsis, haemorrhage and bile leak. If ERCP is not possible, for example, due to previous partial gastrectomy or duodenal stenosis, or if it fails for some other reason, then percutaneous biliary intervention will be tried. In addition, there are strong arguments for using percutaneous biliary intervention as the primary mode of palliation for malignant hilar strictures, i.e. proximal lesions that involve one or more of the common hepatic duct or right or left hepatic ducts.[46]

Percutaneous biliary drainage

The first step in undertaking any percutaneous biliary tract intervention is to gain access to the bile ducts. This is done by first performing a percutaneous transhepatic cholangiogram (PTC). Having ensured that the blood clotting is normal and prophylactic antibiotics have been administered, the patient is placed on the X-ray table in the supine position with their right arm raised above their head. The right upper quadrant is imaged by fluoroscopy and a suitable point for skin puncture is selected. Local anaesthetic is administered along with intravenous sedation and/or analgesia. A thin (22 or 21G) Chiba needle is advanced into the liver, and is then gradually withdrawn whilst contrast is gently injected. Several passes of the Chiba needle may be required in order to access a bile duct, although if the biliary tree is dilated it is rare to fail.

Once the bile ducts have been opacified a suitable guidewire is inserted through the Chiba needle. Occasionally it proves necessary to reposition the needle prior to guidewire insertion. The Chiba needle is exchanged for a coaxial dilator system, allowing insertion of a larger guidewire. If biliary drainage alone is to be performed, it is possible at this stage to insert a pigtail drainage catheter over the guidewire into the bile duct, to provide external drainage of bile; this option may be chosen, for example, if there is cholangitis which requires treatment before definitive therapy.

If it is possible to pass the guidewire through the ampulla of Vater, it is possible to use an internal/external biliary drain. This device has drainage holes along a greater length than the standard external drainage catheter such that, when positioned with the pigtail in the duodenum, drainage holes lie above and below the papilla. This allows much of the bile to drain internally, while retaining access to the biliary tree for future intervention. Internal/external biliary drains tend to be more secure, and can be useful for providing internal drainage whilst making decisions regarding management.

Biliary stenting

Both plastic and metallic stents are available for relief of biliary obstruction. At ERCP the vast majority of stents used are plastic, as they are relatively cheap. However, due to the fact that they are of much smaller diameter than metallic stents they have a much greater tendency to block. There is evidence that, when stents are being employed for the palliation of malignant biliary strictures, metallic stents are in fact more cost effective than plastic devices because of the lower reintervention rate.[47,48]

When placing stents percutaneously, some consideration needs to be given to the size of the device being placed across the liver parenchyma. At 12 French in diameter, the plastic stents placed at ERCP are considered by many operators to be too large to be inserted through the liver, so many percutaneously placed stents are only 10 French in diameter, with a consequent reduction in lumen size. It is advantageous to use self-expanding metallic stents percutaneously (Fig. 38.12A,B); these not only have the advantage of a small delivery system size (7 French), but they also provide a much larger lumen (10 mm or the equivalent of 30 French).

The other factor in deciding whether to use a metallic or plastic stent is the cause of the biliary stricture. If metallic stents are used in benign strictures, for example, those caused by chronic pancreatitis, most will occlude over a period of months due to the overgrowth of epithelial cells through the stent mesh. As a result, one can face great difficulties in management, and it is better where at all possible to manage such patients by ERCP and regular elective stent

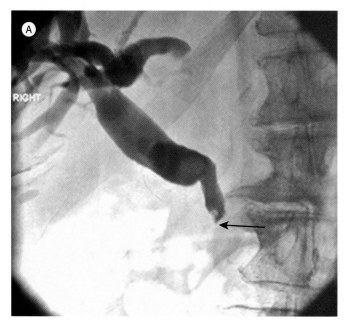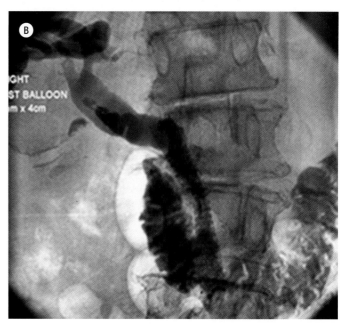

Figure 38.12 (A) Obstructed common bile duct – cholangiogram performed via catheter positioned in the biliary tree. Complete obstruction of the distal common bile duct has been demonstrated (arrow). (B) stenting bile duct obstruction – the obstruction has been relieved by the deployment of a 10 mm diameter self-expanding metallic stent

changes. In malignant biliary strictures, the reduced reintervention rate and delivery system size associated with metallic stents makes a compelling case for their use.

Dilation of benign biliary strictures

There are a wide variety of potential causes for benign biliary strictures. However, in the western world the majority are iatrogenic, either as a result of trauma to the bile ducts at the time of laparoscopic cholecystectomy or occurring at anastomoses formed between the small bowel and the biliary tree, either at the time of liver transplantation or biliary bypass for the management of biliary strictures or surgery for pancreatic carcinoma. Benign biliary strictures may also be caused by chronic infection associated with bile duct calculi.

Decision making and management in this patient group can be complex, and requires a multidisciplinary approach. Even relatively mild strictures can cause stone formation, cholangitis and cirrhosis. Surgery has traditionally been used but ERCP has become increasingly important in the management of such patients, and good long-term results with plastic stents and repeated stent changes have been reported.[49,50] Where ERCP is not possible, perhaps because of previous surgery, percutaneous treatment may be required. Plastic stents are frequently employed, and balloon dilation of strictures is reported as being very successful. However, several treatments may be required in order to achieve a satisfactory result; if percutaneous therapy is to be used

this will require long-term placement of a biliary drain which is inconvenient for the patient.[51]

NON-VASCULAR INTERVENTIONAL TECHNIQUES: UROGENITAL TRACT

The most widely undertaken procedure in the urogenital tract is percutaneous nephrostomy. Having gained access to the urinary tract it is also possible to introduce ureteric stents to relieve obstruction and use balloons to dilate strictures. Percutaneous nephrolithotomy (PCNL) is also used in the treatment of renal calculi. In recent years, increasing numbers of uterine artery embolisations (UAEs) have been performed for the treatment of uterine fibroids.

Percutaneous nephrostomy

Percutaneous nephrostomy is usually performed to relieve urinary tract obstruction. An alternative approach is to place retrograde ureteric double 'J' stents cystoscopically. However, nephrostomy has advantages in certain situations such as malignant obstruction and if there is infection present (pyonephrosis).

The procedure itself can be carried out using either fluoroscopy or US alone or a combination of the two, which may ensure more confidence. The patient is placed prone on the fluoroscopy table with the side to be treated slightly elevated. A US scan is performed to identify the hydronephrotic kidney; it is usually possible to identify calyces, and select one for puncture. Wherever possible one aims to puncture a posterior lower pole calyx, as the arrangement of intrarenal vessels at this site means that the risk of bleeding complications is lower with this approach. The skin and deep tissues are infiltrated with local anaesthetic and intravenous sedation is administered. Then, a suitable needle is introduced into the collecting system under US guidance.

After the collecting system has been successfully punctured a stiff or superstiff guidewire (for example 'Amplatz') is introduced; if at all possible the guidewire is directed down the ureter to give the most secure position. It is impossible to see this reliably on US, and is best visualised on fluoroscopy, hence the combined US and fluoroscopic method is most often preferred. Once the operator is satisfied with the guidewire position a suitable nephrostomy catheter (typically 8 French in diameter) is introduced, fixed to the skin and attached to a drainage bag.

If the cause for the obstruction is self limiting, such as a small ureteric calculus, the nephrostomy may only be required for a few days then removed. Similarly, it may be removed after definitive treatment such as ureteroscopy and stone removal has been carried out. In other situations further intervention may be required either at the same time as nephrostomy insertion, or on another occasion. This will be discussed in the following sections.

Minor complications requiring no additional therapy are fairly common, and virtually every patient will develop transient mild haematuria. Severe bleeding necessitating transfusion or other intervention is reported as occurring in 1-3% of cases.[52]

Ureteric stent insertion

Ureteric obstruction may arise from a variety of causes. Antegrade stenting via a nephrostomy track is only rarely required for temporary causes such as calculi. However, causes such as strictures or obstruction caused by malignancy or radiotherapy can rarely be stented retrogradely, and antegrade ureteric stenting is of immense value in this patient group.[53,54]

The stents used have a pigtail shape at either end and are made of plastic. They need to be changed every few months, although this does not require repeat nephrostomy; once the obstruction has been crossed it is almost always possible to change stents retrogradely. The principles behind antegrade ureteric stenting are relatively simple. Having gained access to the upper urinary tract by performing a nephrostomy, an angiographic catheter and guidewire are manipulated into the ureter and through the obstruction. The guidewire is exchanged for an 'Amplatz' stiff guidewire and a suitable size of stent is introduced over it. In order to achieve a suitable angle for stent insertion it may prove necessary to gain access via middle or even upper pole calyx, as attempting to push the stent forwards from a lower pole puncture can lead to a loop forming in the proximal guidewire which is then pushed into the upper pole region. If stenting from a lower pole puncture, a peelaway sheath advanced into the proximal ureter will normally remedy this problem without having to resort to a further puncture.

Balloon dilation of ureteric strictures

Benign strictures in the native ureters may occur for a variety of reasons including calculus disease, radiotherapy and surgical trauma. In renal transplants, ureteric strictures may be due to periureteric fibrosis, anastomotic fibrosis or ischaemia. Diffuse strictures caused by chronic rejection or necrosis cannot be successfully dilated with balloons. The procedure is identical in many respects to that of ureteric stent insertion, except for the fact that a high pressure balloon is placed across the stricture and dilated, followed by insertion of a stent. The stent is then removed some weeks later. Good long-term results can be anticipated in up to 50% of benign ureteric strictures.[55]

PCNL

PCNL was developed in the mid 1970s and, as it became accepted, largely replaced open surgery for urinary tract stones. Despite the subsequent development of extracorporeal shockwave lithotripsy (ESWL) and ureteroscopic techniques, PCNL is still used for the management of urinary tract stone disease.

PCNL may be carried out either in the operating theatre with a mobile image intensifier, or in the radiology department; in either instance the patient is placed under general anaesthetic. It is important to establish which calyces contain stones on preoperative imaging; the appropriate calyx for puncture is then selected. Initially the urologist performs a cystoscopy and passes a ureteric catheter into the proximal ureter. The patient is then turned prone, and the collecting system is opacified with contrast medium injected through the ureteric catheter. The chosen calyx is then punctured and a guidewire introduced and placed within the ureter.

A peelaway sheath is introduced over the guidewire, which allows the insertion of a second 'Amplatz' superstiff guidewire. This provides two guidewires, one for dilating the track and the other as a safety guidewire to prevent access being lost. The track is dilated to 30 French in diameter using either coaxial metal dilators or a balloon system, followed by insertion of a 30 French working sheath. This allows the introduction of a nephroscope, baskets and mechanical lithotripters for the breaking up and removal of calculi. This part of the procedure is undertaken by the urologists, so teamwork is very important.

After successful stone removal the working sheath is removed and a large nephrostomy tube left in situ for 1–2 days. Success rates for stone removal are high. The mortality rate for such large bore access to the urinary tract is low (less than 0.3%).[56] Significant bleeding is more likely than with smaller bore tubes, but can usually be managed by inserting a balloon dilation catheter into the track to provide tamponade. If tamponade over a few days fails, angiography and embolisation may be needed.

UAE for uterine fibroids

Embolisation in general has been described earlier in this chapter, however, UAE for uterine fibroids merits special consideration under genitourinary therapies.

The technique was first described in the mid 1990s, and has been taken up enthusiastically by many radiologists and patients alike. It is attractive as an alternative to hysterectomy, as it is a day case procedure, whereas hysterectomy is a major surgical procedure with a prolonged period of recovery often required. There are other clear resource benefits such as reduction in hospital bed and nursing care requirements when compared to hysterectomy.

The technique involves selective catheterisation of both uterine arteries and embolisation is achieved using polyvinyl alcohol particles. A tightly collimated beam should be employed and where pulsed fluoroscopy is employed, the slowest pulse rate compatible with adequate visualisation should be used. If at all possible, formal angiographic runs should be avoided, but where these are necessary they should be kept as short as possible. This is because the patients who undergo this examination are relatively young females.

Initial reports regarding UAE were very enthusiastic, claiming few if any complications and great success both for reducing the size of the fibroids themselves and in treating the associated symptoms. However, as experience with the technique has grown it has become apparent that it is not without its complications. All patients experience pelvic pain of varying severity after the procedure, and some professionals advocate patient controlled analgesia in the post-procedure period to counter this. Perhaps the most worrying, though thankfully relatively uncommon, complication is sepsis. Although deaths are reported, they are rare and it should not be forgotten that hysterectomy has a significant morbidity and mortality. There is currently a randomised trial underway in Scotland which should clarify many of the issues surrounding this therapy and allow patients and clinicians to make informed decisions about treatment.

REFLECTION ON INTERVENTION AND THERAPIES

This chapter illustrates the immense breadth of procedures undertaken by interventional radiologists today. Although there is much commonality between the techniques employed, for example the use of catheter and guidewire manipulation, ever increasing amounts of clinical knowledge are required for the safe application of these techniques. As a result, there has, in many cases, been a tendency for individuals to subspecialise further within interventional radiology, for example to concentrate on vascular radiology alone. In some cases, organ specialists undertake the interventional procedures relevant to them. A good example of this is in musculoskeletal radiology, where specialists often undertake bone biopsy and even vertebroplasty; there is insufficient space to describe all of the available techniques in this chapter – hence their omission.

Another issue facing interventional radiologists is that as techniques become more complex, the clinicians looking after the patient will have less knowledge of them, making subsequent patient care more difficult. This is especially the case where junior staff care for a patient on the ward after the procedure. There is thus a strong case for greater clinical involvement of interventional radiologists by performing ward rounds and maybe even outpatient clinics, both to assess patients prior to treatment, and follow them up afterwards. Such clinical involvement should also allow for improved quality of patient consent, given the direct communication with the expert in the interventional procedure, rather than a representative from a different specialist area.

In the author's opinion it is essential that we grapple with these issues, or face the prospect of these techniques being performed by others in the future. Although some might argue that this would be appropriate, the unique knowledge of imaging which is brought to these procedures by interventional radiologists must improve the quality of their conduct, although this would be difficult to measure.

References

1. Van Andel G, et al. Percutaneous transluminal dilatation of the iliac artery: long term results. Radiology 1985; 156:321–323.
2. Wolfe, et al. Surgery or PTA for peripheral vascular disease; a randomised controlled trial. Journal of Vascular and Interventional Radiology 1993; 4:639–648.
3. Ballard J. Aortoiliac stent deployment vs. surgical reconstruction. Journal of Vascular Surgery 1998; 28:94–103.

4. Lofberg A-M, et al. Percutaneous transluminal angioplasty of the femoropopliteal arteries in limbs with chronic critical lower limb ischaemia. Journal of Vascular Surgery 2001; 34:114–121.

5. Shaw M, et al. The results of subintimal angioplasty in a district general hospital. European Journal of Vascular and Endovascular Surgery 2002; 24:524–527.

6. Perkins J, et al. Exercise training versus angioplasty for stable claudication: long and medium term results of a prospective, randomized trial. European Journal of Vascular and Endovascular Surgery 1996; 11:409–413.

7. Whyman M, et al. Is intermittent claudication improved by percutaneous transluminal angioplasty? Journal of Vascular Surgery 1997; 26:551–557.

8. Brown K, et al. Infrapopliteal angioplasty: long term follow-up. Journal of Vascular and Interventional Radiology 1993; 4:139–144.

9. Tetterooe E, et al. Randomised comparison of primary stent insertion versus primary angioplasty and selective stent insertion in iliac artery occlusive disease. Lancet 1998; 351:1153–1159.

10. Bosch J, Hunink M. Meta analysis of the results of PTA and stent placement in aortoiliac occlusive disease. Radiology 1997; 204:87–96.

11. Bosch J, et al. Iliac arterial disease: cost effectiveness analysis of stent placement versus PTA. Radiology 1998; 208:641–681.

12. Van de Ven P, et al. Arterial stenting and balloon angioplasty in ostial atherosclerotic renovascular disease: a randomised trial. Lancet 1999; 353(9149):282–286.

13. Reidy J, Taylor P. The use of stent grafts in thoracic aortic disease. Cardiovascular and Interventional Radiology 2000; 23:249–251.

14. Faries P, et al. A multicentre experience with the Talent endovascular graft for the treatment of abdominal aortic aneurysms. Journal of Vascular Surgery 2002; 35:1123–1128.

15. Fifth report on the registry for endovascular treatment of aneurysms. The Vascular Surgical Society of Great Britain and Ireland and the British Society of Interventional Radiology 2001.

16. Katz D, et al. Operative mortality rates for intact and ruptured abdominal aortic aneurysms. An eleven year state wide experience. Journal of Vascular Surgery 1994; 19:804–817.

17. Lameris J, et al. Percutaneous placement of Hickman catheters: comparison of sonographic guided and blind techniques. American Journal of Roentgenology 1990; 155:1097–1099.

18. Girard P, et al. Medical literature and vena cava filters: so far so weak. Chest 2002; 122:963–967.

19. Decousus H, et al. A clinical trial of vena caval filters in the prevention of pulmonary embolism in patients with proximal deep vein thrombosis. New England Journal of Medicine 1998; 338:409–416.

20. Morice M-C, et al for the RAVEL study group. A randomized comparison of a Sirolimus-eluting stent with a standard stent for coronary revascularization. New England Journal of Medicine 2002; 326:1773–1780.

21. Sousa J, et al. Two year angiographic and ultrasound follow-up after implantation of Sirolimus-eluting stents in human coronary arteries. Circulation 2003; 107:381–383.

22. Duerk J, et al. A brief review of hardware for catheter tracking in magnetic resonance imaging. MAGMA 2002 Jan; 13(3):199–208.

23. McLean G, et al. Radiologically guided balloon dilatation of gastrointestinal strictures. Radiology 1987; 165:35–43.

24. Starcke E, et al. Esophageal stenosis: treatment with balloon catheters. Radiology 1984; 153:637–640.

25. Sabharwal T, et al. Balloon dilation for achalasia of the cardia: experience in 76 patients. Radiology 2002; 224:719–724.

26. Cowling M, et al. The use of self-expanding metallic stents in the management of malignant oesophageal strictures. British Journal of Surgery 1998; 85:264–266.

27. Cwiekiel W, et al. Malignant esophageal strictures: treatment with a self expanding nitinol stent. Radiology 1993; 187:661–665.

28. Saxon R, et al. Treatment of malignant esophageal obstructions with covered metallic Z stents: long term results in 52 patients. Journal of Vascular and Interventional Radiology 1995; 6:747–754.

29. Earlam R, Chunha-Melo J. Oesophageal squamous cell carcinoma: 1. A critical review of surgery. British Journal of Surgery 1980; 67:381–390.

30. Earlam R, Chunha-Melo J. Oesophageal squamous cell carcinoma: 2. A critical review of radiotherapy. British Journal of Surgery 1980; 67:457–461.

31. Herskovic A, et al. Combined chemotherapy and radiotherapy compared to radiotherapy alone in patients with cancer of the oesophagus. New England Journal of Medicine 1992; 326:1593–1598.

32. Adam A, et al. Palliation of inoperable esophageal carcinoma: a prospective randomized trial of laser therapy and stent placement. Radiology 1997; 202:344–348.

33. Morgan R, et al. Malignant esophageal fistulas and perforation: management with plastic-covered metallic endoprostheses. Radiology 1997; 204:527–532.

34. Hicks M, et al. Fluoroscopically guided percutaneous gastrostomy: analysis of 158 consecutive cases. American Journal of Roentgenology 1990; 154:725–728.

35. Wills J. Percutaneous gastrostomy: applications in gastric carcinoma and gastroplasty stoma dilatation. American Journal of Roentgenology 1986; 147:826–827.

36. De Baere T, et al. Percutaneous gastrostomy with fluoroscopic guidance: Single centre experience in 500 consecutive cancer patients. Radiology 1999; 210:651–654.

37. Cowling M, et al. Self expanding metallic stents in the treatment of pyloric dysfunction after gastric pull-up operations. European Radiology 1999; 9:1123–1126.

38. Binkert C, et al. Benign and malignant stenoses of the stomach and duodenum: treatment with self-expanding metallic endoprostheses. Radiology 1996; 199:335–338.

39. Feretis C, et al. Palliation of malignant gastric outlet obstruction with self expanding metal stents. Endoscopy 1996; 28:225–228.

40. Wong Y, et al. Gastric outlet obstruction secondary to pancreatic cancer: surgical vs endoscopic palliation. Surgical Endoscopy 2002; 16:310–312.

41. Yim H, et al. Clinical outcome of the use of enteral stents for palliation of patients with malignant upper GI obstruction. Gastrointestinal Endoscopy 2001; 53:329–332.

42. Mainar A, et al. Colorectal obstruction: treatment with metallic stents. Radiology 1996; 198:761–764.

43. Dauphine C, et al. Placement of self expanding metal stents for acute malignant large bowel obstruction: a collective review. Annals of Surgical Oncology 2002; 9:574–579.

44. Aviv R, et al. Radiological palliation of malignant colonic obstruction. Clinical Radiology 2002; 57:347–351.

45. England R, Martin D. Endoscopic and percutaneous intervention in malignant obstructive jaundice. Cardiovascular and Interventional Radiology 1996; 19:381–387.

46. Deviere J, et al. Long-term follow-up of patients with hilar malignant stricture treated by endoscopic internal biliary drainage. Gastrointestinal Endoscopy 1988; 34:95–101.

47. Prat F, et al. A randomised trial of endoscopic drainage methods for inoperable malignant strictures of the common bile duct. Gastrointestinal Endoscopy 1998; 47:1–7.

48. Davids P, et al. Randomised trial of self expanding metal stents versus polyethylene stents for distal malignant biliary obstruction. Lancet 1992; 340:1488–1492.

49. Draganov P, et al. Long term outcome in patients with benign biliary strictures treated endoscopically with multiple stents. Gastrointestinal Endoscopy 2002; 55:680–686.

50. Born P, et al. Long term results of endoscopic and percutaneous transhepatic treatment of benign biliary strictures. Endoscopy 1999; 31:725–731.

51. Gabelmann A, et al. Metallic stents in benign biliary strictures: Long term effectiveness and interventional management of stent occlusion. American Journal of Roentgenology 2001; 177:813–817.

52. Farrell T, Hicks M. A review of radiologically guided percutaneous nephrostomies in 303 patients. Journal of Vascular Interventional Radiology 1997; 8:769–774.

53. Chitale S, et al. The management of ureteric obstruction secondary to malignant pelvic disease. Clinical Radiology 2002; 57:1118–1121.

54. Sharma S, et al. A review of antegrade stenting in the management of the obstructed kidney. British Journal of Urology 1996; 78:511–515.

55. Lucey B, et al. Miscellaneous visceral renal intervention. Seminars in Interventional Radiology 2000; 17:367–372.

56. Segura J, et al. Percutaneous removal of kidney stones: review of 1000 cases. Journal of Urology 1985; 134:1077–1081.

VASCULAR IMAGING OF THE HEAD AND NECK

Patricia Fowler, Andrew Layt

The role of conventional angiography in the examination of the vasculature of the head and neck has changed substantially over the last decade. The advent of computed tomography angiography (CTA) and advances in magnetic resonance imaging (MRI) techniques have led to a reevaluation of the role of conventional approaches. In this chapter, consideration will be given to methods made possible by recent technological developments as well as those employed where access to this technology is not available.

INDICATIONS FOR VASCULAR EXAMINATION

Cerebral aneurysm

This is the most common indication for cerebral angiography. Aneurysmal rupture occurs in 10 per 100 000 population[1] and the presence of asymptomatic aneurysms is thought to be in the region of 2% of the population.[2] A ruptured aneurysm presents the commonest cause of subarachnoid haemorrhage in adults. The most common type is the congenital berry or saccular aneurysm which accounts for over 90% of intracranial aneurysms.[3] Typically, defects develop by the pressure of systolic waves causing herniation of the vessel wall.[2]

The average age of presentation is 50 years. Below this age presentation is more common in men than women with this reversing from 50 years upwards.[1] Most cerebral aneurysms are under 1 cm in diameter but they can range from 0.2 to 3 cm.[2] The majority (75%) are located in the anterior circulation with 25% in the posterior circulation,[4] the most common site (45%) being around the anterior communicating arteries.[2] The risk of bleeding generally increases with size.[5]

Clinical presentation of rupture includes:

- sudden severe headache[6]
- rapid loss of consciousness[6]
- vomiting[7]
- photophobia[5,7]
- nuchal rigidity[6]

Photophobia and nuchal rigidity result from meningeal irritation as a result of blood in the subarachnoid space.

Complications include:

- rebleeding – the highest rate of rebleeding occurs on days one or two. Fifty percent of patients rebleed during the first 6 months if the patient is not treated immediately following the initial subarachnoid haemorrhage[8]
- vasospasm with cerebral ischaemia[8]
- hydrocephalus due at least in part to obstruction of arachnoid villi by blood products.[9] This may be temporary

Arteriovenous malformation (AVM)

AVMs are the second commonest cause of subarachnoid haemorrhages in adults. They result from developmental abnormalities of arterial and venous vessels leading to the formation of fragile vascular walls[2] as well as the lack of development of a capillary bed.[9] Typically they are made up of three parts: a core of dysplastic vessels known as a nidus, arterial feeding vessels and draining veins.[10] The associated vessels are hypertrophic and hyperplastic. AVMs are typically 3–4 cm in diameter[2] and are usually symptomatic by the age of 50 years.[10]

Clinical presentation:

- intracranial haemorrhage[7,9]
- seizures[7,9]
- headache[9]
- progressive neurological deficits[9]

Points of note:

- A subarachnoid haemorrhage occurs when blood escapes into the subarachnoid space, which is the space between the arachnoid and pia mater. In this space it mixes with the cerebrospinal fluid
- A subdural haemorrhage describes the presence of blood between the dura and arachnoid mater
- An extradural haemorrhage is a bleed outside the dura mater, between the dura mater and the bony skull
- Subarachnoid haemorrhage may arise from a ruptured intracranial aneurysm, bleeding AVM or infrequently as a result of trauma. In contrast, subdural and extradural haemorrhages usually occur as a result of trauma

Stroke

Occurs in 2 per 1000 of the general population[2] and may be divided into two main categories:

- ischaemic   85%
- haemorrhagic   15%[2]

Ischaemic stroke

This type may lead to regional infarction or to small isolated areas known as lacunar infarcts. It occurs as a result of a regional lack of blood supply to the brain and can be due to occlusion of an artery by any mechanism such as thrombosis, emboli or dissection. Thrombus may form intracranially or more commonly at the region of the carotid bifurcation, a common site for atheromatous disease and from where distal emboli frequently occur.

Haemodynamic ischaemic stroke occurs following:

- a reduction in perfusion for any reason
- dissection of the vessels in the neck particularly following trauma

Vasospasm, a common complication of subarachnoid haemorrhage, may also lead to ischaemic stroke. This process can also be a complication of the use of some recreational drugs.

Haemorrhagic stroke

This may result from bleeding into the brain tissue and may be the outcome of aneurysm rupture, AVM or head injury. It can also be spontaneous, for example as a result of hypertensive bleed. Cocaine and heroin abuse also increases the risk of cerebral haemorrhage and may lead to stroke.

Clinical presentation:[9]

- vomiting
- sometimes headache
- deficits in the body area related to associated cerebral involvement. Associated pressure on the brain may lead the patient's condition to deteriorate rapidly and patients can present in coma

Tumour

Presurgical examination of the layout of the vascular supply to tumours is now more usually undertaken by magnetic resonance angiography (MRA). However, preoperative devascularisation (embolisation) is used in some centres.

IMAGING METHODS

Digital subtraction angiography (DSA)

DSA remains the gold standard in the examination of the cerebral vasculature for many abnormalities. It is advantageous to utilise a biplane C-arm mounted fluoroscopic system rather than a single-plane system, to enable reduction in examination time and the amount of radiological contrast medium administered. Bi-plane is preferred for diagnostic use, and is considered essential for interventional use. The introduction of 3D rotational angiography has proved particularly useful in the depiction of intracranial aneurysms, providing the facility to rotate the resultant angiographic image to display the vessels under examination to their best advantage. It should now be considered a standard requirement for neuroangiography.

Procedure

Fully informed consent must be obtained. Patients who are acutely ill may be unable to give consent, and may be treated as an emergency. Those undergoing diagnostic investigation may later undergo interventional treatment, and will need to give their consent for this separately. Preparation is as for standard peripheral angiography, with the addition of a baseline neurological observation. Studies are routinely carried out with the patient awake, or with mild sedation. General anaesthesia may be used in the case of a patient who is unwell, or unable to cooperate, or where diagnostic angiography may proceed to interventional treatment.

Arterial access is normally gained via the femoral artery. The catheter and guide wire are advanced via the aorta and each cerebral vessel is selectively catheterised. Catheters for cerebral angiography have preshaped tips to facilitate vessel access. More than one catheter type may be used if vessels are tortuous or stenosed and a different shape is required. The catheter is often connected, via a 3-way tap, to a pressurised saline flush, which is maintained throughout the procedure to minimise the risk of thrombus formation in the catheter.

Physiological monitoring is maintained throughout the procedure, with neurological observations at 15-minute intervals. Neurological and catheter site observations are made every 30 minutes for 4 hours after the procedure. Bed rest is necessary for 4 hours post procedure, and during this time neurological and catheter site observations are made every 30 minutes.

Complications
- Stroke – risk of between about 0.1 and 1%. This may be transient and result from vessel dissection, arterial spasm or embolus
- Haematoma around the catheterisation site
- Allergy to local anaesthetic or contrast media

Technique
Cerebral angiography
The routine examination is the '4-vessel angiogram' (right and left internal carotid arteries, right and left vertebral arteries). Both internal carotid arteries are selectively catheterised, with the tip of the catheter placed above the carotid bifurcation in the internal carotid artery. Often only one vertebral artery is selectively catheterised as the termination of the contralateral vertebral artery may be filled by reflux, so demonstrating both posterior inferior cerebellar arteries with a single injection. Some centres include selective injections into both external carotids particularly if a dural fistula is suspected.

It is prudent to examine first the vessel most suspected of having an abnormality, in case the procedure needs to be terminated before completion. Non-selective runs, for example with the catheter in the common carotid artery, may be performed if vascular access is difficult, but the quality of the study will be degraded by the superimposition of vessels.

Limited studies, for example of a single vessel, may be performed at follow-up.

A standard set of projections will be taken for each patient. This will vary slightly, depending on the radiologist's preference and the angiographic equipment used.

Internal carotid artery (Figs 39.1, 39.2, 39.3)
Typical standard projections are shown in the following table.

Projection	Positioning guidelines	Field of view
Occipitofrontal	Petrous ridge viewed at the top of the orbit. Vertex at the top of the field of view	17 cm
Anterior oblique	From the OF position, oblique image intensifier to the side under examination 20–25°	17 cm
Lateral	Anterior of the skull at the top of the field, include from the skull base to the vertex, with as much of the rest of the cranium as possible	22 cm

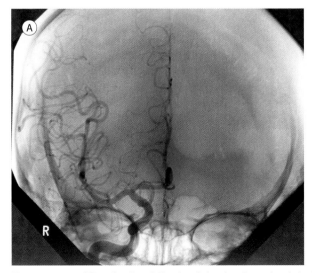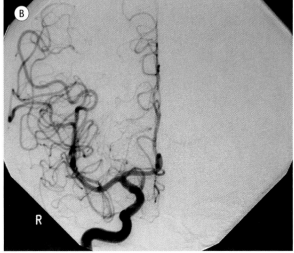

Figure 39.1   OF projection following injection into the right internal carotid artery: **(A)** unsubtracted and **(B)** subtracted

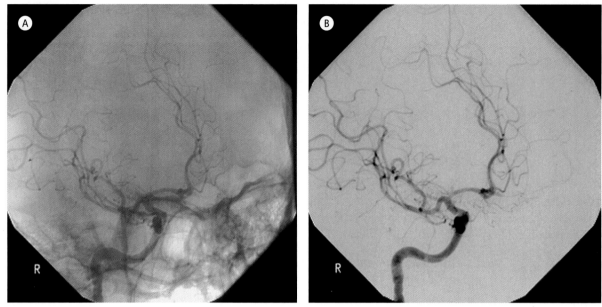

Figure 39.2   AO projection following injection into the left internal carotid artery: **(A)** mask and **(B)** subtracted image

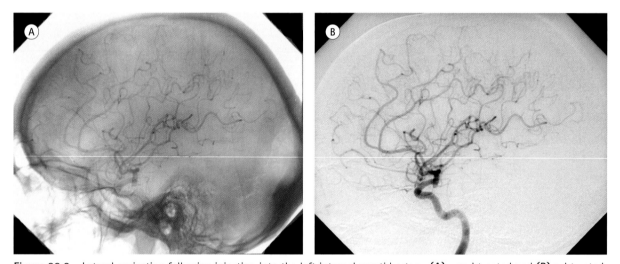

Figure 39.3   Lateral projection following injection into the left internal carotid artery: **(A)** unsubtracted and **(B)** subtracted

Vertebral artery (Figs 39.4, 39.5, 39.6)

Typical standard projections are shown in the following table.

Projection	Positioning guidelines	Field of view
FO 30° (Townes)	Posterior clinoids viewed through foramen magnum. Foramen magnum positioned at the lower third of the field	17 cm
OF 20°	Petrous ridge at bottom of orbits. Include occiput in field of view	17 cm
Lateral	Include all of the occiput. Position with C2 at the bottom of the field of view	22 cm

Final positioning adjustment is made under fluoroscopic control.

Supplementary projections (see the following table on p. 485) may be taken to exclude or demonstrate pathology. These will be dependent on the patient's anatomy.

It is often difficult, with limited projections, to distinguish normal vessels from those with pathology, because the arteries are complex 3D structures. For example, a normal vascular loop may be superimposed over another vessel and mimic an aneurysm. Supplementary projections will allow a full understanding of the anatomy, including which vessels supply or drain any abnormality. It is important to demonstrate fully the morphology of aneurysms to determine the optimum treatment. Of particular interest is the ratio of diameter of the aneurysm body to the neck and

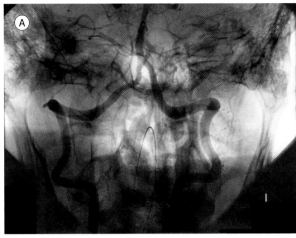

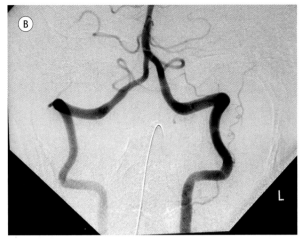

Figure 39.4   FO 30° projection following injection into the left vertebral artery: **(A)** mask and **(B)** subtracted

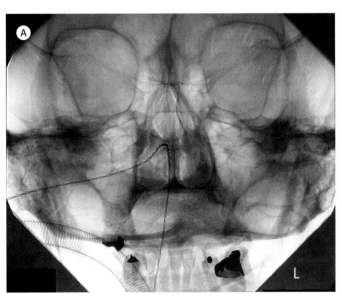

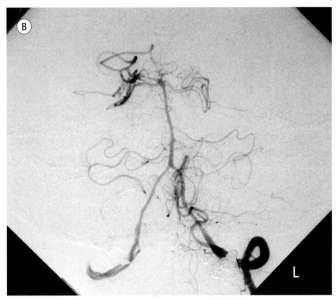

Figure 39.5   OF 20° projection following injection into the left vertebral artery: **(A)** mask and **(B)** subtracted

Supplementary projection	Positioning guidelines	Field of view
Orbital oblique	From the standard anterior oblique projection, angle caudally to project the petrous ridge at the bottom of the orbit	17 cm
Reverse oblique	Anterior oblique 20–25° to the side opposite to the vessel under examination	17 cm
Submentovertical	Raise the patient's chin as much as possible (the head support may be removed) and angle cranially as much as the equipment will allow	17 cm

the relationship of normal vessels to the aneurysm. The choice of projections, and the use of supplementary projections, is modified if 3D rotational angiography can be performed.

Neck vessels
Examination of the extracranial portion of the arteries may be performed. The catheter is placed in the proximal vessel, and injections are made as described above. A common indication is atheromatous stenosis of the carotid bifurcation. Standard projections for the common carotid artery are lateral and 20° anterior oblique.

Hard copy imaging

If hard copy is to be produced, a representative selection of images from each run should be included. This should include the arterial images that best demonstrate the vessel,

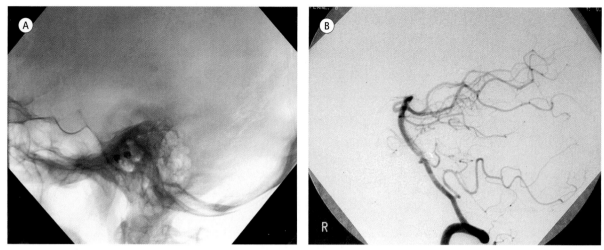

Figure 39.6   Lateral projection following injection into the left vertebral artery: **(A)** unsubtracted and **(B)** subtracted

and venous images. Each sheet of film should have an image included without subtraction to allow orientation with bony landmarks.

3D rotational angiography

Rotational angiography is performed, using suitable equipment, by rotating the C-arm around the vessel of interest during contrast injection administered by injector pump. A series of projections is acquired which can be reformatted on a workstation to produce a 3D representation of the vessel. This can be performed as digital subtraction angiography (DSA) or as a simple non-subtracted acquisition.

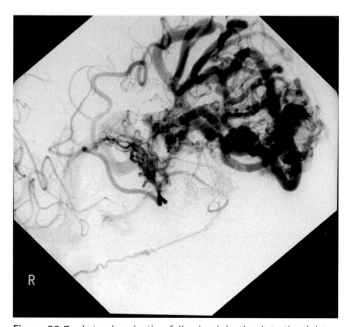

Figure 39.7   Lateral projection following injection into the right common carotid artery. Subtracted image demonstrating an arteriovenous malformation

The catheter is positioned in the vessel as for a conventional angiogram. The vessel of interest is positioned at the isocentre under fluoroscopic control. The rotational run consists of 2 main parts: the C-arm rotates to acquire a series of projections immediately prior to contrast injection, to form the DSA mask; this acquisition series is then repeated during injection of the contrast bolus. The resultant data set consists of a series of subtracted images taken at intervals around the vessel.

A typical set of parameters (Siemens Neurostar) for demonstration of cerebral aneurysms is:

- 200° rotation from left anterior oblique (LAO) to right anterior oblique (RAO)
- 8-second acquisition
- 2.5° per image
- 80 images
- 25 mL contrast injected over 10 seconds, starting 1 second before acquisition and finishing 1 second after to ensure constant opacification

Manipulating the 3D reformat of the images on a workstation allows the vessel to be viewed from any angle, without the need for further acquisitions. An appreciation of the morphology of the vessel, and any abnormality, can be gained, which can add significantly to the information gained from conventional projections. It allows the operator to determine the optimum working projection, that is, the C-arm position, at which to perform embolisation.

The ability to perform rotational angiography with 3D reformatting often removes the need for conventional supplementary oblique projections to be taken. The standard projections may be limited, depending on radiological preference, to frontal, lateral and rotational acquisitions for each vessel. Alternatively, the rotational acquisition may be used only where an abnormality is demonstrated conventionally.

CTA (Figs 39.8, 39.9)

CTA relies on a volume acquisition, the slice thickness dependent on the particular vessels of interest. A radiological contrast medium is introduced intravenously via an automatic injector, the dose being dependent on the speed of flow and diameter of the vessels of interest. The data obtained is reviewed as a maximum intensity projection (MIP) or a 3D surface rendered image. Post-processing facilities enable extraction of surrounding data and this together with 360° rotation of the 3D image enables optimum visualisation of the vessels under examination.

MRA (Fig. 39.10)

The use of MRI is more difficult in emergency situations where it may not be easy to establish whether or not a patient is contraindicated for the examination, and also for those who are critically ill, because of limited patient access. If suitable there are several imaging options available. These are time-of-flight (TOF) angiography, phase contrast angiography (PCA), and more recently, contrast-enhanced MRA (CE-MRA). Each takes a different approach and has advantages and disadvantages in the investigation of the cerebral vessels.

Doppler ultrasound

Doppler ultrasound is utilised in the examination of the carotid arteries in the neck particularly following transient ischaemic attacks (TIAs) or for those at risk of stroke. The aim of the investigation is to examine patency of the carotid arteries especially in the region of the bifurcation where plaque may build up. This region is of particular interest in Doppler

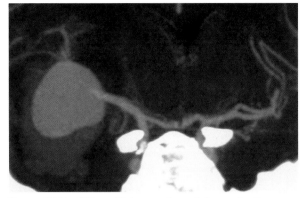

Figure 39.9   CTA multiplanar reformat demonstrating aneurysm

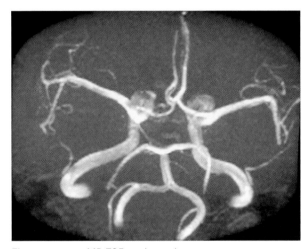

Figure 39.10   MR TOF angiography

ultrasound because it is an area of turbulence as the flow divides between the external and internal carotid arteries. The peak velocity and the relative changes in systole and diastole in different sections of the common, internal and external carotid arteries are indicators of the degree of patency.

Transcranial doppler ultrasound

This approach provides a method of gaining information on the direction and velocity of flow of the cerebral vasculature.[11] It is limited to a small acoustic window and the biggest limitations remain its inability to provide anatomical information or information on surrounding brain tissue. It has been found that its use may be enhanced by the introduction of specially designed contrast agents.[12,13]

AIM OF IMAGING METHODS

• *Aneurysms:* to demonstrate the aneurysm neck and adjacent vessels to inform the choice of appropriate treatment methods: surgery or endovascular therapy

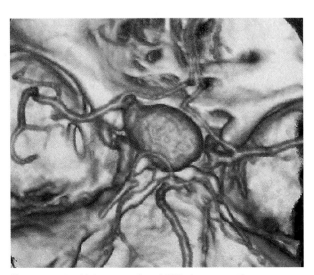

Figure 39.8   Volume rendered CTA demonstrating aneurysm

- *Arteriovenous malformations:* to gain information on the layout of the vascular anatomy to inform treatment decisions
- *Stroke:* to establish the type of stroke and define the area of the vasculature involved, and to more accurately assess the endovascular anatomy of vessels particularly in the context of vasculopathies

Imaging methods employed

Aneurysms

Cerebral angiography supplemented with 3D rotational angiography enables a more exacting presentation of anatomical details than other approaches,[14,15] is a reliable means of demonstrating aneurysms of less than 3 mm in size and does not suffer from the flow artefacts present in MRA.[16] CTA provides a non-invasive and lower cost alternative to DSA,[17] however, its use is dependent on the available technology and, in some centres, acceptance by radiologists and surgeons. The sensitivity of CTA has now approached that of DSA.[18,19] DSA with 3D capabilities remains the gold standard, although some centres make a treatment decision solely on the information provided by CTA.

Vasospasm may occur as a complication of subarachnoid haemorrhage and will affect treatment decisions. It typically occurs 3–10 days following aneurysmal rupture.[5] In the imaging of vasospasm, CTA is more suited to the critically ill patient. CTA demonstrates anatomical configuration independent of the possible flow artefacts associated with MRA. Vasospasm may also be investigated by single photon emission computed tomography (SPECT) by means of measuring regional cerebral blood flow.[20]

Arteriovenous malformations

In the management of AVMs, the layout of the vascular anatomy will influence treatment decisions. Information is required on the size and location of the nidus as well as the feeding and draining vessels. MRI and CT both have a role in providing information on location of the AVM, with MRA and CTA providing additional information on the vascular anatomy. It has been shown that use of volume rendered views may increase the diagnostic confidence in MRA.[21] In preoperative assessment of AVMs there is a role for the range of imaging methods but DSA remains the definitive procedure and provides optimum resolution for differentiation between vessels.

Stroke

CTA and MRA both have important roles. Diffusion weighted (DW) and perfusion weighted (PW) MRI both have the capability of yielding information that will assist in patient management and treatment. DW imaging will provide a hyperintense signal of areas of ischaemia, because of the accumulation of intracellular water in the area of the ischaemic tissue.[22] Early ischaemic changes can be detected by perfusion-weighted imaging, the deficit in perfusion representing the area involved.[22] Where MRA is not available, CTA as well as CT perfusion studies provide a reliable alternative.

THE FUTURE

The gold standard for the demonstration of vascular abnormalities remains conventional catheter angiography. However, many conditions can now be adequately demonstrated using alternative techniques that are less invasive and quicker.

Continuing refinements in MRA mean that the use of this investigation will expand. With a range of different angiographic sequences available, this non-invasive, non-ionising technique is ideal for imaging many vascular abnormalities, with the exception of acute haemorrhage. The current provision of MR scanners in the UK means that rapid access to this investigation may be restricted. Acutely ill patients may be unable to cooperate with MRI scanning, and the restrictions of the MRI environment produce difficulties in imaging high-dependency patients.

The introduction, and now widespread installation, of multislice CT scanners, has changed the way in which many vascular pathologies are imaged. Their ability to produce high speed, high resolution CT angiography over a wider anatomical area than single slice helical scanners means that this has become a primary investigation for patients presenting with conditions such as subarachnoid haemorrhage or stroke. Advances in hardware and processing software mean that diagnostic confidence in CTA compared to conventional DSA is high. Even relatively small vascular abnormalities, such as small aneurysms, can be demonstrated. This investigation can be performed on patients presenting from the A&E department, leading to rapid diagnosis, with demonstration of the morphology of vascular abnormalities, and subsequent expedition of effective treatment.

CTA is not suitable for all conditions: degradation from metallic artefacts makes it unsuitable for patients with vascular clips or coils, and its demonstration of abnormalities such as small vessels in slow-flowing AVMs is inferior to conventional angiography. DSA will remain the investigation of choice for such conditions.

DSA will continue to be performed where the results of other techniques are equivocal, but its use as a diagnostic tool will lessen. The acceptance of the efficacy of interventional radiological treatment over conventional neurosurgery for many intracranial vascular abnormalities[23] means that the DSA room will become more dedicated to treatment than diagnosis.

Acknowledgements

Neuroradiology Department, King's College Hospital NHS Trust, London.

Thanks are extended to Dr Timothy Cox, Consultant Neuroradiologist, The National Hospital for Neurology and Neurosurgery, London and Dr Neil Deasy, Consultant Neuroradiologist, King's College Hospital, London for their helpful comments.

References

1. Stoodley M, Weir B. Aneurysms and arteriovenous malformations. In: Asbury A, et al, eds. Diseases of the nervous system: clinical neuroscience and therapeutic principles, vol.2. 3rd edn. Cambridge University Press; 2002:1392–1404.
2. Stevens A, Lowe J. Pathology. 2nd edn. Edinburgh: Mosby; 2000.
3. Toole J. Cerebrovascular disorders. 5th edn. London: Lippincott Williams and Wilkins; 1999.
4. Lindsay K, Bone I. Neurology and neurosurgery illustrated. 3rd edn. Edinburgh: Churchill Livingstone; 1997.
5. Wiebers D, et al. Unruptured intracranial aneurysms: natural history, clinical outcome, and risks of surgical and endovascular treatment. Lancet 2003; 362:9378:103–110.
6. Fitzgerald M, Folan-Curran J. Clinical neuroanatomy and related neuroscience. 4th edn. Edinburgh: Saunders; 2002.
7. Ellis S. Clinical neurology: essential concepts. Oxford: Butterworth Heinemann; 1998.
8. Chicoine M, Dacey R. Clinical aspects of subarachnoid hemorrhage. In: Welch K, et al, eds. Primer on cerebrovascular diseases. San Diego: Academic Press; 1997: 425–432.
9. Porth C. Pathophysiology. 6th edn. New York: Lippincott-Raven; 2002.
10. Lawton M, Spetzler R. Surgical management of acutely ruptured arteriovenous malformations. In: Welch K, et al, eds. Primer on cerebrovascular diseases. San Diego: Academic Press; 1997:511–519.
11. Allan P. The carotid and vertebral arteries and transcranial colour Doppler. In: Allan P, et al, eds. Clinical Doppler ultrasound. London: Churchill Livingstone; 2000.
12. Hansberg T, et al. Effects of the ultrasound contrast-enhancing agent Levovist® on the detection of intracranial arteries and stenoses in Chinese by transcranial Doppler ultrasound. Cerebrovascular Diseases 2002; 14:105–108.
13. Drost D, et al. Sonovue® (BRI), a new long-acting echocontrast agent improves transcranial colour-coded duplex ultrasonic imaging. Cerebrovascular Diseases 2002; 14(1):27–32.
14. Hochmuth A, et al. Comparison of three-dimensional rotational angiography with digital subtraction angiography in the assessment of ruptured cerebral aneurysm. American Journal of Neuroradiology 2002; 32(7):1199–1205.
15. Sugahara T, et al. Comparison of 2D and 3D digital subtraction angiography in evaluation of intracranial aneurysms. American Journal of Neuroradiology 2002; 23:1545–1552.
16. Cloft H, et al. Risk of cerebral angiography – patients with subarachnoid haemorrhage, cerebral aneurysm and arteriovenous malformation: a meta-analysis. Stroke 1999; 30:317–320.
17. Villablanca J, et al. Detection and characterization of very small cerebral aneurysms by using 2D and 3D helical CT angiography. American Journal of Neuroradiology 2002; 23(7): 1187–1198.
18. Cloft H, Kallmes D. Detection and characterization of very small cerebral aneurysms by using 2D and 3D helical CT angiography. American Journal of Neuroradiology 2003; 24(1):154; author reply 154–156.
19. Leclerc X, et al. Symptomatic vasospasm after subarachnoid haemorrhage: assessment of brain damage by diffusion and perfusion-weighted MRI and single photon emission computed tomography. Neuroradiology 2002; 44:610–616.
20. Mallouhi A, et al. Investigation of cerebrovascular disease with MR angiography: comparison of volume rendering and maximum intensity projection algorithms – initial assessment. Neuroradiology 2002; 44:961–967.
21. Moonis M, Fisher M. Imaging of acute stroke. Cerebrovascular Diseases 2001; 11:143–150.
22. Molyneux A, et al. International subarachnoid aneurysm trial (ISAT) of neurosurgical clipping versus endovascular coiling in 2143 patients with ruptured intracranial aneurysms: a randomised trial. Lancet. 2002; 360(9342):1267–1274.

SECTION

8

ADDITIONAL IMAGING METHODS

COMPUTED TOMOGRAPHY

Barry Carver

INTRODUCTION

Radiography produces 2D images of 3D objects, it is important to remember that they are shadow projections (Ex Umbris Eruditio). This inevitably means that structures are superimposed and the structure that is the object of imaging may be obscured from view. To address this problem, focal plane tomography was developed shortly after the First World War, blurring out layers above and below the region of interest, to provide an image of the required structure but again it is 2D and prone to equipment and operating problems. The ideal is a technique which allows for 3D rendition of images.

The advent of X-ray computed tomography (CT) has had a great impact on medical imaging, primarily because CT solves this fundamental limitation of radiography by eliminating the superimposition of imaged structures.

CT uses a rotating X-ray source coupled to a bank of detectors to produce diagnostic images of the body. The basic premise of CT is that the attenuation pattern of the X-rays can be measured during rotation and spatially located; the sum of attenuation at each point can then be calculated and displayed. Since its inception at the beginning of the 1970s CT has now become a major technique in the routine diagnosis of disease and scanners can be found in almost all district general hospitals in the UK.

Advantages of CT include:
- Axial acquisition of cross-sectional images: with modern isotropic imaging, data can be post processed into multiple planes or rendered volumes, producing 2D or 3D images. Magnetic resonance (MR) is truly multiplanar as scans are acquired directly in different planes without the need for reconstruction; however the quality of CT isotropic reconstructions is high.

- Cross-sectional imaging has excellent low contrast resolution (LCR), which is superior to other imaging methods with the exception of MR, which matches and in some cases exceeds the LCR of CT.
- CT images also show good high contrast (spatial) resolution, and excellent bone detail. MR does not image bone directly due to the lack of free hydrogen within cortical bone.
- Digital imaging: this enables the manipulation of images, as well as post processing to other planes; the applied algorithm and windows can be adjusted to better visualise specific tissues. The application of filters and digital processing can enhance content, e.g. the use of edge enhancement for looking at bone.
- CT is generally well tolerated by patients, certainly more so than MR, which is less well tolerated due to noise and claustrophobia. Contraindications for MR due to safety requirements do not apply to CT.
- CT is still more readily available than MRI and radionuclide imaging (RNI), being in situ in the vast majority of district general hospitals (DGHs) in the UK.

Disadvantages of CT include:
- Ionising radiation dose: CT is undeniably an extremely high dose technique, many examinations being amongst the highest, if not the highest doses, in use in medical imaging. Multiple examinations may approach the thresholds for deterministic radiation effects.
- Metallic artefacts cause loss of image detail; this effect is much reduced by software corrections on many modern scanners.
- Soft tissue structures surrounded closely by bone can be difficult to image, e.g. in the posterior fossa, where the soft tissue contrast of MR is superior. This is again a problem largely overcome in the latest generation of scanners.

- Misregistration artefact can be caused by relative movement of the body structures from the acquisition of single slice to the next, e.g. due to inconsistencies in the patient's respiratory pattern. If misregistration occurs then the reconstruction will be meaningless, as the same portion of anatomy could be portrayed at different positions in the reconstructed image. With the advent of single breath hold scanning this is now less of a consideration. However many centers, when scanning two areas such as the chest and upper abdomen, will overlap the two acquisition blocks to ensure no loss of information due to breathing differences between the two acquisitions. The dose implications of this technique are worthy of consideration.

In some quarters there is an attitude that CT can be undertaken by anybody, including non-radiographically qualified staff such as departmental assistants. It can be argued however that, along with every other branch of imaging, CT is operator dependent. Image quality is dependent on factors that should be adjusted for each examination and more important for each patient. In addition, due to the high dose burden, all operators of CT equipment should be trained and skilled in optimising CT examinations,[1] indeed specific additional training requirements are mandatory in some countries such as the USA.[2]

EQUIPMENT CHRONOLOGY

1874 Sir William Crookes constructs the cathode discharge tube. During his experiments over the next few years he discovers fogging of photographic plates stored near discharge tubes.

1895 Wilhelm Roentgen discovers X-rays whilst investigating gas discharge using a Crookes' tube.

1935 Grossman coins the term 'tomography' describing his apparatus for looking at detail in the lungs.[3]

1951 Godfrey Hounsfield starts work at EMI, initially working on early computers.

1956 Ronald Bracewell uses Fourier transforms to reconstruct solar images. At the same time Alan Cormack starts to work on solving 'line integrals'.

1958 Korenblyum and colleagues in Ukraine work on obtaining thin section X-ray images using mathematical reconstructions.

1961 William Oldendorf produces an image of the internal structure of a test object using a rotating object. He was unable to make further progress due to the lack of available equipment to provide the computation that would have been required.

1963 Cormack publishes a paper on mathematical reconstruction methods.

1965 David Kuhl, one of the pioneers of RNI, produces a transmission image using a radioactive source coupled to a detector.[4]

1967 Bracewell produces a mathematical solution for reconstruction with fewer errors and artefact than found with Fourier.
Hounsfield & Ambrose come together to develop CT head scanning. Hounsfield uses an iterative algebraic technique rather than more complex mathematical formulae.

1971 The first clinical CT scanner is installed at Atkinson Morley Hospital under the supervision of James Ambrose. The first patient is scanned on 1 October. The first scanners were somewhat crude and took several minutes to produce each slice, which were of fairly poor quality. However, at the time, even these crude images were revolutionary, enabling a first non-invasive glimpse within the skull, at the soft tissue contents.

1972 Ambrose & Hounsfield discuss the clinical use of CT at the British Institute of Radiology annual conference.[5] Clinical images are shown at RSNA.

1973 Hounsfield & Ambrose publish papers describing the design and clinical applications of the CT system.[6,7]
EMI scanner becomes commercially available.
Hounsfield starts work on the second generation scanner.

1974 Hounsfield produces abdominal images with a 20-second acquisition time.

1975 EMI CT 1010 second generation scanner becomes available, soon to be followed by the CT 5005 – the first EMI body scanner.
In the next few years, third generation scanners become available but have problems with artefact; a problem solved by General Electric (GE). Fourth generation scanners were later introduced to avoid the artefact problems initially suffered by the third generation machines.

1979 Hounsfield & Cormack are awarded the Nobel prize for medicine.

1983 The first 2-second scanner introduced by GE (CT 9800).

1985 Electron beam CT developed.

1989 Siemens introduce spiral (helical) CT, using slip ring technology to enable the tube to rotate continuously without the need to go back to unwind its cables.

1992 Elscint Twin scans 2 slices simultaneously, which is a return to a method used by the original EMI scanners.

1998 Multislice CT initially incorporating 4 slices is
on introduced, GE, Picker, Siemens and Toshiba

displayed systems at RSNA. Since then 8,16,32,40 and now 64 slice machines have become available. Sub second scan times enable body areas to be scanned in a single breath hold. Toshiba are currently working to develop '4D CT', utilising 256 detector rows to provide functional and real time 3D imaging.[8] Advancements have in many cases had to wait on the development of computer systems robust enough to cope with the huge quantities of data generated, a problem initially encountered by Oldendorf.

As mentioned above, CT systems have been classified according to the motion of the X-ray tube and detectors during scanning. There have been several generations of CT scanner, which are described here in brief.

First generation scanner

The first generation CT scanner utilised a single pencil beam of X-rays being measured by a single detector. In order to cover the area of interest, the movement required is a combination of translation and rotation. In the initial position, the tube/detector assembly moves across the scan field of view (translation) and a series of measurements of transmitted intensity are made. It then rotates 1° to its next position before commencing another translation.

This is a very time-consuming method and typical scan times were of the order of 4 to 6 minutes per slice acquisition. The early scanners attempted to compensate by having two detectors to perform 2 slices at once, a technique now resurrected in the latest generation of spiral scanners that offer 'new' multislice acquisition.

- Advantages: it was the first of its kind and offered the first opportunity for axial imaging of the head
- Disadvantages: mechanically complex, slow scans, which were only practical for scanning the head of patients who could be adequately immobilised using a water bag. The water bag was used to reduce the range of information required as its density is closer than air to that of tissue

Second generation scanner

The second generation used the same principles of movement as the first generation, i.e. a combination of translation and rotation, but utilised several new innovations. Instead of a pencil beam, a narrow fan beam was now utilised, being measured by a bank of detectors. The fan beam is still not sufficient to cover the entire area of interest so translation and then rotation is still required, but because more information is being gathered at each position, multiple degree rotational incrementation is possible.

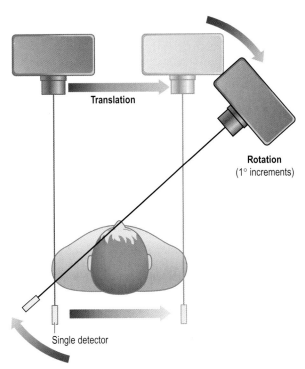

Figure 40.1 Schematic of first generation scanner

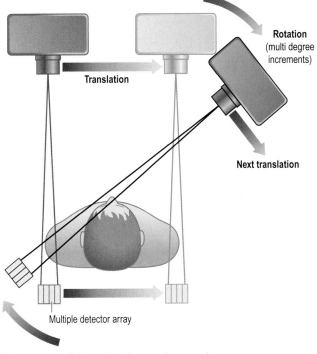

Figure 40.2 Schematic of second generation scanner

- Advantages: as several detectors were being utilised, scanning times were significantly reduced and quality was increased. Typical scan times of the order of 20 to 80 seconds per slice were achievable. Again 2 slices were acquired simultaneously on the EMI 1010 with a fixed slice thickness of 13 mm
- Disadvantages: The maintenance of the translate–rotate movement renders these scanners still mechanically complex

Third generation scanner

Also known as a rotate–rotate scanner, this model was the first to do away with the requirement for translation across the patient by utilising a wide fan beam of X-rays. A large number of detectors (up to 1000) are used to allow for the increased beam width, and the tube and detectors are rigidly coupled and rotate jointly about the patient. Rotation only is required as the fan beam covers the entire body. It is this configuration that is still the most commonly used, even in the latest multislice equipment.

- Advantages: the greater number of detectors plus the rotation only movement allows shorter scan times, typically of the order of 2 to 8 seconds. The width of the fan beam can be adjusted (collimated) to limit the beam to the area under examination. Use of the rotation only movement renders this type of unit mechanically simpler than its predecessors.
- Disadvantages: detectors were expensive, therefore more detectors equals more cost. Also more processing power

is required, as more information is gathered at one time. Initially problems were encountered with circular artefacts but this was overcome by adjusting the detectors

Fourth generation scanner

This scanner was similar to the third generation scanner; again using a wide fan beam, but with a complete circle of detectors around the patient. In this case only the tube rotates, with the detector ring being stationary.

- Advantages: mechanically simpler due to having fewer moving parts. Scan times reduced and now taking 1 to 10 seconds
- Disadvantages: the high number of detectors equals high cost. There were also greater calibration difficulties. As the tube is rotating within the detector ring, the detectors are further away from the patient leading to a greater penumbral effect

Electron beam computed tomography (EBCT)

A completely different concept, the electron beam is directed to the anode rotating around the patient, and is again linked to a bank of detectors. As mechanical rotational movement is now not utilised, quick (sub second) scans are possible. EBCT has been used for gated cardiac studies for some time. This was the only CT technology which could provide high quality cardiac imaging for several

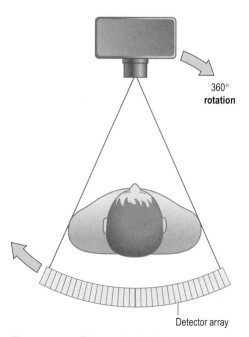

Figure 40.3 Schematic of third generation scanner

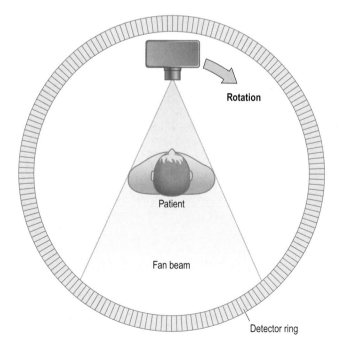

Figure 40.4 Schematic of fourth generation scanner

years, but the latest generation of multislice (64 slice) equipment can now match EBCT in cardiac studies.

Spiral/helical CT

Helical scanners are also described as volume acquisition or spiral scanners, for clarity the term helical will be used throughout this chapter.

In the 1990s, 'conventional' CT began to be replaced by helical scanners. Due to cost, availability, and equipment replacement programmes, it was only in the late nineties that these became the norm in the UK. Ironically, this occurred just as this technology itself was superseded with the introduction of multislice helical scanning.

Helical scanning differs from conventional CT in the method of data acquisition. Instead of a single 360° rotation that produces a single slice followed by an incremental table movement, in helical scanning, a volume of data is acquired.

One of the main advantages of this method of continuous data acquisition is its speed. As a large volume of data can be acquired very rapidly, a series of images that would take several minutes to acquire in conventional 'slice by slice' mode, can now be obtained in seconds.

This is due to both the use of slip ring technology, enabling continuous rotation of the X-ray tube around the gantry (without the cables which previously had to be 'unwound' by a return rotation prior to the next slice being obtained), and also improvements in the design of the tube and its drive motors enabling sub second acquisition times.

This rapid data acquisition means that large areas of the patient can be imaged within a single breath hold, eliminating one of the major problems for image reconstruction and interpretation: misregistration. Respiratory misregistration can be completely eliminated, and the short scan times make it less likely that patient movement becomes a factor.

Multislice CT

The latest advance in scanner design is the multidetector volume acquisition scanner – ironically a return to one of the features of the original EMI scanner – multiple detector arrays. The difference is that the first EMI scanner had two rows of one detector, whereas the latest multislice scanners have tens of thousands of detector elements. The majority of scanners are of the third generation type with rotating tube and detector array.

Large volumes can be rapidly imaged with thin slice widths enhancing the diagnostic capacity of CT. Large numbers of thin slices can be reconstructed to produce high quality volume rendered images, with the elimination of 'stair step' artefacts, and the reduction of partial volume artefacts.

Advantages of multislice include:
- Speed of acquisition – sub second rotation speeds are now the norm
- In comparison to single slice helical, multislice enables the same acquisition in a shorter time, or larger volumes to be scanned in the same time, or for thinner slices to be scanned
- All manufacturers have sub millimetre scan capabilities. Toshiba have detectors that are 0.5 mm, matching the pixel size to produce a voxel which is the same size in each dimension: termed isotropic (Fig. 40.9). Isotropic and near isotropic voxels enhance the 2D reformatting ability of the scanner, enabling high quality multiplanar reconstructions from an axial data set. 3D reformats produced are also excellent, with none of the problems of possible misregistration and information loss inherent in MR due to its longer scan times

EQUIPMENT

The X-ray tube

The advent of spiral scanning with its continuous rotation means that huge demands are placed on the X-ray tube used in modern scanners. The tube needs to provide high output, whilst dealing effectively with dissipation of the heat produced. Air conditioning is generally required to maintain a comfortable temperature within the scan room and to assist with heat dissipation. Large anode discs in metal or ceramic tube envelopes are common, the anode usually being mostly graphite with a tungsten/rhenium target track.

Beam shaping filter

In any CT scanner the X-ray beam produced is in fact heterogeneous, having a range of energies. Filters are applied to the beam on exiting the tube to reduce the range of energies. Filters also shape the beam to produce a more uniform result at the detectors in order to reduce the dynamic range required in the detector electronics.

Collimators

In a single slice system, a pre-patient collimator will limit the beam to the prescribed slice width at the centre of rotation; a post-patient collimator will then limit the beam incident on the detectors to the slice width. For example, pre-patient collimation to 4 mm will result in a 4 mm slice being produced.

In a multislice system, the beam is again collimated at the centre of rotation but the result will differ. For example, in a 4 slice system the 4 mm collimation given above will result in 4 × 1 mm slices being obtained.

Table

The table is an important element in CT. They are usually of carbon fibre construction with rise and fall action, this gives strength without interfering with the resultant image, and facilitates patient handling. The table must be able to provide a wide range of movement at various speeds. Accuracy of movement is vital as any inconsistency would have detrimental effects on the image produced.

Table-tops are generally curved, except for those tables used in radiotherapy planning where a flat table-top is essential to allow CT simulation. Simulation needs to reproduce accurately the patient's position on the flat treatment table. Consequently scanners used for both purposes will often have interchangeable table-tops for diagnostic and planning sessions.

Detectors

Modern detectors are of the solid state type, mostly employing ultra-fast ceramic detector elements. An incident beam causes scintillation; the photon produced is then converted to an electrical signal by a photodiode and sent on to the electronics. The detector array is formed by a series of individual elements as shown in Figure 40.5.

Different manufacturers have differing approaches to the format of detector arrays, with 4 slice machines being available as fixed matrix, adaptive, or mixed arrays. Each of the major manufacturers has taken a different approach to 16 slice and as can be seen in Figure 40.6, the choice of array format affects the minimum slice width available, the number of slices available at minimum width, and the range of slice widths available.

Data acquisition system (DAS)

The DAS 'reads' the measurements from the detector array, converts these analogue signals into digital format, and transmits the digital signal to the computer systems for reconstruction into the presented images.

The DAS needs to be able to deal rapidly with a vast amount of data being generated every second; in current computing technology there is a limit to how much data

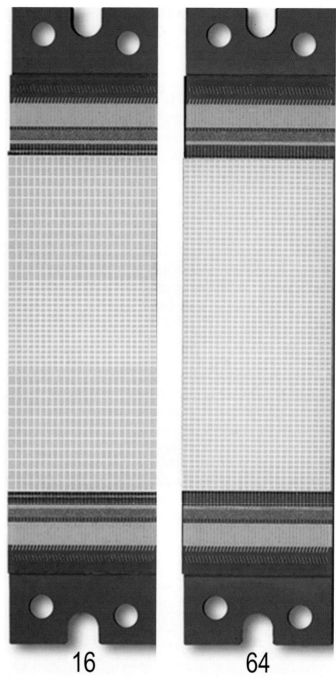

Figure 40.5 Aquilion 16 and 64 detector arrays. Both provide up to 32 mm coverage per rotation. The 16 slice detector has 16 × 0.5 mm elements centrally, with 12 × 1 mm elements either side, enabling acquisition of 16 × 0.5 mm or 16 × 1 mm or 16 × 2 mm slices per rotation. The 64 slice detector provides 64 × 0.5 mm slices per rotation. Reproduced with permission from Toshiba

can be handled at the necessary transfer rates. Development of these systems is advancing rapidly but they have been a limiting factor to the speed of development of larger multislice arrays.

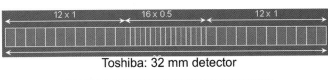

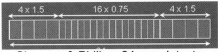

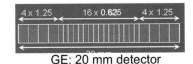

Figure 40.6 Comparison of 16 slice detector arrays

Computer system

The computer system processes operator input to set scanning parameters, patient information, and archiving instructions. It also receives the information from the DAS which is then processed to form the image. A wide range of post-processing options are available on modern scanners which again take place within this system, or alternatively on dedicated workstations. High speed, high capacity computers are required to perform these tasks at speeds that were unthought of only a decade ago.

Archiving requires some consideration; although archiving systems have greatly increased in capacity (and decreased in cost) in recent years the amount of data generated has followed the same pattern. Only selected reconstructions are generally sent for storage and access on PACS systems; raw data, if stored, is often on high capacity optical discs.

PHYSICAL PRINCIPLES OF SCANNING

What happens to a homogeneous X-ray beam as it passes through an object? The X-ray photons interact with the material through which they pass and are attenuated by it. If the intensity of the emerging beam is measured, we know the initial intensity hence the attenuation within the object can be measured.

With the X-ray tube of a CT scanner in one position, a narrow X-ray beam passes through the patient and the attenuation along the line taken by a particular beam through the patient can be calculated from the intensity of the emergent beam measured by a detector. The X-ray intensity transmitted through an object along a particular path contains information about all the material it has passed through, but does not allow the distribution of the material along the path to be discerned.

For the energies used in CT the attenuation of the beam is due to:

- Absorption: photoelectric
- Scattering: Compton (mainly)

Attenuation due to photoelectric absorption is strongly dependent on the atomic number of the material (α Z^3).

Attenuation due to Compton scattering does not depend upon atomic number, but on the number of free electrons present. The number of electrons per gram of an absorber is remarkably constant over a wide range of materials, however because their density varies considerably, the number of electrons per metre does show variation across a range of biological materials.

If we consider the simplistic case of a homogeneous beam passing through the medium, the attenuation within the tissues follows the Lambert–Beer law.

The Lambert–Beer law states:

$$I = I_0 e^{-\mu x}$$

Where: μ = linear attenuation coefficient
I_0 = original intensity
I = transmitted intensity
x = thickness of material.

In CT we are interested in measuring the linear attenuation coefficient. Solving the Lambert–Beer equation for LAC, we get:

$$\mu = \frac{1}{x} . \ln\left(\frac{I_0}{I}\right)$$

I is measured by the detectors, I_0, x are known, hence μ can be calculated.[9]

As mentioned earlier, the X-ray beam produced is in fact heterogeneous, having a range of energies. Filters are applied to the beam on exiting the tube to reduce the range of energies incident on the detector array.

A narrow beam is required for accurate localisation of the attenuating tissues. Readings are then taken from multiple angles to give a series of values of linear attenuation of the beam along intersecting lines through the patient. For example, in Figure 40.7, a bony object would have the same attenuating effect on 'beam 1' whether at position 'A' or 'B'. However, from 'beam 2' it is possible to localise the structure to position 'B'.

In general, then, the transmitted intensity depends on the sum of the attenuation coefficients for all points along the path of the beam. Thus, the log transmission measurement is sometimes referred to as a 'ray sum' or 'line integral' of the attenuation along the path.

A radiograph can be considered to be composed of many such ray sums, produced unidirectionally, hence superimposing all structures encountered by the beam. Because

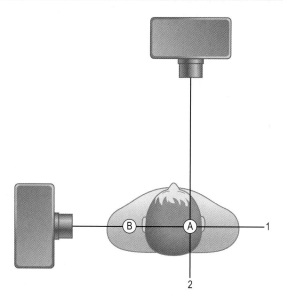

Figure 40.7   Localisation of position

of the differences in transmitted intensity, interfaces between bone, tissue and air are well demonstrated. The differences between adjacent soft tissues are not sufficient for good differentiation and hence they are less well demonstrated.

To demonstrate soft tissues we need to eliminate superimposition by taking ray sums from multiple directions, these ray sum measurements can then be mathematically reconstructed to generate an axial image formed by estimating the distribution of the linear attenuation coefficient within the irradiated volume. The image produced can then be digitally manipulated to maximise contrast enabling adequate visualisation of subtle changes in tissue density. The ability to produce such images is the main strength of CT as an imaging modality.

The information acquired by the detectors is passed to the computer. Once this data is committed to the computer memory it can be manipulated by the resident software to produce an image which is reconstructed on the screen of the viewing console. Reconstruction takes place via the application of a complex mathematical algorithm to the data obtained, usually a filtered back projection. Consideration of the detail of this mathematical process is beyond the scope of this chapter, but is well described in texts such as Seeram.[9]

Image reconstruction in its simplest form consists of recalling the digital information fed to the computer from the detectors via the DAS, and converting this information to an analogue voltage signal which controls the electron sweep within the display monitor.

Helical image reconstruction is more complex: because the table is continuously moving only one ray sum lies in the scan plane, the rest of the 'slice' information is interpolated from the acquired volume. 360° and 180° interpolations are used. As seen in Figure 40.8 a 360° interpolation requires data from two tube rotations for slice reconstruction. 180° interpolation allows smaller slice widths to be accurately reconstructed.

Multislice is more complex again, as it uses two or more data samples to produce each point within a projection, but the basic principles are the same. There is, however, an additional complication in that the more slices that are scanned, the wider the beam becomes in the z direction (along the patient length), meaning the beam ceases to be a narrow fan as seen in conventional and helical scanners; in multislice, the volume of data is the volume between two cones (Fig. 40.9). Each of the manufacturers has different mathematical methods for 'cone beam' correction; the complexity of the multislice reconstruction process is again beyond the scope of this chapter but is addressed in specialist texts.[9]

The amount of movement within the data set is governed by the table movement, and is measured as the scan pitch. Helical pitch is defined as:

Pitch = 'table travel per rotation/nominal slice width'

There are two definitions for pitch quoted in multislice, each of which provides a different number to represent pitch; it is therefore important to know which definition is in use when comparing techniques:

Pitch = 'table travel per rotation/X-ray beam width'
or
Pitch = 'table travel per rotation/detector width'

The data is stored within the computer as a matrix of intensities. The image produced consists of a matrix of cells with various brightness levels on the display monitor; the brightness of each cell is related to the intensity detected.

Each image square (or PICture ELement) is called a pixel. The value of the number represented in each cell is rela-

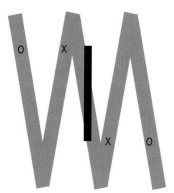

Figure 40.8   Diagrammatic representation of interpolation of helical data. 180° interpolation – X to X; 360° interpolation – 0 to 0

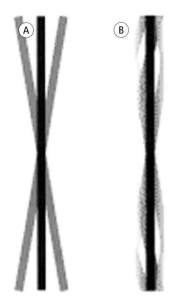

Figure 40.9 Cone beam problem. **(A)** A wide X-ray beam is required to give full coverage of the detector elements. The beams produced at opposing angle form a cone, the slice profile is sharp at the centre but spatial resolution is lost at the edges due to 'cone beaming'. **(B)** For example, Toshiba's TCOT algorithm calculates these complex angles to provide a more accurate slice profile

Figure 40.10 Pixel and voxel

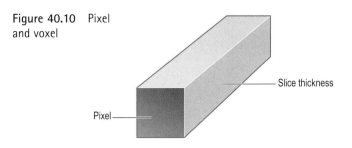

tive, and is used to define image contrast. In CT the numeric information contained in each pixel is a CT number (or Hounsfield unit: HU) and is expressed relative to the density of water. The detector array is calibrated to give a zero value for water.

Each of these 2D picture elements represents a volume of patient data, the volume element, or voxel, and is equal to the pixel size x slice thickness. If the voxel is the same size in each direction then it is called isotropic. This is the ideal for multiplanar reconstruction as the blocks are effectively the same when viewed from any direction, hence maximising the quality of reconstructions. (Fig. 40.10)

The size of image matrix used is determined by the characteristics of the equipment, and the storage capacity of the computer. The size of the image matrix is important as the more squares there are to form the image, the greater will be the image definition.

Measurement of the CT number of an object in an image can be useful for tissue characterisation, as by comparing it to known values such as those in the table below we can get a feel for the composition of the material (although a definitive tissue diagnosis cannot be made).

Windowing

The displayed image will comprise areas of high X-ray attenuation, shown in white; and low attenuation, shown in black. The intervening soft tissues will be shown in various shades of grey according to their individual attenuation properties.

As CT is sensitive to small changes in density, use can be made of the variation in shades of grey represented on the image to give better contrast discrimination. The image can be viewed on a variety of chosen settings to better view the particular structures of interest. This is termed 'windowing'.

The window level is set to the tissue of interest – this will place the tissue of interest in the midpoint of the grey scale. The window width is set to enable the required range of tissues to be viewed, and straddles the window level evenly. For example, a window width of 400 set with a window level of 40 will include tissues with HU values from -160 to 240. Anything below -160 will appear black, whilst anything above 240 will appear white. The shades of grey on the image will divide the 400 units to be demonstrated. A typical monitor displaying 16 grey shades will display these window settings as shown in Figure 40.11.

Hounsfield unit values for a range of tissues	
Tissue type	*Hounsfield unit*
Air	-400+
Fat	-95
Water	0
CSF	10
Oedema	20–30
Clotted blood	30
White matter	30
Grey matter	35–55
Muscle	40–80
Kidney	50
Liver	60
Fresh blood	70
Calcification	~125
Cortical bone	1000

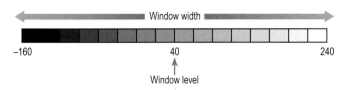

Figure 40.11   Windowing: grey scale

As window width is increased, each grey scale shade represents a greater number of attenuation values, so more tissues are seen, but with a reduction in image contrast. Thus the image appears flat, i.e. it has an overall grey appearance. Lower window widths enable tissues of closer attenuation values to be discriminated so small changes in density may be seen. The image will be of high contrast; i.e. it has more black and white. Low widths make the noise inherent in the image appear more apparent.

Introduction of contrast media can raise the attenuation values of soft tissue structures. It is important then to adjust the window level accordingly to ensure the tissues of interest remain in the centre of the grey scale and that structures which need to be visualised remain within the range of the selected window width.

Thresholds can be set using specific HU values to produce a range of data sets to provide a variety of image types on modern scanners, e.g. maximum intensity projections (MIP). Colourised images can also be produced on the workstation to delineate different structures, particularly in 3D, and surface rendered images, for example.

IMAGE QUALITY

It has previously been stated that CT can be considered to be an operator or user dependent modality; this is because the user has a direct influence on the quality of the images produced and, as will be discussed later, the radiation dose administered to the patient. Given the potential for the administration of high doses within CT, adequate training of appropriately qualified staff is essential.

The greatest influence on image quality results from the choice of scanning factors; which includes mA, scan time, slice thickness, and kVp. These parameters essentially determine the number of photons emitted from the X-ray tube and registered on the detector, which in turn determines the noise level, which has a detrimental effect on image quality.

Noise is superimposed over the whole image as a uniform grainy appearance and is dependent on the number of photons reaching the detectors (signal to noise ratio). Several factors influence the noise level on the image, the primary ones being slice thickness, patient size, and applied mAs. In order to obtain good quality images, noise should be kept to a minimum. However, there is a trade-off to be made: images can be produced with almost no noise, but at the cost of increased dose as the noise level is related to the applied mAs. Noise varies as $(1/\text{dose})^{1/2}$, and consequently doubling the mAs applied (and therefore patient dose) only reduces noise by factor of about 1.4.

The influence of slice thickness has changed, particularly with the higher end scanners (16 or more slices). Conventionally thick slices would be used for general soft tissue use. More photons contribute to image quality so noise is lower, a larger area is covered more quickly, the dose is reduced, and examination time is faster. Thinner slices were reserved for areas where high resolution was required; fewer photons contribute to the image, therefore noise level is higher, and to achieve a similar image quality to the thicker slice, the dose administered needs to be increased to improve the signal to noise ratio. More slices are also needed to cover the same area so dose is increased but resolution improves.

With the latest multislice units, the beam collimation is equivalent to a thick slice on a single slice unit (Fig. 40.12) so we have the benefits of a thick slice but can reconstruct very thin slices from this irradiation of the patient. For example, if we consider a 16 slice scanner with a detector array of 0.5 mm elements, an 8 mm collimation (thick slice on a standard helical scanner) can yield 16×0.5 mm images (very thin slice).

Reconstruction algorithms or filters are applied to the image reconstruction in conjunction with factors such as slice thickness so that optimal image quality is obtained. They too affect the amount of noise and spatial resolution in the final image.

Increasing kVp provides greater penetration, hence this should be considered when scanning areas of higher attenuation; this can be utilised instead of, or as well as, increases in applied mA, depending on the anatomical area being examined.

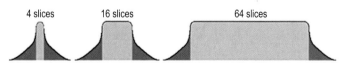

Figure 40.12   Multi slice z axis dose profiles. In single slice scanners the X-ray beam is a close match to the imaged width. 'Overbeaming' occurs in multislice scanners as there is a non-uniform beam distribution but each detector requires equal beam intensity. The 'overbeamed' portion of the dose profile (generally a few mm – dark shading) can be seen for each scanner type. As the number of slices increases the proportion of excess radiation decreases with respect to the total profile, so the greater the number of slices the greater the 'overbeamed' dose efficiency

Artefacts are patterns on an image that are not on the original object. There are many causes of CT artefact such as motion, metal, beam hardening, and partial volume effect. Motion artefacts have been greatly reduced due to the rapid acquisitions available in multislice, in particular. The ability to scan whole body areas in a single breath hold has great advantages.

Some metals absorb X-rays producing radiation shadows; this results in a streak artefact in the reconstructed CT image. Where practicable, all metal objects such as jewellery, coins and clothing with metal fasteners should be removed in order to prevent this effect. This must however be balanced against the psychological needs of the patient. Only if the objects are likely to be situated within the scan field should they be removed. There is no need to change every patient into a hospital gown and indeed it is better for patient comfort and dignity if they can remain dressed where possible.

Beam hardening artefact appears as a streak artefact on the image. As the X-ray beam is heterogeneous on entering an object, particularly if it is high density, the lower energy photons are absorbed. This increases the effective energy of the beam, so adjacent soft tissues are more easily penetrated. This is also seen in non-circular areas such as the shoulder and pelvis where the attenuation is greater along the long axis, producing directional noise. This can be addressed by adaptive filters and correction software.

Partial volume artefact is caused by structures being partially included in the scan thickness. Each voxel represents an average attenuation value for the structures in that slice; if a high attenuation structure (e.g. bone) is partially included in a voxel, that voxel will have an average value higher than its surroundings, producing an error in reconstruction. This is avoided by the use of thinner slices (structures are then less often partially included) or volume artefact reduction software provided by several manufacturers.

CT SAFETY: DOSE

In a little over 30 years, CT has progressed from giving the first glimpse of imaging of cranial contents to the potential to replace planar radiography. However, with all CT examinations, the overriding concern is that of dose to the patient.

In 1989 in the UK it was reported that 20% of the dose from medical examinations was from CT, which at the time accounted for just 2% of examinations.[10] By 1998 this had grown to 40% of the dose and 4% of examinations.[11] By 2000 there were in the region of 34 000 scanners world-wide accounting for 5% of examinations and 34% of the dose.[12] In the USA, even higher figures have been quoted with CT accounting for up to 11% of examinations and 67% of the collective dose.[13]

The introduction of multislice scanners produced an increase in patient dose as the first scanners of this type were less dose efficient than single slice equipment due in a large part to 'overbeaming' (Fig. 40.12). With the production of more efficient detectors and increasing numbers of slices creating a greater effective slice width, this dose increase has been reduced.

Concern is warranted as tissue doses resulting from CT are amongst the highest used in diagnostic imaging. Repeat examinations can produce dose levels which approach and may exceed levels at which increased incidence of cancer has been observed,[1] hence the arguments put forward regarding hormesis and reduced risk from radiation exposure[14,15] do not apply to CT.

Effective dose equivalent (EDE) is, in many circumstances, the quantity used to describe patient dose, but due to the complex manner of its calculation it is difficult to assess for individual patients in CT. There is a requirement for recording of doses and those typically used in CT are the computed tomography dose index (CTDI), and dose length product (DLP), both of which can be used for approximation of EDE.

The first line of approach to dose reduction is to ensure appropriateness of the examination, CT must be the imaging modality best suited to answer the clinical question. In the UK there is a requirement for all complex examinations, such as CT, to be vetted and justified by a consultant experienced in the imaging modality.[16] Given the greater capabilities of modern scanners, there is a wider variety of examinations and techniques available; multiphase contrast examinations should not be routine and should be used only for those clinical situations for which they are the most appropriate.

The operator can have a significant effect on administered dose, with up to 50% reduction achievable by use of appropriate parameters, including auto exposure control, reinforcing the case for appropriate training.[1] Automatic exposure controls include mA modulation to match beam quantity to patient body part. This can be achieved in a variety of ways; two scout views can be used to assess the patient size, and then vary the mA slice by slice during the scan. Another alternative is using feedback from the previous rotation to determine the signal received by the detectors and alter the mA accordingly.

Patient dose can be increased by failure to alter scan parameters to match the individual patient, especially in children, who should not be scanned using adult protocols.

COMMON CLINICAL APPLICATIONS

CT is widely used in imaging virtually every anatomical region and the full range of clinical applications of CT is a text in itself. The following section therefore considers major areas for discussion; it is not intended to be a thorough evaluation of all CT applications. The use of CT in paediatrics is necessarily limited by the radiation burden, which is more significant due to the greater radio sensitivity of children's tissues. This is a specialist topic that will not be considered in detail within this chapter.

It would be inappropriate to attempt to be prescriptive regarding detailed protocols for examinations. In any case the differences in requirements of single slice compared to 4 slice and in turn both of these to 64 slice are such that this would not be possible.

As CT is a user dependent modality, protocols vary widely and must take into account local preferences. In view of the high radiation burden associated with CT, any local variations should, however, fall within the framework of accepted best practice, with evidential support, rather than being simply an individual clinician's preference. Differing techniques for the same examination in different institutions have been reported as having the potential to increase (or reduce) doses by a factor of greater than four;[17] this amount of variation is clearly unacceptable and needs to be addressed.

The objective of the individual examination must always be considered, the objective being to provide the referring clinician with sufficient diagnostic information to enable the appropriate clinical management of the patient. Contrast enhancement is a good example of this; with modern scanning equipment it is possible to perform an initial unenhanced scan followed by multiphasic studies. Initial unenhanced images may not aid the answering of the clinical question and can therefore be omitted; the number of phases of contrast-enhanced scans should then be limited again to those that will address the clinical question for each individual patient.

In the evaluation of major trauma, CT is invaluable, particularly if multislice equipment is available, as it facilitates rapid and thorough evaluation of the head, neck, thorax, abdomen and pelvis. This should not however be used as a 'routine' screening tool for all major trauma; clinical justification for the inclusion of each body area is as essential as in all other circumstances. If used in this way, there is the danger that imaging replaces clinical acumen. Hadley has shown, in a study of a major trauma centre in the USA, that application of 'routine' imaging involving CR and CT led to 73% of examinations being performed 'unnecessarily'.[18] This has clear implica-

tions for over-irradiation of patients and could lead to litigation.

■ Preparation for the examination

Due to the association of CT with cancer (CT – cancer test) it is important to remember that preparation is both mental and physical. A good explanation of the procedure can allay patient's nervousness, which may be due not only to fear of the examination but also its result.

The patient may be changed into a hospital gown, depending on departmental protocol, but if this is not necessary in order to remove artefacts from the scan field then consideration should be given to scanning the patient without having to undress to avoid depersonalisation.

Any checks required for intravenous (IV) contrast administration should be made as appropriate. Here again there is a wide variety of local practice, particularly around administration to asthmatic patients, and to diabetic patients taking Metformin.

For abdominal scanning the patient may be starved for several hours prior to the scan to avoid the appearances of food in the stomach, although starving may increase associated anxiety. An oral contrast medium is commonly given to outline the bowel, which is typically administered at least an hour before scanning to allow transit. Increasingly, negative contrast is used, e.g. water, often for looking at the stomach, and this is finding increasing popularity in other abdominal examinations. Water has the advantages of being cheap, readily available and well tolerated by the patient.

■ 'Scout'

For almost all examinations the first image taken is a scout (also called topogram, digital image, scan projection radiograph, scanogram). The X-ray beam and detectors are kept stationary as the patient moves through a thin, collimated beam of radiation. Dependent on anatomy and equipment, this projection may be performed as an AP, lateral, or both.

The scout is used for localisation and scan selection. Gross abnormalities may be demonstrated; also presence of metal or other artefacts may be seen. The combination of two scouts can be used on some equipment for calculation of mA modulation to reduce dose. This requires some thought on the part of the operator, for example when performing cranial CT and not utilising mA modulation, is it appropriate to perform two scouts? The reason for each aspect of every examination needs to be considered in order that the 'as low as reasonably achievable' (ALARA) principle is maintained.

Use of IV contrast

The high speed of modern multislice equipment enables contrast enhancement to be viewed in multiple phases: arterial, portal venous, venous, and delayed. As previously stated the selection of which phases are to be performed should be dictated by the clinical question to be answered.

Non-ionic media delivered via a pressure injector is the norm; coupled with scanner software, accurate timing of contrast delivery is relatively straightforward. Again the dose implications of such methods must be considered; for example, if observing contrast build up in a region of interest, is it necessary to begin observation scans at the same time as starting the injection? Can the interscan delay be made longer to produce fewer of these scans but maintain an optimal start for the diagnostic scan?

CT angiography is made possible; multiplanar reconstruction, maximum intensity projections, 3D and surface rendered images are easily created on the typical workstation now common (Fig. 40.13). Large areas of anatomy can be demonstrated in a manner that is less invasive than conventional angiography, using less contrast and providing extra luminal information of the surrounding tissues and organs.

The brain

CT is the investigation of choice in the trauma setting where bony injury and intracranial haemorrhage (ICH) are more readily demonstrated, and also for the investigation

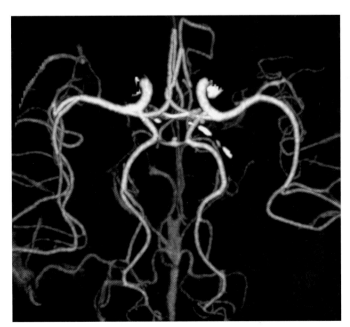

Figure 40.13 CTA: circle of Willis. Reproduced with permission from Toshiba

of acute stroke and paranasal sinus disease, although MR should be used for the staging of neoplasia prior to resection. Perfusion imaging is becoming available for the demonstration of blood flow, particularly in the immediate investigation of stroke; as described in Chapter 39, the size of infarct and volume of ischaemic, but viable brain tissue can be determined.[19]

In head injury, CT is the investigation of choice where there is a suspicion of a clinically important brain injury. The Canadian Head CT rule[20] has been adopted by both the National Institute for Clinical Excellence[21] and the Royal College of Radiologists (RCR) for their guidelines.[22]

Patients presenting with acute stroke should be scanned as soon as possible, certainly within 24 hours of onset, as per the national clinical guidelines for stroke.[23] The information required for appropriate treatment is whether or not the stroke is haemorrhagic, as this informs treatment options. This guidance post dates the RCR[22] guidelines, and is designed to facilitate swift, appropriate treatment for this group of patients. Research has shown that rapid intervention can have significant results.

It *must* be remembered that:

'Stroke is a medical emergency. With active management in the initial hours after stroke onset ischaemic brain may be saved from infarction.'[23]

Common indications
- Trauma
- Acute stroke
- Transient ischaemic attack (TIA)
- Space occupying lesion (SOL)
- Acute severe headache (suspected subarachnoid haemorrhage (SAH))
- Sinus disease

The use of CT for vascular studies of the head is covered in Chapter 39.

Typical protocol
Lateral scan projection radiograph (SPR) from the skull base to vertex is commonly taken and used for planning axial slices/volume. In multiple trauma cases, the cervical vertebrae may be included.

In general, thinner slices are acquired through the posterior fossa which is often not well visualised on CT. MR is superior if posterior fossa pathology is suspected. Whilst cranial CT is still commonly performed using sequential scans, thin spiral scans can be performed, and reformatted into the required slice thickness. 64 slice in particular demonstrates the posterior fossa well; thin slices are combined for viewing and provide good axial demonstration of this area. Isotropic or near isotropic multiplanar reconstructions are also readily produced.

Patient positioning for cranial CT is the subject of debate. Many centres adopt the 'supraorbital baseline'; slices are planned parallel to a line running between the external auditory meatus (EAM) and the superior orbital ridge. The reasoning for this is to reduce the dose to the lens of the eye by not scanning through the globe. In practice, this is often badly performed as can be seen by the eyes being present on the lowermost images of many scans. This baseline exacerbates the problems of visualisation of the posterior fossa which is not well demonstrated.

The commonest alternative is Reeds baseline, extending from the EAM through the inferior border of the orbit. Whilst irradiating the orbit, it does better demonstrate the posterior fossa, and the path of the optic nerve. This method is in use in several specialist neurocentres. The use of Bismuth shields, as seen in Figures 40.14 and 40.15, to protect the eyes during scanning has been suggested and seems worthy of consideration.[24]

Whichever baseline is to be used, thought needs to be given to patient positioning in order to minimise the use of gantry angulation, which is to be avoided due to the potential to increase patient dose.[25]

Cranial CT is usually performed without the addition of contrast media. A second scan post administration of

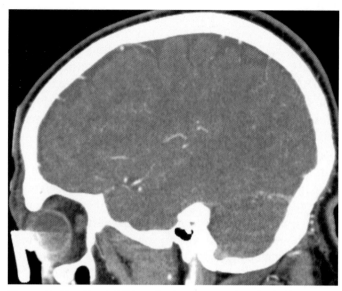

Figure 40.15   Cranial CT: sagittal reconstruction. Again Bismuth shielding is seen without artefact affecting visualisation of brain. Reproduced with permission from Toshiba

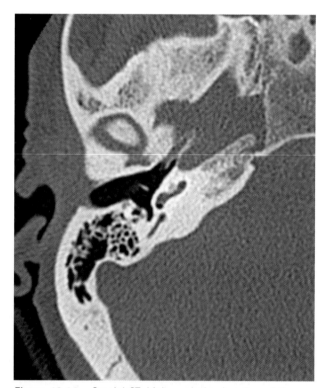

Figure 40.16   Cranial CT: high resolution imaging of the temporal bone. Reproduced with permission from Toshiba

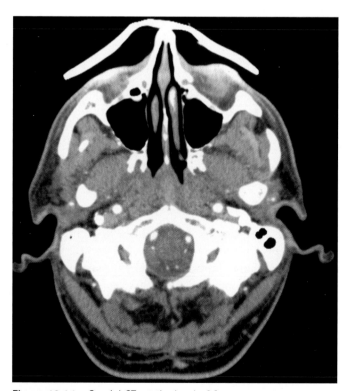

Figure 40.14   Cranial CT: at the level of foramen magnum. Note use of Bismuth eye shields and lack of artefact remote from shielding. Reproduced with permission from Toshiba

contrast is useful in some acute circumstances. The exception to this is in scanning for metastases when a single contrast-enhanced scan is usual; referral for MRI should also be considered subject to availability.

Cranial CT reporting by radiographers is a recent role development which has been demonstrated to be a feasible means for addressing radiologist shortages and of providing waiting list reduction. Studies have shown high accuracy rates are achievable after a suitable course of training,[26,27] and radiographers have taken on this role in some centres.

With multislice technology in particular, there is no longer any requirement for additional direct coronal scanning for paranasal sinuses, as reconstructions can be obtained in any plane. The effect of this when looking at fluid levels does, however, need to be considered.

Spine

CT is of limited application other than in the case of trauma. Its use is mandatory in cases of cervical spine trauma where plain film findings are equivocal or have failed to demonstrate the cervico-thoracic junction. CT is increasingly replacing plain film imaging, particularly in cases of major trauma and/or when the patient is undergoing cranial CT. In the case of thoracic or lumbar trauma with neurological deficit, CT can be used to demonstrate bony detail.

MRI is the investigation of choice for spinal pathology because of its greater soft tissue resolution and its ability for multiplanar imaging of the cord.

The neck

CT may be used for the staging of tumours in the neck; MR is better in this area and should be used where available. Other investigations are generally used for the diagnosis of lesions in the neck, although carotid studies can be performed, as shown in Figure 40.18.

The chest

Justification for the CT examination of young females should be particularly robust considering the potential for breast cancer induction. Consideration should be given to the application of breast shielding which has been shown to achieve a breast dose reduction of more than 50% without compromising the demonstration of the thoracic contents.[28]

Staging of both chest primary lesions and metastatic spread from other primary sites in association with a chest radiograph, is a commonly seen utilisation of CT in this body area. Generally the thorax and upper abdomen are scanned; this is to enable assessment of upper abdominal lymphadenopathy and to view the adrenals and liver, particularly for metastatic spread. CT has high accuracy rates and can facilitate biopsy. The introduction of positron emission tomography (PET) will have an impact in this area, particularly when used in conjunction with CT (see Fig. 40.43).

Nodal disease is well visualised. Specific sites in which nodes are often seen are the aortopulmonary window in the subcranial and perihilar regions and retrocrural area. Multiplanar reconstructions can be helpful in interpretation, as can the use of varying window settings, and advanced techniques such as maximum intensity projections (MIPs).

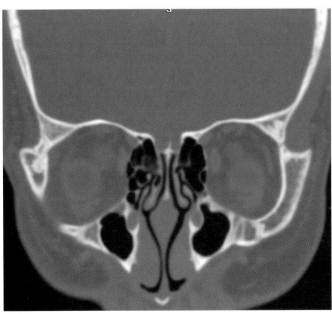

Figure 40.17 Cranial CT: coronal reconstruction used for viewing sinuses or facial bones. Reproduced with permission from Toshiba

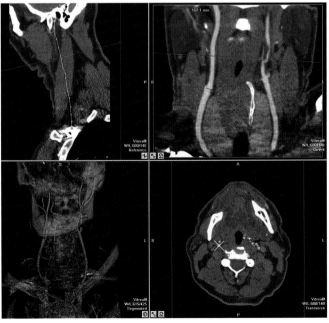

Figure 40.18 Neck CT: workstation images of carotid study. Reproduced with permission from Toshiba

High resolution CT (HRCT) is used for detailed evaluation of the lung parenchyma. When scanning using thin slices on high end multislice equipment, utilising lung windows effectively provides 'free' HRCT imaging, which again can be reconstructed into any desired plane.

There is debate on the use of 'low dose' CT as a screening tool.[29] Whilst CT may increase detection of early tumours, there is a high rate of detection of nodules which require follow up with standard dose high resolution CT to classify them as benign, or otherwise, and prevent the requirement for unnecessary intervention (approximately 23% of screened patients had nodules, and 2.7% had a malignancy in one large study).[30] The requirement for a second scan with 'normal' dose rates makes such screening costly, both financially and in terms of dose burden, particularly to asymptomatic patients. If patients with benign nodules are then followed up with interval scans the potential for extremely high dose burdens is clear.

It has been suggested that there is no difference in survival rate between patients with solitary lesions of 1 cm or 3 cm on diagnosis.[31] Further evaluation of the utility of CT screening is suggested and would seem appropriate. There are, however, already screening centres offering a CT screening service for chest and other body areas, even with self referral, which is of some concern without evidence of benefit, particularly given that multiple examinations will inevitably involve a high cumulative dose with the attendant risks thereof.

Rapid scan times enable visualisation of the entire thorax in a single breath hold, eliminating the previous problems associated with respiratory misregistration. Utilising software to optimise the timing of IV contrast injections the area can be scanned in arterial phase, enabling demonstration of vascular structures in the thorax. CT is rapidly becoming the examination of choice for the investigation of pulmonary embolus. High accuracy rates are achieved and the examination can be coupled with an examination of the upper legs for underlying deep vein thrombosis (Fig. 40.21).

Cardiac CT

Another use for fast scan times is in imaging of the heart. This has been described as the ultimate goal for multislice CT. Electrocardiogram (ECG) gating techniques enable high quality imaging of the heart and associated vascular structures in as little as five cardiac cycles. Image quality now matches and in some cases exceeds that of EBCT, and availability of multislice scanners has certainly become more widespread than EBCT has been.

Coronary artery calcium scoring has been in use for some time, and is used to provide an indication of the presence and amount of atherosclerotic plaque, enabling the detection of potential disease prior to the development of symptoms such as angina and dyspnoea. High resolu-

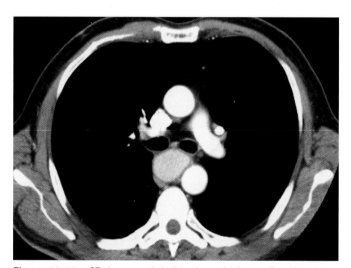

Figure 40.19   CT thorax: axial slice through thorax. Excellent arterial contrast enhancement is seen on this image. Reproduced with permission from Toshiba

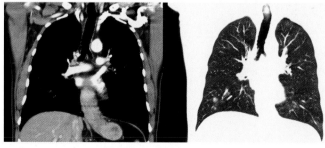

Figure 40.20   CT thorax: coronal reconstructions viewed on 'soft tissue' and 'lung' windows. Reproduced with permission from Toshiba

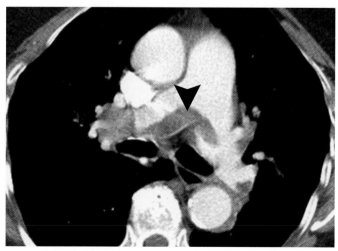

Figure 40.21   CT thorax: PE scanning demonstrating saddle embolus (arrowed)

tion, non-contrast scans are obtained and volumetric analysis used to produce a calcium score. This score can then be compared with a database of known scores adjusted for age and gender, and appropriate advice given on risk of coronary artery disease (Fig. 40.22).

The information gained from calcium scoring does not give a direct measure of arterial narrowing, but has good correlation with the severity of underlying disease. It does not rule out the presence of soft non-calcified plaque, but soft plaque evaluation is now becoming available. Dissection, aneurysm, and coarctation of the aorta can also be assessed, as well as the structure of the heart itself. Such structural information can also be obtained using MRI, which should be considered as an alternative where available (Figs 40.23, 40.24).

Gastrointestinal tract

Oesophageal perforation may be demonstrated on a contrast swallow; however use of CT will enable the additional demonstration of complications in surrounding tissues. CT is also used for staging of oesophageal and stomach tumours; the primary tumour may be visualised and any local or nodal spread demonstrated. Water is useful as a negative oral contrast in this case as it enables visualisation of the stomach wall which may be partially obscured by the use of positive oral contrast media (Fig. 40.25).

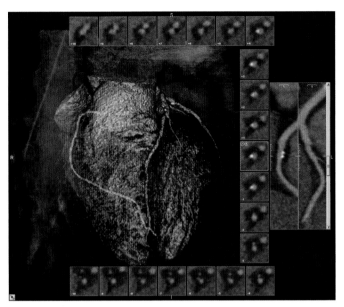

Figure 40.23 Cardiac CT: CT angiography. High quality 3D reconstruction from a 32 slice scanner. The sternum and great vessels can be seen semi-transparent on this image. Curved reconstructions demonstrate the selected vessel which can be viewed 'sliced' in any direction. Reproduced with permission from Toshiba

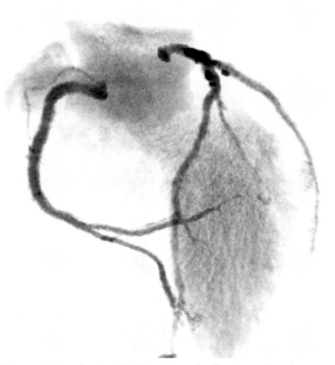

Figure 40.24 Cardiac CT: CT angiography. The image here is manipulated to provide an 'angiographic' appearance. Reproduced with permission from Toshiba

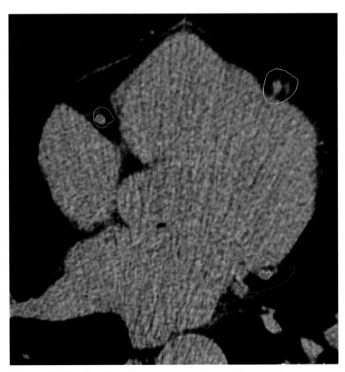

Figure 40.22 Cardiac CT: coronary artery calcium scoring. Regions of interest around coronary arteries can be seen. Reproduced with permission from Toshiba

In adults with acute abdominal pain, CT may be used to establish the cause and level of obstruction. Colonic lesions are well demonstrated by CT colonoscopy, with full and thorough preparation results compared with direct colonoscopy. The use of advanced reconstruction techniques such as virtual colonoscopy allows for comparable images but with the advantage of visualisation of involvement external to the lumen. CT is becoming the investigation of choice for frail patients as it may be better tolerated than barium enema or colonoscopy because of its less invasive nature. CT also facilitates staging of lesions within the same examination (Figs 40.26, 40.27, 40.28).

Abdomen

Abdominal CT is a common examination that has a high diagnostic yield, but equally a high radiation dose burden. It is the examination of choice for nodal staging of many malignancies, including lymphoma. Whilst CT is generally

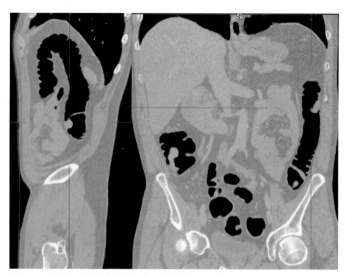

Figure 40.27   CT of GIT: colon. Sagittal and coronal reconstructions from Figure 40.26. Reproduced with permission from Toshiba

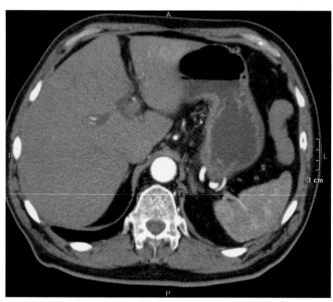

Figure 40.25   CT of GIT. Use of water as negative contrast enables visualisation of the stomach wall. Reproduced with permission from Toshiba

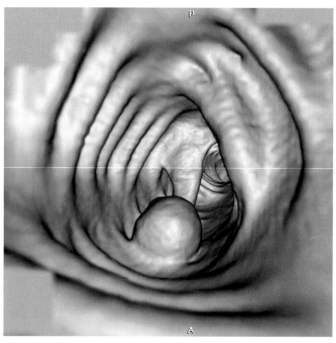

Figure 40.28   CT of GIT: virtual colonoscopy. Prone reconstructions from patient in Figure 40.26, demonstrating the polyp within the bowel, hanging from its stalk. Reproduced with permission from Toshiba

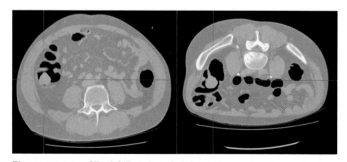

Figure 40.26   CT of GIT: colon. Axial scans can visualise pathology external to the colon. A polyp is seen in the ascending colon. On the prone view the polyp has moved anteriorly under gravity and its stalk can be seen. Reproduced with permission from Toshiba

thought to be the 'better' examination in cases of suspected abdominal mass, sepsis or pyrexia of unknown origin, ultrasound should be performed first. Ultrasound may yield the required information to answer the clinical question without the high radiation dose associated with abdominal CT. Both imaging methods may be used to facilitate biopsy or drainage.

Liver

CT is far more sensitive than ultrasound (US) and is commonly used for staging prior to resection, although US is again usually the first line investigation for diagnosis. Three phase post-contrast techniques are particularly useful for diagnosis and presurgical staging of liver metastases, which are the most frequently occurring malignant tumours of the liver. Many liver lesions look similar precontrast and can look similar at different timings following injection. The use of precontrast scans has been questioned for some time; both its utility and dose implications must be considered. The soft tissue contrast sensitivity of MR makes it the investigation of choice for staging of primary lesions, and if available, should be considered for the evaluation of metastases.

CT can also be used in the investigation of cirrhosis, demonstrating fatty infiltration, and also to characterise possible haemangioma. The use of MRI should be considered in these cases.

Kidneys and adrenal glands

The adrenals are commonly scanned in association with the thorax for bronchial staging as they are a common site for metastatic spread from a lung primary (Fig. 40.30). There is potential for unenhanced CT of the kidneys, ureter and bladder (KUB) region to replace the intravenous urogram (IVU), it is already the investigation of choice for renal colic and detection of calculi. It should be performed with reduced exposure factors as it has been shown that diagnostic accuracy can be maintained with a low dose protocol.[32]

Contrast enhanced CT is the investigation of choice for renal masses, again it is usual for US to be the first line investigation, but CT can detect smaller lesions. MRI may be used in staging of advanced disease where it is superior to CT. CT is the examination of choice in renal trauma, in which case a post-contrast two phase examination is indicated.

Pancreas

US is better in thin patients and CT is better in larger individuals where the peripancreatic fat is useful for delineation. IV contrast enhancement is used to assess necrosis in the immediate post-acute phase of pancreatitis, and is better than US for follow up, but due to the dose implications, US should be used for monitoring chronic conditions. For pancreatic tumours, CT is required for staging, whilst both US and CT may be used to facilitate biopsy (Fig. 40.31).

Musculoskeletal system

CT is classified as a specialised examination by the RCR guidelines.[22] It has an important place in musculoskeletal imaging due to its ability to demonstrate occult and complex fractures, and bone healing. For example, CT can be used to clarify a clinically suspected scaphoid fracture,

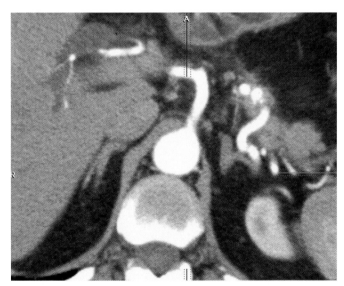

Figure 40.30   CT adrenals. Reproduced with permission from Toshiba

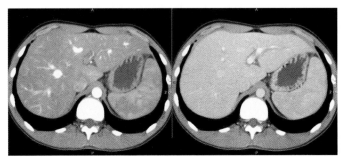

Figure 40.29   CT liver: arterial and venous phases. Reproduced with permission from Toshiba

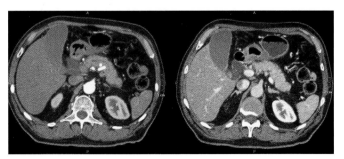

Figure 40.31   CT pancreas: arterial and venous phases. Reproduced with permission from Toshiba

but MRI is better where it is available. Conventional radiography is still the first line technique for the detection of fractures and dislocations. RNI is sensitive though not specific for the detection of occult or stress fractures and metastatic disease. US and MRI are the investigations of choice for associated soft tissue injuries.

CT is used for orthopaedic surgical planning, clarification of complex fractures and demonstration of develop-

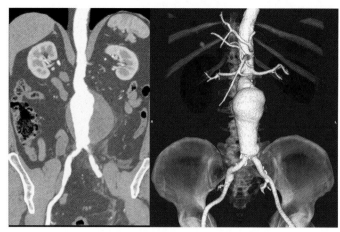

Figure 40.34   CTA: abdominal aortic aneurysm. Curved MIP demonstrating extent and location of aneurysm. 3D image demonstrates non-involvement of renal arteries. Reproduced with permission from Toshiba

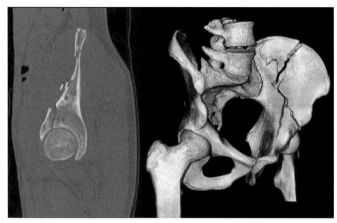

Figure 40.32   CT pelvis. A combination of oblique reconstructions and surface rendered images are used here to clarify a complex fracture. Reproduced with permission from Toshiba

Figure 40.35
CTA: peripheral angiography. Coverage from renal arteries to ankles shown on this MIP. Reproduced with permission from Toshiba

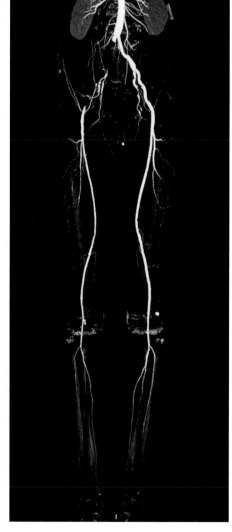

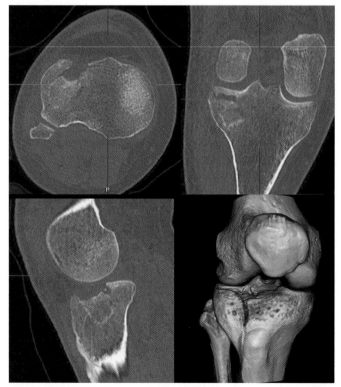

Figure 40.33   CT knee. Tibial plateau fracture, well demonstrated by axial scan, coronal and sagittal reformats, and surface rendered 3D image. Reproduced with permission from Toshiba

Figure 40.36
CTA: peripheral angiography. Using image reformatting, a single volumetric acquisition can be used to view key areas from different planes/angles, and with or without semi-transparent bone for positional reference. Reproduced with permission from Toshiba

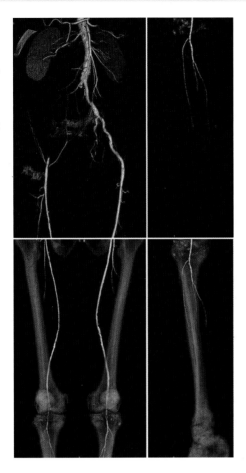

mental deformities. Areas of particular value are the tibial plateau, calcaneus, and pelvic fractures. CT can also be utilised for leg length measurement and assessment of scoliosis. If scout views are used for measurement they have the advantage of being obtained using a non-divergent beam, rendering measurement more accurate.

CT angiography

CT has long been used to image vascular structures, but the advent of multislice technology has opened up a new range of examinations, which are now achievable due to increased speed, coverage, and reconstruction techniques. The aorta is commonly scanned for dissection and aneurysmal disease; coronal reconstructions, MIPs, or 3D images can clearly resolve questions, e.g. regarding renal artery involvement (Fig. 40.34).

Peripheral angiography can be performed in a far less invasive manner than traditional angiography (Figs 40.35, 40.36); the dose advantages of magnetic resonance angiography (MRA) should be considered where this technique is available. This is an area where the ability to scan faster with more slices may be disadvantageous, as it is possible to scan faster than the travel of the contrast bolus.

THERAPY

CT has many applications within radiotherapy. Tumour staging has already been mentioned, but recent years have seen the growth of the use of CT for treatment planning.

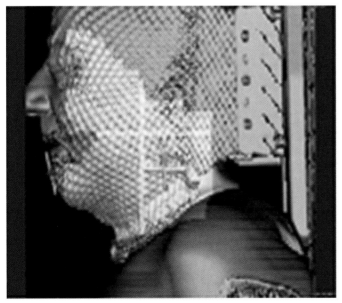

Figure 40.37   Prosoma. Skin surface image reconstructed from CT data set. This demonstrates the radiotherapy light field to aid treatment set up verification. Reproduced with permission from OSL

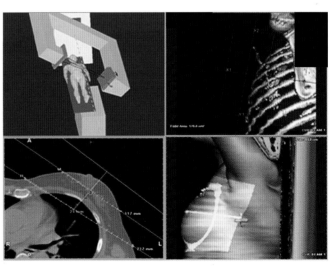

Figure 40.38   Prosoma. CT simulation of radiotherapy for breast cancer. Reproduced with permission from OSL

CT simulation uses CT data sets to plan the delivery of radiotherapy treatment beams (Fig. 40.37).

The patient is scanned using immobilisation devices which are used on the treatment table which is flat; consequently, the scan table used for planning must also be flat as it is vital for planning accuracy that the positions are exactly duplicated (Fig. 40.38).

A new development is tomotherapy,[33] the use of megavoltage CT for delivery of therapy treatments. The megavoltage beam can be used to image the tumour as it responds to treatment; its size, shape, and position may alter and the megavoltage images obtained can be used to replan the treatment, enabling more effective use of the delivered doses (Figs 40.39, 40.40).

FUTURE DEVELOPMENTS

New technology is being launched on at least an annual basis, the latest launch at RSNA 2005 being a dual source system from Siemens. Developments such as this have made CT the most rapidly evolving imaging technology. No sooner has spiral CT been replaced by quad multislice, than it in turn has been replaced by 8 slice and now 64 slice machines. 256 slice (4D)[8] machines are being considered in the near future, with the possibility of flat

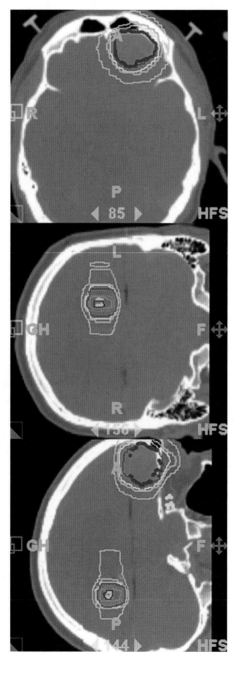

Figure 40.39 Tomotherapy. Dose distribution for small intracranial stereotactic type lesion. Reproduced with permission from OSL

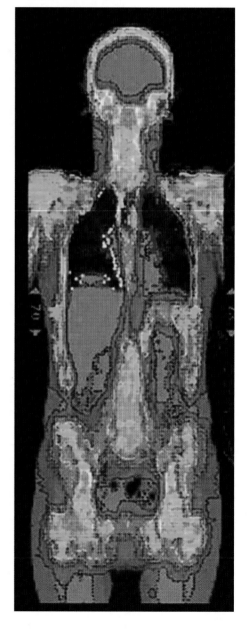

Figure 40.40 Tomotherapy. Dose distribution for total body irradiation prior to bone marrow transplant. Reproduced with permission from OSL

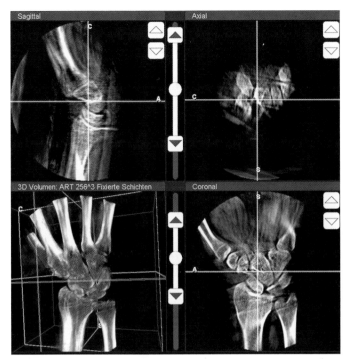

Figure 40.41 Vario 3D. Multiplanar and 3D images reconstructed from images taken during rotation of the C-arm. Reproduced with permission from Xograph

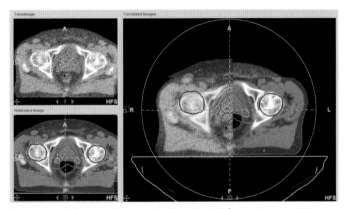

Figure 40.42 Tomotherapy. Verification CT ('tomoimage': MV acquisition) fused with planning CT ('reference image': kV acquisition) at the planning console. These are images the radiographer will use and evaluate on the treatment machine on a daily basis. Reproduced with permission from OSL

plate digital detector systems raising the possibility of single rotation scanning of a body area. This could produce a data set of an anatomical area, e.g. the chest, from which could be reconstructed a chest image plus lateral and obliques as required, as well as slices in any plane, 3D and MIP reconstructions – all from a single rotation. This would have a similar acquisition time to standard chest X-ray.

C-arm CT systems are being developed for use in operating theatres; the system has the same footprint as a

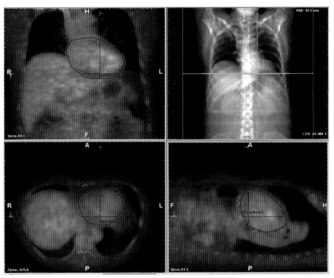

Figure 40.43 Prosoma: CT-PET image fusion. The image fusion aids delineation of tumour volume for radiotherapy. Reproduced with permission from OSL

standard image intensifier system. The system can be used as a standard image intensifier; the CT function is selected and a series of images taken at fixed angles as the intensifier C-arm rotates around a preselected isocentre (Fig. 40.41).

These advances in medical imaging technology are being driven by the rapid advances in computing and associated technologies. Already we can look to the image registration of various cross-sectional studies, for example, the registration of CT and MRI images may enable bony and soft tissue structures and their relationships to be better demonstrated than is possible with each individual modality.[34] CT and PET images can be combined to provide anatomical and functional information simultaneously. Kilovoltage and megavoltage images are combined within tomotherapy (Fig. 40.42).[33]

This is an exciting and challenging time to be working with this dynamic imaging modality.

References

1. ICRP. Managing patient dose in computed tomography. ICRP Publication 87. Elsevier; 2000.
2. American College of Radiology. ACR practice guideline for performing and interpreting diagnostic computed tomography (CT). ACR; 2002.
3. Grossmann G. Lung tomography. British Journal of Radiology 1935; 8:733.
4. Kuhl D. Transmission scanning. Radiology 1966; 87:278–284.
5. Ambrose J, Hounsfield G. Computerised transverse axial tomography. British Journal of Radiology 1972; 46:148.
6. Hounsfield G. Computerised transverse axial scanning (tomography), Part 1: description of system. British Journal of Radiology 1973; 46:1016.

7. Ambrose J, Hounsfield G. Computerised transverse axial scanning (tomography), Part 2: clinical applications. British Journal of Radiology 1973; 46:1023.

8. Toshiba Medical Systems. 4D CT. www.toshibaeurope.com/Medical/medicalp.asp?PageID=1131&PRODUCT_ID=1624

9. Seeram E. Computed tomography: physical principles, clinical applications, and quality control. 2nd edn. Philadelphia: Saunders; 2001.

10. Shrimpton P, et al. Survey of CT practice in the UK. Part 2: Dosimetric aspects. NRPB-R249. London: HMSO; 1991.

11. Rehani M, Berry M. Radiation doses in computed tomography. British Medical Journal 2000; 320:593–594.

12. UNSCEAR. Report to the general assembly, Annex D: Medical Radiation Exposures. New York: UN; 2000.

13. Mettler F, et al. CT scanning: patterns of use and dose. Journal of Radiological Protection 2001; 20:353–359.

14. Cameron J. UKRC 2004 debate: moderate dose rate ionising radiation increases longevity. British Journal of Radiology 2005; 78:11–13.

15. Feinendegen L. UKRC 2004 debate: evidence for beneficial low level radiation effects and radiation hormesis. British Journal of Radiology 2005; 78:3–7.

16. The Ionising Radiation (Medical Exposure) Regulations. Statutory Instruments 2000, no. 1059. London: HMSO; 2000.

17. Shrimpton P, et al. Reference doses in computed tomography. Radiation Protection Dosimetry 1998; 80:55–59.

18. Hadley J. Over utilization of imaging in the acute trauma setting. In RSNA scientific assembly and annual meeting program. Oak Brook Ill: RSNA 2004; 372.

19. Wintermark M, et al. Comparison of admission perfusion computed tomography and qualitative diffusion and perfusion weighted magnetic resonance imaging in acute stroke patients. Stroke 2002: 33:2025–2031.

20. Steill I, et al. The Canadian CT Head rule for patients with minor head injury. Lancet 2001; 357:1391–1396.

21. NICE. Head injury – triage, assessment, investigation and early management of head injury in infants, children and adult guideline. National Institute for Clinical Excellence. June 2003. (www.nice.org.uk)

22. RCR Working Party. Making the best use of a department of clinical radiology. Guidelines for doctors. 5th edn. London: Royal College of Radiologists; 2003.

23. Intercollegiate stroke working party. National Clinical Guidelines for Stroke. 2nd edn. London: Royal College of Physicians; 2004 (June).

24. Hopper K, et al. Radioprotection to the eye during CT scanning. American Journal of Neuroradiology 2001; 22:1194–1198.

25. Murphy U. Dose implications of gantry tilt in cranial computerised tomography. Radiography Ireland. 6(3):137–139.

26. Carver B. Meeting service needs: cranial CT reporting by radiographers. In proceedings of UKRC 2004. BIR Congress Series 2004; p. 10.

27. Carver B. Is Cranial CT reporting by radiographers a feasible option to assist radiologist workload and provide a route for radiographer role extension? In RSNA scientific assembly and annual meeting program. Oak Brook Ill: RSNA 2004:553.

28. Hopper K, et al. The breast: in plane x-ray protection during diagnostic thoracic CT: shielding with bismuth radioprotective garments. Radiology 1997: 205:853–858.

29. Ellis J, Gleeson F. Lung cancer screening. British Journal of Radiology 2001; 74:478–485.

30. Henschke C, et al. Early lung cancer action project: a summary of the findings on baseline screening. The Oncologist 2001; 6:147–152.

31. Patz E, et al. Correlation of tumour size and survival in patients with Stage 1A non-small cell lung cancer. Chest 2000; 117:1568–1571.

32. Meagher T, et al. Low dose computed tomography in suspected acute renal colic. Clinical Radiology 2001; 56:873–876.

33. www.tomotherapy.com/intro/index.html

34. Panigraphy A, et al. Registration of three-dimensional MR and CT studies of the cervical spine. American Journal of Neuroradiology 2000; 21:282–289.

MAGNETIC RESONANCE IMAGING

John Talbot

INTRODUCTION

Magnetic resonance imaging (MRI) is still considered a relative newcomer to the field of diagnostic imaging. In fact, it was first identified as a possible imaging modality in 1969 and was developed almost over the same time-scale as computed tomography (CT).

MRI uses a combination of magnetic fields and radio waves to produce diagnostic images of the body. The basic premise of MRI is that a radiofrequency pulse is applied to the hydrogen nuclei within the patient's tissues which causes them to change their energy state and net magnetic alignment to an external magnetic field. As the nuclei lose this energy to realign with the field, their transmitted energy can be measured and spatially located. This technique uses a series of radio wave applications and magnetic field gradient applications known as a pulse sequence. The timing of these applications determines tissue contrast because molecular behaviour differs between various tissue types, particularly fat and water.

Since its inception at the beginning of the 1980s, MRI has now become a first line technique in the routine diagnosis of disease and scanners can be found in most district general hospitals.

Like CT, MRI is a cross-sectional imaging modality acquiring user-definable slices having variable size (field of view) and thickness. MRI does however have certain advantages over CT:

• MRI uses non-ionising radiation rather than X-rays. To be precise, MRI utilises radio frequencies between 6 to 127 MHz depending upon the power of the scanner. This portion of the electromagnetic spectrum is approximately the same as that used by domestic cordless telephones and is therefore clearly very safe.

• MRI has very marked soft tissue contrast. MRI is unique among diagnostic modalities in that the signal that forms the image is generated by the body tissue itself. Radiographs and CT rely on X-rays passing through, and being attenuated by, the area under investigation. Although the user has control over the penetrating power and intensity of the beam, the resulting image is still essentially a shadow of the anatomy. MRI on the other hand has multiple user-definable parameters which exploit the molecular behaviour of the tissues and can dramatically modify tissue contrast in much the same way as nuclear magnetic resonance (NMR) spectroscopy can differentiate between individual elements in a chemical substance.

• MRI acquires images in any given plane without having to change the position of the patient. Although CT data can be post-processed into many different planes and rendered volumes, the acquisition plane is still essentially axial.

• MRI can obtain both structural (morphological) information and *functional* information. Functional MRI (fMRI) exploits the fact that MRI can detect minute changes in the chemical composition of body tissues such as the amount of haemoglobin vs. deoxyhaemoglobin. The principle of fMRI imaging is to rapidly acquire a series of images of the brain and to statistically analyse the images for differences between them. This is usually done after a baseline scan and the patient is asked to perform a physical or mental task during acquisition.

Because of these advantages, the use of MRI has exponentially increased over the last 10 years, not to replace CT but to sit comfortably alongside it. There are currently over 10 000 scanners in use world-wide performing tens of millions of scans. MRI is a multibillion dollar industry employing huge numbers of people including radiographers, technicians, radiologists, physicists, imaging scientists, biomedical engineers, pulse sequence designers and service engineers. Interestingly, researchers are currently developing MRI scanners for use on board manned space craft and the international space station.[1]

EQUIPMENT CHRONOLOGY

The chronology of MRI charts the discovery and development of a physical phenomenon known as NMR.

1845   Michael Faraday investigated the magnetic properties of dried blood.

1938   In the 1930s American physicist Isidor Rabi researched into methods of observing atomic spectra. During his work he demonstrated that the spin state in a molecular beam can be reoriented in a magnetic field. He received the Nobel prize in physics in 1944 'for his resonance method for recording the magnetic properties of atomic nuclei'.[2]

1946   The process of NMR was discovered by the independently operating research teams of Felix Bloch (Stanford University) and Edwin Purcell (Harvard University).

1948   Nicolaas Bloembergen presented his theory of relaxation times, based on experiments in Purcell's laboratory.

1950   Irwin Hahn 'accidentally' discovered spin echoes while working on relaxation experiments. He cursed the signal as an 'annoying glitch.'

1950s– NMR was used in the field of analytical chemistry
1960s   where NMR spectroscopy revolutionised the non-destructive analysis of the composition of chemical compounds. These techniques tested very small samples that were placed inside high field magnets having a very narrow bore only a few centimetres wide. Paramagnetic reagents were used in NMR spectroscopy and can be thought of as the forerunners of modern MRI contrast media.

1966   Richard Ernst showed that Fourier transform gives increased sensitivity of magnetic resonance (MR) spectroscopy.

1969   Dr Raymond Damadian (SUNY Downstate Medical Centre) used NMR spectroscopy in research into sodium and potassium in living cells. This led him to his first experiments with NMR and caused him to first propose the possibility of an NMR body scanner.[3]

1971   Following animal studies on rats, Damadian discovered considerable differences in the NMR signals emitted by healthy tissues and tumours. He authored a paper entitled 'Tumor Detection by Nuclear Magnetic Resonance',[4] and although this work was met with scepticism from many quarters Damadian maintained his idea of the MR body scanner.

1972   Damadian filed the first of his patents for an MRI body scanner. The patent described how liquid helium could be used to create a super-cooled electromagnet housed within a cylindrical cryostat. The patent also described how the nuclei of hydrogen atoms in the body would react to the resultant magnetic field, and how a 3D spatial localisation method could encode the signals into a scan.

1973   The journal *Nature* published an article written by Professor Paul Lauterbur, Professor of Chemistry at the State University of New York, entitled 'Image Formation by Induced Local Interaction; Examples Employing Magnetic Resonance'.[5] Lauterbur, described a new imaging technique for which he coined the term zeugmatography (from the Greek meaning 'to join together'). This alluded to the principle of his technique which involved the joining of two magnetic fields in the spatial localisation of two test tubes filled with normal water sitting in a bath of heavy water. Lauterbur used a static main magnetic field over which he applied a weaker gradient field. He then used a back projection method (as used in CT) to produce an image of the two test tubes (Fig. 41.1).

This landmark imaging experiment was of great importance for two reasons. First, it was the first time that NMR had given spatial information rather than just spectroscopic information. Second, it had never previously been possible to distinguish between heavy water and normal water using analytical techniques.

Ironically, the journal editor nearly declined to publish the paper on the grounds that it was 'not of sufficiently wide significance for inclusion'. Professor Lauterbur received a Nobel prize for this and other work in the field of MRI in 2003.

1973   In the same year Professor Peter Mansfield was beginning his studies into NMR at the University of Nottingham in the UK. He initially worked on studies of solid objects, such as crystals. However, one year later, Mansfield and collaborator Alan Garroway filed a patent and published a paper on image formation by NMR.[6]

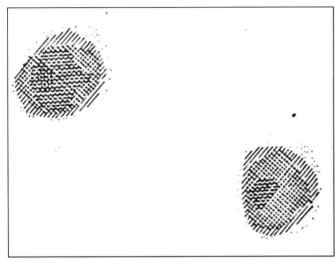

Figure 41.1 The first use of spatial encoding with NMR by Professor Paul Lauterbur. The shaded areas represent the spatial position of two tubes filled with water.[5] Image reproduced by kind permission of Professor P. Lauterbur and *Nature*[5]

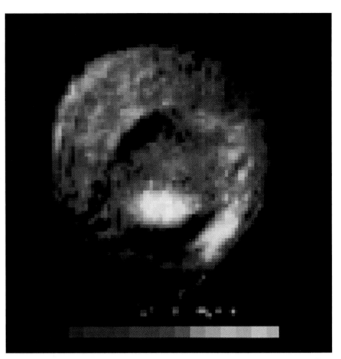

Figure 41.2 First human MRI scan by Mansfield and Maudsley.[7] Axial cross-section through a finger. Image reproduced by kind permission of Professor Mansfield

1975   Richard Ernst proposed MRI using phase and frequency encoding, and the Fourier transform. This technique is still the basis of spatial encoding in the modern MRI scanner. Peter Mansfield and another colleague Andrew Maudsley who were also working in the field of spatial encoding proposed a technique which could produce in vivo imaging.

1976   Professor Mansfield et al began to study ways of fast imaging using NMR and an improved picture display. They produced the first in vivo image of human anatomy, a cross section through a finger (Fig. 41.2).[7]

1977   Raymond Damadian aided by graduate students, built a prototype NMR body scanner consisting of a homemade superconducting magnet. The magnet itself was made of nearly 50 km of niobium-titanium wire spun onto a cylinder, a technique still used today. The magnet bore itself was 134 cm in diameter, big enough to allow the positioning of a human body. To ensure superconductivity the magnet was super-cooled using liquid helium but unlike today's systems the boil off and leakage was so great that refills cost $2000 per week.

The receive coil was constructed from cardboard and copper wire and designed to be worn around the body like a corset, very much like modern phased array wrap-around body coils. The patient transport system was little more than a wooden tray. After an abortive first attempt to scan Damadian, one of his research assistants, Laurence Minkoff, was placed into the scanner. The receive coil was positioned around his thorax and the scan procedure itself took nearly 5 hours. The result was a rudimentary image, reconstructed from the data acquired using crayons. It showed a 2D view of Minkoff's chest including his heart and lungs.[8] Meanwhile in the UK, Professor Mansfield et al published two papers on imaging using NMR and a paper on multiplanar image formation.[9,10,11]

1978   Following on from earlier images of small body parts, Professor Mansfield presented his first image through the abdomen. He also published animal studies showing how NMR could be used in the diagnosis of tumours.

Professor Paul Lauterbur began work on finding a suitable MRI contrast agent in this year using paramagnetic reagents in an animal study.[12]

1979   The Mansfield team continued their studies into the NMR imaging of tumours, specifically carcinoma of the breast.

1980   In the late 1970s and early 1980s, many groups took up the challenge to produce a commercially viable MRI system. This needed to be large enough to scan a human but also to have sufficiently good field homogeneity to produce diagnostic images. These pioneers included the group from the Hammersmith (Professor R. Steiner and Professor G. Bydder) working in conjunction with Picker

Ltd at Wembley (Dr I. Young), two independent groups in Nottingham (Professor P. Mansfield and Dr W. Moore), and in Aberdeen (Professor J. Mallard and Dr J. Hutchinson).

1981   Peter Mansfield and his team introduced the concept of real-time moving images by NMR and presented a paper critically evaluating NMR imaging techniques.[13]

Philips medical systems produced their first scanner.

Schering applied for a patent for an MRI contrast agent Gadolinium diethylenetriamine penta-acetic acid (DTPA).

1983   The first commercial MR scanner in Europe (from Picker Ltd) was installed in 1983 at the Department of Diagnostic Radiology at the University of Manchester Medical School (Professor I. Isherwood and Professor B. Pullen).

1984   MRI contrast agent Gadolinium DTPA (Magnevist, Schering) was tested on humans.

1985–   In the latter half of the 1980s, NMR applications
1990   and refinements really began to evolve rapidly and included dynamic imaging, cardiac applications, more efficient shimming methods, echo-planar imaging, active magnetic shielding and surface coil improvements.

Gadolinium DTPA was licensed for use in brain and spine imaging. Approval for use in other body areas followed.

1990–   Since the advent of commercial scanning, MRI
present   equipment has been constantly modified and improved. These improvements have not just been in the physical construction but also in the design of the software used to produce the pulse sequences used in scanning.

Instrumentation and pulse sequence design will be discussed more fully in the following sections, but while still in the historical context of MRI, it is worth mentioning here some of the advances that have been made in the design of MRI scanners over recent years.

In the field of medical imaging the word 'nuclear' has been dropped from the term 'nuclear magnetic resonance imaging'. This is because the word 'nuclear' is associated by many patients with nuclear power, nuclear war and radioactivity in general. This was unnecessarily off-putting in the context of a scan that did not use ionising radiation.

Whilst there are variations such as 'open' magnets, and Fonar's Erect system,[14] most modern scanners still have the same basic design featuring a closed bore super-conducting magnet orientated horizontally, allowing the patient to be positioned supine within the field. There have, however, been many modifications and improvements to the original design since the advent of clinical scanning and these include improved bore dimensions, magnetic shielding, reduced scan times and archiving, which are discussed in more detail below.

Improved bore dimensions

- Early scanners had a very long narrow bore that would totally surround the patient during the scan procedure. Modern machines tend to have a much shorter, wider bore of around 1 m or less. This allows many procedures to be undertaken with the patient's head outside the equipment, which reduces the incidence of claustrophobia that previously had been a considerable problem for many subjects.

Magnetic shielding

Another important modification to the superconductive magnet design is in the method of shielding the fringe field. Early machines were not shielded and the main magnetic field was therefore not confined to the magnet room itself. The fringe field, as it is known, could even extend beyond the boundaries of the building. This is a problem because certain implanted medical devices are adversely affected by a strong magnetic field, particularly cardiac pacemakers. To maintain the magnetic field within a reasonable area (or footprint) magnetic shielding was first achieved by bolting large metal plates around the gantry of the scanner or within the walls of the magnet room. Later machines featured an active shielding system that utilised electromagnetic coils positioned around each end of the main magnet and producing an equal but opposite effect. This led to a much smaller and (for the patient) less intimidating gantry design.

Reduced scan times

Scan times have also reduced significantly over the last 20 years. A standard brain protocol would have taken about 1 hour to perform in the late 1980s. The same protocol today could be achieved in under 10 minutes. From an equipment point of view, this advance in scan speed has been possible due to improvements in gradient coil design and receiver coil construction combined with a trend towards higher magnetic field strengths.

Another important factor in scan speed and image quality is pulse sequence design. The principles behind fast scanning were understood as long ago as 1977 when Mansfield et al described a technique known as echo-planar imaging (EPI). As with many other MRI advances it took several years for the hardware to catch up with the theory. Spin echo imaging, which is the mainstay of MRI protocols, had very good image quality, but was very time consuming to perform. The introduction of EPI, gradient echo and fast spin echo (FSE) sequences served to reduce scan times still further with only minimal trade-offs in image quality.

Archiving

The digital revolution has not only improved the speed of computing, but has led to a huge array of archive media such as optical, compact and versatile discs. The tape streamer or hard drive used to store patient data on early systems would require changing after only a handful of patients. Now with the use of 250 GB hard drive arrays it is possible to keep months of patient examinations 'live' on the system for image retrieval and film printing.

SCIENCE AND INSTRUMENTATION

MRI scanners can be categorised in terms of field strength. The unit used to measure MRI field strength is the Tesla (T). 1 T equals 10 000 Gauss; note that the Earth's magnetic field varies from 0.2 to 0.7 Gauss.[15] Clinical scanners are generally described as high, mid or low field systems:

- High field (1.0 to 2.0 T)
- Mid field (0.5 T)
- Low field (below 0.15 to 0.5 T)

Research scanners are often of higher strength than clinical scanners and can be as much as 4.0 T or more in strength. These machines are typically used for applications such as fMRI and spectroscopy.

The magnet design can also vary; the types commonly available are:

Permanent magnets

Early magnet design utilised superconducting electromagnets at the heart of the system, but since then some companies have developed permanent magnet devices. These systems do not feature a closed cylindrical bore but instead have two opposing permanent magnets constructed from a highly magnetic alloy of aluminium, nickel and cobalt (alnico). The patient lies on a couch between the two and the main magnetic field is usually orientated in the vertical plane.

The main advantage of these scanners is the relatively open design, often allowing the patient's head to remain outside the scanner for many examinations and allowing a high degree of access for interventional procedures.

A second advantage is the ability to accommodate obese patients who would not physically fit inside a closed bore magnet.

From a cost point of view, these scanners are cheap to run and maintain as they do not require expensive cryogen fills.

The disadvantages to open magnet design include the fact that it is difficult to achieve field strengths above 0.35 T, and that the magnet must be maintained in a temperature controlled environment to maintain the correct operating frequency. Permanent magnets are also very heavy and therefore may be difficult to site, requiring strong foundations for the magnet room. The only advantage in siting these magnets is that their fringe field is fairly compact.

Resistive magnets

These machines use an electromagnet to generate a magnetic field. An electromagnet is typically constructed from a coil of wire through which current is passed. They are usually lighter and smaller in design than open systems and have the advantage that they may be switched off when not in use. The field is typically orientated horizontally along the bore of the magnet.

Because the coil is not super-cooled, there are cost implications in having to supply power when in use. This is offset by the fact that they do not require cryogen refills.

The main disadvantage of these systems is that the field strength is limited by the amount of current that can be applied to the coil without causing overheating due to resistivity in the windings.

Superconducting magnets

Superconducting magnets are also electromagnets but are super-cooled with cryogens. The wire used in the windings of a superconductive system is made from an alloy of niobium and titanium. This material is superconductive which means that at extremely low temperatures (nearly absolute zero or -270° centigrade) the resistance to electrical current drops to virtually zero. The advantage of this is that a very high current can be applied to the windings without any associated heating which allows the production of a very powerful magnetic field. The current will also continue to flow indefinitely while the coils are maintained at a low temperature. To achieve this, the coils are bathed in liquid helium.

Helium boil-off was reduced in early scanners by insulating the cryostat in a separate bath of liquid nitrogen and finally a layer containing chilled water. Modern scanners tend not to require liquid nitrogen and have improved the cryostat to such a degree that helium refills are now only required every few years rather than months. This is a big cost saving as a full cryogen refill can cost over £30 000.

The process of applying an electric current to create the magnetic field is known as ramping. Once the magnet is ramped to the required field strength, the supply can be disconnected and the current will continue to flow through the windings for as long as the low temperature is maintained. The magnetic field of a closed bore superconductive scanner is orientated horizontally along the magnet bore.

Other designs

Other magnet designs include 'niche' scanners, small bore portable units for imaging the limbs and 'double doughnut' superconducting systems that allow direct access to the patient during scanning. Niche scanners tend to be about the same size as a refrigerator and have a very narrow bore that allows the positioning of extremities. The double doughnut design consists of two short cylindrical electromagnets situated slightly apart, allowing a surgeon to stand between the two during a procedure. This also demands the use of non-ferrous surgical equipment to avoid projectile hazards due to strong magnetic attraction.

◼ The closed-bore scanner

The MRI scanner itself consists of a large cylindrical super-cooled electromagnet mounted inside a covered gantry. The magnet is sandwiched between other components that are responsible for radiofrequency transmission/reception and spatial encoding.

These individual components when viewed in transverse cross-section, form concentric circles as shown in Figure 41.3.

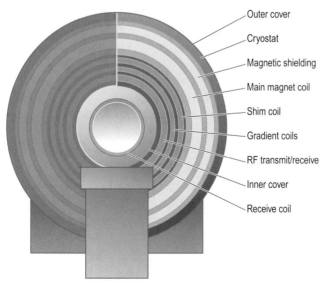

Figure 41.3 The components of a closed bore MRI scanner in transverse cross-section

Working from the outermost structure inwards the important components are the: outer cover, cryostat, magnet, shim system, gradient system, radiofrequency transmitter/receiver and receive coils. These are discussed in more detail below.

Outer cover

This is a plastic or fibreglass shell protecting the scan components from damage and dust.

Cryostat

The cryostat is essentially a large Dewar flask, made of non-ferrous metal. It contains the cryogens used for maintaining superconductivity of the magnet. The cryostat is equipped with a chimney-like vent known as the quench pipe to allow the expulsion of helium gas in the event of a quench. A quench is a phenomenon whereby the cryogen liquid boils off rapidly to gas and it occurs if the coils of the magnet become resistive and start to heat the cryogens or if particles of ice fall into the cryogen bath. One litre of liquid helium produces approximately 600 L of gas and a full cryogen bath can liberate over 800 000 L of gas in a fairly short explosive burst. This gas must be safely vented away from the patient and other personnel because although non-toxic, it can quickly displace oxygen in the magnet room and other areas. There have been rare cases where suffocation has occurred as a result of cryogen leakage. There is usually a button located in the magnet room that can be used to quench the system in the event of an emergency. It should be noted from a safety viewpoint that the magnetic field can take several minutes to reduce.

Magnet

Inside the cryostat is the main electromagnet. This reel-like structure resembles a much larger and wider version of a car wheel with the tyre removed. Around the centre of this assembly are the windings that generate the main magnetic field. These are formed by a continuous piece of niobium titanium alloy wire several km in length, which is wound onto the reel evenly and carefully under the control of a technician. The coils are bathed in liquid helium to maintain superconductivity and are briefly attached to a power supply to initiate the magnetic field. This main magnetic field is known as B_0 and is of very high power and homogeneity, typically between 0.5 and 4 T depending upon the number of windings used and current applied. There is an exponential relationship between the number of windings used and the field strength. Keeping all other factors the same it requires 4 × the windings to double field strength. At each end of the magnet outside the main coil there are separate windings that form the active shielding system designed to reduce the size of the fringe field.

Shim system

Moving further towards the centre of the scanner, the next layer consists of the shim coil, another electromagnet. This is a resistive coil that is not inside the cryostat. As stated previously, MRI demands a homogeneous magnetic field. Homogeneity is measured in parts per million (ppm). Perfect homogeneity is impossible to achieve and the raw magnetic field of the main MRI magnet is homogeneous to approximately 1000 ppm. This can be further improved by a process known as shimming. Shimming is achieved in two ways, known as active and passive shimming.

Passive shimming is performed by the placement of metal discs (or shims) inside small circular apertures in a hollow fibreglass former or non-ferrous trays encircling the magnet bore. The former has typically over 200 of these circular pockets, each designed to hold several shims. The placement of the shims is calculated by software after scanning a phantom or test object and is usually only performed once when the system is first set up for use.

Active shimming uses the shim coil, a resistive electromagnet that can be activated every time a pulse sequence is performed and can therefore correct for any field inhomogeneity caused by the introduction of different sized patients into the magnet bore.

After shimming, the magnetic field homogeneity should be better than 10 ppm, which equates to a difference in precessional frequency of less than 4 Hz over a 22 cm spherical volume. A full explanation of precessional frequency can be found later.

The homogeneous volume of the magnet bore in closed bore scanners can be described as an imaginary sphere of approximately 50 cm diameter, centred at the very midpoint of the bore in all three directions – the point known as the magnetic isocentre.

Gradient system

The main difference between MRI and NMR spectroscopy is the ability to determine the spatial origin of the signal returned by a sample. Spatial encoding is performed by the application of gradients to the main magnetic field. The gradient coils form the next layer in the construction of the MRI scanner and consist of three separate electromagnets orientated inside a cylindrical structure encircling the bore.

Each element of the gradient set can be individually activated by the application of an electric current sent from the gradient amplifiers. This results in the generation of a secondary field superimposed onto the main magnetic field on either side of the isocentre and producing a linear slope in magnetic field strength from end to end. The orientation of the elements in the gradient coil allow the gradient to be applied in any plane.

Using conventional coordinate nomenclature, the three orthogonal planes are given the labels X, Y and Z. For a patient lying in the magnet in the head-first supine position the X, Y and Z directions are as follows:

- X direction – left to right
- Y direction – posterior to anterior
- Z direction – inferior to superior

Activating the gradient coils in isolation allows selection of sagittal, coronal and axial slices. Activation of the different gradient elements in tandem can produce imaging planes with any degree of obliquity, i.e. parasagittal, paracoronal and paraaxial. These imaging planes are achieved without having to reposition the patient.

When purchasing a scanner, it is worth investigating the various specifications of gradient system offered by the manufacturer. The speed and power of gradients vary and there is usually a cost implication when purchasing high-speed power gradients because they require better gradient amplification and sometimes require water cooling due to resistivity effects. This cost is often justified because the increased scan speed will allow higher throughput, and increased temporal resolution for dynamic studies. Increased gradient strength will allow better spatial resolution, thinner slices and a smaller minimum field of view. For applications such as fMRI, spectroscopy, perfusion and diffusion imaging, power gradients are strongly recommended.

Gradient strength is usually measured in milliTesla (mT) per metre, i.e. how much the magnetic field strength in mT changes over distance in metres. At the time of writing, standard gradient systems deliver around 15 mT/m whereas power gradients for clinical use deliver around 65 mT/m. Research systems such as those found in universities may provide a gradient strength of up to 80 mT/m. The limiting factor for gradient strength in clinical applications is the point at which physical side-effects occur. Volunteers undergoing research scans at high gradient power/speed report unpleasant temporary side-effects such as migraine-like visual disturbances known as magnetophosphenes and peripheral nerve stimulation causing involuntary contractions of the muscles in the extremities. These effects are caused by the induction of electrical currents in nerve fibres and stop when the gradients are switched off.

Another important point to mention about gradient systems is that they are responsible for the noises made during scanning. MRI scans can be very loud, reaching over 100 decibels for some pulse sequences.[16] The reason for this noise is that the gradient coils carry current and are situated in the main magnetic field. Faradays law of electromagnetic induction states that a conductor lying in a magnetic field will move if unrestricted. The MRI gradient system is subject to a current of rapidly changing polarity and will therefore vibrate vigorously against its mountings. The higher the power and speed of the gradient set, the louder and more unpleasant the noise becomes.

This acoustic noise problem has been tackled by the use of ear defenders, music systems and special noise cancelling headphones. Manufacturers have also tried to reduce gradient noise by sealing the gradient system in a vacuum.

Radiofrequency (RF) transmitter/receiver

The final component layer consists of the RF transmitter, another electromagnetic coil whose task is to transmit and receive radiofrequency pulses. This device is colloquially known as the 'body coil'. The purpose of this transmitter is to produce a secondary electromagnetic field at 90° to the main magnetic field which is achieved by applying an alternating electric current to the coil. The frequency of this alternating current is matched to the precessional frequency of hydrogen nuclei within the patient, allowing a transfer of energy from the secondary field to the oscillating nuclei, a process known as NMR.

The body coil is capable of transmitting RF on all MRI systems but RF transmission is also performed by separate detachable coils on many systems. These are typically the head and knee coils.

Receive coils

Although the body coil is capable of receiving RF, it has inherent image quality problems due to signal to noise ratio issues. It is situated quite a distance away from the area under investigation and tends to receive a comparatively high level of random electrical noise compared to useful signal. For this reason, manufacturers provide an array of purpose-built receiver coils designed to be positioned in close proximity to the area under investigation.

The three main types of receive coils are:

Surface coils

These coils are typically circular or elliptical in shape and consist of a wire antenna encased in a padded protective jacket. They can either be generic in that they can be positioned closely to *any* area of anatomy or specifically designed to fit a region of interest. An example of a specific surface coil is a traditional spine coil which is encased inside a plastic mattress cover and has an external handle to allow positioning under different vertebral levels. Generic surface coils are positioned close to the skin surface over the region of interest such as the temporomandibular joint or wrist.

Surface coils receive less electrical noise than the body coil and because of their close proximity to the patient, have a good inherent signal to noise ratio. The main disadvantage to their use is the fact that they can only receive signal from a depth equal to their own radius, so a 12 cm wide coil will only image structures to a depth of 6 cm below the surface of the skin. For uniform signal reception, a volume coil is needed.

Volume coils

Volume coils are designed to encircle the entire region of interest, usually the head, elbow, wrist, knee, ankle or foot. Their design often resembles a cylinder or cage and the head coil often incorporates a mirror or prism allowing the patient to see an unrestricted view down the magnet bore. Volume coils detect signal uniformly across the region of interest without the signal fall-off associated with surface coils and have a better signal-to-noise ratio (SNR) compared to the body coil.

Phased array coils

These consist of a number of smaller receive coils ganged together. The signal detected by each element of the array is incorporated into one large field of view. Phased array coils give the best of both worlds in that they offer the coverage of the body coil but with the good SNR of a surface coil. The elements themselves can be deselected or selected depending upon the anatomical coverage sought. For example, a phased array spine coil might have five distinct elements, only one of which would be switched on for a cervical study. A cervicothoracic study may require three elements to be activated and a scan for the whole spinal cord may need all five elements in use. There are currently phased array versions of coils used for most anatomical areas.

◼ Quadrature detection

Many coils these days benefit from a feature known as quadrature detection. This increases SNR by detecting signal from two physical orientations simultaneously (known as the real and imaginary components of the signal).

◼ Patient transport system

In early scanners the patient was physically hoisted into position on a wooden table-top. The patient couch has now evolved into a sophisticated mechanism that allows accurate positioning of the region of interest using laser positioning devices.

Table movement itself is also more sophisticated allowing different speeds and having the capability to centre the imaging volume to isocentre for every pulse sequence. With the advent of phased array coils the current trend is to position the patient with various coils in situ and perform scans of multiple regions without repositioning the patient. An example of this is magnetic resonance angiography (MRA) where a single injection of contrast agent is imaged as it passes in a bolus through the entire arterial system from the abdomen to the lower extremities. This kind of scan requires fast acquisition and also very rapid table movement between areas of interest.

When purchasing a scanner it is well worth investigating the option of a detachable patient table. Detachable tables offer the advantage of a non-ferrous (safe) patient trolley that can quickly remove the patient from the scan room in an emergency and can aid throughput by positioning non-ambulant patients in readiness for their procedure whilst the previous patient is still being scanned on a second table.

MRI SAFETY

The scope of MRI safety considerations is very wide and there are books and websites devoted to this complicated topic.[17] This section provides a brief overview, not a complete safety strategy, and practitioners working (or intending to work) in the field of MRI should seek further information before entering the MRI environment. Unit guidelines and hospital health and safety procedures should also be consulted.

Radiofrequency pulses

From a radiation protection viewpoint, MRI can be said to be a very safe modality. The electromagnetic radiation used is non-ionising and causes no tissue damage. RF applications do, however, deploy energy into the body tissues (measured in watts per kilogram) and this causes a heating effect. Most of the body systems can be adversely affected by overheating so the scanner requires information about the patient weight to ensure that safe levels are not exceeded.

Magnetic fields

The magnetic fields used in MRI are of considerable danger to the patient due to:

- Projectiles attracted to the main magnetic field
- Damage to implanted devices by the main magnetic field
- Torque applied to implanted devices and foreign bodies by the main magnetic field
- Damage to implanted devices due to gradient magnetic fields
- Damage to implanted devices due to RF magnetic fields

Projectiles

Projectiles have caused a number of deaths and injuries to patients since 1980. Ferromagnetic objects such as wheelchairs, stretcher poles, floor polishers, oxygen cylinders and ancillary equipment have a strong attraction to the main magnetic field and may be dragged from the floor into the magnet bore. Ferromagnetic objects may reach a speed of up to 40 miles per hour and follow a complex trajectory through the scanner and cause serious trauma to a patient (and damage to the equipment costing hundreds of thousands of pounds to repair).

Implanted devices

Implanted devices such as pacemakers may be adversely affected by a strong magnetic field and cease to function properly. There have been a number of deaths caused by patients entering the proximity of an MRI scanner with a pacemaker in situ. Other non-MRI compatible implanted devices such as artificial heart valves, breast implants and stents may experience violent deflection causing injury.

The application of rapidly fluctuating gradient magnetic fields and RF pulses can induce currents in conductive elements of a device causing damage. Electromagnetic induction can occur in any looped conductor. For this reason it is a good idea to keep any cables away from the patient's skin and to ensure that the patient does not lie in a position where the arms and legs are crossed.

Foreign bodies

Items such as shrapnel and other metal fragments may experience a torque or attraction to the main magnetic field. This could lead to haemorrhage or damage to internal organs. Deflection of intraoccular foreign bodies could also cause damage to the retina.

To prevent patients with contraindications from entering the scan environment it is common policy to administer a screening form on attendance. There is currently no British standard MRI safety screening form, but the British Association of MR Radiographers offer the following advice:

> 'The MR safety questionnaire should be designed to determine if there is any reason that the patient or individual would undergo an adverse reaction if they were to undergo an MRI investigation.'[18]

They suggest that the questionnaire should be designed to obtain information concerning:

- Relevant previous surgery
- Prior injury from metallic foreign bodies
- Pregnancy
- Electrically, magnetically or mechanically activated devices

Further consideration should be given to:

- Permanent colouring techniques
- Body piercing
- Previous reaction to contrast agent
- Breast-feeding
- Last menstrual period

A set of example questions is also available from their website.[18]

It is good practice to inform patients of contraindications at the time of their appointment letter. This will prevent inconvenience to the patient and gaps in workflow if an individual cannot be scanned.

For further safety information on the wide ranging topic of MRI safety visit: http://www.mrisafety.com

THE PHYSICAL PRINCIPLES OF MRI

As already stated, the basic mechanism of MRI is that a radiofrequency is applied to the hydrogen nuclei within the patient's tissues which causes them to change their energy state and net magnetic alignment to an external magnetic field. As the nuclei lose this energy to realign with the field, their transmitted energy can be measured and spatially located. This technique uses a series of radio wave applications and magnetic field gradient applications, known as a pulse sequence. The timing of these applications determine tissue contrast because molecular behaviour differs between various tissue types, particularly fat and water.

Resonance

Resonance is the transfer of energy from one oscillating body to another. In NMR this refers to the transfer of energy from an electromagnetic wave (radio wave) to the nucleus of an atom. To understand how this process works, let us first look at the properties of electromagnetic waves and atomic nuclei.

Electromagnetic waves

Electromagnetic waves form a broad spectrum comprising different kinds of radiation. They all travel at the speed of light but have different wavelengths and therefore occur at different frequencies. This means that if one plotted the waveforms on a graph or oscilloscope, some would have more cycles per second than others. Frequency is measured in Hertz, 1 Hz = 1 cycle per second. The electromagnetic spectrum encompasses waves with frequencies between 10^2 Hz (radio waves) through microwaves and visible light to high energy waves of the frequency 10^{24} Hz (X-rays and gamma rays). High energy ionising radiation can be dangerous as it damages biological tissue whereas the lower energy components of the spectrum such as radio waves do not.

Atomic nuclei

In the traditional Bohr model of the atom (proposed by Niels Bohr in 1913)[19] there is an arrangement of subatomic particles called protons, neutrons and electrons. Protons and neutrons (collectively called nucleons) are bound together to form a nucleus, with the electrons existing in discreet orbits around the nucleus like satellites around a planet.

All of these particles can be described in terms of mass, electric charge and movement:

- Electrons have negligible mass, are negatively charged, spin on their own axes in either direction and orbit the nucleus
- Protons have measurable mass, are positively charged and spin on their own axis in either direction
- Neutrons also have mass, have no electrical charge and spin on their own axes in either direction

Nuclei can have different numbers of protons and neutrons and elements are given a mass number referring to the number of nucleons present and an atomic number that reflects the number of protons present.

If a nucleus has an even number of nucleons (such as helium which has two protons and two neutrons) the nucleus will have a positive electrical charge (due to the protons) but because the nucleons can spin in either direction the clockwise spins will cancel out the anticlockwise spins. The nucleus will therefore have a net positive charge but no net spin.

If a nucleus has an odd number of nucleons (such as lithium which has three protons and four neutrons) there will be a net positive charge and a net spin. This is because there will be an unpaired spinning proton in the nucleus. Whenever there is an electrically charged spinning particle, a magnetic field will be generated by that particle. Nuclei having an odd mass number therefore have an induced magnetic field.

The hydrogen nucleus

The nucleus used in clinical MRI imaging (morphological not spectroscopy) is that of the hydrogen atom. Hydrogen is chosen because its nucleus is a solitary proton with spin, charge and therefore magnetism. Hydrogen is also the most common element in the universe and forms nearly 50% of the human body.

Quantum theory states that different atomic nuclei exist in one of several possible energy states. The number of possible energy states of an individual nucleus varies depending upon the element in question. The single hydrogen proton can only spin in one of two possible directions; its magnetic field can therefore only be generated in one of two possible orientations and it exists in one of two energy states.

Normally the orientation of these tiny magnetic vectors is distributed randomly but when subjected to an external magnetic field such as that found inside an MRI scanner (known as B_0) the magnetic vectors of the nuclei will line up with B_0. Approximately half of the nuclei will align with their magnetic vector, pointing in the same direction as the main magnetic field (called spin-up) and the other half will align in the opposite direction (spin-down). The nuclei can absorb energy from, and emit energy to B_0 and therefore flip between the two energy states constantly. However the nuclei have a slight 'preference' for the low energy spin-up state. This means that over a few seconds the ratio between spin-up and spin-down nuclei will change and there will be slightly more spins in the low energy/spin-up orientation than in the high energy/spin-down orientation (Figs 41.4, 41.5).

The net magnetic vector

In MRI we look at the behaviour of the combined (net) magnetism of all the hydrogen nuclei within a sample of tissue. Looking at the combined magnetic vectors of all the spins in bulk, we get an overall magnetic vector known as the net magnetic vector or NMV. As more of the hydrogen nuclei shift their magnetic vector into the parallel orientation, the net magnetic vector changes over this short period of time to become aligned with B_0. This is because, at the outset, the populations of spin-up and spin-down nuclei are equal and their magnetic fields cancel out. Over time, however, more spins attain the spin-up orientation and the NMV becomes aligned accordingly. The resulting magnetisation is said to be 'longitudinal' or in the +Z direction. The time taken for the NMV to make this shift is known as T1 and is an important factor in image

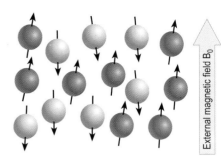

Figure 41.5
Magnetic vectors of hydrogen nuclei in an external magnetic field

External magnetic field B_0

contrast (to be absolutely precise, T1 is defined as the time taken for 63% of the longitudinal magnetisation to recover into the +Z direction). When the populations of spins have reached a steady ratio the system is said to be at equilibrium.

The actual ratio between spin-up and spin-down nuclei is very small; in approximately every million spins there are only three extra spin-up nuclei. This still equates to billions of extra spin-up nuclei in a tissue sample and it is these nuclei alone that give the signal and contrast on an MRI scan.

The number of these extra nuclei available to contribute to the image increases with field strength. This is because it requires more energy to oppose a higher field than a weak field and the spin-up and spin-down populations will reflect this. High field scanners therefore have an inherently better SNR than low field systems. Because these extra spin-up nuclei are the ones that have significance where image production is concerned, we will simply refer to them as the 'spins'.

Precession

When we described motion in the atom earlier, we only mentioned spinning and orbiting. There is another important kind of motion involved in NMR known as precession. When the nuclei are subjected to an external magnetic field, they not only spin on their axes but they also wobble slightly. This is often described as being analogous to a spinning top. If we set a gyroscope spinning on a table-top, it will spin at hundreds of revolutions per minute. It will also be seen to wobble in a circular path at a much slower rate. If we imagine a line drawn through the vertical axis of the gyroscope, this imaginary line will prescribe a cone shape as the gyroscope wobbles. This movement is known as precession and is due to gravity. The speed at which the gyroscope wobbles is also related to gravity; on the moon with less gravity the gyroscope would precess more slowly (fewer turns per minute) than on the earth.

The spinning hydrogen nuclei also precess, not due to gravity but due to the presence of the external magnetic

Figure 41.4 Magnetic vectors of hydrogen nuclei in random alignment

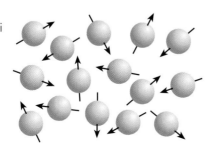

field. If the field strength is increased, the nuclei will precess at a faster rate, if the external field is reduced they will precess more slowly. Remember the speed at which they *spin* remains the same, it's the speed at which they *wobble* that alters.

Phase and frequency

The precessional speed and orientation of a spinning nucleus can be described in terms of frequency and phase. The frequency of precession (i.e. how many wobbles per minute) can be calculated by an equation first published by physicist Joseph Larmor (1857–1942) and it is the only equation used in this chapter!

The Larmor equation states:

$$\omega = \gamma B_0$$

where: ω is the angular precessional frequency of the proton

γ is the gyromagnetic ratio of the nucleus

B_0 is the external field strength.

Every nucleus has its own fixed gyromagnetic ratio expressed in Hertz/Tesla. For hydrogen this is 42.6 MHz/T, so at a field strength of 1 T the hydrogen nuclei will be precessing at a frequency of 42.6 MHz (at 1.5 T it will be 63.9 Mhz and so on).

Knowledge of the precessional frequency for hydrogen at a particular field strength is important because in order to resonate the nuclei it is necessary to apply an electromagnetic wave at a matching frequency and this will differ depending upon the magnet used.

Phase is a term that can be used to describe the orientation of the magnetic vector of a nucleus compared to other nuclei nearby. Let us return to the gyroscope analogy. We stated earlier that the vertical axis of a precessing gyroscope (or nucleus) prescribes a cone shape. If we look at the gyroscope from above, the top of the gyroscope can be seen to move in a circular path as it wobbles about its axis. That is to say, its orientation goes from a 12 o'clock position round to 3 o'clock, 6 o'clock, 9 o'clock and finally ends up back at 12 o'clock. If we set a number of gyroscopes spinning at the same time, it is unlikely that they would all precess in synchronisation. One might be at 12 o'clock while its neighbour is at 3 o'clock.

At equilibrium the nuclei are all precessing at the same frequency because they are all in the same magnetic field strength but they are out of synchronisation when it comes to the orientation of their vectors. The orientation of a single vector around its cone shaped path is known as its phase position, and at equilibrium the spins can be said to be out-of-phase with each other (Figs 41.6, 41.7).

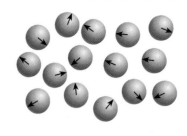

Figure 41.6 The magnetic vectors of hydrogen nuclei, out of phase. (These spins are depicted as being viewed from 'above', i.e. we are looking from a direction parallel to the main magnetic field.) Dephased magnetic vectors cancel out resulting in a loss of signal

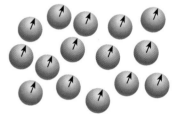

Figure 41.7 The magnetic vectors of hydrogen nuclei, in phase. The combined magnetic effect of all these spins is known as the net magnetic vector (NMV)

Signal

To construct an image it is necessary to receive signal from the region of interest and spatially encode it. MRI signal is in the form of a weak electromagnetic wave emitted by the spins following excitation by an RF pulse.

This weak signal is generated by the positively charged nuclei as they precess. Their NMV results in a moving magnetic field that will induce a current in an antenna (or conductive loop) placed in close proximity.

> The maximum signal is generated when the NMV is 90° to B_0 and the contributing individual vectors are in phase.

At equilibrium the NMV is aligned in the same direction as B_0 and the spins are out of phase. Signal is therefore not generated.

To generate signal we use resonance. When we apply an RF pulse at the Larmor frequency, energy is transferred to the nuclei within the sample. This has two important effects:

1. First the surfeit of nuclei in the low-energy, spin-up direction will absorb energy and become high-energy, spin-down nuclei. If the right amount of RF is used the population of spin-up and spin-down nuclei will become equal. The effect of this is that the NMV will change orientation and precess at 90° to B_0 where it can be detected with a suitable antenna (receive coil). This magnetisation is said to be in the transverse plane, i.e. the RF pulse has converted longitudinal magnetisation into transverse magnetisation. Because it has changed the angle of the NMV by 90° the pulse used is known as a 90° RF pulse (Fig. 41.8).

Figure 41.8 The NMV following a 90° RF pulse

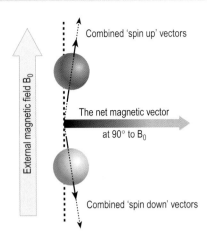

External magnetic field B₀

Combined 'spin up' vectors

The net magnetic vector at 90° to B₀

Combined 'spin down' vectors

2. The second effect of the RF pulse is that it forces the magnetic vectors of the spins to precess in phase. This is important as the signal from out-of-phase spins cancels out and cannot be detected by the receive coil. In-phase spins result in an NMV that precesses at the Larmor frequency at 90° to B₀ and produces maximum signal in the receive coil.

A useful analogy here is to imagine a row of playground swings with children sitting on them. If a row of parents stand pushing the swings and they all push at the same time and with the same frequency (let us say, one push every 2 seconds) the children will swing to and fro in synchronisation. They will all be up in the air at the same time and they will all start to swing down again at the same time. This is analogous to being in-phase.

When the parents stop pushing, the children will slowly fall out of synchronisation, i.e. some of them will be up in the air while others will be at the low point of their swing. This is analogous to the spins losing their phase coherence.

The time taken for the spins to lose (63% of) their phase coherence is known as T2 and is another important factor in image contrast.

Contrast

So far we have seen how signal from hydrogen nuclei can be generated within a tissue sample and detected by a receive coil. In order to make a diagnostic image, however, we need to be able to create contrast between different structures/tissues/pathologies.

There are three principle factors affecting contrast on an MRI image and these are:

• T1 recovery
• T2 decay
• Proton density

T1

It was mentioned earlier that when we apply a 90° RF pulse to the sample, any longitudinal magnetisation is converted into transverse magnetisation. It is also true to say that any (residual) transverse magnetisation will be tipped into the longitudinal plane. The reason that this factor can be used to produce contrast on the image is that different tissues have different rates of T1 recovery.

The most marked difference is between the recovery rates of fat and pure water. Following a 90° RF pulse, fat recovers its longitudinal magnetisation quickly. This is due to the fact that it has large molecules with relatively slow Brownian motion that can dissipate energy quickly. This means that in fat, the spin population loses the absorbed energy quickly and regains its low-energy, spin-up condition.

Pure water, on the other hand, has high energy molecules with rapid Brownian motion that cannot dissipate energy readily. Pure water nuclei therefore retain the absorbed energy and the magnetic vector associated with pure water remains in the transverse plane for longer than that of fat.

If we rapidly apply a second 90° RF pulse to the sample, the fully recovered NMV from fat will once again be flipped into the transverse plane – giving maximum signal. The partially recovered water vector, however, will be flipped into the longitudinal plane and will subsequently return only a limited signal (Fig. 41.9).

If we allowed more time between RF pulses, fat and water would have time to recover their longitudinal magnetisation and would both be flipped by 90° by successive RF pulses causing a loss in T1 contrast.

The time between RF applications is known as the TR (time to repetition), a T1-weighted image uses a short TR (e.g. 300 milliseconds) and will exhibit bright fat and dark fluid.

Figure 41.9 Fat and water vectors during rapid TR. Fat vector is repeatedly flipped to 90° but water is flipped to beyond 90° and the signal becomes saturated

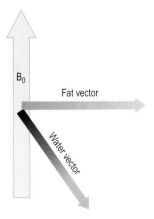

B₀

Fat vector

Water vector

T2

Following the removal of the 90° RF pulse, the spins dephase rapidly. This is due to two processes. The main cause of dephasing is field inhomogeneity. Even with a field homogeneous to 4 ppm there will be a fluctuation in field strength across the imaging volume. The introduction of a human body into the field will also further spoil the homogeneity as water molecules are slightly repelled by an external field (known as diamagnetism). The secondary cause of dephasing is the fact that the nuclei themselves have magnetic fields and these fields interact over time, attracting and repelling each other. These are known as spin-spin interactions.

The reason that T2 is an image contrast parameter is that different tissues lose phase coherence at different rates. The most marked difference here is between solids and pure water molecules. Following the removal of the 90° RF pulse, the magnetic vectors of tightly packed nuclei in solid structures such as bone undergo many spin-spin interactions and dephase readily and quickly. The widely spaced molecules in water contain hydrogen nuclei that undergo fewer spin-spin interactions and therefore their magnetic vectors stay in-phase for longer than those in solid bone.

Contrast is therefore obtained by waiting for a certain time period after the application of the 90° RF pulse before sampling the returning signal. Any tissues that have lost phase coherence will appear darker than tissues whose spins are still in phase.

Although not strictly a solid, fat contains nuclei that are more closely spaced than water and that therefore returns an intermediate signal.

The time period between the 90° RF pulse and the collection of the signal is known as the TE (time to echo), a T2-weighted image uses a long TE (e.g. 100 milliseconds or above) and will exhibit bright water, very dark solid bone and medium intensity from fat.

Proton density

The term proton density refers to the number of hydrogen nuclei present within a given volume of tissue. To compare extremes, think of air and water. There are more hydrogen nuclei in the fluid-filled ventricles of the brain than in the nearby air-filled paranasal sinuses. A proton density weighted image will therefore have varying degrees of signal from different tissues. A proton density image is obtained by using parameters that reduce T1 and T2 contrast, i.e. a long TR to reduce T1 effects and a short TE to reduce T2 effects.

Weighting

When describing the contrast of an MRI image the term 'weighting' is used to indicate that the contrast is weighted or heavily influenced by one of the above parameters. Image contrast never results purely from one of these parameters alone as all images are affected by T1, T2 and proton density to some degree. For example, the air-filled sinuses will appear as dark as a melanoma metastasis on a T2-weighted scan but the lack of signal from the sinuses has nothing to do with T2 contrast and everything to do with proton density.

Spatial encoding

Having generated signal and determined the contrast required, the final stage of the procedure is to spatially encode the signal so that we can reconstruct it into a diagnostic image. Spatial encoding using gradient magnetic fields was first proposed by Lauterbur in 1973[5] and is still used in scanners today. The principle being that spins across the imaging volume can be assigned a particular spatial location depending upon their frequency of precession or phase position. Spatial encoding for a 2D slice is achieved by the use of three gradients that perform the following functions:

- Locating the slice position
- Encoding the position of the spins in the vertical axis of the image
- Encoding the position of the spins in the horizontal axis of the image

Slice position

Determining the slice position is the first part of spatial encoding. As mentioned in an earlier section of the chapter, resonance can only occur if the energy source exhibits the resonant frequency of the target. An example of this would be to obtain two tuning-forks both tuned to the same note, place one of them in a stand and strike the second against an object to start it resonating. If the resonating fork is held in close proximity to the silent fork the transfer of energy between the two would induce resonance in the first tuning-fork even though there had been no physical contact. The important factor is that they must be tuned to exactly the same note (frequency). This experiment would not work if a tuning fork playing the note A was held close to a tuning fork tuned to the note B.

The aim of slice selection is to resonate a thin section of tissue rather than the entire patient. Let us assume that we wish to image a single slice through an abdomen on a patient who is lying supine and head first in the scanner.

The resonant frequency of the hydrogen nuclei can be calculated using the Larmor equation and similarly if a gradient is applied at a known strength, the precessional frequencies of the spins along the length of the gradient can also be calculated. If a gradient is applied over a certain volume (centred at the magnetic isocentre), the mid part of the gradient will remain at centre frequency, while spins at the ends of the gradient will vary from being at a slightly lower than centre frequency to a slightly higher than centre frequency. If we were to apply an RF pulse at the centre frequency we would only resonate the spins at the isocentre. The spins at either end of the slope would not be affected as their frequencies do not match the transmitted frequency. If we were to apply an RF pulse at a slightly higher frequency we would only resonate spins at a spatial location towards the higher end of the gradient (Fig. 41.10).

To achieve an axial slice we would therefore apply a gradient in the Z direction during transmission of the 90° RF pulse.

In reality, it is not quite that simple because we also need to select a slice thickness, so a range of frequencies are applied (called the transmit bandwidth) to excite a narrow band of spins along the corresponding part of the gradient.

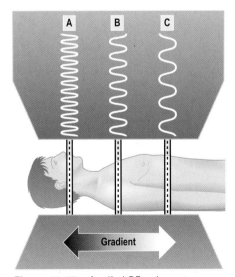

Figure 41.10 Applied RF pulses at different frequencies resonate different slice positions along a magnetic field gradient. Radiofrequency A only resonates spins having the precessional frequency corresponding to the position of the topmost slice. Radiofrequency B is at the centre frequency and only resonates spins at the isocentre. Radiofrequency C only resonates spins having the precessional frequency corresponding to the position of the lowermost slice

Phase encoding

Having selected the slice, we now need to locate the signal returning from within that field of view in 2D. Let us imagine that we wish to encode the signal from the horizontal axis of the image (left to right on a supine patient). To do this, another gradient application is performed called the phase encoding gradient. (Note that the phase encoding gradient can also be used to encode signal along the vertical part of the image depending upon certain other factors). The gradient coils are used to apply a gradient in the X direction causing the precession of the spins to speed up or slow down depending on their location. The gradient is then turned off. In the absence of the gradient, the spins return to the centre frequency, but because of the time spent inside the gradient, their phase positions will have shifted along this axis. Spins at the isocentre were still at the centre frequency during the gradient application so their phase position will be unchanged – let us say at 12 o'clock. Spins that were briefly precessing more rapidly than those at isocentre might have a phase position of 5 o'clock. Spins that were situated at the lower-than-centre frequency portion of the slope might have a phase position of 7 o'clock (Fig. 41.11).

The phase encoding gradient is actually applied many times during the pulse sequence at different strengths and polarities. The phase shift changes each time and the system uses the data collected to uniquely identify every column of voxels within the imaging volume in this axis. The resolution of the image is determined by the number of phase encodings performed, typically 128, 256, 512, or

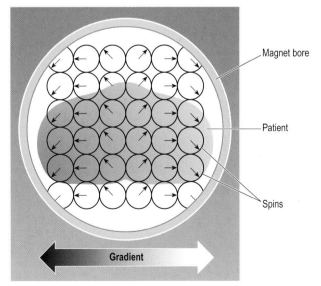

Figure 41.11 The application of a secondary gradient across the field of view changes the precessional frequencies of the spins. When it is turned off, the phase positions of some columns of spins will be advanced or retarded compared to the spins that remained at the centre frequency (isocentre)

1024 pixels. A 512 matrix will therefore require 512 RF applications (512 repetitions) and because the TR is of fixed length, a scan having a matrix of 512 will take twice as long to perform as a scan having a matrix of 256.

Frequency encoding

Having applied the previous two gradients, we have selected the slice position and collected data enabling spatial location and resolution along the horizontal axis of the image. The signal originating from the vertical axis of the image is encoded by a third gradient application known as the frequency encoding gradient. (Note that when planning a scan, phase and frequency directions are interchangeable.)

The frequency encoding gradient is applied at the same time as the signal is collected. This superimposes a range of different precessional frequencies in the spins along the horizontal axis of the region of interest. Once again the spins at isocentre will remain at the centre frequency, but the spins at each end of the gradient will either precess more quickly or more slowly depending upon the magnetic field slope. The net effect of this is that the receive coil detects a range of frequencies at time TE (Fig. 41.12).

Having acquired the signal, the system computer uses a mathematical calculation on the collected data known as the Fourier transform (devised by Jean Baptiste Joseph Fourier, 1768–1830) that essentially separates the individual frequencies and their intensities. Because the applied gradient is linear in nature, each intensity measured will be in a linear arrangement corresponding to its spatial position of origin.

A useful analogy is to imagine playing the note 'middle C' on a piano and asking a concert pianist to name the note. Middle C is the central note on the keyboard and on hearing the sound he would hopefully be able to identify it as middle C. He has received a frequency (261.63 Hz) and has assigned it a spatial location (the middle). You can think of middle C as the central frequency in MRI with all of the other white notes representing the range of frequencies along the gradient axis.

The Fourier transform is also used to separate the intensities and locations of pixels in the phase direction by applying it to the data collected over the duration of the scan.

■ Pulse sequences

The succession of RF pulses and gradient applications used in spatial encoding is known as a pulse sequence. Pulse sequences can be divided into two main categories known as spin echo and gradient echo. The main difference between the two is that spin echo pulse sequences use a 180° RF pulse to rephase the signal lost by field inhomogeneity. Gradient echo uses a magnetic field gradient to produce an echo but does not correct for field inhomogeneity dephasing. Gradient echo is typically faster than spin echo but is prone to artefactual appearances.

Figure 41.13 shows the order of events in a typical spin echo and gradient echo pulse sequence.

These basic pulse sequences have been enhanced and developed to include new contrast mechanisms and methods of rapid acquisition; these include inversion recovery sequences, FSE, driven equilibrium, single shot imaging and echo-planar imaging. Further description of MRI pulse sequences can be found in the clinical applications section of this chapter.

■ Contrast media

Despite the excellent soft tissue capabilities of MRI and its inherently good contrast to noise ratio, development of contrast media for MRI began in tandem with the first scans in 1978.

MRI contrast media can be broadly classified into two main categories:

- Positive contrast agents
- Negative contrast agents

Positive contrast media – T1 agents

Positive contrast agents produce an increase in signal intensity in affected tissues. In MRI the principal positive agents contain gadolinium as their active ingredient. In its native state gadolinium is a silver metal named after a Finnish chemist Gadolin. Like many other metals, gadolinium is mined for use in industry and its medical

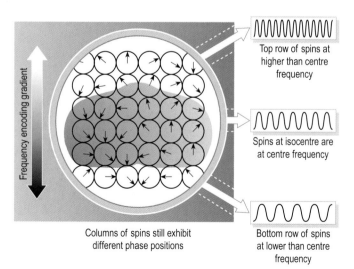

Figure 41.12 Another gradient application at 90° changes the precessional frequency of the spins. Some rows of spins will be precessing more quickly or more slowly than those remaining at the centre frequency (isocentre)

Top row of spins at higher than centre frequency

Spins at isocentre are at centre frequency

Bottom row of spins at lower than centre frequency

Frequency encoding gradient

Columns of spins still exhibit different phase positions

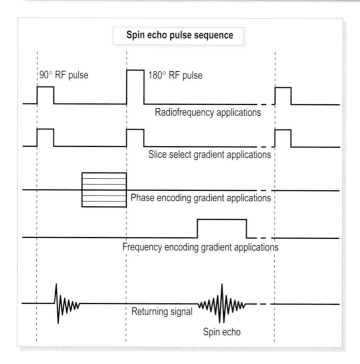

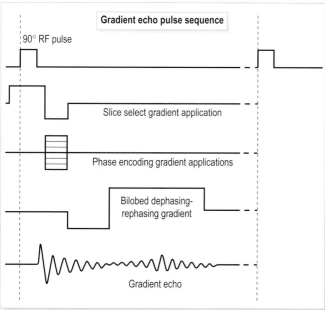

Figure 41.13 Spin echo and gradient echo pulse sequence diagrams. Note that the gradient echo uses another magnetic field gradient application to produce an echo of signal rather than a 180° RF pulse

application forms only a small percentage of its global use. It is a lanthanide element at number 64 in the periodic table. At room temperature gadolinium is paramagnetic. This is to say that it aligns to and adds to an external magnetic field. Gadolinium is toxic and therefore is attached to a chelate or ligand to produce a contrast agent.

Its mechanism as a contrast agent relies on the fact that it causes T1 shortening at fairly low doses. This ability is due to the presence of seven unpaired electrons that form dipolar bonds with hydrogen nuclei in the tissues (blood). The result of this is that the molecular tumbling rate of water is reduced, allowing a more efficient energy exchange. With a rapid TR, water is able to recover much of its longitudinal magnetisation between RF pulses; this results in more magnetisation available to be flipped into the transverse plane. The outcome is that water combined with Gadolinium chelate behaves more like fat and is therefore hyperintense on a T1-weighted image.

Negative contrast media – T2 agents

Negative contrast agents produce a decrease in signal intensity in affected tissues. In MRI the principal negative agents contain iron oxide as their active ingredient. These compounds consist of microcrystalline magnetite cores, coated with dextranes or siloxanes. This impervious coating prevents the iron from binding with the body tissues.

At room temperature, iron oxide is superparamagnetic. This is to say that iron oxide has a higher magnetic susceptibility than gadolinium. Iron oxide is toxic and therefore the particles used in contrast media are coated in an impervious layer to prevent absorption by the tissues.

Its mechanism as a contrast agent relies on the fact that it causes T2 shortening at fairly low doses. The signal loss seen in areas of uptake is due to magnetic susceptibility effects. Spins in cells containing the superparamagnetic iron will have a slightly higher precessional frequency than those surrounding them. This results in dephasing at the boundaries of these microscopic areas and a net loss of signal. This is because transverse magnetisation must be coherent (i.e. in phase) to produce maximum signal, and effects that cause dephasing will reduce the signal intensity.

■ Uses of MRI contrast media

Although MRI has the inherent ability to distinguish between types of soft tissue, there are times when contrast media use is unavoidable.

Lesion conspicuity

The use of contrast media can greatly increase the conspicuity of certain lesions. This is of particular importance where the presence of lesions would alter the treatment given in a dramatic way. For example a patient having a single cerebral metastasis would be considered as a suitable candidate for surgery. If more than one metastasis were present however, surgery would not affect the patient's longevity and would be an unnecessary trauma. Small cerebral metastases can be difficult to appreciate on an MRI scan and therefore positive contrast agents would be considered to increase their conspicuity.[20]

Lesion characterisation

Certain lesions are difficult to characterise using the inherent contrast parameters of MRI.

For example, a neurofibroma returns a high signal on T2 weighting and a low to intermediate signal on T1. Other lesions such as proteinaceous cysts would also have similar contrast characteristics. Cystic lesions, however, do not tend to enhance whereas a neurofibroma does.

Lesion extent

On unenhanced T1-weighted images the boundaries of some lesions are not clearly defined. T2 weighting demonstrates pathology very well but there is often a lot of associated oedema affecting the surrounding tissues that can distort the appearance of a lesion. The true size, shape and position of a lesion is usually better appreciated on a T1-weighted, contrast-enhanced image.

MRA

Early methods of blood vessel imaging using MRI used flow dependent techniques that did not require an injection of contrast agent. Inflow angiography and phase contrast studies produced contrast that relied on the flow of spins relative to their surroundings. These techniques suffered from many shortcomings such as overestimation of stenosis, the ability to only image flow in a particular direction and small fields of view.

The use of gadolinium has reduced most of these problems. Contrast enhanced MRA allows a larger field of view, gives a more anatomical picture of the anatomy, more accurately reproduces the size of stenoses and shortens acquisition time to a matter of seconds.

Other considerations when deciding whether to use contrast include:
- *Throughput:* on low field systems having longer acquisition times or only having conventional spin echo rather than fast spin echo, it may be quicker to make a diagnosis using contrast where the alternative would be to perform a number of more time consuming sequences to make the same diagnosis. An example might be acoustic neuroma, T1 pre and post gadolinium (10 minutes) vs. a high resolution T2-weighted scan (20 minutes)
- *Medicolegal:* many centres in the USA give contrast as part of the routine set of pulse sequences used for every patient in case something is missed
- *Dynamic studies:* in some body areas such as the liver and breast, where different kinds of lesion may exhibit different rates of contrast uptake, a diagnosis is more readily made by dynamic scanning. This uses a series of short sequences performed after injection of gadolinium chelate and studies the uptake curve and appearance of

lesions in the arterial, venous and delayed stages post injection. This can give more information than a simple pre- and post-contrast scan

■ Gadolinium safety

The number of adverse reactions to gadolinium chelates is very small. In a paper written in 1989 following 5 000 000 injections of Gadolinium DTPA there were only 15 severe reactions. Nausea and vomiting occurred in 207 cases.[21]

For most products, the recommended intravenous gadolinium dose should not exceed 0.2 millimoles per kilogram patient weight. Such is the safety profile of gadolinium compared to iodinated media that some centres are using it as a contrast agent for digital subtraction angiography.[22]

COMMON CLINICAL APPLICATIONS

MRI is now used in imaging virtually every anatomical region and the full range of clinical applications in MRI is therefore well beyond the scope of this chapter. The following section will cover only the most commonly requested examinations and it is intended that the protocols suggested will act as a basic guide. MRI protocols vary widely and must take into account the preferences of the reporting radiologist, the time available, the compliance of the patient and the field strength and capabilities of the scanner hardware/software. Please do not alter your scan protocols without consulting other users or backing up the originals! The recommended pulse sequences are generic and are commonly found on equipment from all manufacturers.

■ Pulse sequences

The pulse sequences recommended in the protocols in the next section of this chapter are described in more detail here:

Three plane localiser

This is usually a low resolution T1-weighted gradient echo sequence chosen purely for speed. It is used to prescribe the slice positions for the other pulse sequences used in a protocol.

T1 weighted (spin echo or FSE)

T1 weighting is characterised by hyperintense fat and hypointense fluid. It is traditionally referred to as an 'anatomical' sequence because it has a short echo time that yields high SNR and is therefore suited to displaying anatomical detail. For T1 weighting, CSE rather than FSE is usually the sequence of choice because T1 scan factors make the sequence inherently fast (short TR).

FSE is faster (see below) but has some associated artefacts and does not offer much of a time saving in T1-weighted imaging.

T1 weighting is used in conjunction with gadolinium enhancement and scans are usually performed before and after administration of contrast agent. This is to ensure that any hyperintensity on the image is due to enhancement rather than being an inherently bright structure such as fat or haemorrhage.

The fact that fat is bright on T1 weighting makes this sequence sensitive to changes in bone marrow including metastasis and avascular necrosis. If the fat content of bone marrow is replaced, the signal level will fall and the affected area will appear hypointense on T1 weighting.

T2 weighted (FSE)

T2 weighting in FSE is characterised by dark muscle and bright fluid. A T2-weighted study is traditionally referred to as a 'pathology' sequence because it demonstrates oedema due to its high water content. It is also one of the reasons that MRI became the must-have modality in neuro departments. The bright 'myelographic' effect of cerebrospinal fluid (CSF) on T2-weighted scans allowed MRI to replace conventional myelography for many patients.

For T2 weighting, FSE is usually the sequence of choice because scan factors (the TR must be long to reduce T1 effects) would make a CSE T2-weighted sequence impracticably slow. CSE T2-weighted sequences can take up to 30 minutes to acquire.

Earlier it was mentioned that spin echo pulse sequences use 180° refocusing pulses to produce spin echoes. In a dual echo sequence the signal from each echo is used to create a separate image. In FSE a number of echoes are collected but all of the signal is used in the same image. By collecting more signal per TR, FSE is faster than CSE and can cut scan time by a factor of 8, 16, 32 or more depending upon the settings chosen. There are two slight trade-offs in contrast weighting and sharpness but these do not have serious implications on image quality. The most noticeable difference in contrast is that fat is much brighter on FSE in comparison to CSE. This can be rectified by using fat suppression. The other difference is that the use of a high turbo factor (long echo train) can cause blurring of the image. This effect is mostly compensated for by the fact that FSE yields more signal per second than CSE and therefore smaller voxels may be used (increasing resolution).

T2 weighting is used in conjunction with superparamagnetic iron oxide contrast agents.

Dual echo (FSE)

This can also be done as a CSE pulse sequence, but takes longer to acquire. Dual echo refers to the fact that two sets of images are obtained simultaneously. Usually one set are T2 weighted and the other set are proton density (PD) weighted. PD weighted images have a short TE, high SNR and are therefore suited to demonstrate anatomical detail. They also have good contrast to noise ratio in areas having soft tissues of differing proton density. A dual echo sequence therefore gives anatomical detail with a different CNR to T1 weighting and T2 pathological information in the same acquisition time.

Dual (multiple) echo can also be used in a technique known as T2 relaxometry where there are a number of echoes at different TE values, allowing regions of interest to be drawn and T2 relaxation curves produced for various tissues.

Single shot (FSE)

Single shot techniques have greatly speeded up acquisition times in MRI. These sequences take FSE to the extreme in that they apply numerous 180° pulses allowing collection of all of the signal for a slice within a single TR. This allows imaging while the patient is free breathing. The snapshot effect of the scan typically freezes motion in areas of the body where movement can otherwise cause artefactual problems. Uses therefore include abdominal imaging and paediatric imaging on non-compliant children. Note that the images are taken one slice at a time and although motion is frozen on each slice, the anatomy may appear at very different positions on each slice.

FLAIR (fluid attenuated inversion recovery)

This is an FSE sequence from the inversion recovery family. Inversion recovery refers to the fact that an additional RF pulse is applied at the beginning of the pulse sequence that tips the NMV by 180°. Following the application of this pulse, the magnetic vectors of the tissues recover their longitudinal magnetisation to a degree before the application of a 90° RF pulse. The purpose of this is to add an additional contrast parameter, known as the tau or 'time from inversion'. Different tissues recover at different rates and by changing the timing of the 90° RF pulse, signal can be nulled (eliminated) from selected structures. In FLAIR, the timing is set to remove any signal from (for example) CSF. Proteinaceous fluid such as that found in pathology will still appear bright, making this an ideal technique for assessing periventricular disease in the brain or increasing conspicuity of the cranial nerves.

STIR (short tau inversion recovery)

This is also an FSE sequence from the inversion recovery family. Inversion recovery refers to the fact that an additional RF pulse is applied at the beginning of each repetition in the pulse sequence. This extra pulse tips the NMV by 180°. After this pulse is turned off, the magnetic vectors of the tissues recover their longitudinal magnetisation to a degree before the application of a 90° RF pulse. In STIR the timing of the 90° RF pulse is set to eliminate any signal from fat. Because the mechanism of STIR relies upon longitudinal magnetisation changes rather than precessional frequency, STIR is a robust method of fat suppression that is effective even in the presence of increased field inhomogeneity. Field inhomogeneity causes a drift in precessional frequency across the imaging volume and this is a factor that can often spoil spectral fat saturation methods (fat sat). STIR sequences are very sensitive to pathology and are starting to be used in whole body MRI screening protocols. STIR is also sensitive to bone marrow changes and trabecular microfracture (bone bruising).

Gradient echo (various weightings)

Gradient echo sequences use a gradient application to dephase and rephase the spins rather than a 180° RF pulse. Contrast is achieved by the use of variable flip angles (i.e. not just 90°) combined with the TR, the TE, and whether or not residual transverse magnetisation is allowed to contribute to image contrast. Shortened TR and TE makes for a faster sequence but with some trade-offs.

Gradient echo sequences are more affected by susceptibility artefact than spin echo, a fact that is exploited in the diagnosis of haemorrhage. The iron content of haemoglobin causes susceptibility artefact and is therefore more readily demonstrated on gradient echo sequences in comparison to spin echo. Susceptibility artefact can be a problem, however, when there is metal close to the region of interest, such as dental fixings. In these areas, spin echo or FSE may be required to reduce the artefact.

T2*-weighted gradient echo is also sensitive to flow, causing flowing spins to appear hyperintense on the images. This feature, coupled with a short minimum TE and TR is exploited in flow dependent MR angiography sequences. The use of flow compensation makes gradient echo the sequence of choice where flow may cause image degradation. This includes the spine (CSF flow) and the joints (blood flow in the region of interest).

Another feature of gradient echo is the ability to use echo times that exploit the precessional frequency difference of fat and water. At 1.5 T the magnetic vectors of fat nuclei precess 220 Hz more slowly than those of water. This means that they will drift in and out of phase with each other over time. Fat and water nuclei will be in phase approximately every 4.2 milliseconds. If the TE is set at a multiple of this factor, signal will be generated from voxels containing fat and water components. If a TE is chosen

when fat and water vectors are out of phase there will be a corresponding loss of signal. This is useful in characterising disease where there is a change in the fat to water ratio (such as fatty infiltration of the liver) or lesions where there is a known fat/water content (such as adenoma).

3D volume scans

Volume imaging typically uses gradient echo sequences with an additional phase encoding gradient applied in the slice selection plane. This allows the acquisition of very thin contiguous slices. 2D techniques require a gap between slices of 20–30% of the slice thickness to avoid an artefact known as cross-excitation. Volume imaging does not require a slice gap and is therefore recommended in 3D reconstruction and volume measurement techniques where a gap between slices would cause distortion and inaccuracy. Because the slice thickness can be reduced in comparison to a 2D scan it is possible to achieve isotropic voxels (cubic having the same dimensions of width, depth and height) This is also useful in image reconstruction as the resolution will be the same in every plane (including the slice select direction). This is also one of the reasons why 3D sequences are used in flow-dependent MRA.

Inflow angiography (also called time-of-flight)

Inflow angiography is a flow-dependent method of imaging the vasculature. It relies upon the use of gradient echo sequences having a rapid TR causing saturation of signal from tissues within the imaging volume but allowing spins entering the imaging volume to emit signal briefly before becoming saturated themselves. The TE is kept short to reduce intravoxel dephasing. The base data therefore demonstrates bright flow on a saturated noisy background. The images are created using a post-processing technique called maximum intensity projection (MIP). This process reconstructs the data from different apparent angles of view and conjoins the most intense voxels to build an anatomical looking representation of the vasculature. The reconstructed images can over-exaggerate the size of stenoses and underestimate the true lumen size of vessels and in reporting inflow MRA procedures it is recommended that the base data is also taken into consideration.

Another shortcoming of this sequence is that it is sensitive to tissues having high signal on T1 weighting. This includes fat and some stages of haemorrhage (methaemoglobin) that may obscure the vessels on a MIP. Time-of-flight sequences are only sensitive to flow in a direction perpendicular to the slice or volume.

Phase contrast angiography (PCA)

Phase contrast MRA uses a subtraction method to differentiate between flowing and stationary spins. The pulse sequence used is gradient echo with an additional gradient application known as the velocity encoding gradient or VENC. The steepness of this additional gradient is a user definable parameter used to differentiate between differing velocities of flow (e.g. between arterial and venous flow). The principle of this technique is that two acquisitions are performed to encode flow along a particular direction.

The first acquisition uses a bipolar gradient that results in the flowing nuclei acquiring an advanced phase position while the net effect on the phase position of stationary spins is zero. The second acquisition uses a flow-compensating gradient such as that used in artefact reduction techniques. This is a bipolar gradient that causes both stationary and moving spins to return signal having zero phase difference. When the data from the two acquisitions is digitally subtracted the resulting images show only the difference, i.e. the flowing spins. This technique can be time consuming, as the VENC may need to be applied in all three orthogonal planes (X, Y and Z) if flow is tortuous. The advantages are in the excellent background suppression and the fact that flow can be mathematically quantified. The subtraction technique means that, unlike time-of-flight images, phase contrast images are not obscured by tissues having short T1 times.

Contrast enhanced MRA (CEMRA)

As outlined above, phase contrast and inflow angiograms have certain image quality and artefact issues. Most of these problems can be resolved by the use of positive contrast media. In CEMRA, a bolus of gadolinium-based contrast media is injected into a vein, usually in the antecubital fossa. When the bolus reaches the region of interest, a T1-weighted, 3D volume, gradient echo sequence is performed while the patient holds their breath/keeps perfectly still.

This technique has the following advantages:

- Shorter RF pulses may be used
- Shorter TR and thinner sections may be obtained under 1 mm
- Large 3D data volumes may be collected in a 20–30 second breath hold
- Larger FOVs are possible than with inflow MRA and PCA because in-plane flow may be imaged, allowing the use of coronal sections

The rationale behind the sequence is that paramagnetic contrast agents shorten the T1 time of blood. This makes it possible to acquire an MRA in which image contrast is due to the differences in the T1 relaxation times between blood and surrounding tissues. This is an advantage because it results in a more anatomical image. Flow-dependent methods such as inflow and phase contrast MRA only

yield signal from moving blood. Vessels containing very slow flow or stationary flow cannot be visualised. Using CEMRA, it is (theoretically) possible to image vessels containing stationary blood *providing it has contrast agent present.*

This means that CEMRA does not tend to suffer from flow-related artefacts such as over-estimation of stenosis, incorrect representation of lumen diameter and saturation signal loss due to in-plane flow.

Ideally, the dose of contrast agent used, must be sufficient to shorten the T1 time of blood in comparison to the background tissues. A short TR can then be used which saturates signal from all structures apart from blood. The background tissue having the shortest T1 is fat, 270 ms at 1.5 T, thus enough gadolinium must be injected per bolus to shorten the blood T1 to under 270 ms. Depending upon the size (blood volume) of the patient and other technical factors this means a dose of between 15 and 40 mL.

It is of vital importance in CEMRA that the acquisition is timed so that data is collected during the short time in which the bolus of contrast is present within the imaging volume. There are various strategies that can be used to ensure this. The most basic method is to give a test injection of 3 mL contrast while performing a dynamic scan through the region to be imaged. This must be done with good temporal resolution (i.e. scanning the same slice repeatedly and as quickly as possible). When the bolus has passed through the region, the workstation software can be used to draw a region of interest and an uptake curve to demonstrate the time taken for the bolus to reach the vessel required. If performing a hand injection, this data can be used to time the commencement of the acquisition in relation to the time of injection.

Various manufacturers have automated this process:

- *BolusTrak* from Philips Medical Systems allows the operator to visually monitor the region of interest using a real time scan. When the bolus is visualised the operator can then immediately commence the main scan sequence from the control panel
- *Care Bolus* from Siemens also allows visualisation of the bolus
- *SmartPrep* from GE uses a small 'tracker' slice situated within the imaging volume to monitor the signal level returned by the inflowing blood. The arrival of the bolus automatically begins the scan

The use of a syringe pump in conjunction with these strategies virtually eliminates human error, and gives a reproducibly robust method of imaging the vasculature.

Moving table-top studies allow the bolus to be chased into the extremities in much the same way as early iodine-enhanced radiographic arteriography.[23]

To sum up the main advantages of this technique:

- CEMRA is capable of imaging of in-plane flow (i.e. it is not restricted to perpendicular flow like inflow MRA)
- Because CEMRA can image in-plane flow, a wider field of view can be achieved in a short time frame. This is because, e.g. the aorta can be imaged using relatively few coronal slices whereas with inflow techniques it would require many axial slices
- Signal is not dependent upon flow (i.e. flow of any speed will yield high signal)

SUGGESTED MRI PROTOCOLS BY BODY AREA

The brain

MRI of the brain can be used to assess structure, pathology and brain function.

MRI of the brain has surpassed CT due to its superior sensitivity and soft tissue contrast, for example, MRI can detect demyelination even in early inflammatory lesions where CT studies have shown no abnormality.

The posterior fossa is well demonstrated on MRI images as MRI does not suffer from the beam hardening artefacts associated with CT scans of this region. Aneurysms and vascular anomalies may be demonstrated using flow-dependent imaging techniques that can demonstrate vasculature without the need for iodinated contrast media. This technique has the additional advantages that it is cheap, very quick to perform, has no risk of side-effects, uses no ionising radiation and is more comfortable for the patient.

The multiplanar capabilities of MRI mean that slices can be acquired in non-orthogonal angles. This allows imaging along structures such as the trigeminal nerve and optic nerve as well as allowing sagittal imaging of the pituitary fossa and coronal imaging of the hippocampus.

The functional capabilities of MRI are still being investigated and developed; functional magnetic resonance imaging (fMRI) is a technique that uses MR imaging to measure the metabolic changes that take place in the cortex of the brain during activation. The areas of the brain responsible for speech, sight, hearing and motor function can vary slightly between individuals. fMRI can be used to assess these areas prior to surgery allowing the resection of tumours without damaging nearby structures that are critical to the patient.

fMRI research is currently looking at applications in the fields of stroke, pain, and the seat of language and memory.

MRI does have some disadvantages in comparison with CT in that it has poorer geometric accuracy, particularly in open scanners and is much less able to assess bone structure. MRI is not ideal for the trauma patient because of projectile hazards from incomplete safety screening and attached monitors, etc. CT provides a more immediate solution and can assess bony head injury more readily.

Common indications
- Haemorrhage
- Infection
- Inflammatory processes/multiple sclerosis
- Ischaemia
- Neurodegenerative disease
- Seizures
- Tumours
- Vascular abnormalities

Equipment needed
Quadrature volume head coil

Routine protocol
The routine protocol may include the sequences shown in the following table and in Figures 41.14, 41.15 and 41.16.

	Weighting	Orientation	Pulse sequence
1	T1	Three planes	Gradient echo (localiser)
2	T1	Sagittal	Spin echo
3	Dual echo T2/PD	Axial/coronal	Fast spin echo

It is important to standardise the imaging planes used for every patient. This is because each individual will lie with the head tilted to a different extent (chin up or chin down). The sagittal localiser will allow the operator to use a common landmark for the prescription of all axial images. This can be along the hard palate or the line joining the anterior to posterior commissures. Slices should be positioned to cover the foramen magnum to vertex.

Additional sequences may be added to the protocol as follows.

Pathology of tumour or infection (Fig. 41.17)

	Weighting	Orientation	Pulse sequence
1	T1	Axial/sagittal/coronal	Spin echo
2	T1 plus gadolinium	Axial/sagittal/coronal	Spin echo

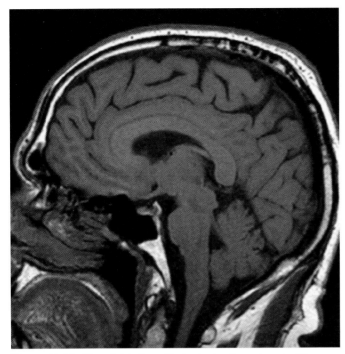

Figure 41.14 T1 weighted, sagittal – brain. Reproduced with permission from Philips Medical Systems

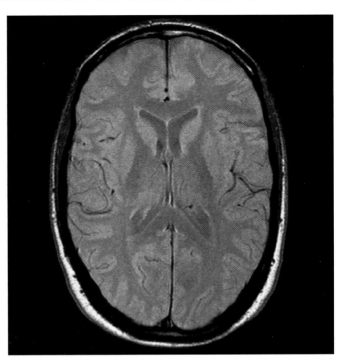

Figure 41.16 Proton density weighted spin echo, axial – brain. Reproduced with permission from Philips Medical Systems

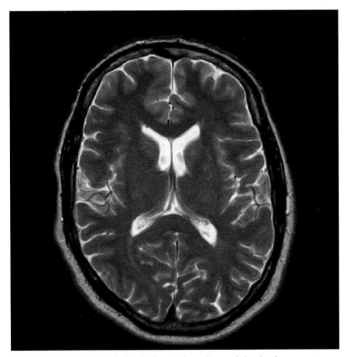

Figure 41.15 T2 weighted, fast spin echo, axial - brain. Reproduced with permission from Philips Medical Systems

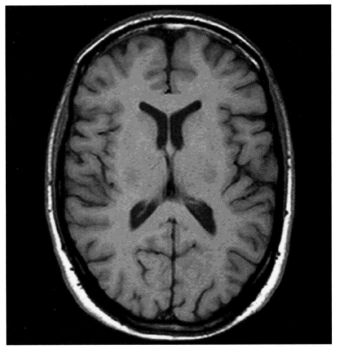

Figure 41.17 T1 weighted, spin echo, axial – brain. Reproduced with permission from Philips Medical Systems

T1-weighted images are used with positive contrast enhancement. Positive extracellular contrast media are able to cross any disruption of the blood–brain barrier. This results in the positive enhancement of brain tumours, infection and other lesions such as active multiple sclerosis plaques.

Multiple sclerosis

	Weighting	Orientation	Pulse sequence
1	STIR	Sagittal	Fast inversion recovery
2	FLAIR	Axial	Fast inversion recovery

Short tau inversion recovery gives a fat suppressed image with bright signal from fluid. Areas of demyelination contain proteinaceous fluid and therefore appear hyperintense. Sagittal imaging allows accurate assessment of the angle of orientation of these areas to the ventricles.

Fluid attenuated inversion recovery uses inversion recovery to suppress signal from the CSF in the ventricles but not the signal from proteinaceous fluid in areas of demyelination. This is useful in defining the extent of periventricular disease (Fig. 41.18).

Epilepsy (Figs 41.19, 41.20)

	Weighting	Orientation	Pulse sequence
1	T2	Coronal thin slices	Fast spin echo
2	T1	Coronal 3D volume	Gradient echo

High resolution T2-weighted scans orientated at 90° to the long axis of the temporal lobe can be useful in assessing hippocampal disease (sclerosis) and structure.

A 3D volume acquisition will allow the measurement of hippocampal volumes as there is no slice gap.

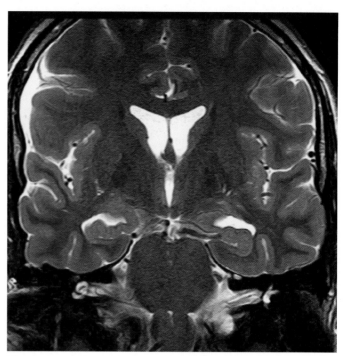

Figure 41.19 High resolution, T2 weighted, fast spin echo, coronal – brain. Reproduced with permission from Philips Medical Systems

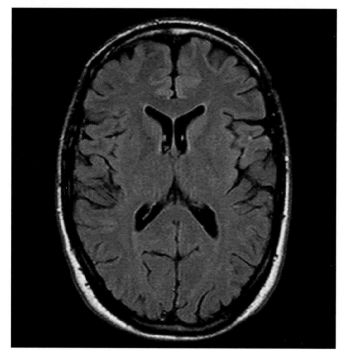

Figure 41.18 Fluid attenuated inversion recovery T2 weighted, axial – brain. Note that an inversion time has been selected to null signal from water so the ventricles appear hypointense despite the T2 weighting. Reproduced with permission from Philips Medical Systems

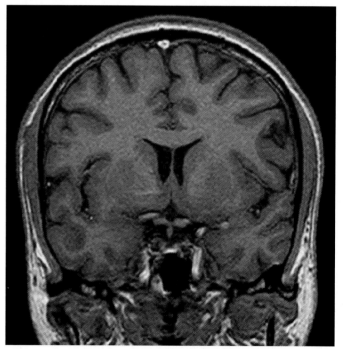

Figure 41.20 T1 weighted, incoherent gradient echo, 3D volume – brain. Reproduced with permission from Philips Medical Systems

Vascular abnormalities and presence of flow (Fig. 41.21)

	Vessels	Orientation	Pulse sequence
1	Arteries/aneurysms	Axial	3D time-of-flight
2	Veins	Sagittal oblique	2D time-of-flight
3	Veins	Axial	Phase contrast

3D time-of-flight gives a high resolution image having isotropic voxels. This allows MIPs having the same resolution along every axis. The field of view (slab thickness) is limited due to saturation effects.

2D time-of-flight can be acquired one slice at a time and therefore allows wider coverage than 3D. Individual slices are not thick enough to cause saturation of slow moving inflowing spins and therefore can be used for venography. Non-isotropic voxels result in lower resolution of the MIP images.

Phase contrast studies allow the encoding of flow in any direction, not just perpendicular flow. The velocity encoding gradient can be selected for arterial or venous flow (Figs 41.22, 41.23).

Assessment of the internal auditory meati (Fig. 41.24)

	Vessels	Orientation	Pulse sequence
1	T2	Axial thin slices	Fast spin echo

or

	Vessels	Orientation	Pulse sequence
1	T1 pre gadolinium	Axial/coronal thin slices	Spin echo
2	T1 post gadolinium	Axial/coronal thin slices	Spin echo

Thin slices 2–3 mm give high resolution images of the acoustic nerves to exclude acoustic neuroma, etc.

On low field systems or systems not having FSE capability it may be faster to use T1-weighted contrast enhanced images.

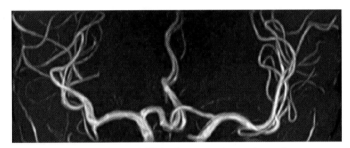

Figure 41.21   3D time-of-flight (post maximum intensity projection) – cerebral angiogram. Reproduced with permission from Philips Medical Systems

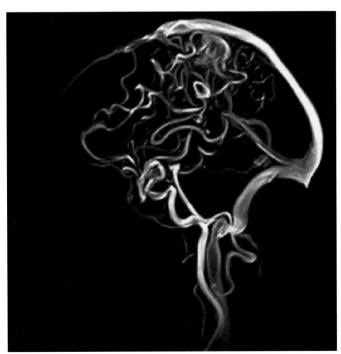

Figure 41.22   Phase contrast angiogram – cranial vessels. Reproduced with permission from Philips Medical Systems

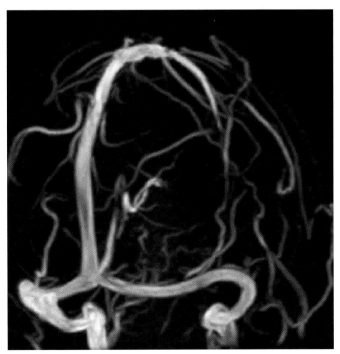

Figure 41.23   Phase contrast venography of the brain. Reproduced with permission from Philips Medical Systems

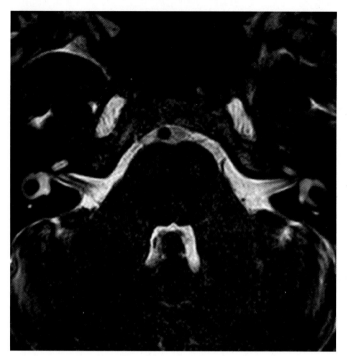

Figure 41.24   High resolution, T2 weighted, fast spin echo, axial – internal auditory meati. Reproduced with permission from Philips Medical Systems

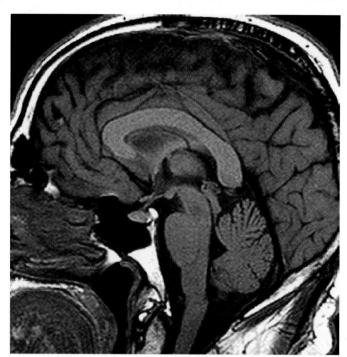

Figure 41.25   High resolution, T1 weighted, spin echo, sagittal – pituitary fossa. Reproduced with permission from Philips Medical Systems

Pituitary fossa (Figs 41.25, 41.26)

	Vessels	Orientation	Pulse sequence
1	T1 pre gadolinium	Sagittal/coronal thin slices	Spin echo
2	T1 post gadolinium	Sagittal/coronal thin slices	Spin echo

The absence of a blood–brain barrier in the pituitary gland and stalk results in homogeneous enhancement after gadolinium chelate injection. A focal hypointense area within the gland immediately after Gd-DTPA is abnormal and is the most common appearance of an adenoma.

Orbits (Figs 41.27, 41.28)

	Vessels	Orientation	Pulse sequence
1	STIR	Axial/coronal thin slices	Fast inversion recovery
2	T1 pre gadolinium	Axial/coronal thin slices	Spin echo
3	T1 post gadolinium	Axial/coronal thin slices	Spin echo

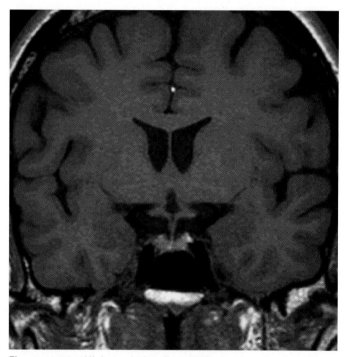

Figure 41.26   High resolution, T1 weighted, spin echo, coronal – pituitary fossa. Reproduced with permission from Philips Medical Systems

STIR saturates the signal from orbit fat improving contrast in assessing the optic nerves. If fat saturation is required on the T1-weighted images chemical fat saturation may be used. Note that this protocol may also be used in imaging the other cranial nerves.

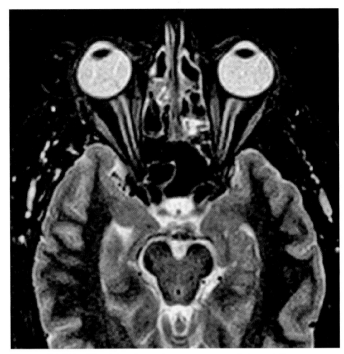

Figure 41.27 Short tau inversion recovery, axial – orbits. Reproduced with permission from Philips Medical Systems

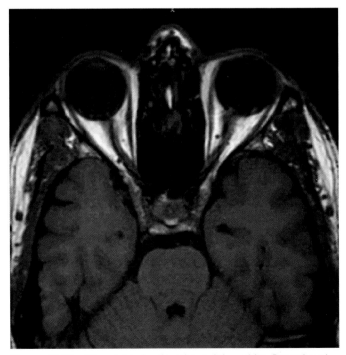

Figure 41.28 T1 weighted, spin echo, axial – orbits. Reproduced with permission from Philips Medical Systems

Spine

The spine is an anatomical area that is inherently suited to MRI. The area is inherently immobile, has good proton density and excellent contrast to noise ratio. Artefactual appearances can occur due to the movement of nearby structures such as the throat, anterior body wall, heart and bowel, but these can usually be reduced by using a saturation pulse. A saturation pulse is a user defined region that is subjected to additional RF pulses to saturate signal. If a region is not emitting signal then it cannot cause artefactual appearances on the image.

MRI is replacing conventional radiography of the spine in many cases because of the wealth of additional information it provides and because of its non-ionising nature.

Common indications
- Congenital abnormalities
- Cord atrophy
- Cord compression
- Degenerative disease
- Demyelination
- Disc disease (new and recurrent following surgery)
- Epidural fibrosis (following surgery)
- Haemorrhage
- Infarction
- Infection
- Metastatic disease
- Tumour
- Vascular malformations

The soft tissue capabilities of MRI make it particularly suited to the demonstration of congenital abnormalities such as chiari malformation, spina bifida, cord tethering, dysraphisms and diastematomyelia.

Changes in bone marrow are also well demonstrated and make MRI a useful tool in the assessment of metastatic disease. Bone marrow is usually of intermediate signal on T1 weighting because of its fat content. Metastatic infiltration has a higher water content and therefore reduces the signal in affected areas.

MRI has a unique sensitivity to demyelinating conditions, T2-weighted sagittal images of the cord are therefore valuable in demonstrating lesions of multiple sclerosis. CT rarely shows such lesions although areas may enhance on delayed scanning after a double dose of iodinated contrast media in advanced cases of disease.

Tumours are well demonstrated on MRI, usually causing a widening of the cord, high signal on T2 weighting and possible enhancement on T1-weighted images. There are several classifications of cord tumour that can be differentiated by close inspection of MRI images in many cases.

The contrast to noise ratio generated on T2 weighting between CSF and cord allows MRI to replace conventional myelography in most cases. Disc disease, cord compression and spinal stenosis will cause indentation of the theca.

Haemorrhage can be detected using gradient echo sequences due to increased susceptibility effects.

■ Cervical spine

Equipment needed
Volume neck coil, phased array spine coil

Routine protocol
The routine protocol may include the sequences shown in the following table and in Figures 41.29, 41.30, 41.31, 41.32 and 41.33.

	Weighting	Orientation	Pulse sequence
1	T1	Three planes	Gradient echo (localiser)
2	T2	Sagittal	Fast spin echo
3	T1	Sagittal	Spin echo
4	T2/T2*	Axial	Fast spin echo/gradient echo
5	T1	Axial	Spin echo

The coronal localiser will allow the operator to orientate the sagittal sections. The field of view should include the posterior fossa to the second thoracic vertebra. The sagittal localiser allows the operator to prescribe the axial slices. Axial slices should cover the intervertebral discs.

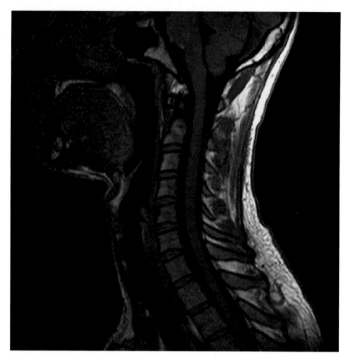

Figure 41.30 T1 weighted, spin echo, sagittal – cervical spine. Reproduced with permission from Philips Medical Systems

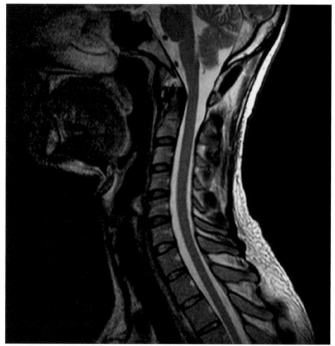

Figure 41.29 T2 weighted, fast spin echo, sagittal – cervical spine. Reproduced with permission from Philips Medical Systems

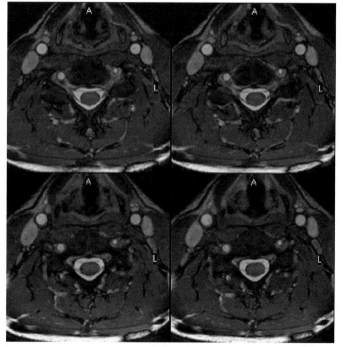

Figure 41.31 T2* weighted, gradient echo, axial – cervical spine. Reproduced with permission from Philips Medical Systems

Additional sequences may be added to the protocol as follows.

Syringomyelia or tumour (Fig. 41.34)

	Weighting	Orientation	Pulse sequence
1	T1 post gadolinium	Sagittal	Spin echo
2	T1 pre/post gadolinium	Axial	Spin echo
3	Short tau inversion recovery	Sagittal	Fast inversion recovery

T1 weighting is used with positive contrast enhancement. STIR images are useful to demonstrate intrinsic signal change within the cord and bone marrow. In cases of syringomyelia, the full length of the lesion must be demonstrated. This may include separate scans of the thoracic and lumbar regions.

Brachial plexus

	Weighting	Orientation	Pulse sequence
1	T2	Coronal	Fast spin echo
2	T1	Coronal	Spin echo
3	T2/PD dual echo	Axial	Fast spin echo

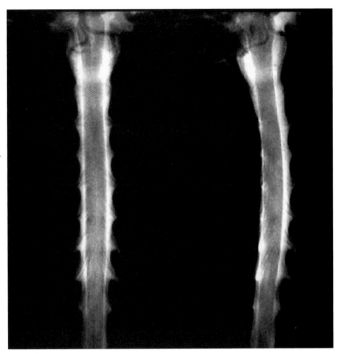

Figure 41.33 Long T2-weighted 'myelographic' maximum intensity projection, cervical spine. Reproduced with permission from Philips Medical Systems

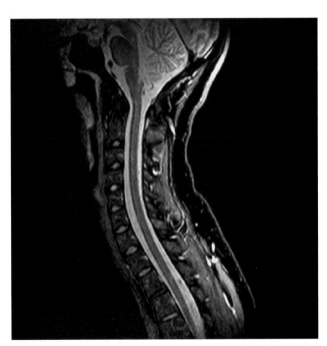

Figure 41.34 Short tau inversion recovery, sagittal – cervical spine. Reproduced with permission from Philips Medical Systems

Slices prescribed from the angle of the mandible to the lung apices. Coronal sections are not usually very useful in routine spine imaging but are very useful when looking for lesions such as neurofibroma. The coronal plane demonstrates the classic dumbbell shape of the lesion that may not be appreciated on sagittal views.

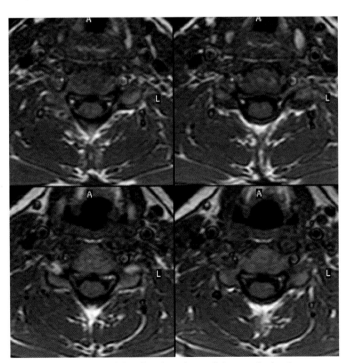

Figure 41.32 T1 weighted, spin echo, axial – cervical spine. Reproduced with permission from Philips Medical Systems

◼ Thoracic spine

Equipment needed
Phased array spine coil

Routine protocol
The routine protocol may include the sequences shown in the following table and in Figures 41.35 and 41.36.

	Weighting	Orientation	Pulse sequence
1	T1	Three planes	Gradient echo (localiser)
2	T2	Sagittal	Fast spin echo
3	T1	Sagittal	Spin echo
4	T2/T2*	Axial	Fast spin echo/gradient echo
5	T1	Axial	Spin echo

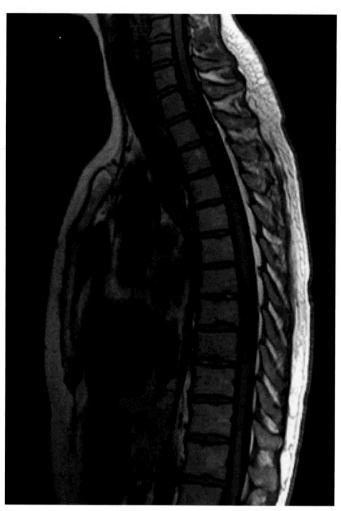

Figure 41.36 T1 weighted, spin echo, sagittal – thoracic spine. Reproduced with permission from Philips Medical Systems

The coronal localiser will allow the operator to orientate the sagittal sections. The field of view should include the seventh cervical vertebra to the first lumbar vertebra. Identification of vertebral level can be facilitated by including the second cervical vertebra on at least one sequence (such as the localiser). The sagittal localiser allows the operator to prescribe the axial slices. Axial slices should cover any relevant intervertebral discs.

Additional sequences may be added to the protocol as follows.

Syringomyelia or tumour

	Weighting	Orientation	Pulse sequence
1	T1 post gadolinium	Sagittal	Spin echo
2	T1 pre/post gadolinium	Axial	Spin echo
3	Short tau inversion recovery	Sagittal	Fast inversion recovery

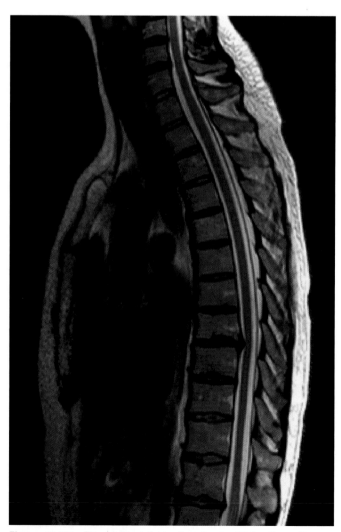

Figure 41.35 T2 weighted, fast spin echo, sagittal – thoracic spine. Reproduced with permission from Philips Medical Systems

T1 weighting is used with positive contrast enhancement. STIR images are useful to demonstrate intrinsic signal change within the cord and bone marrow. In cases of syringomyelia, the full length of the lesion must be demonstrated. This may include separate scans of the cervical and lumbar regions.

Scoliosis

	Weighting	Orientation	Pulse sequence
1	T1	Coronal	Spin echo

Scoliosis causes the spine to curve out of the sagittal plane and therefore a coronal data set will provide better coverage and more readily understandable anatomical information.

■ Lumbar–sacral spine

Equipment needed
Phased array spine coil

Routine protocol
The routine protocol may include the sequences shown in the following table and in Figures 41.37, 41.38 and 41.39.

	Weighting	Orientation	Pulse sequence
1	T1	Three planes	Gradient echo (localiser)
2	T2 or STIR	Sagittal	Fast spin echo or fast inversion recovery
3	T1	Sagittal	Spin echo
4	T2	Axial	Fast spin echo
5	T1	Axial	Spin echo

The coronal localiser will allow the operator to orientate the sagittal sections. The field of view should include the 12th thoracic vertebra to the tip of the coccyx. The sagittal localiser allows the operator to prescribe the axial slices. Axial slices should cover any relevant intervertebral discs.

STIR may be used instead of T2 sagittal images, particularly if the examination is limited replacement for radiographic evaluation. STIR is often described as a 'search and destroy' sequence due to its sensitivity to pathology.

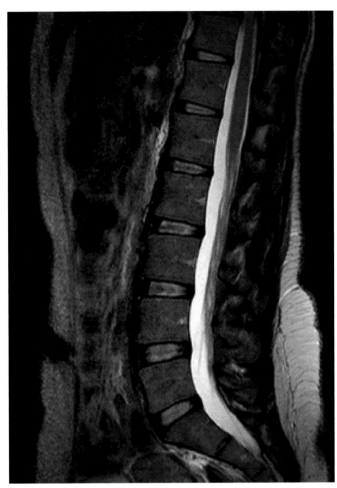

Figure 41.37 T2 weighted, fast spin echo, sagittal – lumbar sacral spine. Reproduced with permission from Philips Medical Systems

Additional sequences may be added to the protocol as follows:

Syringomyelia or tumour

	Weighting	Orientation	Pulse sequence
1	T1 post gadolinium	Sagittal	Spin echo
2	T1 pre/post gadolinium	Axial	Spin echo
3	Short tau inversion recovery	Sagittal	Fast inversion recovery

T1 weighting is used with positive contrast enhancement. STIR images are useful to demonstrate intrinsic signal change within the cord and bone marrow. In cases of syringomyelia, the full length of the lesion must be demonstrated. This may include separate scans of the cervical and thoracic regions.

Figure 41.38 T1 weighted, spin echo, sagittal – lumbar sacral spine. Reproduced with permission from Philips Medical Systems

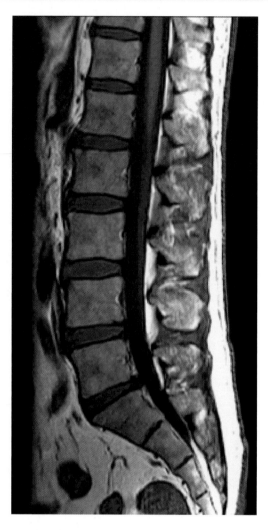

Musculoskeletal system

MRI has an important role in the diagnosis and treatment of musculoskeletal disorders. MRI accurately depicts soft tissue injuries such as muscle, ligament and meniscal tears as well as cartilage and bone injuries. Muscle has an intermediate to slightly long T1 relaxation time and short T2 relaxation time. It appears relatively hypointense on both T1 and T2-weighted sequences, particularly FSE T2.

The fat planes allow identification of individual muscles due to fat's hyperintensity on T1 weighting. Injured muscles have associated oedema and haemorrhage, which cause prolongation of the T1 and T2 relaxation times of the injured tissue so T2-weighted images with fat saturation (or STIR images) demonstrate tears. Water-bearing oedematous tissue is hyperintense in comparison to the relatively hypointense muscle and saturated signal of fat.

T1-weighted imaging may be useful in providing information about haemorrhage, which has changing intensity with time, due to the altering state of the haemoglobin component (oxyhaemoglobin, deoxyhaemoglobin, intracellular methaemoglobin, extracellular methaemoglobin and haemosiderin).

This knowledge is invaluable in formulating the optimum treatment plan for a patient. The sensitivity of MRI is such that it can detect injuries, such as rotator cuff tendonitis and bone bruising. These injuries are ideally treated conservatively so an MRI scan can spare the patient unnecessary surgery. MRI is also an ideal modality to diagnose bone and soft tissue tumours, infection, and avascular necrosis of bone.

MRI studies may now also include MR arthrography. This technique involves the injection of a dilute solution of gadolinium chelate into the joint capsule (1 in 100 dilution). This is followed by T1 fat saturated images. The joint capsule is distended by the high signal gadolinium and allows better visualisation of the intraarticular structures.

Conventional radiography is still the first line technique for the trauma patient in detecting fractures and dislocations of bone, but has limited soft tissue capability. CT still has an important place in musculoskeletal imaging due to its ability to demonstrate bone, occult fractures, complex fractures and bone healing. RNI can detect occult fractures and metastatic disease. All of these techniques involve ionising radiation.

Ultrasound is ideally suited to the demonstration of soft tissue injury in the musculoskeletal system. Its other advantages include easy accessibility, portability, quick scan time, and high patient tolerance. The dynamic nature of

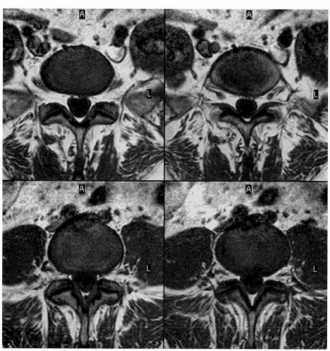

Figure 41.39 T1 weighted, spin echo, axial – lumbar spine. Reproduced with permission from Philips Medical Systems

ultrasound can result in a more directed examination, specific to the individual case being scanned. The disadvantages of ultrasound include the fact that it is highly operator dependent, and considerable experience and training is required to perform consistent, high quality studies.

Shoulder

The shoulder joint allows a wide range of movement at the cost of having a shallow socket. It is therefore susceptible to a range of soft tissue injury involving the ligaments and tendons of the rotator cuff.

Common indications
• Rotator cuff disease
• Labral injury
• Biceps tendon disruption

Equipment needed
Dedicated phased array shoulder coil, surface coil or wrap around coil

Routine protocol
The routine protocol may include the sequences shown in the following table and in Figures 41.40, 41.41 and 41.42.

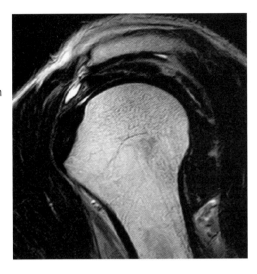

Figure 41.40
T2 weighted, fast spin echo, sagittal – shoulder joint. Reproduced with permission from Philips Medical Systems

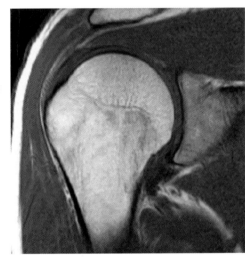

Figure 41.41
T1 weighted, spin echo, coronal – shoulder joint. Reproduced with permission from Philips Medical Systems

	Weighting	Orientation	Pulse sequence
1	T1	Three planes	Gradient echo (Localiser)
2	T2/proton density dual echo	Sagittal	Fast spin echo
3	T1	Coronal	Spin echo
4	Proton density, fat saturation	Coronal	Fast spin echo/ gradient echo
5	T2*	Axial	Gradient echo
6	T1	Axial	Spin echo

The axial localiser will allow the operator to orientate the coronal sections parallel to the supraspinatus muscle. The field of view should include the entire joint and rotator cuff.

The parasagittal sections may be prescribed from the paracoronal data to ensure perpendicular orientation. MR arthrography may be performed in examinations of the shoulder joint.

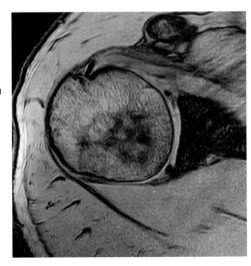

Figure 41.42
T2* weighted, gradient echo, axial – shoulder joint. Reproduced with permission from Philips Medical Systems

Elbow

The elbow is a very stable joint, however, elbow dislocations and fractures are common.

Complex elbow injuries involve related fractures and/or neurovascular injuries. MRI is not particularly useful in acute trauma where conventional radiography can be used to assess bony injury. In the subacute setting, however, MRI is invaluable in assessing soft tissue damage.

From a practical viewpoint the elbow can be difficult to image due to its lateral position. Comfortable patient positioning is therefore of high importance.

Common indications
- Ligament and tendon injury
- Articular cartilage injury
- Occult fractures
- Assessment of neurovascular structures

Equipment needed
Dedicated phased array elbow (extremity) coil, surface coil or wrap around coil

Routine protocol
The routine protocol may include the sequences shown in the following table and in Figures 41.43, 41.44 and 41.45.

	Weighting	Orientation	Pulse sequence
1	T1	Three planes	Gradient echo (localiser)
2	T1	Sagittal, thin slices	Spin echo
3	T1	Coronal, thin slices	Spin echo
4	T1	Axial, thin slices	Spin echo
5	T2, fat saturation	Axial, thin slices	Fast spin echo
6	T2, fat saturation	Coronal, thin slices	Fast spin echo
7	T2*	Sagittal 3D volume	Gradient echo

The axial localiser will allow the operator to orientate the sagittal and coronal sections. The field of view should include the entire joint, the distal humerus and the proximal radius and ulna.

MR arthrography may be performed in examinations of the elbow joint.

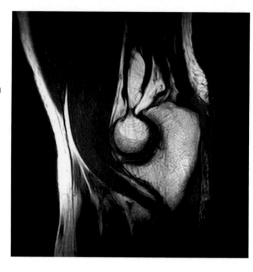

Figure 41.43
T1 weighted, spin echo, sagittal – elbow joint.
Reproduced with permission from Philips Medical Systems

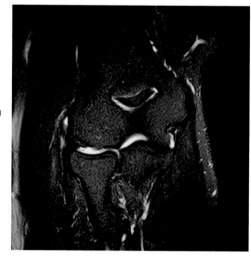

Figure 41.44
T2 weighted, fast spin echo with fat saturation, coronal – elbow joint.
Reproduced with permission from Philips Medical Systems

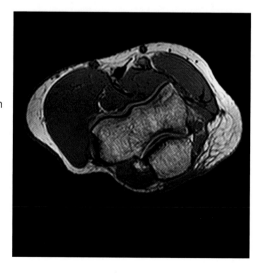

Figure 41.45
T1 weighted, incoherent gradient echo, axial – elbow joint.
Reproduced with permission from Philips Medical Systems

Wrist

In the wrist, dislocations and fractures are common.

MRI is not particularly useful in acute trauma where conventional radiography can be used to assess bony injury. In the subacute setting, however, MRI is invaluable in assessing soft tissue damage and instability due to ligament damage. As an anatomical area, the wrist is not particularly amenable to MRI. Bone and ligaments have low proton density and there is a fair amount of flow from veins and arteries.

Common indications
- Ganglia
- Carpal tunnel syndrome
- Occult fractures
- Assessment of ligaments
- General pain/repetitive strain injury

Equipment needed
Dedicated phased array wrist (extremity) coil, surface coil or wrap around coil

Routine protocol
The routine protocol may include the sequences shown in the following table and in Figures 41.46, 41.47 and 41.48.

	Weighting	Orientation	Pulse sequence
1	T1	Three planes	Gradient echo (localiser)
2	T1	Coronal, thin slices	Spin echo
3	T2*	Coronal 3D volume	Gradient echo
4	Proton density, fat saturation	Coronal, thin slices	Fast spin echo
5	Dual echo T2/ proton density	Axial, thin slices	Fast spin echo
6	Short tau inversion recovery	Coronal, thin slices	Fast inversion recovery

The sagittal localiser will allow the operator to orientate the coronal and axial sections. The field of view should include the entire joint, carpal bones and distal ulna and radius.

MR arthrography may be performed in examinations of the wrist joint.

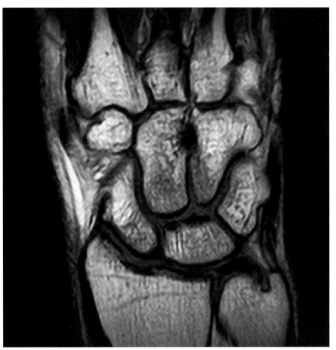

Figure 41.46 T1 weighted, spin echo, coronal – wrist joint. Reproduced with permission from Philips Medical Systems

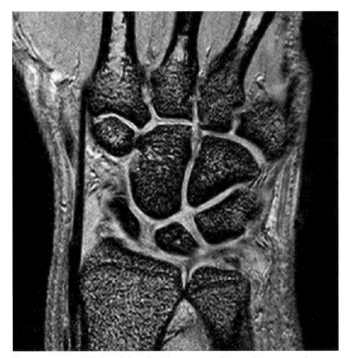

Figure 41.47 T2* weighted, coherent gradient echo, coronal – wrist joint. Reproduced with permission from Philips Medical Systems

Hip

Hip pain is a very common clinical problem and can have a wide number of causes, some musculoskeletal and some not related to the joint itself (e.g. sciatica, hernia or aneurysm).

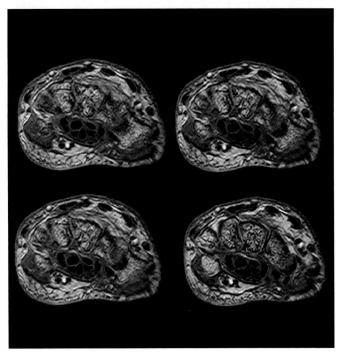

Figure 41.48   T2* weighted, coherent gradient echo 3D volume – wrist joint. Reproduced with permission from Philips Medical Systems

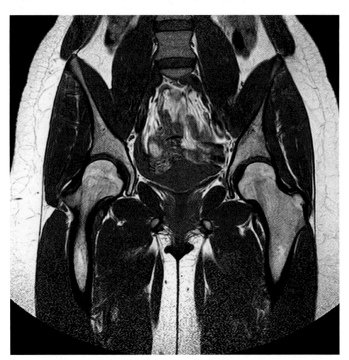

Figure 41.49   T1 weighted, coronal – hip joints. Reproduced with permission from Philips Medical Systems

As an anatomical area the hip is very amenable to MRI as it has a high proton density and is easily immobilised.

Common indications
- Avascular necrosis
- Bone marrow disorders
- Occult fractures
- Neoplasm
- Osteomyelitis

Equipment needed
Phased array torso coil

Routine protocol
The routine protocol may be bilateral or unilateral (having a reduced field of view). It may include the sequences shown in the following table and in Figures 41.49 and 41.50.

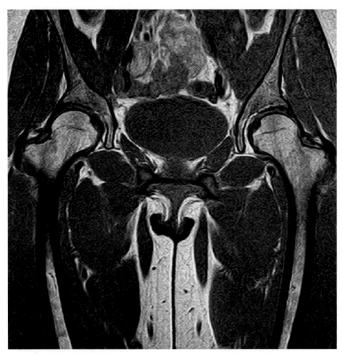

Figure 41.50   Proton density weighted, coronal – hip joints. Reproduced with permission from Philips Medical Systems

The field of view should cover the area from above the acetabulum to below the lesser trochanter.

▮ Knee

The knee joint is the most commonly imaged joint in the body. Plain radiography of the knee is of little value

	Weighting	Orientation	Pulse sequence
1	T1	Three planes	Gradient echo (localiser)
2	T1	Coronal	Spin echo
3	Proton density	Coronal	Fast spin echo
4	Dual echo T2/ proton density	Axial	Fast spin echo
5	T2*	Axial, thin slices	Gradient echo

unless there has been a direct trauma to the joint causing bone fracture. MRI can accurately demonstrate the soft tissue structures of the knee and detect quite subtle damage to these components.

Common indications
- Arthritis
- Bone bruising (trabecular microfracture)
- Cartilage injury chondromalacia
- Cruciate ligament damage
- Evaluation of knee pain
- Infection
- Neoplasm
- Patellar disorders/maltracking

Equipment needed
Quadrature volume knee coil

Routine protocol
The routine protocol may include the sequences shown in the following table and in Figures 41.51, 41.52, 41.53, 41.54, 41.55 and 41.56.

	Weighting	Orientation	Pulse sequence
1	T1	Three planes	Gradient echo (localiser)
2	Proton density	Sagittal	Spin echo
3	T1	Sagittal	Spin echo
4	Proton density	Coronal	Fast spin echo
5	T2	Axial	Fast spin echo
6	T2*	Sagittal/volume	Coherent gradient echo

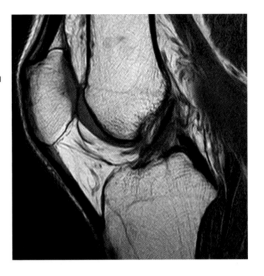

Figure 41.52
T1 weighted, sagittal – knee joint. Reproduced with permission from Philips Medical Systems

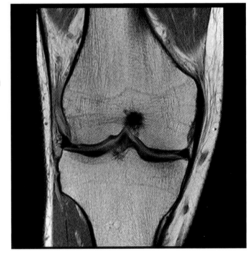

Figure 41.53
Proton density weighted, coronal – knee joint. Reproduced with permission from Philips Medical Systems

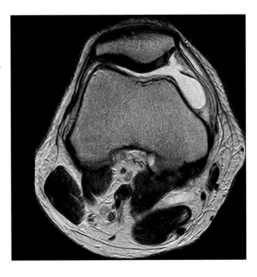

Figure 41.54
T2 weighted, fast spin echo, axial – knee joint. Reproduced with permission from Philips Medical Systems

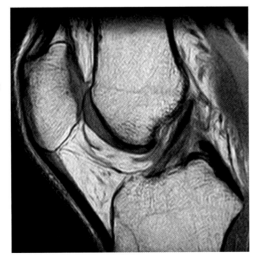

Figure 41.51
Proton density weighted, sagittal – knee joint. Reproduced with permission from Philips Medical Systems

The field of view should cover the entire joint and should include the skin surfaces laterally and medially.

Figure 41.55
T2* weighted,
coherent
gradient echo,
sagittal –
knee joint.
Reproduced with
permission from
Philips Medical
Systems

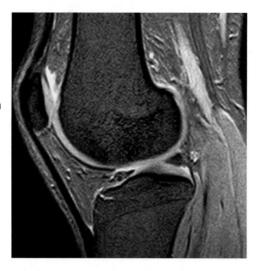

Figure 41.56
Short tau
inversion
recovery, sagittal
– knee joint.
Reproduced with
permission from
Philips Medical
Systems

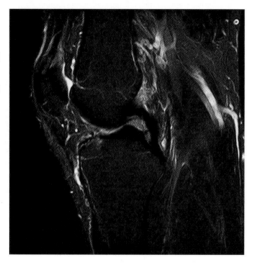

Routine protocol

The routine protocol may include the sequences shown in the following table and in Figures 41.57 and 41.58.

	Weighting	Orientation	Pulse sequence
1	T1	Three planes	Gradient echo (localiser)
2	T1	Coronal	Spin echo
3	Short tau inversion recovery	Coronal	Fast inversion recovery
4	T1	Sagittal	Spin echo
5	T2	Sagittal	Fast spin echo
6	Short tau inversion recovery	Sagittal	Fast inversion recovery
7	Dual echo proton density/T2	Axial	Fast spin echo

ABDOMEN

The commonly imaged areas in abdominal MRI include the liver, the pancreas, the kidneys and adrenal glands and the reproductive system. With the advent of new hardware and pulse sequences the trend seems to be towards breath hold and free breathing scans. T2 weighting can be achieved using single shot FSE, T1 weighting by gradient echo.

Ankle

Plain X-rays of the ankle are of use when ruling out fracture or joint instability.

MRI can demonstrate the soft tissue components of the joint.

MR arthrography can be performed in the ankle joint to demonstrate ligament tears and intraarticular lesions.

Common indications
- Arthritis
- Bone bruising (trabecular microfracture)
- Cartilage injury chondromalacia
- Ligament damage
- Infection
- Neoplasm

Equipment needed
Phased array extremity coil or knee coil

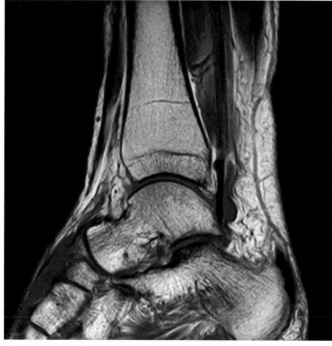

Figure 41.57   T1 weighted, sagittal – ankle joint. Reproduced with permission from Philips Medical Systems

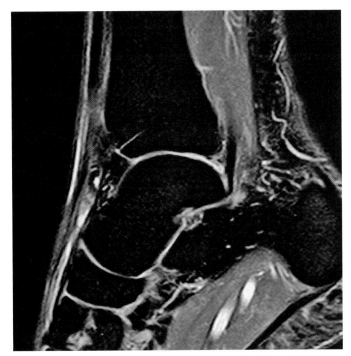

Figure 41.58 Short tau inversion recovery, sagittal – ankle joint. Reproduced with permission from Philips Medical Systems

Liver

Liver MRI is commonly used for the detection and characterisation of focal liver lesions, especially tumours. On a T1-weighted sequence the signal intensity of normal liver is greater than muscle or spleen, less than subcutaneous fat and approximately the same as the pancreas. On T2-weighted sequences normal liver tissue is of relatively low signal due to short T2 relaxation time and is less intense than spleen. Focal lesions in the liver generally enhance following administration of gadolinium Gd-DTPA. Because the liver is a common site for metastatic disease, the imaging of metastases is a very common indication for liver MRI. Metastases generally appear at a lower signal intensity than normal liver tissue on T1-weighted images but due to the presence of oedema they are usually hyperintense on T2-weighted sequences. They can also have haemorrhagic components which appear as inhomogeneous areas at varying intensities depending upon the age of haemorrhage and the weighting used. Super paramagnetic iron oxide agents can be used to enhance the contrast to noise ratio between metastases and healthy tissue in T2-weighted imaging. Iron oxide nanospheres are not phagocytosed by malignant cells and therefore cause the metastases to maintain their signal intensity whereas the healthy liver tissue decreases dramatically in signal intensity.

Common indications
- Characterisation of benign/malignant lesions
- Assessment of diffuse liver disease, e.g. fatty liver, haemochromatosis
- Visualisation of biliary tree in obstructive jaundice

Equipment needed
Phased array torso coil
Respiratory compensation/triggering

Routine protocol
The routine protocol may include the sequences shown in the following table and in Figures 41.59, 41.60 and 41.61.

	Weighting	Orientation	Pulse sequence
1	T1	Three planes	Gradient echo (localiser)
2	T1 pre gadolinium	Axial, breath holding	Incoherent gradient echo
3	T1 dynamic post gadolinium	Axial, breath holding	Incoherent gradient echo
4	T2	Axial, breath holding	Single shot fast spin echo*
5	T2 post SPIO contrast	Axial, breath holding	Single shot fast spin echo*
6	T1	Axial/coronal breath holding	Gradient echo
7	T2	Axial/coronal free breathing	Single shot fast spin echo*
8	T1 fat and water in phase	Axial	Gradient echo
9	T1 fat and water out of phase	Axial	Gradient echo

*If single shot is not available/preferred, FSE with respiratory gating may be utilised.

Free breathing single shot FSE is usually performed with respiratory gating to ensure that each slice is acquired at the same point in the respiratory cycle.

In and out-of-phase imaging can help to diagnose fatty liver as voxels containing fat and water will decrease in signal intensity on the out-of-phase image (Fig. 41.61).

Many liver lesions look similar pre contrast and can look similar at different timings following injection. Dynamic scanning can help to differentiate between these lesions. Dynamic contrast enhanced studies are performed following positive contrast agent injection, typically in the arterial, portal, venous and delayed phases. Fat satura-

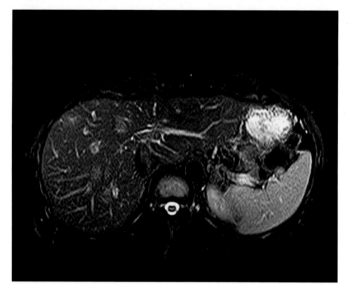

Figure 41.59   T2 weighted, single shot – liver (patient free breathing). Reproduced with permission from Philips Medical Systems

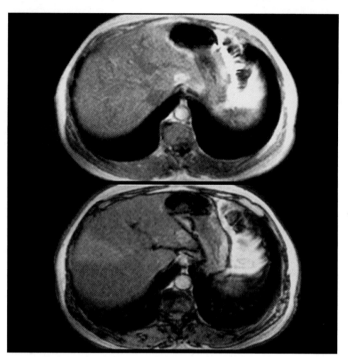

Figure 41.61   In and out-of-phase imaging in the liver. Reproduced with permission from Philips Medical Systems

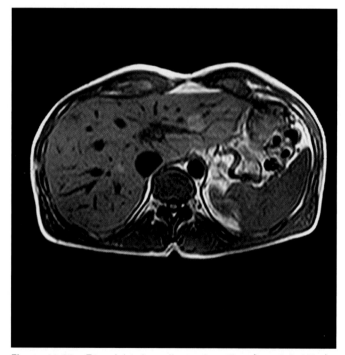

Figure 41.60   T1 weighted, gradient echo – liver (breath holding). Reproduced with permission from Philips Medical Systems

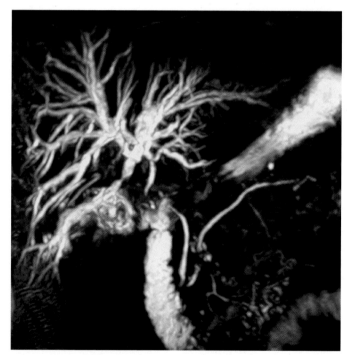

Figure 41.62   Heavy T2 weighting and maximum intensity projection – biliary tree. Reproduced with permission from Philips Medical Systems

tion may be used following contrast injection to help improve the contrast to noise ratio.

Dual echo sequences, because they have long echo times, may be useful in characterising haemangiomas as they remain hyperintense on late echoes.

The biliary tree may be imaged using T2-weighted sequences having very long echo times (Fig. 41.62). This provides an image resembling an endoscopic retrograde cholangiopancreatogram, but without the need for any

intervention or contrast media. A very long echo time results in a scan where only water spins are still in phase. The data can also be post processed using MIP to give multiprojectional images.

Pancreas

The pancreas can be seen on a Tl weighted image as a medium-signal-intensity structure, with an intensity similar to that of the liver, surrounded by hyperintense fat. With increased age the homogeneity of the pancreas decreases due to parenchymal atrophy. The margins of the gland may be smooth or lobulated and the pancreatic duct is shown as a low-signal-intensity structure on Tl weighted images. Narrow slice thickness is required to show the duct as it is less than 2 mm across. Fat suppression imaging leaves the pancreas as a homogenous high-signal structure which has a greater signal intensity than any of the surrounding structures. The pancreatic duct may also be demonstrated on magnetic resonance cholangiopancreatogram (MRCP).

Common indications
• Evaluation of pancreatitis
• Neoplasms
• Trauma

Equipment needed
Phased array torso coil
Respiratory compensation/triggering

Routine protocol
The routine protocol may include the sequences shown in the following table and in Figure 41.63.

	Weighting	Orientation	Pulse sequence
1	T1	Three planes	Gradient echo (localiser)
2	T1 (+/- fat saturation)	Axial, breath holding	Incoherent gradient echo
3	T1	Axial, respiratory compensation	Spin echo
4	T2	Axial, breath holding	Single shot fast spin echo*
5	T1 fat and water in phase	Axial	Gradient echo
6	T1 fat and water out of phase	Axial	Gradient echo

*If single shot is not available/preferred, FSE with respiratory gating may be utilised.

On T1-weighted images, the normal pancreas has higher signal intensity than any other abdominal organ.

Fat-saturated T1-weighted sequences are useful for distinguishing normal from abnormal pancreatic parenchyma because distracting bright signal from intraabdominal fat is removed. For patients unable to hold their breath, respiratory compensated spin echo sequences may be performed.

Breath holding, in and out-of-phase, T1-weighted gradient echo images display similar anatomical information as spin echo sequences but with the additional bonus of signal suppression due to fat and water phase opposition. This technique, which is also used in the liver, can help in distinguishing between some common lesions and tumours in this anatomical area. These include adenoma (in the adrenal area), focal fatty change in the pancreas and renal cell carcinoma metastasis in the pancreas.[24,25,26,27,28,29]

Kidneys

The diagnosis of malignant renal masses requires visualisation of the mass and usually positive enhancement with gadolinium based contrast media. Typically, T1-weighted gradient echo sequences are used.

For renal transplant assessment, T2-weighted sequences and contrast-enhanced 3D gradient echo sequences give anatomical information about causes of graft dysfunction. These may be supplemented by dynamic contrast renography and MRA.

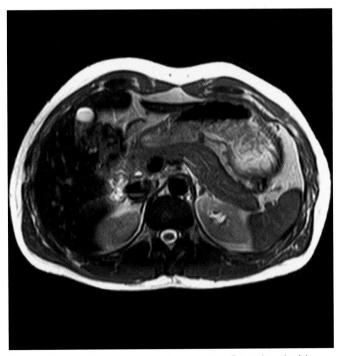

Figure 41.63   T2 weighted, axial – pancreas. Reproduced with permission from Philips Medical Systems

Common indications
- Adrenal gland assessment
- Neoplasms
- Renal transplant

Equipment needed
Phased array torso coil
Respiratory compensation/gating

Routine protocol
The routine protocol may include the sequences shown in the following table and in Figures 41.64, 41.65 and 41.66.

	Weighting	Orientation	Pulse sequence
1	T1	Three planes	Gradient echo (localiser)
2	T1	Coronal	Spin echo (respiratory comp)
3	T1	Axial	Spin echo (respiratory comp)
4	T2	Axial, breath holding	Single shot fast spin echo*
5	T1 fat and water in phase	Axial	Gradient echo
6	T1 fat and water out of phase	Axial	Gradient echo

*If single shot is not available/preferred, FSE with respiratory gating may be utilised.

If renal angiography is needed (Fig. 41.67)

	Weighting	Orientation	Pulse sequence
1	T1	Coronal 3D volume	Incoherent gradient echo

■ Pelvis

The pelvis presents an ideal area for MRI imaging. It has a high proton density, good inherent contrast to noise ratio and is easily immobilised using compression.

Common indications
- Anal fistulae
- Assessment of prostate gland (male)
- Fibroids (female)
- Location of undescended testis (male)
- Neoplasms (prostate, cervix, uterus, ovaries, bladder, rectum

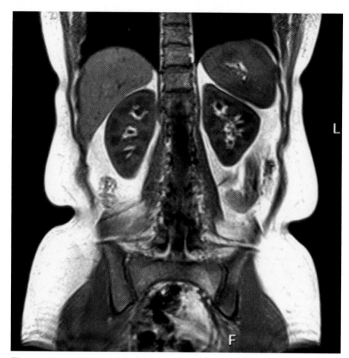

Figure 41.64 T1 weighted, coronal – kidneys. Reproduced with permission from Philips Medical Systems

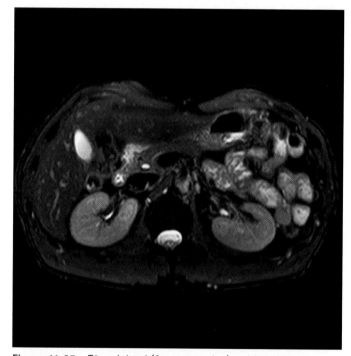

Figure 41.65 T2 weighted (fat suppression), axial – kidneys. Reproduced with permission from Philips Medical Systems

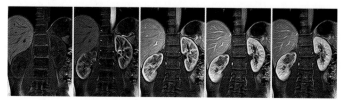

Figure 41.66 T1-weighted dynamic study, coronal – kidneys. Reproduced with permission from Philips Medical Systems

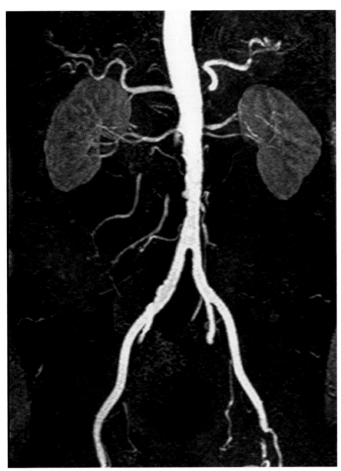

Figure 41.67 Renal contrast enhanced MRA. Reproduced with permission from Philips Medical Systems

Equipment needed
Phased array torso coil, compression band

Routine protocol
The routine protocol may include the sequences shown in the following table and in Figures 41.68, 41.69 and 41.70.

	Weighting	Orientation	Pulse sequence
1	T1	Three planes	Gradient echo (localiser)
2	T1	Axial	Spin echo
3	T2	Axial	Single shot fast spin echo*
4	T2	Coronal	Single shot fast spin echo*
5	T2	Sagittal	Single shot fast spin echo*

*If single shot is not available/preferred, FSE with respiratory gating may be utilised.

For anal fistulae

	Weighting	Orientation	Pulse sequence
1	T2 (fat suppressed)	Coronal	Fast spin echo
2	T2 (fat suppressed)	Sagittal	Fast spin echo
3	T2 (fat suppressed)	Axial	Fast spin echo

Short tau inversion recovery may be used instead of fast spin echo.

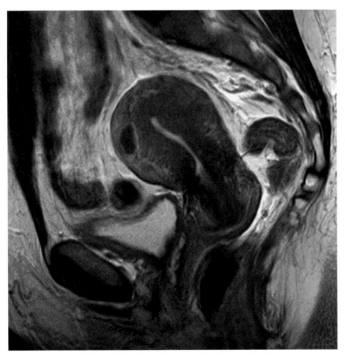

Figure 41.68 T2 weighted, sagittal – female pelvis. Reproduced with permission from Philips Medical Systems

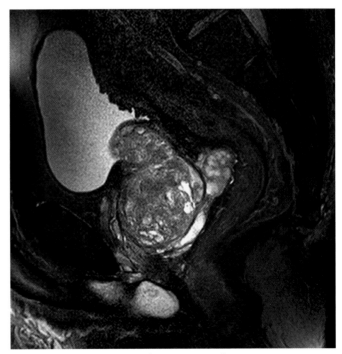

Figure 41.69 T2 weighted (fat suppression), sagittal – male pelvis. Reproduced with permission from Philips Medical Systems

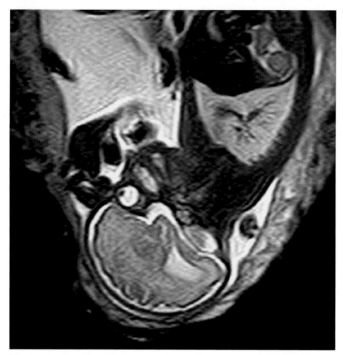

Figure 41.70 T2 weighted, sagittal - fetus. Reproduced with permission from Philips Medical Systems

CONCLUSION

It must be said that it is difficult to do justice to the modality of MRI in a single chapter. I hope that the reader will excuse a certain amount of oversimplification and omission, but this has been necessary to give a reasonable flavour of the modality in a limited number of words.

Acknowledgements
I would like to thank the following for their help in producing this work: Professor Sir Peter Mansfield for historical data and published papers, Dr Graham Plant for proof reading, Gillian Phillips for practical advice on current protocols, Philips Medical Systems.

References

1. Wosik J, et al. Institute for Space Systems Operations: Annual Report 2001. http://www.isso.uh.edu/publications/A2001/112-wosik.htm
2. http://nobelprize.org/physics/laureates/1944/
3. Wakefield J. The 'Indomitable' MRI. Smithsonian magazine. June 2000. http://www.smithsonianmag.com/smithsonian/issues00/jun00/object_jun00.html
4. Damadian R. Tumor detection by nuclear magnetic resonance. Science 1971; 171(976):1151–1153.
5. Lauterbur P. Image formation by induced local interaction; examples employing magnetic resonance. Nature 1973; 242(5394):190–191.
6. Garroway P, et al. Image formation in NMR by a selective irradiative process. Journal of Physics C (solid state physics) 1974; 7:457.
7. Mansfield P, Maudsley A. Medical imaging by NMR. British Journal of Radiology 1977; 50:188.
8. Damadian R, et al. FONAR image of the live human body. Physiological Chemistry and Physics 1977; (9):97–100.
9. Mansfield P, Maudsley A. Planar spin imaging by NMR. Journal of Physics C (solid state physics) 1976; 9:L409–411.
10. Mansfield P, Maudsley A. Line scan proton spin imaging in biological structures by NMR. Physics in Medicine and Biology 1976; 21:847–852.
11. Mansfield P. Multi-planar image formation using NMR spin echoes. Journal of Physics C (solid state physics) 1977; 10(3):L55–L58.
12. Lauterbur P, et al. Augmentation of tissue water proton spin-lattice relaxation rates by in vivo addition of paramagnetic ions. In: Dutton P, et al, eds. Frontiers of biological energetics. New York: Academic Press; 1978:752–759.
13. Ordidge R, et al. Rapid biomedical imaging by NMR. British Journal of Radiology 1981; 54:850–855.
14. http://www.fonar.com/standup.htm
15. Philips. Basic principles of MR imaging. Philips Medical Systems.
16. Ezzeddine B. Active noise cancellation system for magnetic resonance imaging. Neuroscience Directions. 1,1 p3. Wallace-Kettering Neuroscience Institute. http://www.wkni.org/directions/dv01i01.pdf
17. http://www.mrisafety.com
18. http://www.bamrr.org.uk
19. Graham D, Cloke P. Principles of radiological physics. 4th edn. Edinburgh: Elsevier; 2003:222.
20. Talbot J, et al. Somerset MRI Course CD ROM Volume 2. 2001.
21. Niendorf H, et al. Safety review of gadopentetate dimeglumine. Extended clinical experience after more than five million applications. Investigative Radiology 1994; 29(Suppl)(2):S179–182.
22. Spinosa D, et al. Gadolinium chelates in angiography and interventional radiology: a useful alternative to iodinated contrast media for angiography. Radiology 2002; 223:319–325.
23. Meaney J. Magnetic resonance angiography of the peripheral arteries: current status. European Radiology 2003; 13(4):836–852.
24. Mitchell D, et al. Benign adrenocortical masses: diagnosis with chemical shift MR imaging. Radiology 1992; 185:345–351.
25. Outwater E, et al. Distinction between benign and malignant adrenal masses: value of T1-weighted chemical-shift MR imaging. American Journal of Roentgenology 1995; 165:579–583.
26. Jacobs J, et al. Pancreatic sparing of focal fatty infiltration. Radiology 1994; 190:437–439.

27. Isserow J, et al. Focal fatty infiltration of the pancreas: MR characterization with chemical shift imaging. American Journal of Roentgenology 1999;173:1263–1265.

28. Outwater E, et al. Lipid in renal clear cell carcinoma: detection on opposed-phase gradient-echo MR images. Radiology 1997; 205:103–107.

29. Carucci L, et al. Pancreatic metastasis from clear cell renal carcinoma: diagnosis with chemical shift MRI. Journal of Computer Assisted Tomography 1999; 23:934–936.

RADIONUCLIDE IMAGING

David Wyn Jones, Julian MacDonald

INTRODUCTION

Radionuclide imaging (RNI), often referred to as nuclear medicine (NM), is performed in most general and specialised hospitals, and is quite unique in its method of delineating pathological processes and its ability to quantify physiological function.

'Nuclear medicine is to physiology as radiology is to anatomy'[1]

RNI is reliant on manufactured radionuclides, together with complex pharmaceuticals, which have been developed over many years of research, to form the commonly available radiopharmaceuticals we use today. Indeed, the very limits of nuclear medicine's effeceivness are governed by the quality, availability and future development of these products. Radiopharmaceuticals used for diagnosis emit radiation in the form of gamma rays, which are energetic enough to penetrate body structures and be detected by recording instrumentation outside the body.

Due to the nature of human physiology any disease or dysfunction can present itself in 'RNI terms' as abnormal or disrupted distribution of radiotracer introduced into the body. The radiotracer is allowed to follow, or become part of, physiological processes in the body that may differ from the norm, showing as disrupted delivery of radiotracer. As a result, abnormalities such as tumours, malfunctioning organs or systems, and trauma or the effects of pathogenic invasion can be identified. The great advantage of RNI is that, except in the case of trauma, physiological changes usually precede anatomical changes.[1]

The ability to accurately detect and, later, image radiotracers in the body, took many years of development, from radiation probes to rectilinear scanners, and to the modern Anger gamma camera in use today. Although the Gamma camera has some theoretical technical flaws, it represents a highly sensitive and versatile method of imaging radioactivity, together with possibilities for quantitation, multiplanar tomographic imaging and parametric imaging.

The use of radioactivity in medical diagnosis is not without risk, but generally most RNI examinations fall into a 'low dose' category, compared with alternative imaging techniques to obtain the same end result. For example, the whole skeleton can be imaged during a bone scan, giving approximately half the radiation burden of a computed tomography (CT) scan of the pelvis. The use of government regulation, examination justification and optimal imaging technique, helps ensure net benefit to the patient.

Radiation protection measures in RNI differ from those in conventional radiology. Methods of protecting staff and patient will be discussed in this chapter, together with relevant UK legislation.

Nuclear medicine has a therapeutic role. Radioiodine thyroid ablation therapy, for example, has been used for many years. Physiological measurement (non-imaging) is another application where a tracer is introduced into the body – and later the radioactivity present in fluid samples can be measured.

The modality is highly reliant on the skills of a multidisciplinary team to provide an effective end result, which is an accurate representation of the processes taking place within the body. A suspected clinical condition needs to be matched to an appropriate nuclear medicine investigation, which usually involves complex medical and scientific decisions. The most obvious decision is whether to proceed, in terms of net benefit from the radiation dose received, and if so, which radiopharmaceutical to use and imaging technique to employ.

In this chapter an overview of a 'typical' RNI service is given, illustrating briefly its development into the medical imaging specialty it forms today. Key aspects will be explored, together with an appraisal of its usefulness in the modern medical 'diagnostic armoury'.

EQUIPMENT CHRONOLOGY

The first milestone in nuclear medicine was the discovery of radioactivity in 1896 by Henri Becquerel. The invention of the cyclotron in the early 1930s provided the means by which usable quantities of radionuclides could be produced. However it was not until the late 1940s that radionuclides became available for medical use. The radionuclide most commonly used in nuclear medicine today, Technetium-99m ($^{99}Tc^m$), was first produced in the late 1930s.

Early work in tracing radioactive materials administered to patients was based around the use of hand-held Geiger counters and scintillation detectors. In the early 1950s, Cassen et al produced a scintillation detector mounted in an automatic scanning gantry, which was probably the first incarnation of the rectilinear scanner.[2]

Commercial machines were available by the late 1950s. These devices allowed the acquisition of an image by tracing a collimated scintillation detector in a rectilinear pattern over the area of interest. Rectilinear scanners, however, were very slow and could not produce images of dynamic processes.

In the late 1950s, Hal Anger developed a scintillation detector, which has since become known as the gamma camera.[3] This device is kept stationary and collects gamma rays over the field of view, resulting in much more rapid image acquisition than the rectilinear scanner and allowing dynamic imaging. At around the same time, the Brookhaven National laboratory was developing the $^{99}Mo/^{99}Tc^m$ generator, which became commercially available in 1960. One of the earliest reported uses of $^{99}Tc^m$ was for brain scanning.[4] Since then much work has been carried out on the development of $^{99}Tc^m$ based radiopharmaceuticals.

Commercial Anger gamma camera systems were available by 1964. RNI technique was further enhanced with single photon emission tomography (SPET). This technique acquires data at a series of angular positions around the patient that allows the production of multiplanar images. Early development of this technique took place in the early 1960s, the first study being published in 1963.[5] At this stage, images were produced by analogue means rather than by computer algorithms, which were developed in 1967 by Hounsfield. These algorithms accounted for attenuation and scatter and converted the emission tomography technique to single photon emission computed tomography (SPECT). At this time reconstruction of data took several hours; however, due to advances in computing,

the same processes today take a few seconds. Rotating gantries were developed in the mid 1970s to allow automatic SPECT acquisitions.

Radiopharmaceuticals were developed during the 1970s that allowed imaging of most organs in the body and cardiac radiopharmaceuticals became available in the 1980s.

Since the 1980s, systems for planar, dynamic, and SPECT acquisition have been commercially available and have been further developed and refined. In the 1990s, rectangular camera heads replaced circular ones to allow imaging of greater areas. Whole-body imaging by scanning the camera head over the length of the body has become routine practice. Multiheaded gamma cameras became available to reduce imaging times and it is now common for dual-headed systems to allow a range of angular head spacing, to optimise the imaging process. For example, camera heads at 90° to each other are used for cardiac imaging. Other refinements have been made such as automatic contouring, where infrared beams allow the camera head to traverse at an optimal proximity to the patient.

In terms of detector technology, improvements have been made in component stability and performance and by digitisation of signals within the camera head. Such developments have improved the uniformity and spatial and energy resolution of gamma cameras, having an ultimate beneficial effect on image quality. In addition, devices became available for producing attenuation correction maps, which can be used to improve the accuracy of SPECT images. Newer systems have utilised built-in X-ray CT scanners to achieve this. These systems also allow nuclear medicine images to be overlaid on CT images to provide both functional and anatomical information.

Positron emission tomography (PET) developed alongside conventional RNI. The idea of imaging positron emitters was proposed in the early 1950s and the first study published in 1953.[6] As cyclotrons became more available, development accelerated due to the availability of positron emitting radionuclides that could be labelled as clinically useful molecules. Even so, PET remained only a research tool until the late 1970s at which point clinical PET systems started to become commercially available. Only in the latter part of the 1990s, however, did PET really start to become routinely used as a clinical tool in the USA; currently the number of systems in the UK for routine clinical PET is still very small, but it is expected to rise rapidly in the near future thanks to Government intervention. PET has been proven to be a very useful functional imaging modality in oncology, cardiology and neurology.

Much work has been done to modify gamma camera systems to carry out PET studies. However, such systems have limited usefulness due to low sensitivity and problems with count-rate caused by having two large detectors rather than many hundreds of separate small detectors as in dedicated PET systems. Uses have been found for gamma camera PET however, for example in cardiology and some oncology studies.

Much more recently, PET systems have been combined with CT systems to provide perfectly registered functional and anatomical images, which are of particular value in oncology.

SCIENCE AND INSTRUMENTATION

Radioactivity

The atoms of some substances are unstable due to an imbalance in the number of protons and neutrons in the nucleus. Such substances spontaneously emit radiation and are said to be *radioactive*. Radiation is emitted from a radioactive atom when it undergoes a *disintegration*, i.e. a transformation or *decay* to another atom. The *radioactivity* of a substance is defined as the number of disintegrations per second. The unit of radioactivity is the Becquerel (Bq); 1 Bq = 1 disintegration per second. As atoms decay over time, the radioactivity of a substance reduces. The time taken for the radioactivity to reduce to a half of its original value is called the *half-life* of the radionuclide.

The radiation emitted by a radioactive substance can be of several types, e.g. alpha particles, beta particles, gamma rays, positrons. For imaging purposes, only penetrating radiation, such as gamma radiation, is of use.

Radiopharmaceuticals

RNI is a functional imaging technique, i.e. it provides images illustrating patterns of growth and biological activity within the organs of interest. This is achieved by imaging the distribution of radioactive tracers, or *radiopharmaceuticals*, which are selected based on their ability to be taken up in the area of interest.

Radiopharmaceuticals consist of two components: The radionuclide which emits the radiation that allows detection of the radiopharmaceutical, and the chemical component which controls its distribution in the body.

Radionuclide component

The following table gives the ideal requirements of the radionuclide for NM use.

Property	Ideal requirements
Radiation emitted	Detection relies upon radiation being emitted from the body and thus requires a penetrating form of radiation, i.e. gamma rays
Energy	The gamma rays must possess sufficient energy to escape the body but, conversely, their energy must be low enough to allow them to be efficiently stopped within the detector
Half-life	The radioactivity must be sufficient to allow good image quality throughout the duration of the imaging period. The half-life must thus be long enough to allow this. Conversely, if the half-life is much longer than the period of imaging, this may result in a higher exposure to the patient than is necessary
Cost and availability	The ideal radiopharmaceutical will be cheap and readily available

In practice, one radionuclide, $^{99}Tc^m$, dominates traditional RNI due to its almost perfect properties. It is an emitter of 140 keV gamma rays with a half-life of 6 hours. It is relatively inexpensive and readily available via a generator system. Generators containing ^{99}Mo are normally supplied weekly and allow $^{99}Tc^m$ to be removed in solution, or *eluted*, on a daily basis. Other commonly used radionuclides and their uses in diagnostic RNI are given in the table below.

Radionuclide	Production method	Principal photon Energy (keV)	Used to image
$^{99}Tc^m$	Generator (parent: reactor)	140.5	Skeleton, lung perfusion, kidneys, brain, thyroid
^{201}Tl	Cyclotron	78	Heart, parathyroid
^{123}I	Cyclotron	160	Phaeochromocytoma, thyroid, brain
^{67}Ga	Cyclotron	93,185,300	Inflammation and infection
^{131}I	Reactor	364	Thyroid
$^{81}Kr^m$	Generator (parent: cyclotron)	191	Lung ventilation

Radiopharmaceuticals for PET comprise of radionuclides that emit positrons. The positrons lose energy in a short distance in the body and annihilate with atomic electrons to produce two 511 keV gamma ray photons (180° apart) that allow coincidental detection of the tracer. Therefore, unlike traditional nuclear medicine, the energy of the radionuclide's emissions is irrelevant. The half-life and the cost and availability, however, are crucial since PET radionuclides have to be produced by cyclotron. The most commonly used PET radionuclide is Fluorine 18 (^{18}F).

Chemical component

The chemical component attached to the radionuclide determines where the radiopharmaceutical travels in the body. There are several ways in which a desirable distribution can be achieved:

- Using a chemical found physiologically in the organ of interest, e.g. iodine for imaging the thyroid
- Using an analogue. This is a chemical that simulates one found physiologically, e.g. thallium is a potassium analogue and thus can be used to image muscle. Similarly fluorodeoxyglucose (FDG) is a glucose analogue and can be labelled to ^{18}F for PET imaging to illustrate areas of high glucose metabolism, which has several clinical uses
- Labelling cells that fight disease thereby targeting the areas of disease, e.g. white blood cells or antibodies

Combinations of radionuclides and chemicals, however, are limited to those that the chemistry allows. The majority of nuclear medicine tests use standard kits containing a powdered version of the chemical component. These are then reconstituted as and when required with the radionuclide solution.

Radiopharmaceuticals are normally administered intravenously but are occasionally given subcutaneously, orally or via inhalation. Once incorporated, the radiopharmaceutical remains in the body for a period determined by the chemical form, the half-life of the radionuclide and the physiology of the patient. The patient will receive a radiation dose that will depend on the radioactivity administered and the residence time (i.e. the time for which the radionuclide is present in the patient). The effective dose, which allows comparison with other imaging modalities using ionising radiation, is determined from the weighted sum of the absorbed doses to each organ. The weighting factors are organ dependent due to their different radiosensitivities.

Instrumentation

The primary piece of instrumentation in an RNI department is the gamma camera, which is the focus of this section. Brief descriptions will also be given of PET scanners and radionuclide calibrators.

The gamma camera

The most fundamental part of any imaging system is the detector. In the case of a gamma camera, the detector is a large rectangular, or circular, crystal of a scintillation material that produces a weak flash of light when radiation is absorbed, due to excitation.

Flashes of light are thus produced when gamma rays emitted by a patient, previously administered a radiopharmaceutical, fall on the detector as shown in Figure 42.1. The light formed in the crystal is detected by photomultiplier tubes (PMTs) which convert the light to electronic signals whose magnitude is determined by the intensity of light reaching the PMT. There are, in fact, many PMTs packed into the space of the scintillator crystal and those around the point of light emission will detect some amount of light depending on their distance from that point. Those closest will detect more light and, in turn, produce a greater electronic pulse and those further away will produce proportionally smaller pulses. The relative magnitude of these

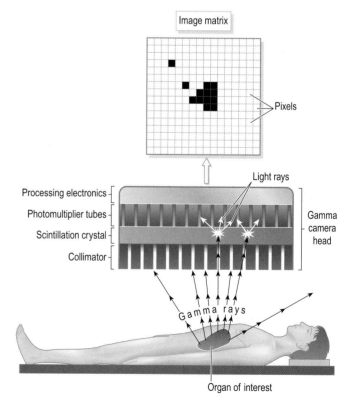

Figure 42.1 Schematic diagram of a gamma camera showing the gamma rays emitted by the patient, the collimator allowing only those aligned with the collimator holes to pass through to the scintillation crystal. Light rays produced by the crystal are detected and quantified to obtain energy and positional information used to assign a count to the correct pixel location in the image matrix

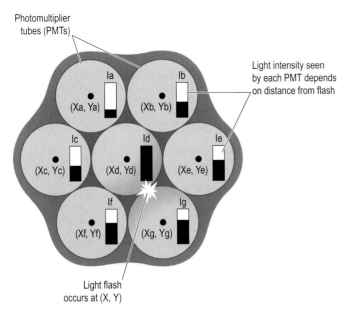

Figure 42.2 The intensity of light detected depends on the distance of the PMT from the position within the crystal that the gamma ray was absorbed and the light flash occurred. These relative intensities are used to reduce a weighted average of the PMT positions (Xa, Ya), (Xb, Yb) etc. to determine the origin of the light flash

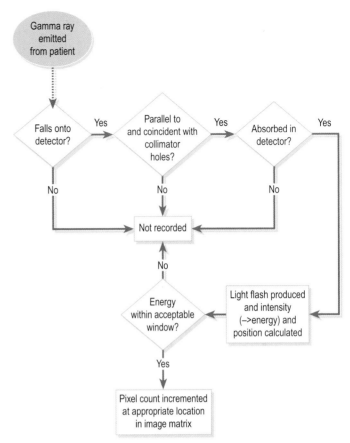

Figure 42.3 The imaging process

pulses can then be used to determine the point of light emission. The pixel count value in a corresponding location in a digital matrix can then be incremented allowing the accumulation of an image (Fig. 42.2).

However, the system so far described does not provide a method of tracing the point of light emission in the detector back to the point of origin of the gamma ray within the patient, which is critical to producing a meaningful image. This is the function of the collimator.

A collimator is essentially a block of attenuating material with a network of holes and is attached to the gamma camera between the detector crystal and the patient. The holes allow gamma rays travelling in a certain direction to pass through to the crystal and be detected. Gamma rays travelling in different directions are attenuated and thus the collimator effectively acts as a filter, only allowing gamma rays travelling in a known direction to contribute to the image. In this way there is a direct one-to-one mapping between the origin of the gamma ray and the position of the pixel within the image matrix (Fig. 42.3).

The detector

The scintillation material used is sodium iodide which contains a small amount of thallium impurity [NaI(Tl)]. The thallium impurity significantly increases the amount of light produced. The properties of the detector affect many aspects of the image including:

- *Thickness.* The thicker the crystal, the more likely the radiation will be absorbed, thus improving efficiency. However, if the crystal is too thick, there will be an increase in the drift of the light photons adding to the uncertainty in the calculated point of interaction and, hence, a worsening in the spatial resolution.
- *Light output.* Different scintillator materials produce different amounts of light per interaction and release the light at different rates. The latter affects the period of processing required to assign the event to a position within the image matrix, the *dead-time*. Ideally a large amount of light is required in a short time. It is also essential that the light intensity produced is proportional to the energy of the radiation absorbed. This allows energy discrimination and, thus, the ability to disregard gamma rays outside a certain energy range, used to reduce scatter.
- *Transparency.* This factor affects the amount of light lost as it passes through the crystal before being detected by the PMTs.

The collimator

Collimators vary in regard to their thickness and the number, direction and diameter of the holes. The most common type of collimator used is the parallel hole collimator in which the holes, as well as being parallel with each other, are perpendicular to the camera face. The number of holes, and hence the thickness of the attenuating material between them, known as the *septa*, is altered to allow imaging for different energies. For example when imaging ^{131}I (^{131}Iodine) gamma rays of 364 keV, a collimator with a smaller number of holes, and correspondingly thicker septa, is essential to prevent penetration of the radiation through the septa.

High resolution and high sensitivity collimators are also generally available and feature variations in collimator thickness and hence hole length. There is a trade-off between resolution and sensitivity such that a high resolution collimator will have a lower sensitivity and therefore take longer to obtain the same number of counts than a high sensitivity collimator and vice versa.

Other geometric arrangements of holes are also available. The holes of a diverging hole collimator fan outwards and allow demagnification of the object, which is useful for large objects. Converging hole or fan beam collimators fan inwards providing magnification of the object and are commonly used in brain imaging. Pinhole collimators have a single aperture at the end of a lead shield that allows magnification of objects near the collimator and demagnification further away. The magnitude of the effect of all these collimators depends on the distance from the collimator and hence distortions in the image will occur. This is particularly the case with the pinhole collimator which can really only be used with thin objects. Nonetheless the pinhole collimator is a very useful way of providing magnified images of, for example, the thyroid gland or small bone joints in children.

The image matrix

RNI images are routinely acquired digitally into an image matrix as shown in Figure 42.1. In this matrix, the field of view of the gamma camera is represented by a square arrangement of pixels. The number of pixels and hence the pixel size can be varied to give a fine or coarse matrix depending on the investigation. Where close assessment of fine anatomical structures is required, a finer matrix, and hence smaller pixel size, is used. Where this is not so important, a larger pixel size is adequate. In general, however, if a finer matrix is used, more counts will need to be collected.

The digital acquisition of data means that images can be analysed or *processed*. Such processing ranges from simple thresholding adjustments to improve contrast, to the generation of curves or quantitative parameters to provide objective assessment of function. This allows reproducibility between different patients and the same patient on follow-up.

SPECT

The majority of RNI studies require the acquisition of static or dynamic planar images, which are acquired with the gamma camera at a fixed position against the patient for the duration of imaging. SPECT imaging, on the other hand, acquires a series of images as the gamma camera rotates around the patient. The image projections can then be mathematically reconstructed to form a 3D data set from which slices through the body or 3D visualisations can be formed, in a similar way to CT. Reconstruction techniques are beyond the scope of this text but are based on backprojection or iterative algorithms.

This imaging technique allows much greater contrast due to the effective removal of overlying structures present in planar imaging. The main applications are in assessing myocardial perfusion, brain functionality and bone lesions.

PET scanners

PET scanning is gaining popularity in the UK but as yet is not part of a routine nuclear medicine service. PET imaging is desirable due to the fact that positron emitting radionuclides are relatively simple to label to biologically active organic molecules. By far the most common PET radiopharmaceutical is ^{18}F-FDG (fluorodeoxyglucose) which provides an image of glucose metabolism that is useful in oncology, cardiology and neurology.

PET tracers emit positrons that annihilate with electrons to form two 511 keV photons which are emitted in opposite directions. PET scanners consist of a ring of detectors in which the two photons are detected coincidentally. The point of emission in the patient must then be somewhere along a line between the two detection events. When sufficient coincident events have been accumulated the distribution in the body can be determined through reconstruction algorithms and a 3D data set is produced which can be used to produce slices through the area of interest. Note that this is a simplified description; in reality the process is much more complex than indicated here.

Image quality

The quality of an image produced by any imaging modality is affected by the amount of noise. In RNI, contributions to noise come from:

- *Insufficient counts in the image.* Statistical noise arises from uncertainties in the number of counts in each pixel of the image. As radioactive decay is a random process, acquired counts follow a Poisson distribution. This means that the uncertainty, measured as the standard deviation of the mean, is equal to the square root of the number of counts. For a pixel with 100 counts, the standard deviation is 10, which is 10% of the mean. Similarly a pixel count of 10 000 has a standard deviation of 1%. The higher the number of counts, the lower the relative uncertainty or noise. Doubling the number of counts improves the noise by a factor of the square root of 2 (~ 1.4). The pixel size has an important impact on this as larger pixels will collect more counts and thus will inherently have less noise.

- *Scatter.* This occurs both within the patient and the detector. Scatter of gamma rays in the patient causes them to change direction. In some cases, a gamma ray may be scattered toward the gamma camera and, if detected, would result in a count being assigned to a wrong pixel within the image matrix, thereby adding to the noise. In many cases, the collimator would filter out such scattered gamma rays but, if the new direction of the gamma ray was parallel to the collimator holes, it would reach the crystal and be detected. This is where the energy discrimination ability is used. The gamma ray will have lost some energy as a result of the scattering interaction. Because the light intensity produced by the scintillator detector is proportional to the energy absorbed, the system can distinguish such scattered gamma rays and disregard them. Unfortunately, however, the various processes involved in the detection process carry their own uncertainties, which means that even unscattered gamma rays may appear to have energies slightly above or below the expected energy, the so-called *photopeak.* This means that there has to be a range or window of acceptable energies set which, in turn, results in some scatter having to be included. In modern systems, with improved and more stable components, the detection uncertainties have reduced, allowing the window of acceptable energies to be narrowed and, hence, more noise to be eliminated and image quality improved.

Quality control

As with any other imaging modality, regular assessment of equipment performance is essential. Some of the parameters assessed routinely for a gamma camera are given below:

- *Uniformity.* The gamma camera has a large field of view and the count-rate observed over its surface for a uniform source should be constant. This is tested either by placing a large uniform source of radioactivity on the collimated camera or by using a small volume source at a distance from the uncollimated detector. An image is acquired in each case and assessed visually and quantitatively for non-uniformity.

- *Energy resolution.* Earlier in this chapter, we discussed the range of apparent energies erroneously assigned to unscattered gamma rays due to the uncertainties involved in the detection process. Energy resolution is essentially a measure of this. A uniform source of radiation is used and data is acquired in the form of a plot of 'the number of gamma rays being assigned a particular energy' against 'energy'. The result is a Gaussian curve centred on the photopeak and the energy resolution is defined as the full width half maximum (FWHM) of that curve. The smaller the value the better, as this means that the energy acceptance window can be narrowed, thereby reducing image noise.

- *Spatial resolution.* This is a measure of the ability of the gamma camera to distinguish objects that are close together. The test consists of imaging a narrow line source and then producing a curve profile through the resulting image. The curve will be a Gaussian curve and the spatial resolution is defined as the FWHM of the curve. The smaller the value the better, as this means that the camera can resolve objects closer together.

Radionuclide calibrators

To ensure an accurate and appropriate radioactivity is administered to the patient undergoing radionuclide imaging, the radioactivity must be measured in a radionuclide calibrator. This is essentially an ionisation chamber that produces a small current dependent on the radioactivity and type and energy of the radiation emitted. Calibration factors must be obtained for particular radionuclides so that the current is then proportional to the radioactivity only and hence the displayed 'radioactivity' readout is accurate. Daily quality control of the calibrator is essential.

RNI PRACTICE

▇ Fundamentals of RNI technique

As discussed earlier, the basic scientific principles of RNI instrumentation necessitate careful application of radiographic technique to ensure optimal image quality. Conventional radiographic positioning principles lend themselves to positioning in RNI. Care must be taken to avoid simulating disease by: poor positioning of the patient in relation to the gamma camera, misuse of radioactive anatomical markers or incorrect use of imaging equipment parameters.

Patient preparation for RNI investigations is paramount for a successful outcome. Many procedures can be ruined by incorrect advice or poor patient compliance prior to the investigation. This can, in part, be remedied by having clear written protocols for each investigation and by providing the patient with unambiguous written instructions on how to prepare for the investigation. The advice can include the cessation of certain drugs, avoidance of particular foods or avoiding intake altogether for certain procedures (to name but a few). This sometimes involves dialogue with the referring clinician, regarding interactions, and carefully relaying advice to the patient. An example of a failed procedure would be the patient who has caffeine on the day of a pharmacological myocardial perfusion stress study. Caffeine has a deleterious action on the effectiveness of pharmacological stressing agent, giving a dubious result when using Dipyridamole. The examination might need to be repeated in this scenario, clearly with associated additional risks from the repeated test.

It is necessary to have a thorough knowledge of human physiology and anatomy to fully understand the complexities of RNI investigations. An understanding of how various radiopharmaceuticals are 'handled' by the body is necessary in order to undertake the appropriate investigation for the clinical question being asked, and to correctly interpret the image appearance. Some image appearances can also represent technical defects in terms of radiopharmaceutical quality or equipment failure.

Supply of unsealed sources for imaging

It is necessary to have a radiopharmacy 'on site' or within a relatively short distance of the imaging department, in order to provide an effective RNI service. Those without 'on site' radiopharmacy facilities usually have a radiopharmaceutical dispensary where daily deliveries from the remote radiopharmacy can be dispensed safely into predetermined activities for patient administration. Some departments even have radiopharmaceuticals delivered predispensed, ready for individual patient use. The latter, however, introduces some lack of flexibility into the service, but is sometimes unavoidable due to constraints of facilities or staff.

Essentially, the radiopharmacy department maintains a stock of pharmaceuticals in the form of 'kits'. These are supplied by manufacturers, and usually contain the required compound in sterile glass vials, ready for reconstitution with the required radionuclide. The radionuclide source is either from the $^{99}Tc^m$ generator, which allows daily elution, or by prior order from the manufacturer, if the radionuclide is produced by other means, for example, by cyclotron.

The radiopharmacy department is usually sited in a 'clean' room where the air is 'ultra filtered' and has a positive pressure. This, together with protective laminar flow cabinets and clothing, ensures the microbial sterility of the manufactured radiopharmaceuticals. Quality tests

are undertaken on the eluate from the $^{99}Tc^m$ generator to check for microbial sterility, and purity – in that it is free of the parent nuclide (^{99}Mo) – and structural alumina from within the generator. Dispensed radiopharmaceuticals are measured according to volume and 'activity' required at a reference time. Calculations are made to account for the physical half-life of the particular radionuclide used and a larger volume is dispensed, allowing for the decay time until administration later in the day. Clearly this indicates that the patient's actual attendance time must be in concordance with the allocated appointment and administration time and this, again, underlines the importance of good advance preparation. In addition to patient explanation, this would include careful explanation to ward personnel if the patient is attending from a ward area rather than from home.

The activity administered to the patient is checked in a calibrator before leaving the radiopharmacy, and it is good practice to double check the activity directly prior to patient administration. Any patient administration must be within agreed diagnostic reference levels (DRLs), and in the UK, these are recommended by the Administration of Radioactive Substances Advisory Committee (ARSAC). It is necessary to scale down adult activities for administration to children, where current best practice is to adopt the advice given in the ARSAC Guidance Notes section 6.5,[7] which maintains the required 'count' density for optimal paediatric images. Although this should lead to similar examination times as adults, this does increase the effective dose (ED) of radiation in comparison. The Committee also discourages the use of administered activities to children less than 10% of the adult recommendation. ARSAC gives an exception to this recommendation when imaging the paediatric brain, which reaches 95% of adult weight by the age of 5 years.

Radiation protection in RNI

Legislation for safe RNI practice is complex, and requires thorough knowledge and careful interpretation of the various regulations and statutory advice.[7,8,9] The purpose of the legislation is mainly to protect the patient, staff, and environment from the detrimental effects of ionising radiation. Practitioners should familiarise themselves with local documents of 'systems of work' in 'Local Rules', which are a requirement for 'non-classified workers' (under the regulations) to work safely in 'controlled areas'.

UK legislation requires the employer to provide the framework for radiation protection and ensure that staff are adequately trained, as well as complying with measures to protect patients from the effects of unnecessary ionising radiation. The Ionizing Radiations (Medical Exposure)

Regulations 2000 [IR(ME)R 2000] ensure best possible patient safety by requiring each individual exposure to be both 'justified' and 'optimised', and insisting that there are measures for 'dose limitation' in place.[9]

Detailed measures, for the practical application of radiation protection in NM are beyond the scope of this text; however the list below shows some common measures for optimising dose reduction:

- Use of DRLs for patient doses (activities)
- Activity measured in calibrators
- Use of syringe shields
- Use of shielding to store unsealed sources (sharps and waste)
- Observation of the inverse square law
- Controlled and supervised areas: limited access
- Patient preparation and aftercare
- Cessation of breast-feeding where recommended
- Avoidance of examination during pregnancy (or suspected pregnancy)
- Scaled down adult doses by weight for children
- Use of contamination monitors, emergency decontamination kits
- Avoidance of ingestion and use of make-up
- Maintenance of strict records
- Use of personal dosimetry
- Safe transport of radioactive materials

In order to justify RNI examinations, there must be an evaluation of risk versus benefit, should the examination be clinically desirable. This evaluation cannot be correctly undertaken without prior knowledge of the radiation burden expected from the examination. The concept of 'effective dose' is used to understand the risk involved and these doses are usually calculated using the medical internal radiation dose (MIRD) schema.[10] Internal radiation doses received are complicated to calculate, however the MIRD system provides a mechanism to estimate dose, taking into account most factors including weighting factors for different organs with varying sensitivities to radiation, the amount of energy deposited and residence time in the organ – to give a whole body 'weighted' dose.

Acquisition of RNI images (data)

The image information leaving the gamma camera head(s) in the form of the X, Y and Z signal is stored in digital form and can be manipulated later, to provide image and quantitative data. The final data output is highly dependent on radiographic technique. Once the patient has been correctly prepared and given the appropriate radiopharmaceutical, the imaging practitioner has to carefully select appropriate imaging factors and correctly position the patient at the predetermined time. Suboptimal images might otherwise be obtained.

An RNI 'study' usually contains a number of predetermined 'frames', and the act of collecting a frame is conventionally referred to as an 'acquisition'. The following represents some of the common factors chosen for the examination by selecting parameters on the 'acquisition platform' of the gamma camera system.

- *Image matrix* – the data is acquired into a predefined image matrix, selected at the outset, and affects the spatial resolution, 'counts per pixel' obtained and number of possible acquired frames (due to computer memory constraints). The matrix is a division of the field of view (FOV) of the gamma camera into predefined pixels. A common example is a 256×256 matrix used for planar imaging.
- *Static frame* (planar imaging) – usually the number of frames required will be selected at the outset and will contain individual images.
- *Dynamic frames* – the number and duration of frames set at the outset – and stored sequentially in time.
- *Whole body acquisition* – this is where the camera traverses the patient at a predetermined rate of motion and length, to acquire a full image of the body.
- *Dual energy acquisition* – the ability of the gamma camera to discriminate incident energies is exploited to produce two simultaneous frames of separate data representing differing images of the distribution of more than one administered radionuclide.
- *Gated acquisition* – the initiation of collection of imaged data into individual frames is controlled by a physiological 'switching' process, e.g. by connecting electrocardiograph (ECG) electrodes to the patient and using 'R' wave pulses to initiate and terminate a sequence of frames. For example: 'gated' SPECT or gated cardiac ventriculography (multiple gated cardiac acquisition (MUGA)).
- *SPECT* – multiple frames of data are acquired at predefined locations around a central axis within the patient. This can be in a 'step and shoot' mode where the camera head(s) rotates a fixed number of degrees, stops, acquires a frame of image data for a predefined period of time, and then moves on to acquire the next frame. A 'continuous' mode allows the head(s) to continually rotate whilst acquiring data at the required angles. The final data can be reconstructed into three orthogonal planes.
- *Termination mode* – a study can have many parameters for terminating individual frames or the whole study.
- *Time* - a fixed time is set for each frame. The system awaits the next frame to be manually started until the predetermined frame limit for the study is reached.

- *Number of counts* - once the system has detected a predetermined number of 'counts' in the entire FOV, then the frame will terminate, and progress is as for 'time' above. A 'count' is taken to be a signal processed by the gamma camera representing an 'allowable' radiation detection event.
- *Number of acquired frames* – this is used to terminate a dynamic study.
- *Length and speed of motion* – these are used to terminate a whole body acquisition.
- *Total number of counts or duration* – these can be used to terminate a gated study.
- *Orientation* – the operator usually selects a 'letter' or a symbol for the required orientation of the image.
- *Magnification* – the image can be magnified at the acquisition stage where the acquisition only uses a small part of the FOV.
- *Energy window(s)* – the operator must select and *verify* that the system is set to acquire data pulses from the gamma camera, which fall into the required energy window for the radionuclide being imaged.

Annotation and orientation for viewing

RNI images need to be correctly orientated for viewing and 'marked' with the appropriate anatomical side. It is common practice to use a cobalt (^{57}Co) 'marker' to identify the correct orientation during imaging, and for later viewing. Another point of note is that contrary to the practice in radiography of denoting a projection by the 'entry' and 'exit' route of the incident radiation (anteroposterior (AP), posteroanterior (PA)), it is correct in RNI to denote the body part directly adjacent to the surface of the collimator, e.g. anterior image or posterior image – not AP or PA. Also, images at 90°, e.g. 'lateral knee', would be correctly annotated as being 'lateral aspect' if the lateral aspect of the knee were adjacent to the collimator. Finally, a study should always have the radiopharmaceutical used and delay time to imaging or frame times marked on the images. Correct annotation is vital for effective image evaluation.

COMMON RNI INVESTIGATIONS

RNI practice involves imaging procedures for most organs and systems of the human body. It is intended here to focus on some common investigations, to illustrate the rationale involved for imaging, and to evaluate their effectiveness. Specific RNI texts should be consulted to understand the whole range available in detail.

Planar skeletal scintigraphy and whole body bone scanning

Summary of indications for skeletal scintigraphy[11,12]
- Metastasis 'screening'
- Lesion localisation for biopsy
- Diagnosis of osteomyelitis before radiographic 'signs'
- Differentiation of osteomyelitis from cellulitis
- Evaluating the painful hip prosthesis for infection or loosening
- Evaluate articular involvement in arthropathies
- Aid in the characterisation of benign bone lesions
- Assessing the 'activity' of compression fractures
- Evaluate bone pain with normal radiographs
- Diagnosis of ischaemic bone disease
- Diagnosis of myositis ossificans
- Delineating a level for preamputation planning
- Delineating healing fractures
- Diagnosis and 'staging' of reflex sympathetic dystrophy (RSD)
- Diagnosis of various metabolic bone disorders such as Paget's disease and osteoporosis
- Costochondritis

Imaging rationale
Isotope bone scanning has been shown to be the most *sensitive* method of imaging diseases of bone, and usually shows abnormal areas much sooner than that shown on radiographs, with an increase of about 50% of calcium in affected areas being required to show changes on a radiograph.[13] Indeed, Alazraki[12] reports that less than 5% of bone scans are normal when radiographs show abnormalities, thus demonstrating the high sensitivity of the imaging modality.

Limitations of the imaging technique are its 'apparent' lack of *specificity* in classifying disease of bone, and the need for scan results to be interpreted with clinical findings and correlated with relevant radiographs, to make a definitive diagnosis. However, 'pattern recognition' can allow a more accurate initial diagnosis, by understanding the characteristic patterns of uptake of ^{99}Tc^m MDP, associated with certain disease processes, for example:[11]

- *Metastases:* often with multiple lesions with random distribution in the skeleton (Fig. 42.4)
- *Rib fractures:* where the focal increase in uptake is linear along the rib cage (Fig. 42.5)
- *Osteomyelitis:* with intense increased uptake on a 3-phase bone scan

Given that there are some instances where a bone scan can be interpreted fairly safely on its own, Smith confirms

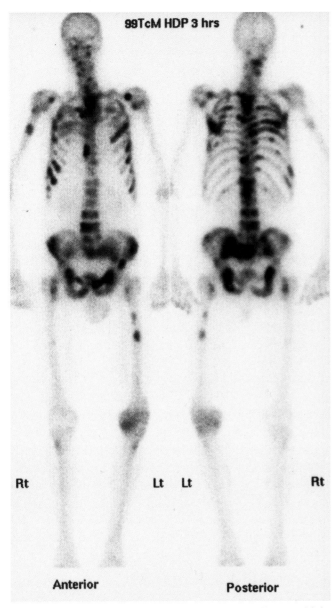

Figure 42.4 Metastatic deposits. This bone scan shows multiple areas of increased uptake of 99Tcm HDP at 3 hours – indicating multiple metastatic deposits in the skeleton. The pattern of uptake suggests a definitive diagnosis

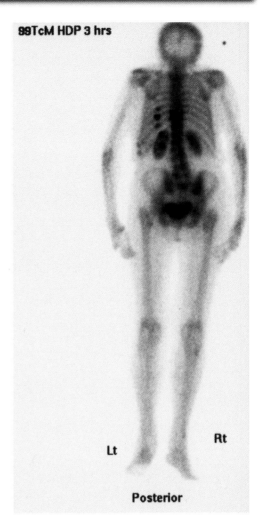

Figure 42.5 Rib fractures. This bone scan shows the typical appearances of rib fractures with the characteristic uptake showing a linear pattern across the left lower posterior ribs

the general non-specificity of the technique by quoting some examples of non-specific abnormal uptake, which need further investigation to clarify their aetiology.[13]

Examples of appearances with non-specific interpretation:

- *Osteomalacia with associated pseudo fractures:* this can be mistaken for multiple metastases in the skeleton or vice versa
- *Simple collapsed vertebrae showing linear increase uptake in spine:* this can be mistaken for discitis or vice versa
- *A solitary spinal lesion can be interpreted as a metastasis:* this could alternatively be due to fracture of the pars

interarticularis; osteoid osteoma; active arthropathy, or primary tumour such as chondrosarcoma

Symmetry, however, is of prime importance in the declaration of a 'normal' whole body bone scan, and it is important that both halves of the skeleton should be mirror images of each other. There should be uniform uptake of the radiotracer in the skeleton, and uptake in organs such as the kidneys and bladder is to be expected. Uptake in the soft tissues of the skeleton can also be an indicator of disease, and should be considered to be a normal area of concern during the interpretation of such an investigation, and care needs to be used when 'windowing' these areas (Fig. 42.6).[11]

It is important not only to recognise increased uptake of radiopharmaceutical due to abnormal 'malignant' osteoblastic activity, but also to be aware of a false negative scan, as in the case of multiple myeloma or renal cell carcinoma.[11] Here the characteristic interpretative sign is that of a 'cold' lesion where there is little or no radioemission from bone. This is therefore, clearly, of prime importance in either justifying the examination – or once

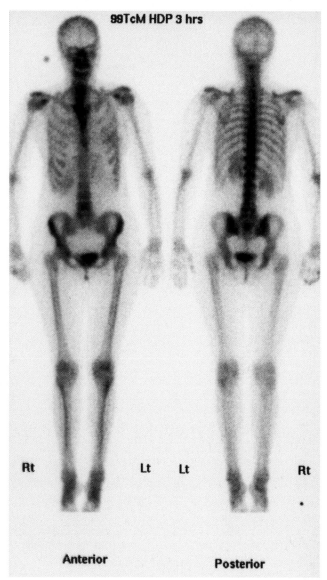

99TcM HDP 3 hrs

Rt   Lt   Lt   Rt

Anterior   Posterior

Figure 42.6 Normal bone scan showing symmetrical uptake throughout the skeleton, with soft tissue visible, and the expected activity in the kidneys, ureters, and bladder

when compared to computed tomography, where examination of a single body area potentially has a higher radiation burden to the patient than that utilised for a whole body bone scintigram.[14]

Practical considerations

^{99}Tc^m methylene diphosphonate (MDP) and ^{99}Tc^m hydroxymethylene diphosphonate (HDP) are both commonly used. They are adsorbed onto the surface of bone by incorporation into the hydroxyapatite crystal formed by osteoblastic activity. Uptake in bone is related to 'delivering' blood flow, extraction rate (by tumours and fractures), and most importantly, osteoblastic activity. There is no appreciable difference in image quality between either form, although it has been suggested that there is higher skeletal uptake with HDP.[15] Peak uptake in bone is shown to be at approximately 1 hour[16] and the usual delay to imaging of 3 hours is related to soft tissue clearance by the kidneys of background activity resulting from non-adsorbed phosphonate. Less than 10% of administered activity is present in the blood compartment at 1 hour, and 2% at 4 hours.[17] Thus it is normal to visualise renal drainage and bladder filling of the tracer, which needs to be emptied prior to imaging. Increased hydration has been conventionally used to improve the object to background ratio of radiotracer to improve image quality; however a recent study showed that increased hydration had little effect on image quality, and that quality is more related to time delay to imaging, and deteriorates with increasing patient age. Increased hydration, however, *is recommended* to reduce the radiation burden to the bladder wall.[18]

▮ Diagnosis of pulmonary emboli

Ventilation/perfusion lung scanning (V/Q) has until recently been the main method of diagnosing pulmonary emboli (PE). Its use has been justified for many years because it is relatively easily available, cost effective, and has low morbidity. More recently, however, there has been greater use of computed tomography pulmonary angiography (CTPA) for the diagnosis of PE. It is recommended that CTPA be performed as the imaging modality of choice in most instances and that a V/Q scan can be considered as the examination of choice where:

- onsite facilities are readily available
- a chest radiograph has been performed and is normal
- clinical examination excludes other concurrent cardiopulmonary disease
- there is a standardised reporting regime[19]

^{99}Tc^m macro-aggregated albumin (MAA) is trapped in the capillaries of the lungs to show normal perfusion, and

undertaken – to consider the above in relation to the clinical history provided.

It is important to image the whole skeleton during skeletal scintigraphy. Localised disease present on planar images can sometimes be related to a systemic problem, and so a whole body bone scan can help to characterise the disease. An example of this would be in the multifocal appearance seen with many arthropathies.[13] It is also important to correlate the abnormal bone scan with radiographs to assess the aetiology of the disease present. Furthermore, the ability of the modality to image the whole skeleton from a single administered dose of radioisotope, justifies its place in diagnostic radiology. As compared to various other imaging techniques, the radiation dose to the patient can be seen to be reasonable, especially any occlusion gives rise to a hypoperfused area appearing as a defect on the image. In order to increase the accuracy of diagnosis, a ventilation scan is also required, where a radioactive gas ($^{81}Kr^m$) or particulate inhalation ($^{99}Tc^m$ Technegas) is used to image the patent airways (dual energy acquisition is possible with $^{81}Kr^m$). This technique relies on a mismatch to suggest the presence of a PE, with the likelihood being greatest when the ventilation scan appears to be normal, thus eliminating effectively other pathological processes in the lung.

Ventilation agents can be expensive, difficult to obtain, and the examination may be difficult to perform on the very ill patient. It is rare for departments to offer a daily facility. These factors, together with the improved diagnostic accuracy of CTPA, render the V/Q scan useful only in limited cases where the availability of CTPA is poor, or the patient is unable to tolerate intravenous contrast media. When performed, the V/Q has been shown to reliably exclude PE when the scan is normal but false positive results occur frequently with abnormal studies.[19]

Endocrinology

Sodium pertechnetate ($^{99}Tc^m$ $NaTcO_4^-$) – the raw eluate of the technetium generator – is readily available and can be used to image the thyroid gland. A delay of 20 minutes post-intravenous administration shows trapping of the pertechnetate ions in the gland. Abnormal tissue can be highlighted as 'cold', hypofunctioning nodules, or 'hot', hyperfunctioning nodules. ^{123}I is also used for imaging the thyroid gland, but gives a higher radiation burden[7] as it is trapped and taken up by the gland. ^{123}I has an advantage in imaging metastatic thyroid deposits in the skeleton, and the theoretical improved detection of retrosternal extension of the thyroid gland, due to its higher emissive energy and lower background activity.

Magnetic resonance imaging (MRI), CT and US are all useful in the anatomical evaluation of the thyroid gland but RNI provides the necessary functional information together with characteristic uptake in various tumours.[20] Whilst US can determine whether a nodule is solid or cystic, the value of RNI is that of characterisation of the function of the nodule. It has been shown that 99% of 'hot' nodules are benign, whereas 10–20% of palpable 'cold' nodules are malignant.[20]

Thyroid scintigraphy is also useful in the evaluation of thyroiditis in its various forms, and the characteristic uptake of radiopharmaceutical can help evaluate the stages of the disease. Thyroid uptake measurements are possible in RNI, where a figure can be quoted of the percentage uptake in the gland at a certain time post administration. This is then useful for comparison with the norm, and helps differentiate Grave's disease from other causes of hyperthyroidism, e.g. subacute thyroiditis – and has a role in the estimation of radioiodine required in thyroid ablation therapy.[20]

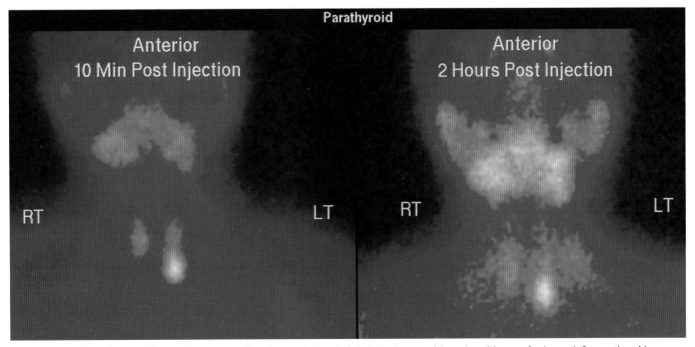

Figure 42.7 $^{99}Tc^m$ Sestamibi parathyroid scan. Showing early 'wash-in' of the tracer with early evidence of a lower left parathyroid adenoma, and the characteristic increased uptake in the tumour in relation to the thyroid on the delayed 'wash-out' image

In the case of hyperparathyroidism, conventional practice was to image abnormal parathyroid glands with $^{99}Tc^m$/^{201}Thallium subtraction techniques, where normal thyroid tissue would be highlighted by technetium and thallium, and abnormal parathyroid tissue highlighted by the digital subtraction of the normal uptake to leave abnormal thallium activity in the parathyroid gland. This is a useful technique but is difficult to perform, requires the use of expensive and poorly available thallium, not to mention absolute patient compliance and results in a high radiation dose (>18 mSv).[7]

Technetium Sestamibi has more recently been successfully utilised in highlighting abnormal parathyroid tissue. It is localised in parathyroid adenomas by concentration in the mitochondria 'rich' tumour, which is related to blood flow.[20] Images are acquired at 15 minutes and 2 hours post administration, as it has been shown that some tumours are more apparent at an early stage (Fig. 42.7).

However, theory dictates that the tracer concentrates in the tumour within 2 hours and the rest 'washes-out' of the normal tissue by then.[20] Parathyroid glands can be ectopic in the neck or mediastinum and are difficult to localise surgically.[21] The radionuclide technique has advantages (over other imaging modalities) in respect of imaging ectopic tissue, as it can image the whole area concerned, giving high sensitivity in the detection of adenomas. Sensitivity has been quoted from as high as 86% for planar studies to 90.5% with SPECT.[22]

The renal tract

There are many radiopharmaceuticals available for imaging the renal parenchyma and drainage system; comparison of the two most commonly used radiopharmaceuticals is discussed here.

$^{99}Tc^m$ MAG-3 is routinely used to image the kidneys, collecting system and bladder. Following intravenous administration it is rapidly removed from the blood circulation by glomerular filtration and tubular secretion, thus effectively representing true renal function. Renal function can thus be imaged with rapid dynamic frames over 30 minutes duration, and a diuretic can be used to differentiate between true obstructive uropathy or non-obstructed dilatation of the renal pelvis.[23] Data analysis can produce time activity curves, which have diagnostic value in themselves, and a figure is usually quoted for relative renal uptake at 2 to 3 minutes. Patients with suspected vesicoureteric reflux can have further imaging whilst voiding, which will show as an activity peak in the ureter. This technique is less traumatic for paediatric patients as direct catheterisation is not necessary as in the conventional radiological method (Fig. 42.8).

In contrast $^{99}Tc^m$, DMSA is used to image the renal parenchyma, where the radiopharmaceutical is absorbed in the proximal convoluted tubules, thus being highly representative of functioning tissue. Its value is in being able to delineate areas of scarring (non-function) caused by infection, and localising ectopic kidneys which may have been absent on an ultrasound (US) scan. Due to its complete binding to the tubules, there is no pelvirenal activity to denigrate the images, and it is especially useful in providing quantitation of relative renal function (Fig. 42.9).[23]

Gastrointestinal (GI) imaging

A novel approach to imaging gastric motility is to radio-label food. Abnormal motility is seen in patients with previous gastric surgery, and has many undesirable symptoms. By exploiting the quantitative abilities of RNI, a 'half-time' can be quoted for emptying gastric contents. The approximate normal half-time is quoted at 40 minutes for a solid meal.[24]

Other problems associated with the GI tract are those of bleeding. Bleeding into the bowel can be imaged with technetium labelled colloid or labelled red cells, where the 'pooling' of activity is representative of a GI bleed. Meckels diverticuli can be a source of bleeding, where acid produced by ectopic gastric mucosa damages the bowel wall. As sodium pertechnetate is naturally taken up by gastric mucosa, this phenomenon can be used to advantage, by highlighting suspect areas of ectopic gastric tissue within the whole abdomen. This enables confirmation of presence and location for subsequent surgical intervention.[25]

Nuclear cardiology

Conventional coronary angiography is used to image patency and location of coronary vessels prior to invasive treatment. RNI has the ability to demonstrate functioning areas of myocardium under strenuous conditions and at rest. The relative ventricular perfusion between stress and rest is useful in differentiating reversible from non-reversible ischaemia. Pharmacological stressing techniques allow the cardiac vessels to be imaged at maximum dilatation, highlighting decreased perfusion due to narrowing caused by arteriosclerosis.

$^{99}Tc^m$ Sestamibi (MIBI) or Tetrofosmin injected intravenously at peak stress, and at rest (on another occasion), will be trapped in the myocardium and will be representative of myocardial perfusion, with minimal redistribution prior to imaging. SPECT imaging then allows tomographic reconstruction in three planes, delineating areas of decreased perfusion due to ischaemia or infarction. It is in great demand, and it should be more widely available (Figs 42.10, 42.11).[26]

^{201}Thallium has the relative disadvantage of redistribution which is undesirable for stress/rest imaging; however

Figure 42.8 ^{99}Tc^m MAG-3 dynamic renogram showing the processed data from the dynamic frames of a 30-minute scan. Normal uptake and excretion can be seen on the curve for the left kidney, compared to the poor function of the right kidney. Here the relative renal function at 2 minutes can be seen to be 81% for the left, and 19% for the right kidney

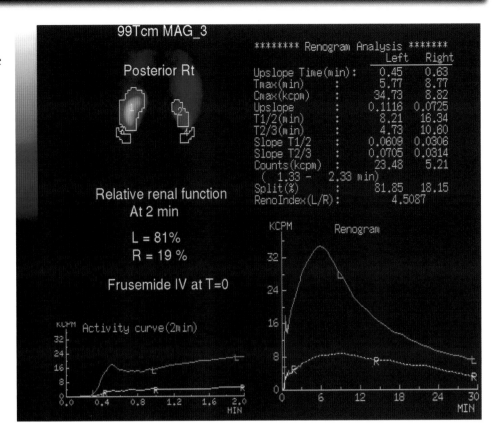

Figure 42.9 ^{99}Tc^m DMSA Static renal scan. These images represent renal function, and any scarring will be demonstrated as in the right kidney here. This represents areas of parenchyma without normal function

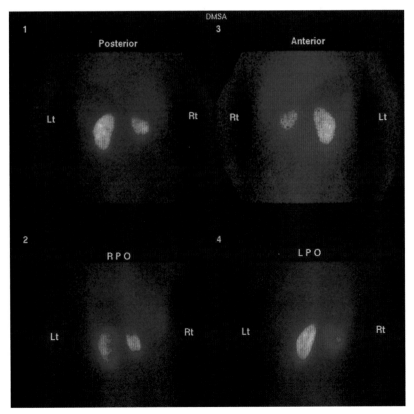

Figure 42.10 $^{99}Tc^m$ Sestamibi (MIBI) Myocardial perfusion scan at rest. Normal scan. These images show the conventional method of displaying the tomographic slices in three planes, horizontal long axis (HLA), vertical long axis (VLA) and short axis (SA). These images show a normal distribution of the tracer at rest – highlighting areas of functioning myocardium

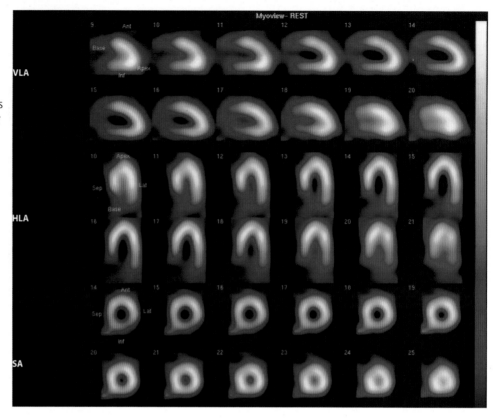

Figure 42.11 $^{99}Tc^m$ Sestamibi (MIBI) myocardial perfusion scan at rest. Abnormal scan. These images delineate areas of non-functioning myocardium with gross disease demonstrated in the infernolateral wall of the left ventricle as compared to Figure 42.10

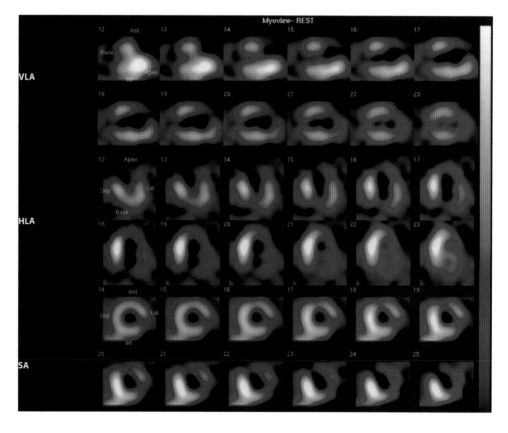

this feature has been exploited in imaging the 'hibernating myocardium', as it diffuses into viable, but apparently dysfunctional, myocardium over a delay of 4 hours. Thus it is possible to delineate areas of suspected hibernating myocardium, to inform subsequent treatment and possible revascularisation.[27]

Other RNI techniques

Radiolabelled white cells, mouse antibodies, $^{99}Tc^m$-HIG and ^{67}Gallium are used for targeting infection. The choice of radiopharmaceutical is usually made in the light of the medical history, and each has its own merit. The basic principle, however, is that the injected radiopharmaceutical will pool in an area of infection, and is especially useful in imaging infected orthopaedic hardware and pyrexia of unknown origin where the whole body may be imaged.

US and CT have largely taken over the role of imaging the liver but $^{99}Tc^m$ HIDA continues to be the method of choice for imaging the biliary tree. US is utilised for imaging calculi in the biliary system, but is not as consistent and specific as a HIDA in the diagnosis of acute cholecystitis. The radiographic cholecystogram in this respect should be considered obsolete.[25] HIDA is also useful in imaging biliary reflux, and in the confirmation of biliary leakage following surgery.

Technetium colloid can be used to image the lymphatic drainage of limbs, where it is not necessary to cannulate a lymphatic vessel directly. The technique is much easier to perform than a conventional lymphangiogram, and satisfactorily delineates areas of stasis.

PET

The poor availability of PET in the UK is largely due to lack of expensive dedicated scanning equipment situated in close proximity to a cyclotron.[18]-Fluorine FDG (^{18}F FDG) has clinical uses in oncology, neurology and cardiology. Being a glucose analogue, it has advantages of imaging glucose metabolism relating to disease and physiology, and the concentrated uptake in tumours linked with efficient coincidence scanning enables a highly sensitive diagnostic investigation to be performed. Its diagnostic advantages should see the modality proliferate in the years to come, as diagnosis and treatment becomes more targeted and cost effective, linked to enhanced patient care.

CURRENT IMPACT AND FUTURE DEVELOPMENTS OF RNI

The role of nuclear medicine within radiology is constantly changing. Examinations such as lung V/Q imaging, for example, which formed the mainstay of RNI work for many years, have recently been greatly reduced in many centres in favour of CT procedures. PET imaging is seen by many as the key area of development in NM. We can therefore expect to see rapidly increasing numbers of PET scanners and cyclotrons over the next few years and the development of new PET radiopharmaceuticals.

Traditional RNI still has an important future; the ability to potentially image any organ or physiological process is a powerful tool. New radiopharmaceuticals and technology will ensure that this functional imaging technique will find new uses as well as retaining the long established gamut of examinations such as bone scanning, renal function analysis and assessment of myocardial perfusion. Developments in radiopharmaceutical design are being made in receptor binding, monoclonal antibodies and labelled peptides and recent commercially available products include:

- ^{123}I-DaTSCAN (Ioflupane) for imaging dopamine transporters for the assessment of Parkinsonian syndromes.
- $^{99}Tc^m$-NeoSPECT (Depreotide), a labelled peptide, for the assessment of solitary pulmonary nodules
- CEA-Scan (Arcitumomab), a labelled monoclonal antibody fragment, for the diagnosis, localisation and staging of colorectal cancer.

Equipment evolution is also an important factor in the future utility of RNI. There are many developments on the horizon which could have a significant impact[28] including:

- Photodiodes to replace PMTs. These solid state devices are much smaller and more robust than PMTs. They also have a greater dynamic range and are significantly more efficient at detecting light.
- Solid state gamma ray detectors to replace scintillation crystals. Solid state detectors offer significantly better spatial resolution. One particular material that shows promise is cadmium zinc telluride (CZT) which also has desirable energy resolution and, unlike many solid state detectors, can be used at room temperature.
- Quantised detector gamma cameras. Instead of one large detector, these consist of many separate detectors positioned in an array. This has been explored both with scintillation materials (CsI – Digirad 2020tc Imager™) and solid-state detectors (CZT). The advantages of quantised detectors include fixed and improved intrinsic spatial resolution, true digital positioning, and application to PET imaging due to increased sensitivity at high count-rates. There is also no degradation in performance at the edge of the field of view as there is for single detector systems.

- New scintillator crystal designs or materials for hybrid SPECT/PET imaging. The stopping power of NaI(Tl) for 511 keV photons produced from positron emission is low. Sensitivity can be increased by using thicker crystals but this degrades the performance for $^{99}Tc^m$. Recent developments in crystal design have been made to improve sensitivity at high photon energies without this degradation at lower energies. One system (Bicron Starbright™) uses a 1 inch, two layer NaI crystal with one layer having slots etched into it to improve spatial resolution which would otherwise be lost due to the additional crystal thickness. The same company has also developed a curved crystal design to reduce distance from the patient with consequent improved spatial resolution. The use of new detector materials for SPECT/PET imaging is also being explored to improve stopping power. One of the most promising is lutetium oxyorthosilicate (LSO) which is already used in many dedicated PET systems. This material has much higher stopping power and a faster light output than NaI.

- Compton 'collimation'. The traditional collimator significantly reduces sensitivity and spatial resolution and imposes an inverse relationship between the two. Electronic collimation through the use of 'Compton cameras' has been researched to overcome this. The basic idea is to have an additional detector between the patient and the main detector. The gamma rays are Compton scattered by the first detector and are subsequently detected by the second detector. The interaction coordinates and the energy deposited are recorded for both detectors. The Compton effect can then be used to obtain the original source location within some uncertainty. Some success has been demonstrated in comparison with traditional collimators.[29]

- It is also worth mentioning that the inevitable increase in computer processing speed with time will also have an impact, particularly in areas of complex calculations such as scatter correction with iterative reconstruction techniques for SPECT/PET and for Monte Carlo simulations. The ability to carry out more calculations in a reasonable time is likely to lead to more accurate algorithms being developed.

In conclusion, developments are being made in radiopharmaceuticals, RNI equipment and computer power which, together, could significantly alter the quality and applications of RNI, ensuring continuing relevance for this unique and sensitive diagnostic service.

References

1. Bailey D, Adamson K. Nuclear medicine: from photons to physiology. Current Pharmaceutical Design 2003; 9:903–916.
2. Cassen B, et al. Instrumentation for I-131 use in medical studies. Nucleonics 1951; 9:46–50.
3. Anger HO. Scintillation camera. Review of Scientific Instruments 1958; 29:27–33.
4. Kuhl DE, Edwards RQ. Cylindrical and section radioisotope scanning of the liver and brain. Radiology 1964; 83:926–935.
5. Kuhl DE, Edwards RQ. Image separation radioisotope scanning. Radiology 1963; 80:653–661.
6. Brownell GL, Sweet WL. Localization of brain tumors with positron emitters. Nucleonics 1953; 11:40–45.
7. Administration of Radioactive Substances Advisory Committee. Notes for guidance on the clinical administration of radiopharmaceuticals and use of Sealed Radioactive Sources 1998.
8. Statutory Instrument 1999 No. 3232. The Ionising Radiations Regulations 1999. HMSO. United Kingdom.
9. The Ionising Radiation (Medical Exposure) Regulations 2000. London: HMSO.
10. Loevinger R, et al. MIRD primer for absorbed dose calculations. Revised edn. 2003.
11. Ryan, PJ, Fogelman I. Muskuloskeletal section. In: Maisey MN, et al. Clinical nuclear medicine. 3rd edn. London: Chapman & Hall; 1998.
12. Alazraki NA. In: Resnick WB, ed. Bone and joint imaging – radionuclide techniques. 2nd edn. London: Saunders; 1996.
13. Sharp PF, et al. In: Smith FW, ed. Practical nuclear medicine. 2nd edn. Oxford: Oxford University Press; 1998.
14. Perkins AC. Nuclear medicine – science and safety. London: John Libbey; 1995.
15. Brown M, et al. Technical aspects of bone scintigraphy. Radiologic Clinics of North America 1993; 31(4):721–730.
16. Mallinckrodt Medical BV. Summary of product characteristics 1996.
17. McKillop J, Fogelman I. Benign and malignant bone disease – clinician's guide to nuclear medicine series (British Nuclear Medicine Society). Edinburgh: Churchill Livingstone; 1991.
18. Klemenz B, et al. The influence of differences in hydration on bone-to-soft tissue ratios and image quality in bone scintigraphy. Clinical Nuclear Medicine 1999; 24(7): 483–487.
19. British Thoracic Society standards of care committee pulmonary embolism guideline development group: guidelines for the management of suspected acute pulmonary embolism. Thorax 2003; 58:470–484.
20. Martin W, et al. In: Sharp P, Gemmell H, Smith F, eds. Practical nuclear medicine. 2nd edn. Oxford: Oxford University Press; 1998:253–271.
21. Coakley A, Wells C. In: Maisey M, et al. Clinical nuclear medicine. 3rd edn. London: Chapman & Hall; 1998:331–381.
22. Billotey C, et al. Advantages of SPECT in Technetium-99-m-Sestamibi parathyroid scintigraphy. Journal of Nuclear Medicine 1996; 37:1773–1778.

23. Testa H, Prescott M. A clinician's guide to nuclear medicine – nephrourology. Amersham: British Nuclear Medicine Society; 1996.

24. Harding L, Notghi A. In: Sharp P, et al (eds) Practical nuclear medicine. 2nd edn. Oxford: Oxford University Press; 1998:181–183.

25. Harding L, Robinson P. Clinician's guide to nuclear medicine – gastroenterology. London: British Nuclear Medicine Society; 1990.

26. National Institute for Clinical Excellence. Technology Appraisal Guidance No.73: Myocardial perfusion scintigraphy for the diagnosis and management of angina and myocardial infarction. London: HMSO; 2003.

27. Pennell D, Prvulovich E. Clinician's guide to nuclear medicine – nuclear cardiology. London: British Nuclear Medicine Society; 1995.

28. Groch MW, Erwin WD. Single-photon emission computed tomography in the year 2001: instrumentation and quality control. Journal of Nuclear Medicine Technology 2001; (29):12–18.

29. Lacasta C, et al. Presented at institute of accelerating systems and applications, international conference on imaging technologies in biomedical sciences: Detectors for PET, SPECT, radiology and for in vitro imaging. 20–24 May 2001.

ULTRASOUND

Rita Philips, Mike Stocksley

INTRODUCTION

Ultrasound scanning is practised by medical staff (e.g. physicians, obstetricians, gynaecologists, paediatricians, orthopaedic surgeons, vascular surgeons) or non-medical ultrasound practitioners (e.g. radiographers, midwives, specialist nurses with appropriate training in ultrasound).

Images are created in real time using contact gel (essential to couple the sound through to the skin surface), gain settings (the controls used to produce an even spread of sound from surface to deep inside the patient's anatomy), focusing zones (depths inside the body at which the sound waves are focused), appropriate frequencies (quoted in MHz – millions of cycles per second) and suitable transducers, sometimes called 'probes' (the hand-held instruments that are placed on the body and produce the sound waves).

When obtaining images, there is no constraint of absolute centring points, and no rigidity of technique to adhere to. Every sonographer will answer a question, often in a slightly different way to another colleague, influenced by their own technique and experience. Images obtained are largely reminders of the real-time examination that has been performed. The images are, for the most part, in grey scale, although examinations of blood flow add colour and on most contemporary machines there is the ability to alter the grey scale to brown, blue, red and yellow scale in order to enhance the individual sonographer's perception of the image.

Ultrasound is a valuable method of imaging, owing to its lack of ionising radiation and ability to provide much useful information without producing clinically significant biological effects. It is therefore ideal for obstetrics, gynaecology and paediatric studies. It can be seen in real time, which is essential for dynamic studies; several sections can be seen in one gentle sweep allowing organs to be seen distinct from one another and pathologies sited correctly. Unlike plain film radiography, ultrasound does not take an image from front to back or side to side with all the inherent overlying structures. Electronic callipers can measure structures directly and accurately as, unlike plain radiography, there is no magnification of the image owing to a sizeable object film distance.

The patient can be scanned in most directions subject to size, shape and gas distribution – ultrasound needs only a change in the position of the transducer unlike those modalities requiring computer reconstruction in order to obtain different planes.

This is not to say that ultrasound has no use for computers, indeed sophisticated computers are used to create 3D and 4D (moving 3D) images for some areas. However these computers are not so unwieldy that all the components cannot be constructed in a small space.

The growing popularity of medical ultrasound over the last 20 years and the increasing detail that it can demonstrate has ensured that the workload is steadily increasing. Recently the number of non-obstetric scans has increased at a greater rate than obstetric scans.[1]

EQUIPMENT AND TECHNOLOGY

Awkward analogue static B-mode scanners in the 1970s used single crystals of fixed frequency that were selected and slotted into the end of an articulated arm linked to a heavy fixed gantry in order to produce static images. Now, digital ultrasound machines are extremely mobile and are seen being moved to the bedside in wards, intensive care units and to the operating theatre table. Even smaller versions are available; latest generations of ultrasound equipment are similar or smaller in size to a laptop computer. These are able to help diagnosis in clinics or theatre within the hospital setting and are of equal, if not more, importance, in the emergency situation in the trauma room or at the scene of a road traffic accident.

Modern equipment has much computer software on board that allows the sonographer to calculate lengths, volumes, estimate fetal weight and growth trends, calculate delivery dates and measure neonatal hip angles.

■ B-mode grey scale imaging

Dynamic images of the highest quality can be obtained in real time, cutting the time per scan by more than a half. Images are now obtained using lightweight probes with linear (used for superficial structures or musculoskeletal scanning), curved linear (used in the majority of cases for abdominal and obstetric scanning), phased sector (some abdominal and paediatric scanning) and transvaginal or transrectal configurations and often with multiple frequencies. The old problem of near field reverberation artefact that obscured some superficial detail unless a water bath or gel blocks were used, has been eliminated with dedicated superficial structure or 'small parts' transducers.

The rule of thumb regarding frequency used is that the higher the frequency, the better the resolution but this is at the expense of transmission of sound into the body. Conversely the lower the frequency, the better the transmission of sound into the body, but the lower the resolution. In practice, an average adult liver is scanned using a 3.5 MHz transducer where the sound needs to reach the posterior part of the liver (15–20 cm in depth approximately) while a thyroid gland or testes would be scanned by a 7.5 MHz transducer (only 2–5 cm of depth is required).

■ Doppler ultrasound

Duplex ultrasound is the combined use of grey scale and spectral, colour, or power Doppler (Fig. 43.1).

Spectral Doppler measures the velocity of moving blood within a small sample of a vessel. It is shown as a display of velocity against time and usually is shown simultaneously next to a grey-scale B-mode image of the sample.

Colour Doppler was introduced in 1982. It gives a real-time image with tissue in grey and blood flow in colour. It uses Doppler ultrasound to analyse the frequency, amplitude and phase information. It measures a velocity of blood cells at each pixel in a chosen area and assigns a colour to a range of velocities, normally red or blue, based on whether the direction of blood is towards or away from the transducer. Blue and red should not be taken as meaning veins and arteries (Fig. 43.2).

Power Doppler assesses the strength of the Doppler signal. It ignores the frequency components, instead con-

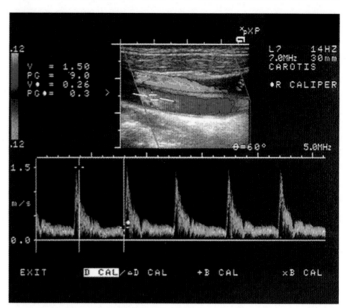

Figure 43.1 Duplex Doppler view of carotid artery. Reproduced with permission from Philips Medical Systems

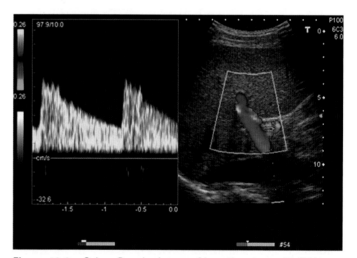

Figure 43.2 Colour Doppler image of hepatic artery with PW Doppler. Reproduced with permission from Toshiba

centrating on the total energy of the Doppler signal. The colour relates to the moving blood volume rather than the direction or velocity of flow. Colour Doppler shows blood flow direction and velocity and is less affected by tissue or probe motion than power Doppler although the latter is slightly more sensitive. Power Doppler can be used where the flow is slow through smaller vessels (Fig. 43.3).

■ Ultrasound images

The first grey scale analogue images were captured by a camera held up to a screen and imaged using high contrast individual Polaroid film. 35 mm photographic film, rolls of photographic paper or film, and later, multiformat

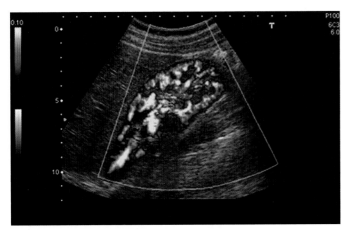

Figure 43.3 Power Doppler image of right kidney. Reproduced with permission from Toshiba

imagers, were also used to record a number of images on paper or X-ray film. Many of these methods were time consuming and laborious. Images had the identity of the patient written on the back of the film before the advent of the character generator that could print the patient's name on the film.

The image, patient details, and scanning factors can now be recorded in a number of ways at the push of a button, for example:

Static imagers
- Laser printer
- Laser imager
- Dye sublimation imager
- Thermal wax transfer
- Ink jet printer

Dynamic imagers
- Video – analogue
- Video – digital
- Cineloop
- CDROMs

Picture, archiving and communication systems (PACS) have enabled all imaging modalities, reports, previous records, examinations and notes to be stored digitally for ease of transfer of information within the hospital and across sites, leading to the so-called filmless, paperless departments. Telemedicine has allowed long distance reporting and opinions to be made when the specialist is not on site.

Images are captured and kept within the recording system of the equipment used such as a hard drive or digital video recorder then transferred or copied to another storage area allowing the images on the equipment's own storage system to be deleted. Rapid access short-term storage is used to store active images being reported or for review. Digital dynamic review is able to digitally store short dynamic real-time clips in order to offer a real-time review of parts of a scan as an alternative to static images. After a period of time, dependent on available space for short-term storage, these images are downloaded to a long-term storage system such as magnetic digital linear tape or optical disk.

Technical advances

Broadband digital ultrasound

This was developed in the 1990s and used digital beam forming technology to control pulses applied to each transducer element. This led to benefits in spatial resolution and contrast allowing display of subtle tissue structures and subsequently to a more confident diagnosis. Broadband technology has led to better image quality.

Harmonic imaging

Harmonic imaging processes the backscattered ultrasound to produce an image from harmonic frequencies rather than the basic frequency used originally.

Multiples of the original transmitted frequency are produced during the passage of the sound wave through the body and they increase in intensity before being attenuated. A filter removes the basic echoes so only the higher frequency harmonic signal is processed. The harmonic beam is narrower than the transmitted beam with less side lobes improving the signal-to-noise ratio. Harmonic signals are not generated near the surface so are spared degradation as they enter the body. They are produced after entering the body and originate from deeper structures, thus harmonic imaging improves resolution in obese subjects (Fig. 43.4A,B).

Contrast media

Contrast media can be used with ultrasound to enhance lesions in the same way as in computed tomography (CT) and magnetic resonance imaging (MRI). Research has taken place in the last 15 years into echo-enhancing ultrasound contrast agents. Thin-shelled microbubbles, (suspended stabilised bubbles or gas bodies) the size of red blood cells (a few microns in diameter), are used to increase the strength of the backscattered ultrasound signal. They resonate at the same lower frequencies used in ultrasound scanning. When insonated, the microbubbles increase the echo signal strength by approximately 1000. About 10 000 000 microbubbles are used in each intravenous injection. Performance of contrast agents is linked to the characteristics of the ultrasound pulses used to insonate the contrast and in processing backscattered signals. There has to be a word of caution here. The introduction of gas bodies has the potential, when activated by ultrasound, to produce some minor biological effects,[2] although there

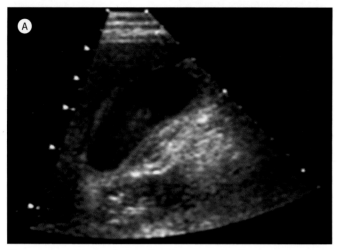

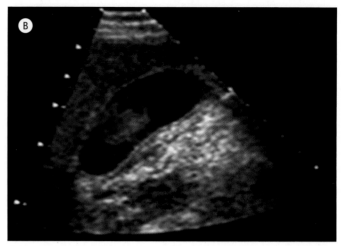

Figure 43.4   Harmonic imaging demonstrating improvement in image of the gall bladder: **(A)** image without harmonic imaging; **(B)** image with harmonic imaging applied

have been no reports of significant adverse reactions in humans. As their use is increasing, the effects must be monitored continually.

Real-time compound imaging

This steers sound at several angles rather than just perpendicular to the probe surface. High level reflectors are enhanced, and low level reflectors and noise are reduced, improving the resultant image. This uses a similar technique of compound scanning to the early static machines where the probe was manually moved in a series of small arcs around the structure in order to build up an improved picture with sound meeting the interfaces at right angles in as many places as possible. It has been used for scanning several structures including the breast.[3]

Extended field of view (EFOV)

Real-time ultrasound has a disadvantage of being limited in the field of view depending on the transducer choice. Using new computer algorithms, a position-sensing image registration based technique allows panoramic images to be produced in real time with no loss in resolution. An echo tracking process that estimates probe motion is available on many modern systems. It is as simple as pressing a button on the transducer and making a long sweep along the region of interest. This innovation is useful for differentiating between pathology and the surrounding structures. It is most useful for superficial structures such as the neck and scrotum where comparison of sides is required, but less useful in the abdominal/pelvic regions except to image large masses (Fig. 43.5).

3D ultrasound imaging

Data is collected as a number of 2D sections which can be reformatted in a variety of ways such as multiplanar reformatting, surface or volume rendering. Power Doppler with 3D imaging can be used with volume rendering to demonstrate blood flow.

COMMON CLINICAL INVESTIGATIONS

◼ Upper abdomen

Ultrasound is very reliable for investigations of the soft tissue organs of the upper abdomen especially in subjects with relatively normal body habitus while CT is often considered better for examining the patient with more adipose tissue. The speed, lack of ionising radiation dose, and low cost of ultrasound usually lead to its initial use.

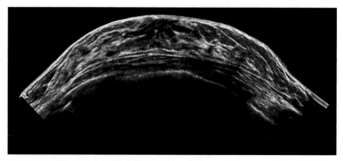

Figure 43.5   Extended field of view – scan of breast. Reproduced with permission from Philips Medical Systems

Liver and bile ducts

Ultrasound has long been utilised in the examination of the hepatobiliary system. Although surrounded by ribs, sternum, intercostal muscles and colonic gas, the liver can be scanned from a number of positions using transducers with a small footprint (the part in contact with the skin) and with a configuration that allows sound to enter through small areas on the surface and to fan out to obtain information at depth in the body. A thorough knowledge of anatomy and technique allows the sonographer to use inter- and subcostal approaches in order to scan the liver. Careful scanning technique is required as there are some areas in the liver that are technically quite difficult to visualise, namely the extreme right lateral border and the left lateral and superior borders.

Ultrasound can be used to help evaluate liver texture, which can be described as homogeneous (normal spread of similar texture), heterogeneous (abnormal spread of different textures), and of high or low reflectivity (brighter or darker than normal). The long promised tissue characterisation by computer has unfortunately never materialised.

The size of the liver based on a right hemidiaphragm to inferior border measurement in the midclavicular line can indicate a large or small liver and liver volume can be calculated. Blood and bile vessels can be assessed for size with electronic callipers and blood flow measured by colour flow Doppler. Diffuse pathology such as cirrhosis and fat infiltration and focal lesions such as simple cysts, haemangiomas and metastases can usually be confirmed or excluded.

Ultrasound should be the initial investigation for suspected focal pathology. It can demonstrate metastases with varying ultrasonic appearances but despite there being some correlation between appearances and primary site (such as highly reflective lesions possibly arising from a gastrointestinal primary), there appear to be too many differential appearances. Some metastases can show the same reflectivity (isoechoic) as normal hepatic parenchyma and may be missed. Where ultrasound is equivocal or surprisingly normal given clinical or biochemical results, CT or MRI can be used to investigate further: also when full staging and planning is required or prior to hepatic resection, although ultrasound is being increasingly used in this situation.

Small haemangiomas in the liver can be seen clearly by ultrasound although CT/MRI show the characteristic features of haemangiomas greater than 1 cm in size more reliably. Colour Doppler can demonstrate blood flow to a metastatic or primary lesion (although this is not always foolproof) but it does not demonstrate any flow to haemangiomas owing to an almost imperceptible flow. Very occasionally, power Doppler will demonstrate a small blood supply to a haemangioma.

In cases of jaundice, ultrasound can confirm surgical jaundice by the presence of dilated intra- and extrahepatic ducts as distinct from medical jaundice that appears essentially normal. The level of obstruction can often be clearly demonstrated by the level at which the ducts or gall bladder is seen to be normal. For example, dilated common hepatic duct and intrahepatic ducts with a normal or small gall bladder and common bile duct would demonstrate a high obstruction of the cystic duct or above, while a fully dilated biliary system would indicate an obstruction at the lower end of the bile duct. If the pancreatic duct was dilated as well, an ampullary/head of pancreas obstruction may be indicated. However, in early cases of obstruction, changes to duct calibre may be subtle.

The common bile duct can be seen and assessed for normality/dilatation but the lower half is often quite difficult to see owing to the gas filled duodenum lying anterior to it. Stones in the lower portion of the common bile duct are also difficult to see for this reason and because there is rarely much bile in a narrow duct to outline a stone. Endoscopic ultrasound (EUS) consists of a small transducer within an endoscope. It is an exceptionally accurate tool in scanning the bile duct for choledocolithiasis[4] and with fine needle aspiration (FNA) has an accuracy of 91% for lymph node staging in cases of cholangiocarcinoma.[5]

Ultrasound is also extremely useful for accurate guidance of a biopsy needle to the area of tissue required for sampling. Two cores from a biopsy needle are taken when cirrhosis is suspected or in the evaluation of a transplant liver in cases of rejection. With focal lesions, a core biopsy is taken in suspected hepatocellular carcinoma and FNA is used for all other lesions. The needle tip is scanned as it enters the body and can be seen in real time as it approaches the lesion or tissue required. Careful technique is required but continual monitoring of the needle tip can avoid the unnecessary penetration of vessels or organs during the procedure (Figs 43.6, 43.7).

Gall bladder

Ultrasound is the method of choice in the initial investigation of the biliary system and has long replaced the oral cholecystogram. Preparation for a hepatobiliary ultrasound scan involves the patient fasting for 6–8 hours in order to fully dilate the gall bladder. For those who lament the loss of the radiographic function test, ultrasound can examine the gall bladder after a fast and after a fatty meal in order to compare the size of the gall bladder pre and post contraction (gall bladder kinetics).[6] Gall bladder volume

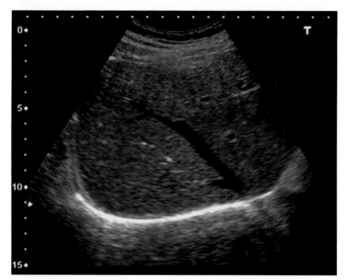

Figure 43.6 Normal liver showing hepatic vein. Reproduced with permission from Toshiba

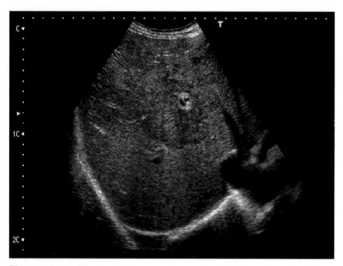

Figure 43.7 Liver with tumour demonstrated. Reproduced with permission from Toshiba

can be calculated using a formula based on 3 measurements although a computer program can be used where available. In addition, variation in shape (Phrygian cap, septate, double), position (intrahepatic, low lying), wall thickness and relevant pathology such as gallstones (the most common), biliary sludge, polyps and tumours, can all be observed.

If the examination is urgent and there has been no time for fasting, a scan of the biliary system can still take place albeit with the caveat that a contracted gall bladder can occur as a result of pathology and also after eating recently.

The flexibility of ultrasound allows patients to be scanned in different positions according to needs, not least to image the organs but to confirm or exclude the adherence of a mass to the inner wall of the gall bladder (stones move freely within the gall bladder lumen unless impacted; polyps and tumours adhere to the lumen).

The ability to turn the patient in the middle of the scan can help to stretch the neck of the gall bladder and allow better visualisation of that area in order to exclude impacted stones. Ultrasound has a sensitivity of >95% and positive and negative predictive values of near 100% in the detection of gallstones.[7] Unlike plain radiography that will only see about 10% of gallstones unless outlined by contrast media as in the oral cholecystogram, ultrasound sees all stones as being similar, irrespective of composition. It takes CT to find out the composition of gallstones although some attempts have been made with ultrasound.[8] Higher frequencies and accurate setting of focussing zones will demonstrate smaller stones and their characteristic posterior shadowing, although the shadow will not be seen if the stone is only partially scanned in the beam thickness.

In 95% of cases of acute cholecystitis, there is often a stone impacted in the neck of the gall bladder. The gall bladder can necrose and perforate if not treated with antibiotics to control inflammation. However, there can be an absence of stones in acute cholecystitis after surgery, extensive burns, major trauma and parenteral nutrition, therefore the absence of stones on an ultrasound scan is insufficient to exclude acute cholecystitis. Radionuclide imaging is more sensitive here.

Cancer of the gall bladder is the fifth most common gastrointestinal malignancy and is associated in many instances with the presence of gallstones. Ultrasound has the ability to identify concomitant gallstones and the irregular wall thickening of a malignancy or bulky polypoidal mass. Colour flow Doppler and B-mode imaging can be used to investigate invasion and obstruction of biliary/portal vessels by tumour and spread to the liver.

The real-time attributes of ultrasound can also be helpful in visualising biliary ascaris that can be seen writhing in the jejunum. Occasionally they move up the common bile duct (CBD) and into the gall bladder causing cholecystitis and obstruction of the ducts.

Pancreas

Ultrasound can discern a normal pancreas, especially in normal sized patients, and can evaluate the lower end of the bile duct through the head of the pancreas. The pancreatic duct can be measured and dilatation excluded or confirmed, dilatation implying distal obstruction. Inflammatory conditions, calcification and pseudocyst formation can be seen, as can tumours in the head and body of the pancreas. Tumours in the tail of the pancreas, while significantly less common, are more difficult to see owing to gas in the stomach. CT and MRI are useful in cases of necrotic and severe pancreatitis.

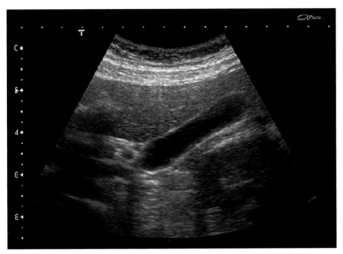

Figure 43.8 Normal gall bladder. Reproduced with permission from Toshiba

The pancreas is harder to see in patients with more adipose tissue, CT will show the anatomy more clearly in these cases. CT will also show calcification in the pancreas more clearly in chronic pancreatitis although EUS has excellent sensitivity when detecting biliary microlithiasis.[9] EUS is good for detecting pancreatic tumours although MRI is best for staging tumours. However, EUS is good at staging many upper gastrointestinal malignancies such as the oesophagus, stomach, duodenum, duodenal ampulla and bile ducts. In addition, EUS can allow safe FNA under ultrasound control.

Spiral CT and EUS have similar accuracy in staging pancreatic cancer.[10] With EUS FNA of pancreatic lesions, the specificity is 94%, sensitivity 86% and accuracy 88%.

Urinary system

In any examination of the urinary system, ultrasound can be used to confirm the presence of two kidneys, which is essential information in the emergency situation where nephrectomy may be a possibility. Electronic callipers can accurately measure the dimensions of the kidney. Differences of 15% or more between each kidney can be significant. Renal volume can be calculated, normal parenchymal thickness can be observed and measured, and normal contours confirmed.

The normal position of the kidneys can be confirmed or, if an ectopic or transplant kidney is present, its location within the abdomen or pelvis can be determined. Variation of kidney shapes and sizes can be observed, from the absent kidney on one side with a corresponding hypertrophy of the contralateral one, to cross-fusion anomalies of which the horseshoe kidney is the most common.

In cases of haematuria, ultrasound (and a plain abdominal X-ray) is used as the first line investigation of the urinary tract; the source of the blood can be from a renal, bladder, or prostate tumour.

Ultrasound is able to see hydronephrosis and its severity as it has 95% sensitivity, and can help in assessing the level of obstruction. The use of colour Doppler can exclude a pseudohydronephrosis, seen on B-mode, caused by prominent renal vessels. Renal stones can be seen on ultrasound especially when the kidney is scanned slowly and carefully, the stones are not too small and they are identified by their highly reflective (white) appearance and posterior acoustic shadowing. They can be clearly seen in the renal pelvis when outlined by urine, but are less obvious when situated in the calyceal system without urine around them as both structures are highly reflective and the stones are indiscernible. The sensitivity of ultrasound in detecting renal calculi is higher than that of abdominal radiography but lower than CT.

Ureteric stones, a common cause of obstruction, are rarely seen on ultrasound as ureters can only normally be seen when leaving the renal pelvis and on their insertion into the bladder (owing to overlying intestinal gas obscuring the mid-ureters). Patency of the ureters can usually be implied by the presence of ureteric jets, the appearance of the passage of urine into the bladder seen at their insertion at the base of the bladder by grey scale or colour Doppler. Colour Doppler can be useful in scanning the renal vascular system and is used to image, with spectral Doppler to analyse, the renal arteries in 80–90% of cases. Obesity and overlying stomach and bowel gas sometimes prevent imaging of the renal vessels, particularly on the left. Colour Doppler is helpful in diagnosing renal vein thrombosis and is the accepted first line of investigation for renal artery stenosis.

Renal lesions can be seen, such as common simple cysts seen in 50% of those over 50 years of age. Ultrasound is used to screen those related to patients with adult polycystic disease. CT and MRI are useful for staging and assessing more complex solid and cystic lesions seen by ultrasound. In suspected renal cell carcinoma, ultrasound is usually the primary imaging modality to confirm tumour presence and size. Colour or power Doppler is used to assess renal vein and IVC tumour involvement. CT/MRI is used subsequently for staging and treatment planning. Small tumours are increasingly being detected incidentally at an early stage on ultrasound scans and subsequently venous invasion is less commonly seen.

If it persists for more than 72 hours, infection of the renal system is investigated by ultrasound to exclude any complications such as abscess or obstruction.

Transplant kidneys can be scanned with a higher frequency because of their superficial position. B-mode real-time scanning is useful in excluding obstruction caused by impinging post-operative haematomas or lymphoceles, and demonstrating fluid collections such as urinomas. Renal vein thrombosis or stenosis can be excluded with colour Doppler ultrasound.

Contrast enhanced CT is superior to ultrasound in determining the extent of post-traumatic abnormalities although ultrasound is often used to assess the kidneys amongst other organs in the trauma situation.

Adequate hydration is essential preparation for demonstrating the bladder. For adults, drinking ½ to ¾ L of water 1 hour before the due time of the scan allows the bladder to distend. Ultrasound can clearly demonstrate the bladder wall and any pathology inside such as tumours (fixed irregular masses), stones or foreign bodies (normally seen with associated posterior shadowing). Ultrasound is useful in being able to measure the bladder wall thickness when distended and when empty, and can demonstrate residual volume after micturition, the volume being calculated using the formula for an ellipsoid (length × width × height × 0.53). Most ultrasound machines can calculate this automatically on demand after measurements have been taken in all three planes. Transitional cell carcinomas (the most common bladder tumour) can be detected along the posterior wall near the trigone. Bladder diverticulae can also be assessed easily with ultrasound and any contents of the diverticulum imaged. Ureteroceles are easily detected by ultrasound and are seen as dilated ends of the distal ureters protruding into the bladder at the region of the trigone.

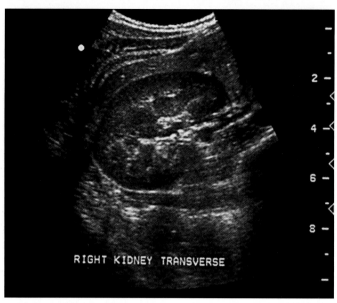

Figure 43.10   Transverse view of right kidney. Reproduced with permission from Philips Medical Systems

Prostate

A common cause of bladder distension in older men is the enlarged prostate.

Any enlargement of the prostate will be seen transabdominally by scanning with caudal direction at the base of the bladder. Scanning in this way will only give an indication about the size of the prostate (it can be measured and translated into a volume and subsequently into a weight). Outline and reflectivity and whether calcification can be seen are almost the limit to transabdominal prostate scanning.

Transrectal sonography of the prostate requiring a specially designed intracavitary probe gives more detail of the prostate gland but despite hopes of it becoming a screening tool for detecting prostate carcinoma, its sensitivity is in the region of 60%. In addition, it is not specific enough to assume that any focal lesion is cancerous so the transrectal scan usually accompanies a prostatic biopsy for accurate sampling. 70% of cancers are hypoechoic (darker) and 30% are hyperechoic (brighter) than the normal part of the gland. 75% are situated in the peripheral zone. Classically, a prostatic cancer should be hypoechoic and in the peripheral zone but only 20–30% of lesions here are actually cancers whereas the rest are inflammatory patches, atrophy, fibrosis and benign prostatic hyperplasia. Digital examination and prostate specific antigen (PSA) tests in addition to biopsy are more common methods of assessing a problematic prostate than using imaging alone. CT/MRI is used for subsequent follow up with confirmed prostatic cancer in order to stage and treat the disease.

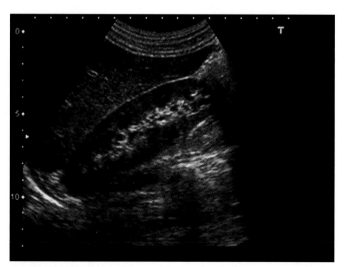

Figure 43.9   Longitudinal view of right kidney. Reproduced with permission from Toshiba

Spleen

The spleen is usually scanned as part of the whole upper abdominal examination in conjunction with the liver in portal hypertension, left upper quadrant pain, suspected splenic infection, and when an enlarged spleen is found at clinical examination. It is also useful as an acoustic window in order to see the tail of the pancreas and upper half of the left kidney. Ultrasound can, like the liver, be used to measure the length of the spleen from the left hemidiaphragm to the inferior border where 13 cm is usually used as an upper limit of normal. In cases of trauma, ultrasound is invaluable for detecting haematoma. It can detect splenic lacerations and ruptures but is less accurate than contrast enhanced CT. However there is the advantage of being able to bring ultrasound to the patient in unstable cases.

Ultrasound is useful in detecting cysts; these are usually the result of trauma and haematoma formation. In Hodgkin's or non-Hodgkin's lymphoma, 25–33% of patients have splenic involvement. There can be diffuse, focal or multifocal appearances, most of which are of low reflectivity. Ultrasound can detect splenomegaly, although this may be absent in one-third of these patients. Of lymphoma patients, up to one-third of enlarged spleens are of a benign nature. Although ultrasound can be used to guide a biopsy needle in the spleen, it is not often performed owing to the spleen being highly vascular and at greater risk of haemorrhage. It can be used to differentiate between a lymphoma and metastasis or to diagnose infection such as candida or tuberculosis.

Lymph nodes

Ultrasound is able to detect lymph node enlargement, depending on location and size. Enlarged lymph nodes are often seen in the upper abdomen, paraaortic region, neck and axilla. For cases of mesenteric lymph node enlargement, ultrasound is useful in differentiating nodes from bowel loops. It can be useful in guiding needles for biopsy.

Aorta and IVC

Ultrasound is used to scan both the great vessels within the abdomen. The inferior vena cava (IVC) is examined with ultrasound and colour Doppler in cases of newly found renal tumours and suspected IVC thrombosis.

However, it is the aorta that is examined in far greater numbers. Ultrasound is useful for the detection and monitoring of abdominal aortic aneurysms and for measuring the diameters and lengths. Extension of the aneurysm to the

common iliac arteries can also be seen if present. Siting of the aneurysm relative to the renal arteries is also possible by ultrasound but is more accurate by CT and MRI, especially in larger patients. Thrombus can be seen clearly.

Doppler can sometimes be used to assess leakage after endovascular stent graft, showing as areas of blood flow outside the lumen of the graft but inside the walls of the aneurysm. Colour Doppler can image aortic dissections by demonstrating flow in both channels, these are sometimes seen on an initial B-mode ultrasound examination, but it is not the modality of choice as intimal flaps can be hard to see. Aortic rupture is also hard to see owing to overlying bowel gas although the presence of fluid in the peritoneal cavity can be seen on ultrasound and is an important indicator suggesting rupture. CT is the modality of choice for detecting a ruptured aorta but the emergency situation often precludes the use of CT and the patient is taken to theatre on clinical evidence with or without ultrasound being performed.

Screening of the aorta with ultrasound has been considered for several years within Europe and the USA. Studies have reported one-time screening of the aorta to be cost effective in 60–65 year olds in the Netherlands.[11] One-time screening is also considered cost-effective in the USA for men aged 65-79 years who smoke or who have smoked[12] and in the UK, for men aged between 65 and 74 years; the cost is at the margin of acceptability after 4 years, substantially improving by 10 years.[13]

Alimentary canal

Often considered difficult to scan by ultrasound because of the gas contained in the bowel, there has been more interest in scanning this area in recent years, especially in

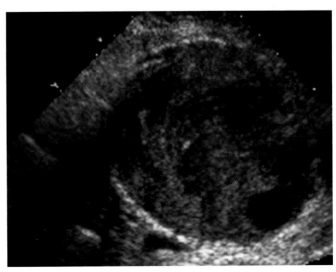

Figure 43.11 Transverse section of abdominal aortic aneurysm

cases involving young and pregnant patients for whom ionising radiation is to be avoided. Higher resolution scanning with recent equipment can enable the layers of the bowel wall to be seen in some cases. Careful compression can sometimes be performed in order to move gas away to reveal fixed diseased segments. Here, thickened bowel wall is usually present, peristalsis is not observed and the lumen can narrow. Colour Doppler can help to demonstrate inflammation of the bowel wall.

Obstruction can be seen by distended, fluid filled bowel loops proximal to an obstruction although these are sometimes obscured by gas filled centrally placed bowel.

Better images have been seen using a retrograde water infusion to distend the colon (hydrocolonic sonography) or ingesting water to see the stomach and small bowel. However, this is not common practice. Flexible sigmoidoscopy, CT virtual colonoscopy, and barium enema are still preferred for imaging the colon.

In cases of intussusception, lack of demonstration of blood flow indicates necrosis and the need for immediate surgery.

Ultrasound, with clinical evaluation, is useful in evaluating pyloric stenosis in infants. It is used in cases of appendicitis. The patient is scanned using a linear high frequency probe and graded compression (pushing gently over the area of pain to move away gas to bring the area of interest closer to the depth seen by high frequencies). This technique has a sensitivity of 89–96% in children and a specificity of 89–98%.[14] The normal appendix is seen in $\frac{1}{4}$–$\frac{1}{2}$ of paediatric patients. Although CT may be more accurate in imaging the appendix, ultrasound has the advantage of being able to see any gynaecological pathologies that might mimic acute appendicitis.

EUS, a combination of high frequency ultrasound (7–12 MHz) and endoscopy, is being increasingly used in the detection and staging of upper gastrointestinal (GI) malignancies including the oesophagus, stomach, duodenum, extrahepatic bile ducts and the pancreas. It can carry out needle aspiration, and tissue samples can be taken from the gut wall, lymph nodes and surrounding organs. The advantage is the proximity at which it can be placed near to the region of interest. This allows a high frequency 12 MHz probe (able to transmit sound only 2.5–3.0 cm) to be used with resultant high-resolution images. EUS is more accurate than CT or MRI in the T-staging of oesophageal cancer.[4] With the additional use of fine needle aspiration (EUS-FNA) the diagnosis can be obtained at the time.

Superficial organs (known as 'small parts')

For these structures, a higher frequency (7.5 MHz and above) small footprint transducer (usually linear array) is used.

Thyroid

Ultrasound can visualise the lobes, isthmus, anterior and posterior muscles and main vessels (common carotid artery and internal jugular vein) during a scan of the thyroid gland. The extended field of view facility available on some equipment is especially good at including all structures on one image as small footprint transducers are traditionally too small to include both lobes on the same image and comparison of texture between one lobe and the other is more difficult. Callipers can measure and confirm the normal size of structures. The largest indication for scanning the thyroid is a nodular thyroid. Ultrasound can differentiate between benign characteristics of a hypoechoic/isoechoic nodule with cystic elements and a malignant characteristic of solid, hypoechoic mass with microcalcifications and cervical lymphadenopathy, especially if those in the jugular chain are round in shape.

Microcalcifications seen by ultrasound show the highest accuracy, specificity and positive predictive value for malignancy as a single sign.[15] Ultrasound and ultrasound guided FNA biopsy increases the effectiveness in diagnosis. Ultrasound is used for diagnosis and staging in malignant cases although CT and MRI are used to assess the local extent of spread (Fig. 43.12).

Parathyroid glands

Normal parathyroid glands are almost never seen with ultrasound. Adenomas are often oval in shape and their long axis lies along the long axis of the patient. They are of low reflectivity and solid and homogenous. They can be round or teardrop in shape. The sensitivity for scanning parathyroid adenomas is 34–92%, with most in the

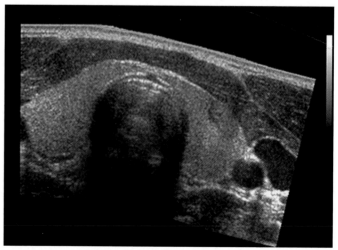

Figure 43.12 Thyroid. Reproduced with permission from Philips Medical Systems

70–80% range.[7] Colour Doppler can demonstrate their hypervascularity but small and deep lesions are difficult to see.

Neonatal head

Ultrasound has the advantage of being mobile and can be used to scan an infant in a special care baby unit either in or out of the incubator. Using a 5 MHz or higher sector probe, the infant brain can be scanned through the anterior fontanelle until between 9 and 15 months approximately, when it closes.

Immediately after birth or for the first 4 days in premature babies, the germinal matrix can haemorrhage owing to its rich vascular supply being disrupted by change in blood pressure. In skilled hands, ultrasound can detect intraventricular haemorrhage, hydrocephalus and some parenchymal bleeds. Monitoring the appearances can detect the occurrence of periventricular ischaemia and periventricular leukomalacia. Fast MRI scans are used when more complex anomalies are investigated.

Neonatal hip

Using a 5.0–7.5 MHz linear probe, confirmation of developmental dysplasia of the hip can be made between 3–6 weeks according to appearances and measurements taken of the acetabulum, femoral head and ileum. Dynamic studies can be performed by real-time ultrasound to demonstrate instability while the hip is manipulated. Partial or complete dislocation can be demonstrated. Radiographs have the obvious inherent problem of ionising radiation compared with ultrasound. They are also difficult to interpret until the infant is 6–12 weeks old as it is difficult to see the cartilaginous head. A radiograph also is only a record of the hip joint at one time with the infant supine; an ultrasound scan of a dynamic physical examination is a far more comprehensive assessment of the hip during a range of movements. Ultrasound can also detect hip effusions and be used to guide a needle into the joint space to drain fluid if required.

Breast

Ultrasound is used to assess the female and male breast when X-ray mammography is not appropriate, either because of the radiation dose or because the structure of the breast is too dense for mammography. Grey scale ultrasound is utilised for the initial evaluation of palpated abnormalities and differentiation between benign and malignant lesions felt or seen on a mammogram. Ultrasound is more useful than mammography for symptomatic breast problems. It is also helpful in the assessment of the breast with implant. Ultrasound is not used in the UK as a routine screening tool owing to its lower sensitivity than mammography.[16] It can, however, be used to screen high-risk younger women unsuitable for mammography as long as the limitations are recognised and understood. Complete evaluation of both breasts using ultrasound is extremely time consuming as a screening tool. Only 40–50% of cancers seen on MRI can be seen with ultrasound.[17]

Microcalcifications with diameters of 0.2–0.5 mm seen on mammography are a sign of ductal carcinoma in situ (DCIS). Breast ultrasound cannot clearly image clustered microcalcifications. They produce no acoustic shadowing at that size at frequencies of 7.5–10.0 MHz although some higher frequency probes (10–15 MHz) are being introduced. Microcalcifications can sometimes be seen within a mass, but when outside, as is often the case with DCIS, they are very difficult to see.

Ultrasound is the localisation technique of choice for breast biopsy. Cyst aspiration can be performed without image guidance, but ultrasound enables direct visualisation of the needle into the cyst and confirmation that the cyst is completely empty after aspiration. It is more accurate when performing biopsy of a tumour within a cyst. Ultrasound guided fine needle aspiration cytology (FNAC) along with clinical examination is considered to be the best approach for a definitive answer to many equivocal situations.

Testes

Ultrasound is the primary modality for the investigation of the scrotum. Using a high frequency, linear array transducer, it is used in the evaluation of the scrotum in epididymitis, inflammation, hydroceles, torsion of the testis, trauma and testicular masses. In cases of torsion, ischaemia

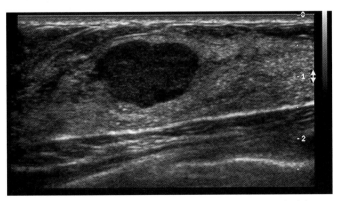

Figure 43.13 Breast containing mass lesion. Reproduced with permission from Philips Medical Systems

is considered relative to the amount of torsion, starting in venous compromise to arterial occlusion. Varicoceles can be seen on grey scale and enhanced by colour Doppler during the Valsalva manoeuvre.

Tumours are usually well seen with ultrasound and are of lower reflectivity than the rest of the testis. Colour Doppler can demonstrate an enlarged flow to the tumour. On occasions, the whole testis is infiltrated with tumour and therefore the texture of both testes should be compared on one image. If a germ cell tumour (the most common testicular tumours in young adult men) is suspected on ultrasound, both ultrasound and CT are used to search for nodal metastases in the retroperitoneum. If biopsies of metastases elsewhere in the body indicate that they are secondary to a germ cell tumour, ultrasound of the testes is indicated and if nothing is seen there, scrotal MRI can be performed. Testicular microlithiasis can also be seen and has a high association with malignancy. Ultrasound can be used to detect an undescended testis, which is important owing to the markedly increased incidence of testicular cancer in these cases. It is usually found in the inguinal canal or within the abdomen although in the latter case, this can be difficult especially in larger adults.

Musculoskeletal

Ultrasound is being used increasingly in the diagnosis of musculoskeletal disorders as higher resolution equipment can give excellent detail of muscle, fat, ligaments, tendons and cartilage. It can be used to image most joints, the shoulder (rotator cuff injuries), wrist, elbow and knee being the most common. The knee is often also imaged with MRI. A high frequency 7.5–10.0 MHz linear array transducer is

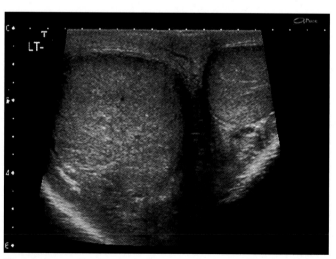

Figure 43.14 Testes with right-sided tumour demonstrated. Reproduced with permission from Toshiba

the probe of choice. Extended view imaging can also be useful in places. Modern equipment provides better spatial resolution than MRI and has the benefit of being able to scan during a dynamic movement.[18]

Good technique is vital in scanning muscle/ligament/tendon as sound not directed at 90° to the muscle will show a pseudo fluid area owing to the reflection strength being less and a consequent reduction in reflectivity (anisotropy). Ultrasound can demonstrate complete tendon and muscle tears, inflammation, differentiate solid/cystic/complex masses and if the mass is vascular. It is less accurate in partial tears and, as usual, is operator dependent. It can help to locate foreign bodies in the extremities and identify fluid collections and guide drainage needles to the site of the fluid collection. Improved colour Doppler can examine small vessels within the extremities.

Carotid arteries

Spectral and colour Doppler are used to assess the carotid arteries in patients with cerebral vascular accidents (CVAs), transient ischaemic attacks (TIAs), if dissection or embolus is suspected, or prior to surgery. The common carotid, the first 2–3 cm of the internal carotid, external carotid and vertebral artery are usually examined. A 5.0-7.5 MHz transducer is used depending on the size of the neck. Flow and flow velocity information can be seen with spectral Doppler. Colour and power Doppler is used to assess stenosis and occlusion and to demonstrate plaque. For total or near total occlusions, magnetic resonance angiography (MRA) should confirm ultrasound findings. Computerised tomographic angiography (CTA) or MRA is used when results are equivocal on ultrasound. Catheter angiography is the gold standard. 3D ultrasound is being used in research to demonstrate plaque dimensions with more accurate measurements.

Leg veins

B-mode grey scale and Doppler ultrasound is a well-established technique for the detection of deep vein thrombosis (DVT), despite conventional venography still being considered the gold standard. Ultrasound has a sensitivity of more than 95% and specificity of 98% for femoral popliteal DVT, although the figures are lower for calf DVT.[7] It is the initial modality of choice for detecting DVT owing to low cost, ease of examination, lack of ionising radiation and ability to demonstrate other causes of leg pain and swelling. It is limited in pelvic or calf veins and in swollen limbs and large body habitus. A 5 MHz or higher linear array probe for grey scale is used; lower frequencies are used for colour Doppler. The noncompressibility of the vein is the most sensitive and specific finding for thrombus. Thrombus can sometimes be seen on grey scale imaging.

Echocardiography

Ultrasound is used to image the heart and surrounding structures. It is helpful in establishing diagnoses and the severity of various acquired and congenital cardiac diseases. It can evaluate cardiac chamber size, wall thickness and motion and the proximal great vessels. Information regarding function can also be derived. Mass lesions in the heart and outside can be detected as can the accumulation of pericardial and pleural fluid. M-mode (one dimensional format), B-mode (2D) and Doppler are all used. Many diagnoses can be obtained from the scan and the other cardiac based tests that the patient undergoes. The position of the heart being surrounded by bone and lung means that the anatomical windows through which the heart is scanned are very small and consequently, dedicated cardiac transducers with small footprints are usually used.

EMERGENCY ULTRASOUND

The non-intrusiveness of ultrasound makes it ideal as an imaging modality in the emergency room in cases of blunt abdominal trauma. Recent advances in reducing size and weight of the equipment have enabled ultrasound to be carried not only to the bedside but also to the roadside in cases of road traffic accidents and on the battlefield. Focused abdominal sonography for trauma (FAST) is now usually performed in place of peritoneal lavage in the detection of intrabdominal haemorrhage, a sign of serious abdominal injury.

A quick scan looks at 6 areas:

- Heart
- Right upper quadrant and subhepatic space
- Right lower quadrant
- Left upper quadrant
- Left lower quadrant
- Midline pelvis

A quick assessment of these areas in a hypovolaemic patient, perhaps with lowered level of consciousness, can save much time in contacting a surgeon if free fluid is found.

Using ultrasound to detect fluid in the abdomen was first described in 1988[19] and although it is used widely in the USA, it was slower to be implemented in the UK. Major organ laceration in liver, spleen and kidney, missing organs or shifted organs can be seen. Ultrasound is less sensitive than CT in detecting parenchymal damage to these organs and cannot detect bowel injuries but it is useful for patients who are hypotensive and cannot be stabilised for CT or to assess stable patients. Bowel gas and body habitus can limit the examination.

In addition to focused scanning in blunt abdominal trauma, ultrasound contributes to other aspects of emergency care such as abdominal aortic aneurysms, foreign body localisation, abscess location and gynaecological emergencies.

Emergency ultrasound in gynaecology

Patients presenting to the A&E department usually do so with acute pelvic pain. The first line of investigation is clinical palpation and a pregnancy test for women of child-bearing age, usually to exclude/confirm a pregnancy, followed by a pelvic ultrasound scan.

The role of ultrasound in these instances is primarily to exclude an ectopic pregnancy by the identification of intrauterine implantation and secondly in the detection of an extrauterine gestation sac or ruptured ectopic pregnancy when pelvic free fluid from a ruptured corpus luteal cyst or ectopic pregnancy may be demonstrated. Quantitative serum beta human chorionic gonadotrophin (hCG) assays and an ultrasound scan are vital for patient assessment and management.

In the case of a non-pregnant patient, acute pain can be the result of ovarian torsion, torted cyst, ruptured ovarian cyst, torted pedunculated fibroid or appendiceal abscesses. This results in haemorrhage, and/or the presence of free fluid in the pelvis, especially in the Pouch of Douglas (rectouterine pouch) or surrounding an ovary. These can be useful ultrasound indicators. In some cases there may be echoes within the free fluid that represent blood or pyogenic material as may be in the case of pelvic inflammatory disease (PID). Patients usually complain of low bilateral abdominal pain. Ultrasound findings include free fluid in the pouch of Douglas along with a hydrosalpinx or pyosalpinx, and tuboovarian abscess.

GYNAECOLOGY

Gynaecological ultrasound is utilised primarily, in the assessment of the uterus, endometrium, ovaries, and the fallopian tubes. Other structures can also be visualised during a pelvic scan such as vagina, cervix, bowel, pelvic vessels and musculature, and the urinary bladder. It is also used in the location of intrauterine contraceptive devices, and the exclusion of post-operative complications such as pelvic haematoma, and abscesses. One-stop gynaecology clinics with ultrasound as a first line investigation have made patient management more streamlined and effective. The use of ultrasound is also invaluable in infertility studies.

Different ultrasound scanning techniques are used for obstetric and gynaecological scans; these include transabdominal, transvaginal, transrectal, intraoperative, transperineal/labial examinations and spectral Doppler and colour flow Doppler examinations.

The endometrium and ovaries are dynamic organs undergoing changes throughout a woman's life, on a day-to-day basis in cases of women of child-bearing age. Therefore before any interpretations and diagnosis can be made, it is imperative that the sonographer is aware of the:

* patient's history: age and menstrual status, i.e. prepubertal, premenopausal, menopausal and recent cycle history
* clinical indications: abdominal distension; palpable pelvic mass; abnormal bleeding per vagina; pelvic pain; dyspareunia, amenorrhoea, dysfunctional menstrual bleeding, and post-menopausal bleeding
* past gynaecological history including any previous gynaecological surgery which must be known, as must medication such as the oral contraceptive pill, hormone replacement therapy (HRT) and tamoxifen, which may have an influence on the appearances of the ovaries and the endometrium

In the case of women of child-bearing age, results of a recent pregnancy test should always be sought to rule out possibility of pregnancy-related complications such as an ectopic pregnancy.

Technique

The two main approaches to pelvic ultrasound examinations are transabdominal and transvaginal scans. The decision as to which one is utilised needs to be evaluated according to the clinical indications, the information required and the suitability of the patient. As a rule, generally, both methods are advised to give a comprehensive approach to the scan, in terms of gross pelvic anatomy, position of the ovaries, presence of large pelvic/abdominal masses, and the detailed assessment of the uterus, endometrium, ovaries and any tubal pathology.

In cases of significant pelvic pathology such as large pelvic masses or suspected malignancy, distant associated pathology should also be excluded. These include hydronephrosis, lymphadenopathy, and the presence of ascites. The combination of both these approaches can also aid in the detection of non-gynaecological pathology such as appendicitis, diverticular disease, inflammatory bowel disease e.g. Crohn's disease, and pathology such as ureteric calculi and bladder tumours in the case of the urinary tract.

Transvaginal scans (TVS)

Due to the proximity of the organs to the transducer, a higher frequency can be used ranging from 6 MHz to 8 MHz. This gives an increased resolution which is essential when evaluating endometrial thickness, or assessing ovarian architecture. The need for a full bladder is eliminated, hence making the examination more comfortable for the patient. Superior images are gained especially in obese patients. However, this examination is not always appropriate as it can be perceived as invasive in terms of privacy for some patients, and due to the intimate nature of the examination, not suitable for minors. It also has an added disadvantage, in terms of a narrow field of view making it difficult to image high and lateral organs, and distinguishing the absolute margins of a large pelvis mass.

Transabdominal scans (TAS)

This mode of scanning offers a wider field of view, is non-invasive and suitable for most patients. However, to visualise the uterus and ovaries adequately, a full bladder is required to displace the overlying bowel gas and lift the pelvic organs out of the pelvic cavity. It also straightens the uterine long axis so that it can lie perpendicular to the transducer ultrasound beam. A transabdominal scan uses frequencies in the range of 3 MHz to 5 MHz depending on the subject characteristics. This can result in a poorer resolution compared to a TVS, especially in the case of an obese patient. This decreased resolution has also the potential to miss small pathologies. Recent advances in transducer technology have allowed an EFOV so that large pathology can be related to other anatomical landmarks.

Assessment of the uterus

The uterus can be assessed on an ultrasound scan for its size, shape and outline as it undergoes normal physiological changes resulting from age.

Ultrasound imaging is useful in diagnosing uterine congenital abnormalities such as bicornuate uterus, didelphic (double uterus) unicornuate and septate uterus and also demonstrating changes in the myometrium. It can indicate the presence of serous, or intramural fibroids. Adenomyosis, the presence of endometriotic deposits within the myometrium, is at times difficult to detect except in the classic cases of an enlarged uterus with low reflective deposits located within the myometrium.

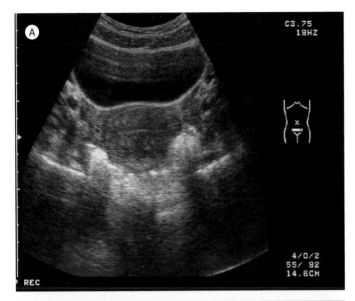

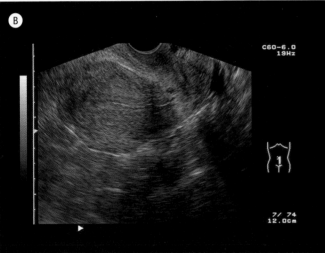

Figure 43.15 **(A)** Transabdominal transverse scan of the uterus; **(B)** transvaginal longitudinal scan of the uterus. Reproduced with permission from Toshiba

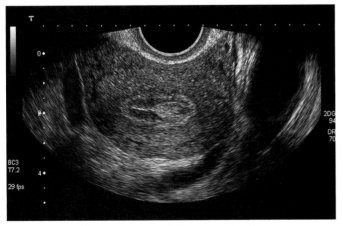

Figure 43.16 Transverse scan of the uterus showing an endometrial polyp. Reproduced with permission from Toshiba

Endometrial assessment

The endometrium is best visualised with a high resolution, transvaginal scan, and should also be assessed with the knowledge of the patient's menstrual history. This is particularly important in the presence of abnormal vaginal bleeding. In a menstruating woman, the endometrial thickness and echo pattern varies according to the menstrual cycle; the upper limit of normal varies with different studies but is in the region of 14–20 mm. Vaginal bleeding in a post-menopausal woman can be a cause for concern as there is a higher incidence of endometrial malignancy, however, in the majority of these women, there will be a benign cause for the bleeding such as hyperplasia or polyps. An upper limit of a total endometrial thickness of 4 mm will reliably exclude any significant endometrial pathology, although in the presence of HRT, this value is more like 8–10 mm and 10 mm in the case of tamoxifen therapy.

While transvaginal ultrasound demonstrates morphological characteristics of the endometrium, (thickness, integrity, presence of intracavity masses, fluid), transvaginal colour Doppler enables the assessment of blood flow velocity and vascular impedance in the cases of endometrial carcinoma and the vascular resistance in the uterine arteries and its branches. It also has the capability of providing additional information such as abnormal endometrial perfusion. The accuracy of TSVs will be further increased with new technological advances such as 3D sonography allowing endometrial volume assessment.[20] Simultaneously imaging the endometrium in all three planes may be invaluable in the morphological evaluation and diagnosis of tumours, and enhance the detection of myometrial tumour spread that is currently assessed by MRI.

Ultrasound and infertility

Diagnostic ultrasound plays a crucial part in the assessment and management of the female reproductive tract. Initially, it is important to evaluate the normality of the uterus, endometrum, ovaries and the patency of the fallopian tubes. Ultrasound is used to exclude the presence of pathology that may be the cause of the infertility. Conditions such as endometriosis, chronic pelvic inflammatory disease, multiple fibroids and endometrial pathology such as polyps may all play a part in the prevention of a successful journey and implantation of the embryo. Ovulatory disorders resulting from ovarian dysfuntion can also be assessed by ultrasound investigations. These include polycystic ovaries and failed luteal phase follicular rupture. It is important to remember ultrasound is not specific in these cases.

Contrast medium studies such as *hy*sterosalpingo *c*ontrast *s*onography (HyCoSy) have been successful in replacing the conventional hysterosalpingogram in the assessment of tubal patency and the uterine cavity.[21,22] Obvious advantages are that it is a safe investigation using non-ionising radiation. Saline can be introduced in the endometrial cavity to outline any pathology such as polyps, submucosal fibroids or adhesions, while contrast medium such as galactose monosaccharide microparticles (Echovist) can be introduced into the uterine cavity, and observed to determine tubal patency.

Ultrasound is a useful tool in monitoring the development of ovarian follicles following stimulation by drug inducement. It can determine the size and number of follicles, the timing of ovulation and assess endometrial response. These observations, along with serum hormonal monitoring, also help prevent ovarian hyperstimulation and avoid the possibility of multiple pregnancies of a large order. In in vitro fertilisation (IVF) studies, ultrasound is primarily used as a guiding tool in the aspiration process of the mature follicles. After successful conceptions/ implantations, ultrasound can be used to determine the number of gestational sacs and embryos and to exclude ectopic pregnancies.

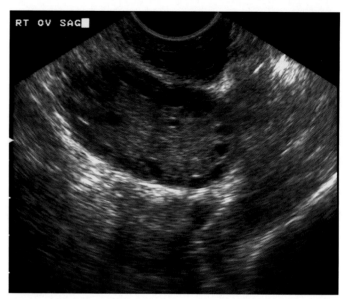

Figure 43.17　Enlarged polycystic ovary. Reproduced with permission from Toshiba

■ Ovarian assessment

The size and texture of the ovaries depend on the reproductive status of the patient, for example in the prepubescent patient, immature follicles can be visualised within the ovaries. After menarche, these follicles can be visualised maturing, with the development of a dominant follicle measuring between 2.0–2.5 cm in diameter before ovulation. In the post-menopausal patient, ovaries appear atrophied with no evidence of follicular activity.

Ultrasound is sensitive in detecting ovarian pathology, however features like wall thickness, echogenicity, posterior enhancement/shadowing and internal architecture, all aid to derive differential diagnosis such as dermoid cysts, endometrioma, Brenner cysts, cystadenomas, and cystadenocarcinomas.

Sonomorphologic scoring systems have been derived looking at these features to assess ovarian tumours.[23] Occasionally, pathology not related to the ovaries can be detected such as paraovarian cysts, pedunculated fibroids and broad ligament cysts. Further assessment of adnexal and tubal masses can be improved using Doppler and 3D ultrasound where the sensitivity and specificity is reported to be 89% and 97% respectively.[24]

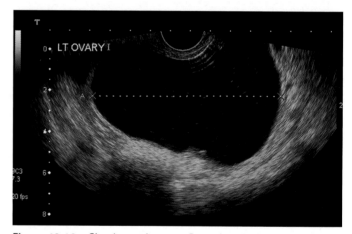

Figure 43.18　Simple ovarian cyst. Reproduced with permission from Toshiba

■ Screening for gynaecological malignancy

Screening for early ovarian cancer in asymptomatic and high risk women using ultrasound and CA125 have been evaluated in the last decade. However, there is as yet no conclusive evidence to suggest an impact on the survival rates. Similarly with endometrial assessment, there is no evidence to date to support endometrial screening.[25,26]

The main pitfalls in gynaecological ultrasound are inadequate patient preparation such as an empty or over-distended bladder in the case of transabdominal scans, or a full or partially full bladder in case of a transvaginal scan resulting in artefacts such as reverberations causing the uterus to appear retroflexed, or increasing the distance between the pelvic organs and the transducer. Inadequate history taking can also lead to misdiagnosis or over-diagnosis.

Bowel shadowing can be problematic in not only obscuring the relevant organs but also mimicking some pathology. In these cases, patience is required to observe the peristalsis in the bowel, or gentle abdominal pressure should be applied to the area of interest to disperse the bowel. Indeed in some cases the opposite may occur where pathology can mimic bowel; this is common in the case of dermoid cysts due to the heterogeneous echo-pattern resulting from the contents of the cyst. Previous adhesions resulting from surgical interventions, PID or the presence of non-ultrasound detectable endometriotic deposits can be problematic in the assessment of pelvic organs due to the resultant immobility.

OBSTETRICS

The scope of prenatal scanning has undergone a significant change since its introduction in the 1980s. The primary use then was to reduce obstetric risk to the mother and child by estimating correctly the gestational age, placental localisation and exclusion of multiple pregnancies. These diagnostic observations enable effective pregnancy management such as monitoring of fetal growth and well-being in the presence of abnormal clinical findings and maternal disease such as diabetes and hypertension. As imaging technology has evolved, along with society's expectations, there has been an increased focus on its use as a screening modality in terms of structural and chromosomal abnormalities through anomaly and nuchal translucency scans. This in turn has the inevitable burden on training and expertise and, more importantly, ethical concerns and prenatal counselling. Current advances in ultrasound (3D sonography, for example) have enabled further fetal detail to be imaged, and in the current climate of high expectations from parents for a 'perfect baby', its potential to be abused is apparent. Although it is important to keep up with these new advances, the balance between 'risk' and 'benefit' must be maintained.

◼ Overview of fetal biometrics

Evaluating large groups of fetuses with normal growth patterns has derived standard tables and curves of fetal measurements. These can be used as a reference to assess fetal gestational age and growth patterns.[27]

Gestational sac

This is the first measurement of early pregnancy. The gestational sac is measured in three planes and a mean sac diameter (MSD) calculated. This measurement is useful between 5 and 8 weeks gestation with an accuracy of +/- 0.5 week and is usually performed in the absence of an ultrasonically demonstrable fetal pole (Fig. 43.19).

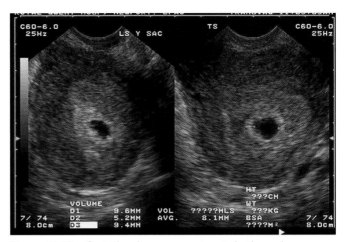

Figure 43.19 Gestational sac measurements in three planes. Reproduced with permission from Toshiba

Crown rump length (CRL)

This is performed by measuring the longest axis of an embryo, and is useful to determine the gestational age, with accuracy being +/- 3-5 days. The main pitfall is including the yolk sac in the measurement, resulting in over-estimation of the gestational age. After the first trimester, there is the potential to under-estimate the CRL due to the flexion of the fetal spine, therefore this measurement is not advised after 14 weeks (Fig. 43.20).

Fetal head measurements – bi-parietal diameter (BPD) and head circumference (HC) (Fig. 43.21)

These measurements are usually best after 12 weeks, and are taken at the widest diameter of the fetal head, transversely across the parietal bones, and are used to determine gestational age. Presence of identifiable landmarks such as the thalami and cavum septum pellucidum makes them a robust measurement for repeatability, although the accuracy decreases with increasing gestational age (14 weeks accuracy is +/- 1 week; 30 weeks is +/- 3-4 weeks).

As head size is dependent largely on fetal brain development, these measurements are less affected by conditions like placental insufficiency and are often spared in fetal growth restriction. When there is evidence of fetal head growth restriction, it is usually associated with symmetrical growth retardation as a result of genetic, toxic, or infectious factors, or microcephaly.

The accuracy of BPD measurement is dependent on the shape of the fetal head, and can result in under- or over-estimation in the presence of fetal head moulding. The fetal head circumference is therefore a more reliable measurement, as it allows for the variation in fetal head shape.

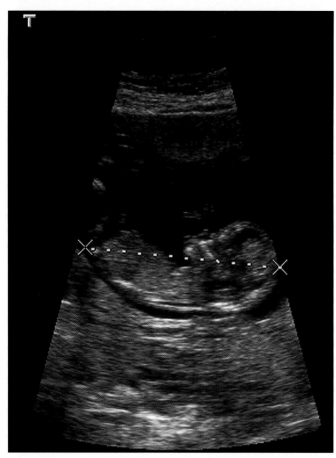

Figure 43.20   CRL measurement. Reproduced with permission from Toshiba

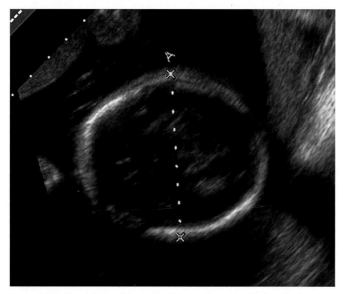

Figure 43.21   BPD measurement. Reproduced with permission from Toshiba

Femur length (FL)

This has the same accuracy as a BPD measurement, and is a reliable measurement after 14 weeks to estimate gestational age. It can be affected by skeletal dysplasias, but on the whole, as with fetal head measurement, inconsistencies are usually associated with intrinsic fetal problems.

Abdominal circumference (AC)

This measurement is obtained as a circumference of the fetal abdomen, through the fetal liver, at the level of the left portal vein and stomach. It is crucial in the assessment of fetal growth and well-being. Deficiencies in the nutrient storage such as subcutaneous fat and liver glycogen will decrease this measurement in the setting of maternal/placental insufficiencies, resulting in a 'starved' fetus. The opposite occurs in conditions such as maternal/gestational diabetes whereby elevated blood glucose levels result in increased metabolic storage and increased fetal subcutaneous fat, causing macrosomia.

Serial AC measurements are required to monitor the fetal growth pattern in such cases in order to plan pregnancy management and, if necessary, early delivery of the fetus. The ratio of head measurement and abdominal measurement is also used to identify symmetrical/asymmetrical growth patterns.

■ First trimester

The main aims of a first trimester scan are:

- to exclude an ectopic pregnancy
- confirm ongoing pregnancy especially in the setting of vaginal bleeding and pain
- establish gestation age and estimated date of delivery (EDD) when menstrual history is inadequate. Factors such as infertility treatment, use of the oral contraceptive, and menstrual history are important in establishing gestational age, vital for post-term pregnancy management.

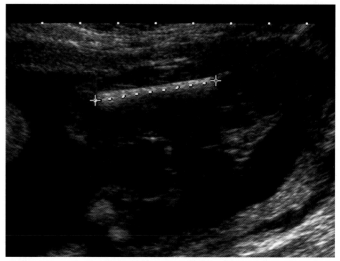

Figure 43.22   FL measurement. Reproduced with permission from Toshiba

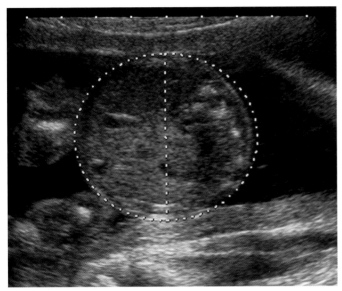

Figure 43.23 AC measurement. Reproduced with permission from Toshiba

Decidual reaction can be visible within the uterus as early as 4 weeks, with the presence of a gestation sac at 5 weeks. The gestation sac should be eccentrically placed with the presence of a yolk sac and amnion within the sac (Fig. 43.24A,B). This observation can help distinguish between a pseudo-sac of an ectopic pregnancy or some fluid collection in the cavity and a true gestation sac.

An early dating scan can also exclude multiple pregnancy, or determine the chorionicity of multiple pregnancies in order to aid appropriate management. Sonographic criteria used in the diagnosis of chorionicity are the number of placental sites, the lambda and T signs and the thickness of the inter-twin membrane[28] (Fig. 43.25A,B).

Early pregnancy assessment

Early pregnancy assessment can be performed in one-stop clinics designed to streamline the service and select appropriate patient management, thus eliminating the need for unnecessary admission. These units are usually carried out as an outpatient service, and are aimed at women with bleeding in the first trimester. Indeed, recent studies advocate the use of conservative management in the case of missed miscarriage, and report a decrease in the incidence of dilatation and curettage (D&C) induced infection, and the prevention of adhesions and Asherman's disease, which can complicate future pregnancies.[29,30]

The role of ultrasound in this situation is to confirm an ongoing intrauterine pregnancy, or diagnose a failed pregnancy such as missed miscarriage or incomplete miscarriage. Follow-up studies for women presenting with bleeding in the first trimester showed that 17% of these women had a subsequent miscarriage, however, in the presence of a yolk sac and fetal heart activity, 95% of pregnancies proceeded to term.[31] Gestational sac volumes (GSV) and mean sac diameters (MSD) can be calculated to aid estimation of gestational age before a fetal pole can be demonstrated. These measurements are also very useful in the diagnosis of an anembryonic pregnancy (blighted ovum) where there is an absence of fetal pole or embryonic parts. Once a fetal pole is visualised, fetal heart pulsations should be demonstrated, and recorded with motion mode scanning. A crown rump length is measured to establish gestational age.

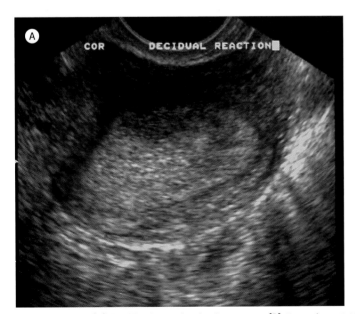

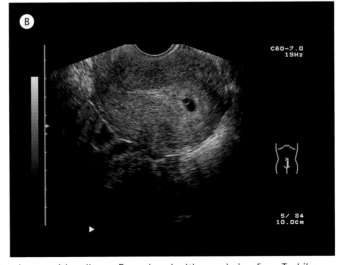

Figure 43.24 (A) Decidual reaction in the uterus; (B) 5-week gestational scan with yolk sac. Reproduced with permission from Toshiba

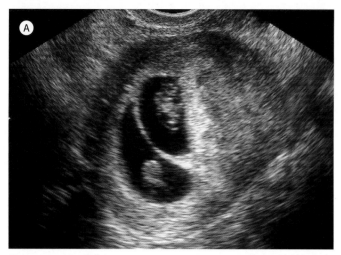
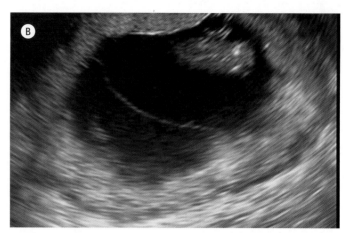

Figure 43.25 (A) Lambda sign for dichorionic, diamniotic (DCDA) twin pregnancy; (B) T sign to show a monochorionic diamniotic twin pregnancy. Reproduced with permission from Toshiba

Early pregnancy assessment guidelines for diagnosing an early pregnancy failure are MSD of 20 mm or more without evidence of embryonic parts, an empty amnion sign, CRL of >6 mm with no heart activity or an absence of growth of the gestational sac or fetal pole after a 7–10 day interval.[32]

Trophoblastic disease such as complete hydatidiform moles and partial moles can also be detected with ultrasound scans in the first trimester. These women present with an enlarged uterus, elevated levels of bhCG, vaginal bleeding and hyperemesis. Typically on ultrasound, the uterine cavity is filled with trophoblastic tissue with swollen villi presenting as cystic areas. There may or may not be a presence of fetal pole depending on a complete or partial mole.

Occasionally, fluid collections around the gestational sac are detected during the ultrasound scan. These can be for reasons such as implantation bleeds, subchorionic, chorioamniotic and intraamniotic haematoma and can be a cause of bleeding in the first trimester. However, the presence of these does not necessarily affect prognosis although such women do experience further or prolonged bleeding in the presence of these findings.

Screening for abnormalities

Between the gestational ages of 11 and 14 weeks, a soft marker of nuchal thickening or nuchal translucency (NT) is considered to be a reliable screening parameter for chromosomal deviations, namely trisomy 21, trisomy 18 and trisomy 13.[33,34] NT is defined as the maximum thickness of the subcutaneous area between the skin and the soft tissues overlying the cervical spine. This shows up as a translucency on the ultrasound scan. NT screening encompasses a whole programme and is a risk assessment programme. This is based on a standardised measurement of the nuchal translucency, providing an individual risk estimate of trisomies 21, 18, 13 by combining maternal age, family history correlated with fetal gestational age and the NT measurement.

More recently, NT measurements are combined with maternal serum screening (MSS) for the combined test in the first trimester, and with the serum integrated test in the second trimester to enhanced detection rate of Down's screening. The detection rate is reported in the region of 89% for Down's syndrome with a false positive rate of <3%.[33,34] Increased NT is also associated with other non-chromosomal conditions such as cardiac defects, and diaphragmatic hernias, and skeletal dysplasias.[35] The observation of a nasal bone in fetuses is also reported to exclude chromosomal abnormalities in 99.5% of fetuses between 11–14 weeks.[36,37]

NT measurements, in multiple gestation, are also useful where conventional methods such as MSS are not applicable. For example, in dichorionic gestations, discordance for NT thickness is a useful marker for chromosome and other abnormalities. In monochorionic gestations, it appears to be a useful marker for potential twin–twin transfusion syndrome.[38]

With increased image resolution, transvaginal ultrasound scans are also reported to be effective in screening for structural anomalies in the first trimester. These include anencephaly, cystic hygromas, hydrops, renal anomalies, anterior wall defects and skeletal dysplasias.[39,40]

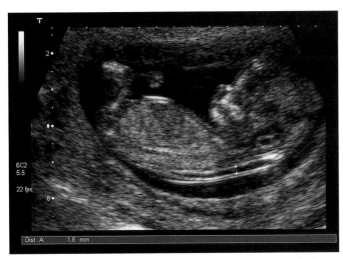

Figure 43.26 Nuchal translucency. Reproduced with permission from Toshiba

Second trimester

Prenatal screening for structural problems in the second trimester is now accepted as a normal procedure. The timing of the second trimester is usually taken as being between 18 to 22 weeks dependant on individual hospital policy. The majority of the screening population will have an apparently ultrasound normal scan given that the prevalence of major structural abnormalities in the UK population is in the region of 1–2%. Some of these abnormalities will not be detected by ultrasound alone. The women invited for the scan should be made aware from the outset of the main purpose of the scan. Bearing in mind advances in technology and knowledge, additional information regarding the detection rate and the limitations of the scan should also be explained to the woman and an informed consent obtained. All women capable of giving consent can accept or refuse any or all of the tests offered. Whatever the reason for an individual choosing or declining testing, the aim should be for each woman to have autonomy and support in the decision she makes for each pregnancy.

The equipment to identify fetal abnormality needs to be of a higher imaging specification than that commonly used in more general ultrasound testing in pregnancy. A range of transducer frequencies of between 3 and 6 MHz and transvaginal transducers in the range of 5–7 MHz are essential. Equipment should be no more than 5 years old unless electronic hardware and software upgrades are available, in which case the most recent relevant upgrade should be no more than 5 years old. A quality assurance programme should regularly monitor equipment performance. The equipment should also have colour flow Doppler capability for the diagnosis of complex cardiac abnormalities.

Many structural malformations can be identified by an ultrasound scan, however a normal scan result does not completely exclude abnormality in the fetus. It simply means that the operator observed no abnormality at the time of the scan. Apart from technical factors, suboptimal scan images may in part be related to maternal and pregnancy factors, for example it is difficult to obtain optimum images if the mother is overweight or if there is too little fluid around the fetus (Figs 43.27, 43.28, 43.29).

The commonest malformations detected by diagnostic ultrasound scanning are those affecting the central nervous system, urinary tract, gastrointestinal system, skeletal system and to a lesser degree the heart. Types of abnormality and their reported detection rates have been listed by the Royal College of Obstetricians and Gynaecologists.[41] If a single malformation is identified, it is important to examine closely all other systems for evidence of any associated anomalies. In some pregnancies, multiple malformations are detected initially by ultrasound scanning. Detailed

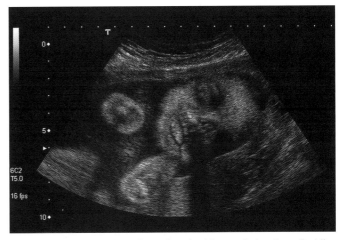

Figure 43.27 Fetal face. Reproduced with permission from Toshiba

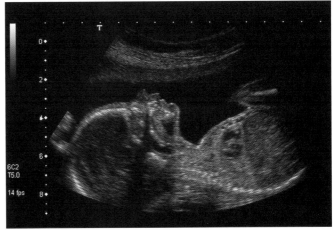

Figure 43.28 Profile of fetal face, thorax and abdomen. Reproduced with permission from Toshiba

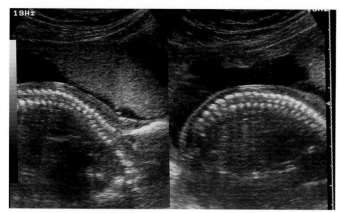

Figure 43.29 Longitudinal image of fetal spine. Reproduced with permission from Toshiba

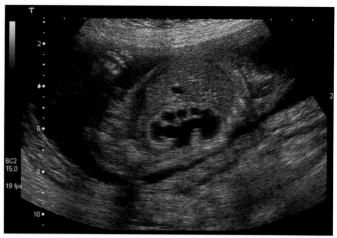

Figure 43.31 Hydronephrosis in fetal kidney. Reproduced with permission from Toshiba

diagnostic scanning should then be undertaken at a fetal medicine unit. Fetal karyotyping techniques, such as amniocentesis, chorionic villus sampling (CVS) and fetal blood sampling may then be performed to give a more definite diagnosis. If the pregnancy is to continue, provision may be required for ongoing care at a specialist antenatal clinic and contacts established with neonatologists and paediatricians.

Doppler studies can provide the sonographer with additional information in the differentiation between normal and abnormal fetal morphology, especially in the case of fetal echocardiography, where duplex Doppler and colour Doppler can enhance the visualisation of the cardiac chambers and major vessels and with the aid of pulsed Doppler spectral analysis, give more information of fetal cardiac haemodynamics. By delineating fetal or cord vessels, certain conditions can be confirmed in the presence of a suboptimal B-mode scan such as in cases of ectopic kidney, cord insertion in the presence of an omphalocoele, cord

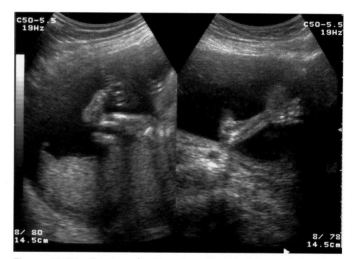

Figure 43.32 Fetal arm and leg. Reproduced with permission from Toshiba

cyst, nuchal cord, single umbilical artery and vasa praevia.

Careful examination of the vasculature of the placenta can aid the detection of placenta praevia, accreta and succenturiate lobes.

Interventional ultrasound guided techniques to obtain fetal tissue

- *Amniocentesis.* This procedure is usually undertaken during the mid trimester between 15 and 17 weeks for fetal karyotype, however it is also done in the third trimester for rhesus incompatibility. It accounts for about 90% of prenatal tests. A needle is inserted under ultrasound guidance through the maternal abdominal

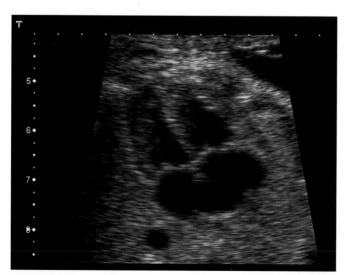

Figure 43.30 Four chamber view of fetal heart. Reproduced with permission from Toshiba

wall and into the amniotic sac around the fetus and a sample of amniotic fluid collected. Cells in the amniotic fluid have been shed from the surface of the fetus and membranes. These cells are then usually cultured for 10 days approximately before performing the prenatal diagnostic tests. Testing may involve chromosomal, biochemical or deoxyribonucleic acid (DNA) analysis. There is a procedure-related fetal loss or miscarriage rate of 0.5–1.0%. The main limitation of amniocentesis is the relatively advanced gestational age at which it is performed and the need to culture cells in the laboratory. Increasingly, fluorescence in situ hybridisation (FISH) analysis may be used for rapid diagnosis of some cases, particularly in women at an advanced gestational age.

- *CVS.* CVS can be performed in the first trimester of pregnancy, usually at 10–12 weeks of gestation. It can be performed transabdominally when a needle is passed through the maternal abdominal and uterine wall or transcervically, when a catheter or biopsy forceps is passed through the cervix into the uterus. Both procedures are performed under ultrasound guidance and the aim of the procedure is to obtain a sample of actively proliferating placental tissue. Both operator preference and the position of the placenta may determine the approach used. DNA analysis, limited cytogenetic analysis and some biochemical studies can be performed on uncultured chorionic villus tissue. Full cytogenetic analysis requires cells to be cultured. Fetal loss rates vary from 1–3%. CVS is particularly useful where DNA analysis is required for e.g. Duchenne muscular dystrophy.

- *Fetal blood sampling.* Cordocentesis or percutaneous umbilical blood sampling under ultrasound guidance are means of obtaining fetal blood cells. These cells can be used for the detection of haematological and some metabolic abnormalities. Chromosome analysis can also be undertaken and this method may be used to clarify some ambiguous chromosome results on amniocentesis or CVS. The fetal loss rate may be 1–3% when experienced personnel perform the procedure.

Chromosomal markers

Anatomical 'soft markers' are structural changes detected at an ultrasound scan which may be transient and in themselves have little or no pathological significance but are thought to be more commonly found in fetuses with congenital abnormalities, particularly chromosomal abnormalities.[34] Common examples are choroid plexus cysts (CPCs), renal pelvic dilatation (RPD), echogenic foci in the fetal heart, short limbs, echogenic bowel and nuchal thickening.

The observations of soft chromosomal markers and their relation to chromosomal abnormalities have been reported since the early 1990s, but to date, there still seems to be controversy regarding the usefulness of these markers. The impact of these soft marker observations has been studied in an unselected population over 6 years.[42] A 4% rise in the detection of fetal malformations was reported; however, the downside was that there was also a 12-fold increase in the false positive rate. Obvious concerns highlighted were resource implications, risk of pregnancy loss following invasive procedures, not to mention the psychological impact on the expectant parents.

Cost effectiveness of antenatal screening

A systemic review of cost effectiveness of antenatal screening highlighted two important factors:[43]

- The skill of the ultrasonographer and the time taken for the scan had a significant influence on the cost effectiveness of any ultrasound screening programme. Furthermore, ultrasonographers who are not properly trained may have a detrimental effect on clinical efficacy and on cost effectiveness
- Ultrasound screening for fetal abnormalities in the second trimester is cost effective, although this result holds only if termination of pregnancy is acceptable

This systematic review emphasises the need for better research on the costs and cost effectiveness of such screening, and the overall benefit in terms of maternal and fetal mortality and morbidity still remains to be a controversial issue.

MRI assessment for fetal abnormalities

Ultrafast MRI sequences have revolutionised the use of MRI for evaluating fetal abnormalities. Reported application currently is in the assessment of fetal brain development[44] and the differentiation of abnormal fetal thoracic and abdominal masses.[45] MRI has the added advantage over ultrasound in the case of reduced liquor volumes, where ultrasound assessment is difficult.

Third trimester

Ultrasound scanning in the third trimester is primarily carried out for fetal surveillance, for clinically small or large for dates gestations, poor obstetric history, multiple pregnancies and maternal conditions such as hypertension and diabetes. It is worth remembering that a one-off morphometric fetal measurement cannot identify the fetus that is constitutionally small for dates, or growth restricted. Serial growth measurements combined with Doppler investigations are needed, along with a fetal non-stress test (NST), and fetal biophysical profile (BPP).

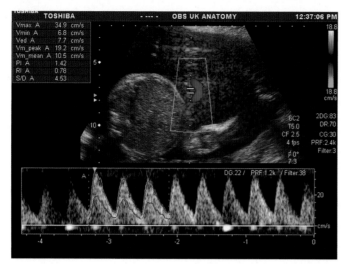

Figure 43.33 Umbilical artery Doppler. Reproduced with permission from Toshiba

From around 1985, Doppler waveform changes were associated with abnormal placental function. Fetal Doppler indices were initially developed for the detection of intra-uterine growth restriction and fetal hypoxia. Fetal growth restriction is a significant factor for increasing umbilical artery Doppler indices, which can identify the growth-restricted fetuses, which are at higher risk of adverse peri-natal outcome. These fetuses are metabolically compro-mised, with conditions of oxygen and nutrient depriva-tion. Vascular redistribution occurs in favour of vital organs such as the fetal brain (brain sparing effect) whereby there is a reduction in the end diastolic flow velocities in the umbilical arteries and an increase in the fetal cerebral vascular end diastolic flow. The use of fetal colour power angiography which demonstrates the hypoperfusion status of various organs has been reported as useful in the evaluation of the growth restricted fetus in the evaluation of circulatory redistribution, however there is not suffi-cient evidence to support its use as a routine test.

Oligohydramnios, (reduced amniotic fluid due to ruptured membranes or chronic fetal compromise and reduction of fetal urine production) and polyhydramnios, (increased amniotic fluid due to overproduction of fetal urine or fetal abnormalities concerning the fetal GI tract) can be diag-nosed by the ultrasonic measurements of either the maximum pool depth, linear amniotic fluid pocket measurements or by an amniotic fluid index where the sum of maximum depth of pools in all four quadrants is calculated.

Placenta praevia can be excluded by the location of placental site in the third trimester, following a low-lying placenta in the second trimester, although only a small percentage (10%) of these remain low at term.[46] A trans-vaginal approach is often useful to locate the margin of a low placenta where the low fetal parts prevent clear visualisation.

Using a tranvaginal approach, cervical length measure-ments, i.e. the distance between the external and internal os provide a useful predictor for the risk of early spon-taneous preterm delivery in high-risk pregnancies.[47] In cases where the cervical length is 15 mm or less at 28 weeks or 32 weeks, there is an increased risk, 90% and 60% respectively, of preterm labour.[48]

Other indications for a third trimester scan are fetal weight estimation and fetal presentation.

3D ULTRASOUND IN OBSTETRICS AND GYNAECOLOGY

3D sonography, originally developed in the 1980s, has only recently gained sophistication and hence significant popularity in prenatal diagnostics. With its multiplanar mode, the main advantages in obstetrics are improved assessment of complex anatomical fetal structures, detec-tion of minor defects, volumetric measurements of organs and a 3D examination of the fetal skeleton,[49] allowing accurate measurements and visualisation of structures otherwise obscured, e.g. nuchal translucency.[50] This improves the accuracy of the diagnosis and increases the spatial resolution of the area of interest. However, fetal movements can cause artefacts, which make its use in fetal echocardiography currently not suitable.

3D ultrasound technology has the added advantage of spatial orientation and additional information derived in terms of accurate volume measurements. It has applica-tions in the field of gynaecology in the diagnosis of uterine anomalies, the assessment of tubal patency, and in detect-ing intrauterine, endometrial and ovarian pathology.[51,52] Because of its advanced technology, and limited avail-ability, current use is confined to research, developmental embryology, and the diagnosis of specific malformations. It is also more time consuming, and the need for highly trained operators and interpretations is vital.

ETHICAL ISSUES

Ultrasound scans are very attractive to women and their partners, providing visual confirmation of pregnancy and enabling early bonding with their babies. However, there are potential implications on the psychological and social consequences for pregnant women such as anxiety, dis-belief, negative attitudes towards the fetus, loss of confi-dence and disappointment when a problem is detected prenatally or in cases of false positives, where there are

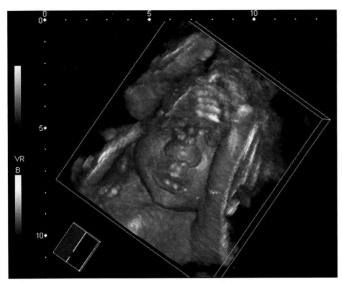

Figure 43.34 3D fetal face. Reproduced with permission from Toshiba

minor anomalies that are of uncertain clinical significance.[53] Conversely, as no screening test is without false negatives, the opposite exists when an abnormality is not detected by ultrasound and there is false reassurance. There is evidence to show that women and their partners are still not made fully aware of the purpose and limitations of the scan.[54,55] Prenatal counselling is vital if couples are to be provided with information that would enable them to make an informed choice with respect to their unborn baby.

PROFESSIONAL ISSUES

In the presence of ever increasing complexities and the widening scope of ultrasound in all fields of medicine, clinical competence, role extension, appropriate education, ultrasound equipment and safety are all important issues that need to be addressed. It is imperative that sonographers understand their responsibilities and the associated medico-legal implications to ensure safe practice.[56] National and local guidelines and policies are developed to standardise practice; these along with regular audit will ensure the provision of a safe and effective ultrasound service.[57,58,59] Where there is an absence of national guidelines within a certain field, it is vital that written local policies and protocols are mutually agreed between all members of the multidisciplinary team to provide a framework in which sonographers can practice. Current literature should be researched to guide the development of such policies and they should be regularly audited, evaluated and updated.

Reporting

The sonographer undertaking the scan should write the report, in a clear language that the requestor of the scan can understand. Misdiagnoses can be made by inaccurate reporting of a scan based on one or two still images of someone else's scan, or by not realising one's own limitations in practice. The support of a clinician (e.g. radiologist, obstetrician or gynaecologist) should always be available for effective team dynamics and safe practice. The images should serve as a reminder of what was seen during the scan, be it normal or pathology. Guidelines have been produced for sonographers in order to maintain standards of reporting, scan contents and writing style.[58]

Health and safety – patients and sonographers

All modern equipment has an output display standard that alerts the operator of the actual output of the ultrasound machine. The two indices usually displayed are the thermal index (TI) that provides an estimation of the potential temperature rise and the mechanical index (MI) that indicates the potential of non-thermal or mechanical bioeffects. All sonographers should be aware of these possible hazards and, by implementing the ALARA principle, keep these indices and the potential for bioeffects 'As Low As Reasonably Achievable' in order to obtain the necessary diagnostic information.[2]

The increase in demand for ultrasound examinations has had a considerable impact on the potential occupational hazard to the sonographer, especially in work-related upper limb disorders and musculoskeletal injuries caused by continuous movements of a repetitive, forceful or awkward nature. These result in trauma to the associated muscles, tendons and ligaments. It has been reported that 80% of 10 000 respondents in the USA and Canada are scanning while experiencing pain and one in five has been affected by a career ending injury. The average time in the profession before experiencing pain was 5 years.[60,61]

Vision fatigue is another hazard identified, which is thought to be linked with regular use of a visual display unit (VDU). Risk assessments of workstations, VDUs and ergonomics of individual sonographers should be carried out within departments, to minimise work-related disorders.[62,63] In addition, all sonographers should be made aware of potential risks and ways to avoid them.

Factors identified to minimise work related disorders are:

- Equipment ergonomics
- Arm and cable supports
- A relaxed grip, (not pen holder grip)

- Appropriate scanning positions
- Use of saddle seats
- Arm abduction <30°
- Appropriate lighting in the room
- Use of slave monitors
- Mini and micro breaks within a long session – the shortage of sonographers and increasing workload, however, make this difficult
- Workload rotations to minimise repetition

SUMMARY

With respect to its position relative to other imaging modalities, the obvious benefits of portability and the lack of ionising radiation make ultrasound the first choice for imaging in many circumstances. The huge improvement in resolution in recent years has enabled ultrasound to become not only a first line imaging source but a high quality one. The low cost per examination makes it attractive in situations involving multiple monitoring scans or screening of families or whole populations. The real-time nature of ultrasound has many uses in dynamic studies, especially in blood flow studies, and in musculoskeletal imaging and in the positioning of stents, biopsy needles and needles for drainage and aspiration. Ultrasound has uses within the operating theatre, and intraluminal ultrasound using extremely small, high frequency transducers is used to obtain high resolution detail of vessel walls.

As is the case with all medical imaging modalities, ultrasound scanning is highly operator dependent. As such, it may look easy to the untrained eye and untrained practitioners use ultrasound with varying levels of success. Operators must be trained to understand the complex nature of ultrasound, recognise artefacts and use equipment safely to obtain optimum images in order to raise the level of diagnostic accuracy. In the right hands, ultrasound is an extremely effective and efficient tool.

The use of ultrasound is growing steadily as any ultrasound department will confirm. Just one such example has been the recent recommendation, owing to the failure rate of up to 35% when no imaging is used, that 2D real-time scanning is used to guide central venous catheters (CVCs) into the internal jugular vein.[64] As 200 000 CVCs are inserted every year in the UK, this suggests a potential additional growth in the use of small, portable scanners and a demand for training for those who will be inserting the catheters.

As long as limitations are recognised, rigorous training is enforced and research and development continues to produce advances in technology, image quality and miniaturisation within a small, user-friendly package, medical ultrasound will continue to be an ever-expanding, useful, imaging modality.

References

1. Department of Health. Hospital activity statistics: imaging and radiodiagnostics. 2003. http://www.performance.doh.gov.uk/hospitalactivity/about_data/kh12.htm
2. ter Haar G, Duck F. The safe use of ultrasound in medical diagnosis. British Institute of Radiology. London; 2000.
3. Entrekin R, et al. Real time spatial compound imaging in breast ultrasound: technology and early clinical experience. Medicamundi 1999; 43(3):35–43.
4. Ryan A, Roberts S. Endoscopic ultrasound of the upper gastrointestinal tract and adnexae. British Medical Ultrasound Society Bulletin 2001; 9(4):24–29.
5. Hoffman B, Hawes R. Endoscopic ultrasonography guided puncture of the lymph nodes: first experience and clinical consequences. Gastrointestinal Endoscopic Clinics of North America 1995; 5:587–594.
6. Bissett R, Khan A. Differential diagnosis in abdominal ultrasound London: WB Saunders; 2002.
7. Middleton W, et al. Ultrasound: the requisites. Missouri: Mosby; 2004.
8. Kapoor B, et al. Prediction of stone composition by ultrasound: implications for non-surgical therapy. British Journal of Radiology 1995, 68:459–462.
9. Norton S, Alderson D. Endoscopic ultrasonography in the evaluation of idiopathic acute pancreatitis. British Journal of Surgery 2000; 87(12):1650–1655.
10. Legmann P, et al. Pancreatic tumors: comparison of dual-phase helical CT and endoscopic sonography. American Journal of Roentgenology 1998; 170:1315–1322.
11. Boll A, et al. Mass screening on abdominal aortic aneurysm in men aged 60–65 years in The Netherlands. Impact on life expectancy and cost-effectiveness using a Markov model. European Journal of Vascular and Endovascular Surgery 2003; 26(1):74–80.
12. Lederle F. Ultrasonographic screening for abdominal aortic aneurysms. Annals of Internal Medicine 2003; 139(6):516–522.
13. Multicentre aneurysm screening study group. Multicentre aneurysm screening study (MASS): cost effectiveness analysis of screening for abdominal aortic aneurysms based on 4 year results from randomised controlled trial. British Medical Journal 2002; 325(7373):1135.
14. Dogra V, Rubens D. Ultrasound secrets. Philadelphia: Hanley and Belfus; 2004.
15. Solbiati L, et al. Thyroid nodules: which sonographic criteria for differentiation between benign and malignant lesions? British Medical Ultrasound Society Bulletin Aug 2001; 9(3):11–19.
16. Wilson A. Contrast-enhanced breast ultrasound: the clinical context. European Radiology 2001; 11(Supp3):E35–E40.
17. Kneeshaw P, et al. Current applications and future direction of MR mammography. British Journal of Cancer 2003; 88:4–10.

18. Sykes C, Connell D. Ultrasound elbows MRI in joint examinations. Diagnostic Imaging Europe 2003; June/July: 31–33.
19. Chambers J, Pilbrow W. Ultrasound in abdominal trauma: an alternative to peritoneal lavage. Archives of Emergency Medicine 1988; 5:26–33.
20. Riccabona M, et al. Three-dimensional ultrasound: accuracy of distance and volume measurements. Ultrasound in Obstetrics and Gynaecology 1996; 7:429–434.
21. Kiyokawa K, et al. Three-dimensional hysterosalpingo-contrast sonography (3D-HyCoSy) as an outpatient procedure to assess infertile women: a pilot study. Ultrasound in Obstetrics and Gynaecology 2000;16(7): 648–654.
22. Dijkman A, et al. Can hysterosalpingocontrast-sonography replace hysterosalpingography in the assessment of tubal subfertility? European Journal of Radiology 2000; 35(1):44-48.
23. Weber G, et al. A new sonographic scoring system (Mainz score) for the assessment of ovarian tumors using transvaginal ultrasonography. Part II. A comparison between the scoring system and the assessment by an experienced sonographer in post menopausal women. Ultrashall in der Medizin 1999; 20(1): 2–8.
24. Kurjak A, et al. Preoperative evaluation of pelvic tumours by Doppler and three Dimensional sonography. Journal of Ultrasound in Medicine 2001; 29(8):829–840.
25. Fung M, et al. Prospective longitudinal study of ultrasound screening for endometrial abnormalities in women with breast cancer receiving tamoxifen. Gynecologic Oncology 2003; 91(1):154–159.
26. Cohen I. Limited value of sonohysterography for endometrial screening in asymptomatic postmenopausal patients treated with tamoxifen. Gynecologic Oncology 2001; 82(2):406–407.
27. Chitty L, et al. Charts of fetal size 1, 2, and 3 head, abdominal and femur length measurements. British Journal of Obstetrics and Gynaecology 1994; 101:125–131.
28. Carroll S, et al. Prediction of chorionicity in twin pregnancies at 10–14 weeks of gestation. British Journal of Obstetrics and Gynaecology 2002; 109:182–186.
29. Condous G, et al. The conservative management of early pregnancy complications: a review of the literature. Ultrasound in Obstetrics and Gynecology 2003; 22(4):420–430.
30. Wiebe E, Janssen P. Conservative management of spontaneous abortions. Women's experiences. Canadian Family Physician 1999; 45:2355–2360.
31. Walker J, Shillito J. Early pregnancy assessment units, service and organisational aspects. In: Gradzinskas J, O'Brien P, eds. Problems in early pregnancy, advances in diagnosis and management. London: RCOG Press; 1997:160–173.
32. Guidelines on ultrasound procedures in early pregnancy. Report of RCR/RCOG Working Party Guideline No 25. London: RCOG; 2000.
33. Snidjers R, et al. UK multicentric project on the assessment of risk for trisomy 21 by maternal age and fetal nuchal translucency at 10–14 weeks of gestation. Lancet 1999; 352:343–346.
34. Nicolaides K, et al. Fetal nuchal translucency: ultrasound screening for chromosomal abnormalities in the first trimester of pregnancy. British Medical Journal 1992; 304:867–869.
35. Hyett J, et al. Using fetal nuchal translucency to screen for major cardiac defects at 10–14 weeks gestation; a population based cohort study. British Medical Journal 1998; 318:81–85.
36. Cicero S, et al. Absence of fetal nasal bone in fetuses with trisomy 21 at 11–14 weeks of gestation: an observational study. Lancet 2001; 358(9294):1665–1667.
37. Vintzileous A, et al. Absent nasal bone in the prenatal detection of fetuses with Trisomy 21 in a high risk population. Obstetrics and Gynaecology 2003; 101(5 pt 1):902–908.
38. Sebire N, et al. Screening for Trisomy 21 in twin pregnancies by maternal age and fetal nuchal translucency thickness 11–14 weeks of gestation. British Journal of Obstetrics and Gynaecology 1996; 103:999–1003.
39. Hernadi L, Torocsik M. Screening for fetal anomalies in the 12th week of pregnancy by transvaginal sonography in an unselected population. Prenatal Diagnosis 1997; 17:753–759.
40. Economides D, Braithwaite J. First trimester ultrasonographic diagnosis of fetal structural abnormalities in a low risk population. British Journal of Obstetrics and Gynaecology 1998; 105:53–57.
41. RCOG Fetal abnormalities: guidelines for screening, diagnosis and management. Report of a joint working party of the Royal College of Obstetricians and Gynaecologists and the Royal College of Paediatricians and Child Health. London: RCOG; 1997.
42. Boyd P, et al. 6-year experience of prenatal diagnosis in an unselected population in Oxford, UK. Lancet 1998; 352(9140):1577–1581.
43. Bricker L, et al. Ultrasound screening in pregnancy: a systematic review of the clinical effectiveness, cost effectiveness and women's views. Health Technology Assessment 2000; 4(16).
44. Twickler D, et al. Second opinion magnetic resonance imaging for suspected fetal central nervous system abnormalities. American Journal of Obstetrics and Gynecology 2003; 188(2):492–496.
45. Hubbard A, Harty M. MRI for the assessment of the malformed fetus. Baillière's best practice and research in clinical obstetrics and gynaecology 1999; 14(4):629–650.
46. Bricker L, Neilson J. Routine ultrasound in late pregnancy after 24 weeks gestation (Cochrane review) The Cochrane Library 2. Oxford; 2001.
47. Welsh A, Nicolaides K. Cervical screening for preterm delivery. Current Opinion in Obstetrics and Gynecology 2002; 14(2):195–202.

48. Heath V, et al. Cervical length at 23 weeks of gestation: prediction of spontaneous preterm labour. Ultrasound in Obstetrics and Gynaecology 1998; 12(5):312–317.

49. Merz E, et al. Volume scanning in the evaluation of fetal malformations: a new dimension in prenatal diagnosis. Ultrasound in Obstetrics and Gynaecology 1995; 5:222–227.

50. Kurjak A, Kupesic S. Three dimensional ultrasound improves measurement of nuchal translucency. Journal of Perinatal Medicine 1999; 27:97–102.

51. Maymon R, et al. Three dimensional vaginal sonography in obstetrics and gynaecology. Human Reproduction Update 2000; 6:475–484.

52. Sladkevicius P, et al. Three dimensional power Doppler imaging in the assessment of fallopian tube patency. Ultrasound in Obstetrics and Gynaecology 2000; 16:644–647.

53. Aksoy S. Antenatal screening and its possible meaning from unborn baby's perspective. BMC Medical Ethics. Epub 2001; May 22; 2(1):3.

54. National Childbirth Trust. The stress of tests in pregnancy: summary of National Childbirth Trust antenatal survey. London: NCT9; 1997.

55. Baillie C, et al. Scanning for pleasure. British Journal of Obstetrics and Gynaecology 1997; 107:1023–1024.

56. Harrison G, Mitcalf R. Trends in litigation activity against sonographers. British Medical Ultrasound Society Bulletin 2003; 11(1)33–36.

57. College of Radiographers. Occupational standards for diagnostic ultrasound. London: College of Radiographers; 1998.

58. United Kingdom Association of Sonographers. Guidelines for professional working standards. Ultrasound Practic. London: United Kingdom Association of Sonographers; 2001.

59. Society of Radiographers. Professional standards to be achieved in diagnostic imaging, radiotherapy and oncology. London: Society of Radiographers; 1996.

60. Baker J, Murphy S. Minimising workplace injuries among sonographers. Innovations in Ultrasound 2001; Nov:23–24.

61. Society of Radiographers. The causes of musculoskeletal injury amongst sonographers in the UK. Society of Radiographers. June 2002.

62. Society of Radiographers. VDUsers FRIENDLY: A guide to dealing with health and safety issues arising from their use. London: Society of Radiographers; 1994.

63. Royal College of Radiologists. Risk management in clinical radiology. London: Royal College of Radiologists; 2002.

64. NHS National Institute for Clinical Excellence. Technology Appraisal Guidance No 49. London; 2002.

GLOSSARY
OF RADIOGRAPHIC TERMS

Abduction	Refers to limbs or digits, when they are moved away from the median sagittal plane or trunk. An abducted thumb is moved away from the rest of the hand.
Adduction	Refers to limbs or digits, when they are brought towards the median sagittal plane or trunk. An adducted thumb is moved towards the rest of the hand.
Anatomical position	The trunk and limbs are extended fully, with the arms slightly abducted at the side. The palms of the hands face forwards. The front of the patient faces forwards.
Anterior	The front of the patient, or body part, when the patient is in the anatomical position.
Anterior oblique	An oblique position, when the anterior aspect of the patient is nearest the image receptor *or* a posteroanterior position with an oblique angle applied in a lateral or medial direction.
Anteroposterior	A position where the anterior aspect of the patient faces the X-ray tube, and the central ray passes through this aspect and exits through the posterior aspect.
Anthropological baseline	Baseline used in radiography of the head (see Chs 16 and 17).
Bucky	Antiscatter device.
Caudal	Relating to the lower part of the body, or feet. Used mainly in conjunction with beam angulation, meaning to direct the beam towards the feet.
Coronal plane	An imaginary line which divides the front and back of the head and trunk vertically. It is perpendicular to the median sagittal plane.
Cranial	Relating to the head. Used mainly in conjunction with beam angulation, meaning to direct the beam towards the head.
Craniocaudal	Mammographic term used when the breast is placed with its inferior aspect on the image receptor and the X-ray beam directed vertically to enter the breast on its uppermost surface, exiting inferiorly.
Decubitus	The patient is in a horizontal position. Used in conjunction with a qualifying term to indicate which aspect of the body is nearest the image receptor, as in 'lateral decubitus', 'prone decubitus'.
Dorsal	The back of the patient or body part; sometimes used instead of 'posterior'.
Dorsiflexion	Flexion of the hand at the wrist when the dorsum of the hand moves in a posterior direction, or flexion of the foot at the ankle when the dorsal aspect of the foot moves towards the ankle.
Dorsipalmar	The hand is placed with its palmar aspect on the image receptor.
Dorsiplantar	The foot is placed with its sole on the image receptor.
Dorsum	The back of the hand or the top of the foot.
Erect	The patient is standing or sitting, with the median sagittal and coronal planes vertical.

611

Eversion	Lateral flexion at the ankle joint. Excessive forced eversion can cause injury in the ankle or other joints.
Extension	Typically, effecting 'opening' or straightening of a joint. For example, the extended elbow will place the arm in a position where the forearm and humerus continue in the same plane. Lumbar or thoracic spine: the patient usually bends backwards. Cervical spine: the head is tipped backwards to lift the chin. Foot: the foot is moved at the ankle so that the toes point downwards or posteriorly (although this is sometimes referred to as plantar flexion).
External	On the outside/towards the outside/ away from the median sagittal plane. Often used in conjunction with describing rotation of a limb, when the big toes or thumbs are turned outwards, away from the trunk or median sagittal plane.
External auditory meatus	Surface marking used in radiography of the head (see Ch. 16).
External occipital protuberance	Surface marking used in radiography of the head (see Ch. 16).
Flexion	Typically, effecting 'closing' of a joint such as bending the knee or elbow and can be described in conjunction with description of the direction of flexion, such as lateral/dorsal/palmar flexion for other body parts, such as the hands and feet. Lumbar or thoracic spine: the patient usually bends forwards but lateral flexion may also be described. Cervical spine: the head is bent forwards to tuck the chin down.
Focus film distance	Distance from the focal spot to the image receptor (known as source image distance in some countries).
Focus object distance	Distance from the focal spot to the body part (known as source object distance in some countries).
Frontooccipital	Refers to positioning of the head, when the X-ray beam enters the frontal aspect and exits via the occiput.
Glabella	Surface marking used in radiography of the head (see Ch. 16).
Grid	Antiscatter device.
Image receptor	A plate, upon which X radiation impinges and creates a latent image. Can be a film which is placed in a cassette, or a radiosensitive structure which converts the image digitally for reproduction on a display screen (see Chs 1 and 2).
Inferior	Below or underneath.
Inferosuperior	A position where the inferior aspect of the body part is nearest the X-ray tube and the central ray passes through this aspect, exiting through the superior aspect. Mainly used in examination of limbs and the shoulder girdle.
Internal	On the inside/towards the inside/ towards the median sagittal plane. Often used in conjunction with describing rotation of a limb, when the big toes or thumbs are turned inwards, towards the trunk or median sagittal plane.
Inversion	Medial flexion of the ankle joint. Excessive forced inversion can cause injury in the ankle or other joints.
Lateral	The outermost side of the trunk or body part, furthest from the median sagittal plane. Can be used in description of rotation of limbs (see entry for rotation). Also a radiographic position/projection where the side of the trunk or body part faces the X-ray tube.
Lateral oblique	Initially a lateral position, the body part is tilted towards the image receptor *or* the lateral patient position is maintained but a tube angle is employed.

Lateromedial — A position where the lateral aspect of the body part faces the X-ray tube and the central ray passes through this aspect, exiting via the medial aspect. Mainly used in mammography but can be used in some limb radiography to describe beam direction.

Left anterior oblique — An oblique position, when the anterior aspect of the left side lies nearer the image receptor than the right side.

Left posterior oblique — An oblique position, when the posterior aspect of the left side lies nearer the image receptor than the right side.

Lordosis/lordotic — The patient is leaning back.

Medial — Towards or nearest the median sagittal plane. Can be used in description of rotation of limbs (see entry for rotation).

Median sagittal plane — An imaginary line which divides the left and right sides of the head and trunk vertically, in the midline.

Mediolateral — A position where the medial aspect of the body part faces the X-ray tube and the central ray passes through this aspect, exiting via the lateral aspect. Mainly used in mammography but can be used in some limb radiography to describe beam direction.

Nasion — Surface marking used in radiography of the head (see Ch. 16).

Object film distance — Distance from the body part to the image receptor (known as object image distance in some countries).

Oblique — The body part position lies between the lateral and anteroposterior or posteroanterior positions. For hands and feet, the palm or sole is raised from the image receptor along one of the lateral aspects.

Occipitofrontal — Refers to positioning of the head, when the X-ray beam enters the occipital aspect and exits via the forehead (frontal bone).

Occipitomental — Refers to positioning of the head, when the X-ray beam enters the occipital aspect and exits via the chin.

Orbitomeatal baseline — Baseline used for skull radiography (see Ch. 16).

Palmar — Relating to the palm of the hand.

Plantar — Relating to the sole of the foot.

Plantar flexion — Flexion of the foot at the ankle when the dorsal aspect of the foot moves away from the ankle.

Posterior — The back of the patient or body part, when the patient is in the anatomical position.

Posterior oblique — An oblique position, when the posterior aspect of the patient is nearest the image receptor *or* an anteroposterior position with an oblique angle applied in a lateral or medial direction.

Posteroanterior — A position where the posterior aspect of the patient faces the X-ray tube, and the central ray passes through this aspect and exits through the anterior aspect.

Pronation — Used when referring to the position of the hand when it is placed palm down.

Prone — The patient is lying horizontally face down.

Right anterior oblique — An oblique position, when the anterior aspect of the right side lies nearer the image receptor than the left side.

Right posterior oblique — An oblique position, when the posterior aspect of the right side lies nearer the image receptor than the left side.

Rotation — Turning the trunk or head laterally in relationship to the median sagittal plane.
External or lateral rotation: turning a limb when the big toes or thumbs are turned outwards, away from the trunk or median sagittal plane.

Internal or medial rotation: when the big toes or thumbs are turned inwards, towards the trunk or median sagittal plane.

Semi prone One side of the patient is partly raised from the prone position, as in the anterior oblique position.

Semi recumbent The patient is leaning back, between the erect and supine positions.

Submentovertical A position of the head where the beam enters below the chin and exits via the top of the skull (vertex).

Superior Above or uppermost.

Superoinferior A position where the superior aspect of the body part is nearest the X-ray tube and the central ray passes through this aspect, exiting through the inferior aspect. Mainly used in examination of limbs.

Supine The patient is lying horizontally on their back.

Tilt Tipping the trunk or head away from the median sagittal plane, anteriorly, posteriorly or laterally.

INDEX